中英对照版

生长因子与创面修复图鉴

Atlas of Growth Factors and Wound Repair

主审　李校堃

副审　林　丽

主编　陈善亮　肖　健　王建波

耿武军　陈　忠　王小尚

科学技术文献出版社
SCIENTIFIC AND TECHNICAL DOCUMENTATION PRESS

·北京·

图书在版编目（CIP）数据

生长因子与创面修复图鉴 = Atlas of Growth Factors and Wound Repair：汉文、英文 / 陈善亮等主编. -- 北京：科学技术文献出版社，2024. 11.

ISBN 978-7-5235-1965-3

Ⅰ. R622-64; R64-64

中国国家版本馆 CIP 数据核字第 20249TE988 号

生长因子与创面修复图鉴（中英对照版）

Atlas of Growth Factors and Wound Repair

策划编辑：孔荣华　　责任编辑：王　霞　　责任校对：王瑞瑞　　责任出版：张志平

出 版 者　科学技术文献出版社

地　　址　北京市复兴路15号　邮编 100038

编 务 部　（010）58882938，58882087（传真）

发 行 部　（010）58882868，58882870（传真）

邮 购 部　（010）58882873

官方网址　www.stdp.com.cn

发 行 者　科学技术文献出版社发行　全国各地新华书店经销

印 刷 者　中煤（北京）印务有限公司

版　　次　2024年11月第1版　2024年11月第1次印刷

开　　本　889 × 1194　1/16

字　　数　795千

印　　张　36.5

书　　号　ISBN 978-7-5235-1965-3

定　　价　368.00元

编委会
Editorial Board

主审简介

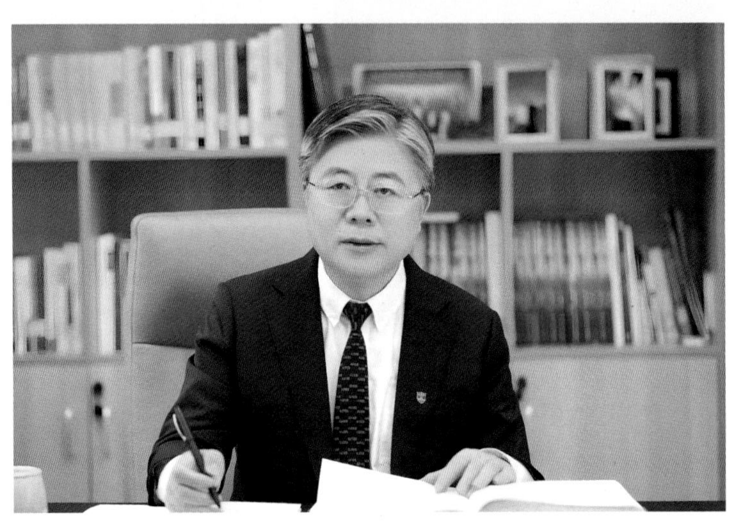

李校堃

第十四届全国人大代表，中国工程院院士，国家教学名师，温州医科大学校长，大分子药物与规模化制备全国重点实验室主任，细胞生长因子与蛋白制剂国家工程中心主任，生物医药省部共建协同创新中心主任。

30余年从事细胞生长因子再生与系统调控研究，在细胞生长因子与疾病研究上取得一系列原创性成果，使我国成为世界上第一个将成纤维细胞生长因子（FGF）研制成功并投产的国家，为烧伤创伤、慢性创面及糖尿病并发症、急性救治及国防战备提供重要治疗手段。先后在*Nature*、*Cell Metab*、*Mol Cell*、*Circulation*等上发表论文200余篇。曾获国家技术发明奖二等奖、国家科学技术进步奖二等奖、教育部自然科学奖一等奖、何梁何利基金科学与技术进步奖、谈家桢生命科学奖、光华工程科技奖和转化医学杰出贡献奖等重要奖项。

Introduction to the Chief Judge

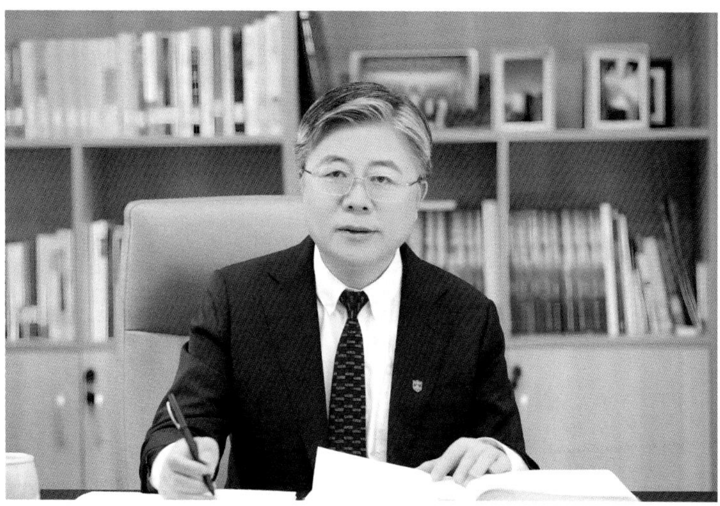

Li Xiaokun

Deputy to the 14th National People's Congress, academician of the CAE Member, national famous teacher, president of Wenzhou Medical University, director of the national key laboratory for macromolecular drugs and large-scale preparation, director of the national engineering center for cell growth factors and protein preparations, and director of the innovation center of the provincial and ministerial co construction association for biomedicine.

He has been engaged in the research of cell growth factor regeneration and system regulation for more than 30 years, and has made a series of original achievements in the research of cell growth factor and disease, making China the first country in the world to successfully develop and put into production fibroblast growth factor (FGF), providing an important treatment method for burn wounds, chronic wounds and complications of diabetes, acute treatment and national defense readiness. Published over 200 papers in *Nature*, *Cell Metab*, *Mol Cell*, *Circulation*, and other journals. He has won the second prize of the State Technological Innovation Award, the second prize of the National Award for Science and Technology Progress, the first prize of the Ministry of Education for Natural Science, the Science and Technology Progress Award of the Ho Leung Ho Lee Foundation, the Tan Jiazhen Life Science Award, the Guanghua Engineering Science and Technology Award, and the Outstanding Contribution Award of Translational Medicine and other important awards.

副审简介

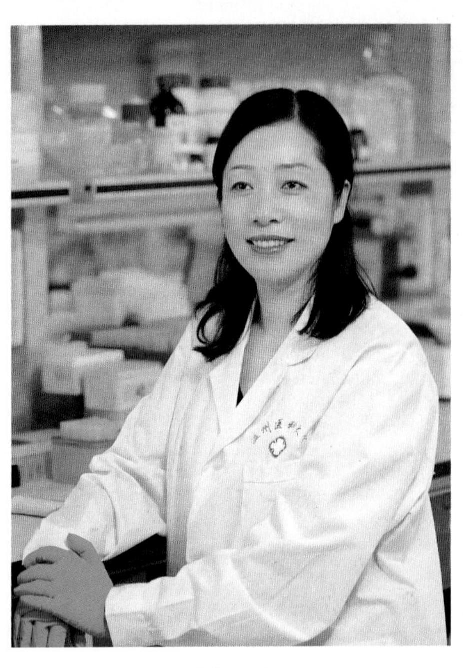

林丽

温州医科大学药学院院长，入选国家百千万人才工程，国家有突出贡献中青年专家，享受国务院政府特殊津贴，浙江省“万人计划”教学名师，兼任浙江省药理学会副理事长等职。主要从事细胞生长因子和神经修复的理论创新及新药转化研究，主持国家级项目10余项。以主要完成人获国家级教学成果奖二等奖2项、国家科学技术进步奖二等奖1项。

Introduction to Deputy Judge

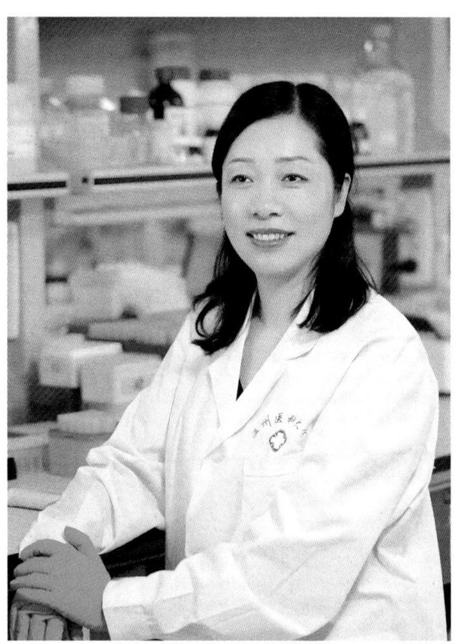

Lin Li

Dean of the School of Pharmacy at Wenzhou Medical University. Selected as a member of the National Hundred, Thousand, and Ten Thousand Talents Project, a young and middle-aged expert with outstanding contributions to the country, a recipient of the State Council Special Allowance, a teaching master of the Zhejiang Province "Ten Thousand Talents Plan", and also serves as the Vice Chairman of the Zhejiang Pharmacological Society. Mainly engaged in theoretical innovation and new drug translation research on cell growth factors and neural repair, leading over 10 national level projects. Received 2 second prizes for national teaching achievements and 1 second prize for national scientific and technological progress as the main contributor.

主编简介

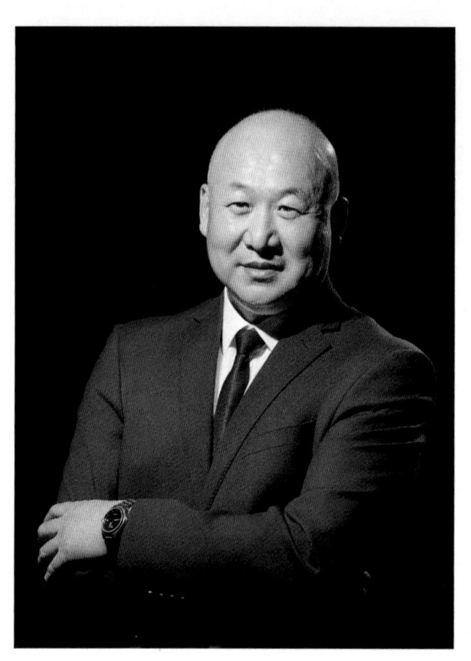

陈善亮

温州曙光中西医创面修复医院院长，手足显微外科主任，创面修复科主任，副主任医师，温州医科大学整合医药研究院生长因子与复杂创面修复临床研究基地主任。温州市龙湾区政协委员会第四、第五届政协委员，农工党温州市龙湾区基层委一支部主任委员。中国康复医学会康复学组委员，浙江省医学会显微外科学分会委员会委员，浙江省医学会手外科学分会委员会委员，温州市医学会手外科学分会委员。《创伤骨科治疗学》主编，《实用手外科杂志》编委。“肤生工程”公益项目副秘书长，长期从事医疗公益事业。2008 年度被农工党中央委员会评为汶川地震抗震救灾优秀党员；2019 年被温州市委宣传部、温州市文明办评为温州好人。2023 年获第四届温州慈善奖——志愿服务奖。

Introduction to the Editor in Chief

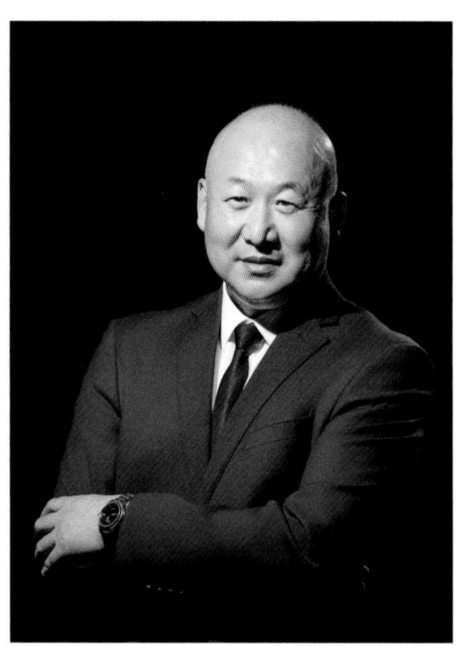

Chen Shanliang

Dean of Wenzhou Shuguang Traditional Chinese and Western Medicine Wound Repair Hospital, Director of Hand and Foot Microsurgery, Director of Wound Repair Department, Deputy Chief Physician, and Director of the Clinical Research Base for Growth Factors and Complex Wound Repair at Wenzhou Medical University Integrated Medicine Research Institute. Member of the Fourth and Fifth Political Consultative Conference Committee of Longwan District, Wenzhou City, and Chairman of the Grassroots Committee Branch of the Agricultural and Labor Party in Longwan District, Wenzhou City. Member of the Rehabilitation Group of the Chinese Rehabilitation Medicine Association, Member of the Microsurgery Branch Committee of the Zhejiang Medical Association, Member of the Hand Surgery Branch Committee of the Zhejiang Medical Association, and Member of the Hand Surgery Branch Committee of the Wenzhou Medical Association. Editor in chief of *Orthopedic Treatment of Trauma* and editorial board member of *Journal of Practical Hand Surgery*. Vice Secretary General of the "F&S CHARITY" public welfare project, engaged in medical public welfare undertakings for a long time. In 2008, he was awarded the title of Outstanding Party Member for the Wenchuan Earthquake Relief by the Central Committee of the Agricultural and Labor Party; In 2019, he was awarded the title of Wenzhou Good Person by the Propaganda Department of the Wenzhou Municipal Committee and the Wenzhou Civilization Office. Won the Fourth Wenzhou Charity Award - Volunteer Service Award in 2023.

主编简介

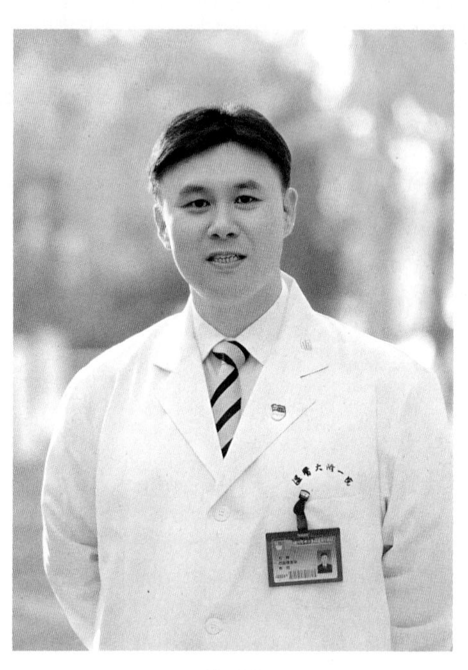

肖健

研究员、博士研究生导师，温州医科大学研究生院院长，国家自然科学基金委优秀青年科学基金项目获得者，入选浙江省“万人计划”科技创新领军人才；研究方向为生长因子与创伤修复，主持国家自然科学基金项目、国家“重大新药创制”重大专项、浙江省杰出青年科学基金项目等20余项。以第一作者或通讯作者在*Advanced Materials*、*Advanced Functional Materials*、*Autophagy*、*Signal Transduction and Targeted Therapy* 等上发表SCI收录论文100余篇，上述论文已被*Science* 等他引7300余次。获授权发明专利41项，主持研发创面修复Ⅱ类医疗器械2项，参与研发国家Ⅰ类新药1项、Ⅲ类医疗器械1项。参与获得国家科学技术进步奖一等奖(2015年）、国家科学技术进步奖二等奖（2018年），主持获得中华医学科技奖二等奖（2020年）、王正国创伤医学奖创新奖（2019年）。

Introduction to the Editor in Chief

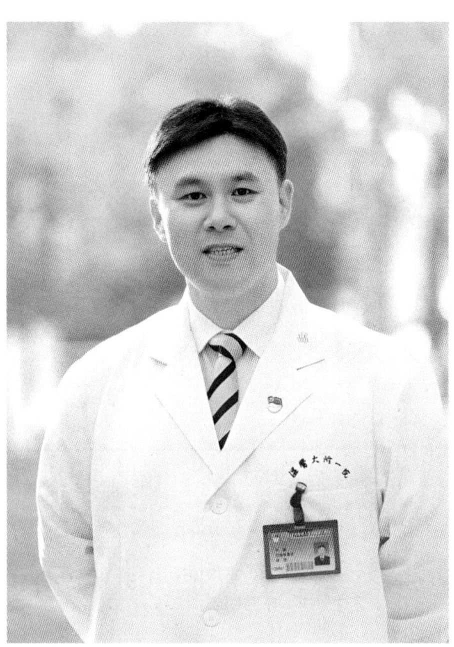

Xiao Jian

Researcher, doctoral supervisor, Dean of the Graduate School of Wenzhou Medical University, recipient of the National Natural Science Foundation of China's Excellent Youth Science Fund project, and selected as a leading talent in scientific and technological innovation under the Zhejiang Province "Ten Thousand Talents Plan"; My research focuses on growth factors and trauma repair, and I have led over 20 projects including the National Natural Science Foundation of China, the National Major New Drug Creation Project, and the Zhejiang Outstanding Youth Science Fund. As the first or corresponding author, I have published over 100 SCI papers in *Advanced Materials*, *Advanced Functional Materials*, *Autophagy*, *Signal Transduction*, and *Targeted Therapy*, among others. These papers have been cited more than 7300 times by *Science* and others. Obtained 41 authorized invention patents, led the research and development of 2 Class II medical devices for wound repair, participated in the research and development of 1 national Class I new drug, and 1 Class III medical device. Participated in winning the first prize of the National Science and Technology Progress Award (2015) and the second prize of the National Science and Technology Progress Award (2018), hosted and won the second prize of the Chinese Medical Science and Technology Award (2020) and the Wang Zhengguo Trauma Medicine Innovation Award (2019).

主编简介

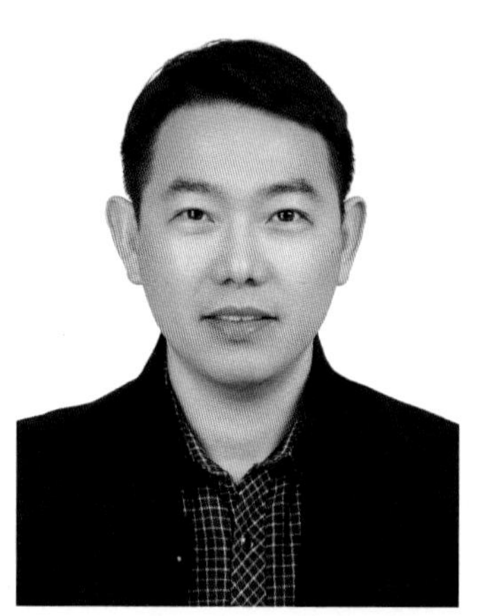

王建波

硕士研究生学历，温州医科大学药学院党委书记、副院长，现任“肤生工程”副秘书长，曾任省网络社会组织联合会理事、温州市网络文化协会副会长、温州市高校清朗网络联合会秘书长等。以“肤生工程”为主题牵头的创新创业项目获“挑战杯”中国大学生创业计划竞赛，“互联网+”全国大学生创新创业大赛国赛、省赛金奖等5项。致力于社会公益和科普活动，建立学院、医院、企业、协会等参与的党建联建社会服务机制，带领学院团队获全国工人先锋号、教育部思政精品项目等国家级荣誉5项。通过浙江省药学会、温州市青少年科技教育协会等组织，将科学家精神、教育家精神和“肤生”精神向社会科普。

Introduction to the Editor in Chief

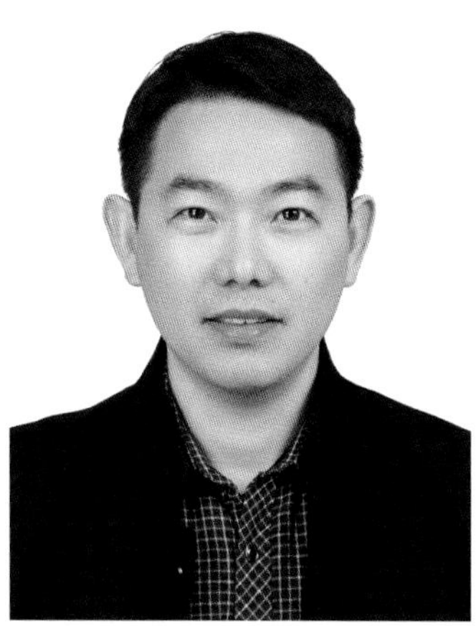

Wang Jianbo

Master's degree holder, Secretary of the Party Committee and Vice Dean of the School of Pharmacy at Wenzhou Medical University, currently serving as the Deputy Secretary General of the "F&S CHARITY". Formerly served as a director of the Provincial Network Social Organization Federation, Vice President of the Wenzhou Network Culture Association, and Secretary General of the Wenzhou University Qinglang Network Federation. The innovation and entrepreneurship project led by the "F&S CHARITY" won five gold medals, including the "Challenge Cup" Chinese Undergraduate Entrepreneurship Plan Competition, the "Internet plus" National Undergraduate Innovation and Entrepreneurship Competition. Committed to social welfare and science popularization activities, establishing a party building and social service mechanism involving colleges, hospitals, enterprises, associations, etc., leading the college team to win 5 national honors such as the National Worker Pioneer Award and the Ministry of Education's Ideological and Political Quality Project. Through organizations such as the Zhejiang Pharmaceutical Association and the Wenzhou Youth Science and Technology Education Association, we aim to popularize the spirit of scientists, educators, and the "skin born" spirit to society.

主编简介

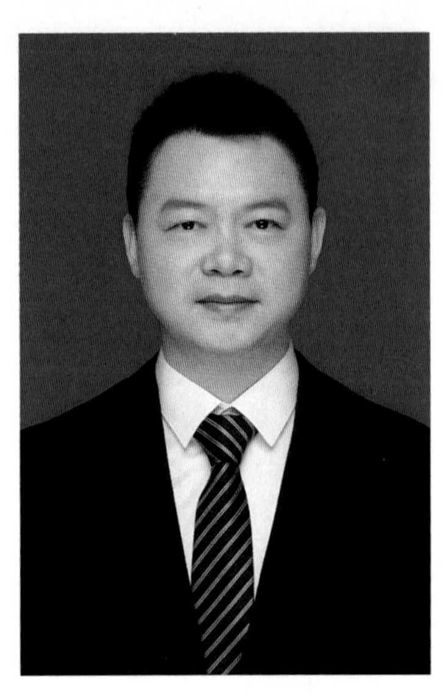

耿武军

教授、主任医师、博士研究生导师 / 博士后导师，瓯江实验室党委委员、副主任，温州市科协副主席（兼），中华医学会麻醉学分会疼痛学组副组长，浙江省医学会疼痛学分会候任主任委员，温州市疼痛与围术期医学重点实验室主任，*Frontiers in Cellular Neuroscience* 客座主编。主持国家自然科学基金项目、浙江省尖兵领雁项目等 16 项；发表 SCI 收录论文 66 篇，主编、参编著作 3 部，获授权国家发明专利 10 项，实施成果转化 3 项。先后荣获 2019 年国医盛典——融贯中西麻醉青年精英奖、教育部 2020 年度高等学校教育研究优秀成果奖（科学科技）一等奖、2022 年度浙江省科学技术进步奖科普成果提名、2022 年度温州市十大杰出青年、2023 人民好医生（疼痛学）青年典范、2024 日内瓦国际发明展银奖等。研究方向：疼痛、麻醉。

Introduction to the Editor in Chief

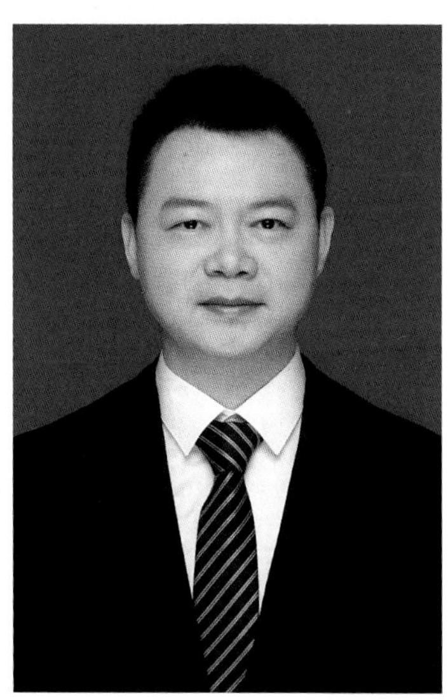

Geng Wujun

Professor, chief physician, doctoral supervisor/postdoctoral supervisor, member and deputy director of the Party Committee of Oujiang Laboratory, vice chairman (concurrently) of Wenzhou Association for Science and Technology, deputy leader of the Pain Group of the Anesthesiology Branch of the Chinese Medical Association, elected chairman of the Pain Credit Committee of Zhejiang Medical Association, director of Wenzhou Key Laboratory of Pain and Perioperative Medicine, and guest editor in chief of *Frontiers in Cellular Neuroscience*. Hosted 16 projects, including the National Natural Science Foundation of China and the Zhejiang Province Vanguard Leading Goose Project; Published 66 SCI indexed papers, edited and co edited 3 books, obtained 10 authorized national invention patents, and implemented 3 achievements transformation. He has successively won the 2019 National Medical Ceremony – Rongguan Chinese and Western Anesthesia Youth Elite Award, the Ministry of Education's 2020 Higher Education Research Excellent Achievement Award (Science and Technology) First Prize, the 2022 Zhejiang Province Science and Technology Progress Award Science Popularization Achievement Nomination, the 2022 Wenzhou Top Ten Outstanding Youth, the 2023 People's Good Doctor (Pain Medicine) Youth Model, and the 2024 Geneva International Invention Exhibition Silver Award. Research direction: Pain and anesthesia.

主编简介

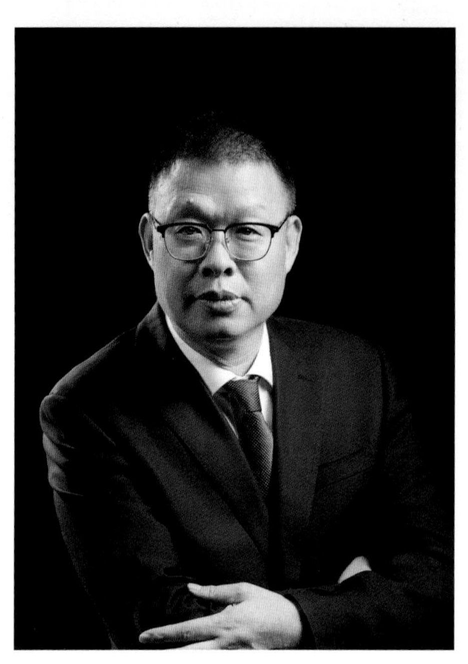

陈忠

主任记者，现为温州都市报陈忠慈善工作室负责人，温州都市报义工队队长，温州医科大学第二临床医学院创新创业导师。“不在新闻的路上，就在慈善的路上”，这是陈忠从业20多年来的真实写照。他采写新闻稿件超200万字，其中采写的200多篇稿件被《人民日报》、新华社转载，采写的新闻作品30多次被评为省、市好新闻奖。这些年来，陈忠策划了在西部造一片温州林、明眸工程、新年新衣温暖行动、慈善大使寻找寒门学子、“一带一路”善行万里、大拇指工程、圆心计划、童心筑梦工程、肤生工程、温心守护等50多项公益慈善活动，累计发动捐款捐物超亿元，超60万人受益，慈善行程遍布中西部地区和温州市各地，行程百万公里，累计志愿服务超1万小时。

Introduction to the Editor in Chief

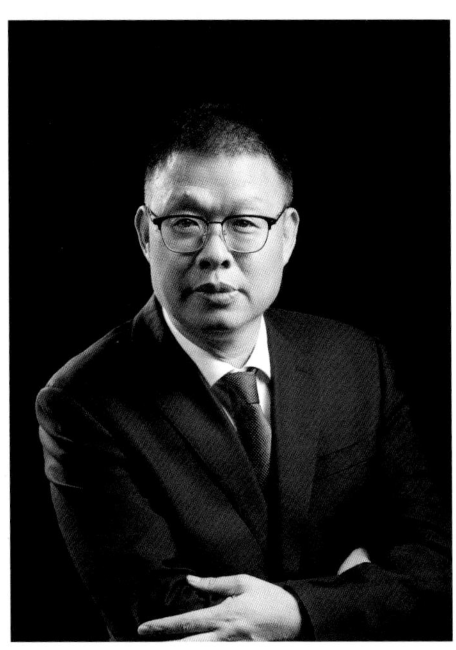

Chen Zhong

Chief journalist, currently in charge of Chen Zhong Charity Studio at Wenzhou Urban Daily, team leader of Wenzhou Urban Daily Volunteer Team, and innovation and entrepreneurship mentor at the Second Clinical School of Wenzhou Medical University. "Not on the road of news, but on the road of charity "is a true portrayal of Chen Zhong's more than 20 years of experience in the industry. He has written over 2 million words of news articles, of which more than 200 have been reprinted by People's Daily and Xinhua News Agency. His news works have been awarded the Provincial and Municipal Good News Award more than 30 times. Over the years, Chen Zhong has planned more than 50 public welfare charity activities, such as building a Wenzhou forest in the west, the Eyes Brightening Project, the New Year's New Clothes Warming Action, charity ambassadors looking for underprivileged students, the "the Belt and Road" Goodwill for thousands of miles, the Thumb Project, the Heart Rounding Plan, the Children's Heart Dream Building Project, the F&S CHARITY, and the Heart Warming Guard. He has launched donations of more than 100 million yuan in total, benefiting more than 600 000 people. Charity trips have spread throughout the central and western regions and Wenzhou City, covering millions of kilometers, and volunteering more than 10 000 hours in total.

主编简介

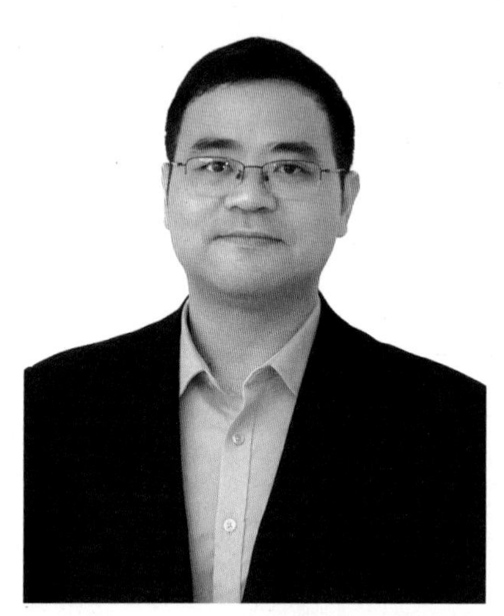

王小尚

讲师，温州医科大学阿尔伯塔学院党委副书记，温州市法学会常务理事，温州医科大学机关工会主席，温州医科大学欧美同学会（留学人员联谊会）副会长。曾任学生辅导员，从事来华留学生教育管理工作十年，获评浙江省优秀辅导员，获浙江省辅导员职业能力大赛二等奖。指导学生参加全国“互联网 +”创业大赛获银奖、全国志愿服务大赛获银奖、浙江省“挑战杯”创业大赛获金奖。所带学生获浙江省最美寝室、省最美春泥团队、全国大学生暑期社会实践优秀团队等荣誉。所带学生中一名毕业生为现任加纳驻华副大使。2018 年 7 月至 2019 年 9 月，在教育部国际合作与交流司借调，参与来华留学教育管理及相关政策修订工作。2020 年 2 月至今，作为主要参与者之一，推动“肤生工程”各项公益慈善活动开展。

Introduction to the Editor in Chief

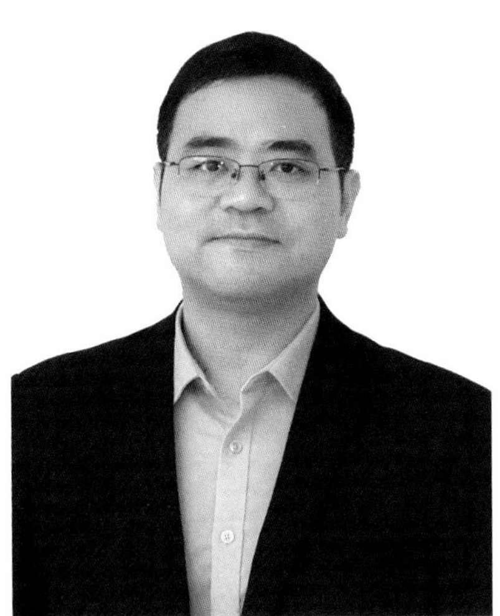

Wang Xiaoshang

Lecturer, Deputy Secretary of the Party Committee of Alberta College, Wenzhou Medical University, Executive Director of Wenzhou Law Society, Chairman of Wenzhou Medical University Union, Vice President of Wenzhou Medical University European and American Alumni Association (Overseas Students Association). Formerly served as a student counselor, engaged in education management for international students in China for ten years, awarded the title of Excellent Counselor in Zhejiang Province, and won the second prize in the Zhejiang Province Counselor Professional Ability Competition. Guiding students to participate in the National "Internet plus" Entrepreneurship Competition won a silver award, the National Volunteer Service Competition won a silver award, and the Zhejiang "Challenge Cup" Entrepreneurship Competition won a gold award. The students I led have won honors such as Zhejiang Province's Most Beautiful Dormitory, Zhejiang Province's Most Beautiful Spring Mud Team, and National Excellent Team for College Students' Summer Social Practice. One of the students under my guidance is a graduate who is currently the Deputy Ambassador of Ghana to China. From July 2018 to September 2019, I was seconded by the International Cooperation and Exchange Department of the Ministry of Education to participate in the management of studying abroad education and related policy revisions in China. Since February 2020, as one of the main participants, I have been promoting various public welfare and charity activities of the "F&S CHARITY".

副主编简介

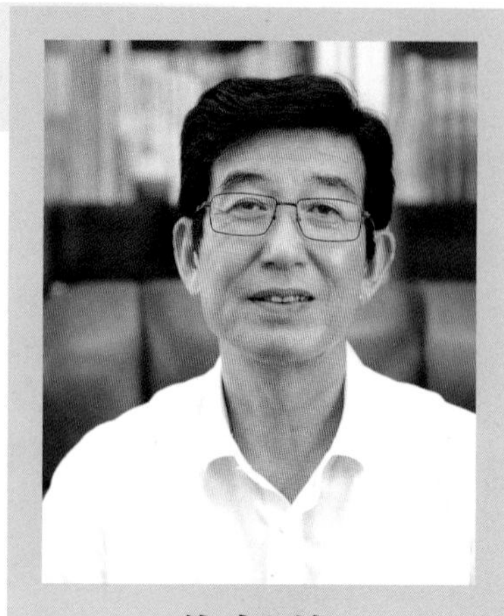

仇杨均

历史学学士学位，在职研究生学历，副研究员，1983 年 6 月加入中国共产党，温州市慈善总会会长。作为一位资深党员和领导者，他不仅在多个政府岗位上有卓越表现，更在慈善领域展现了无私与爱心。自 2021 年 7 月担任温州市慈善总会会长以来，他提出“有为慈善、品牌慈善、实力慈善、全民慈善、阳光慈善”的理念，积极推动慈善事业发展，倡导社会各界参与公益，帮助弱势群体。近年来，温州市慈善总会先后荣获“2021 年度浙江省品牌社会组织”称号、浙江省“优秀慈善组织”称号、第二届“长三角慈善之星”称号和第四届温州慈善奖慈善事业突出贡献奖，第四次蝉联“5A 级社会组织”等。

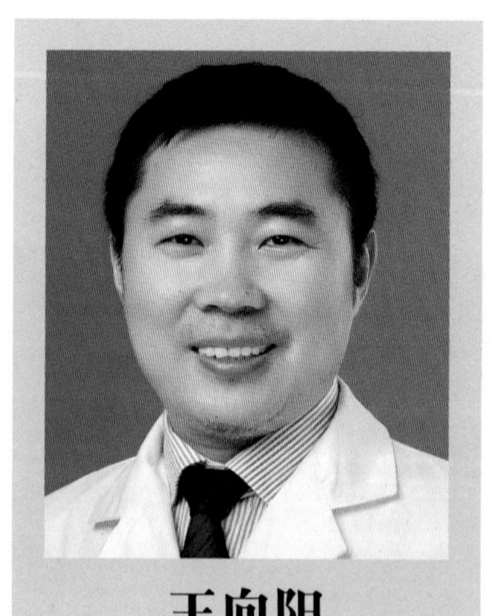

王向阳

主任医师，教授，博士研究生导师，毕业于上海交通大学医学院，博士学位，温州医科大学附属第二医院育英儿童医院骨科建设委员会主任，浙江省儿童青少年脊柱健康指导中心执行主任，国家临床重点专科学科带头人，全国十佳中青年骨科医师奖获得者。创建了“育英脊梁工程”慈善基金和“脊良正姿”联盟。主持国家自然科学基金项目 5 项，浙江省自然科学杰出青年基金、浙江省“领雁”重点研发项目，省部共建项目、浙江省钱江人才项目等 8 项，以第一作者和通讯作者发表 SCI 和 EI 收录论文 150 余篇，主编《脊柱内固定解剖学》及参编著作 15 部。以负责人或主要研究者获国家科学技术进步奖二等奖、中华医学科技奖一等奖、浙江省科学技术进步奖一等奖和上海市科技进步奖一等奖。

Introduction to the Deputy Editor in Chief

Qiu Yangjun

He has a bachelor's degree in history, an on-the-job postgraduate degree, an associate researcher, joined the CPC in June 1983, and is the president of Wenzhou Charity Federation. As a senior party member and leader, he has not only shown outstanding performance in multiple government positions, but also demonstrated selflessness and love in the field of charity. Since taking office as the President of Wenzhou Charity Federation in July 2021, he has put forward the concept of "proactive charity, brand charity, strength charity, public charity, and sunshine charity", actively promoting the development of charity, advocating the participation of all sectors of society in public welfare, and helping vulnerable groups. In recent years, the Wenzhou Charity Federation has successively won the titles of "2021 Zhejiang Province Brand Social Organization", "Excellent Charity Organization", "Second Yangtze River Delta Charity Star", and "Outstanding Contribution to Charity" at the Fourth Wenzhou Charity Award. It has also won the "5A level Social Organization" award for the fourth time.

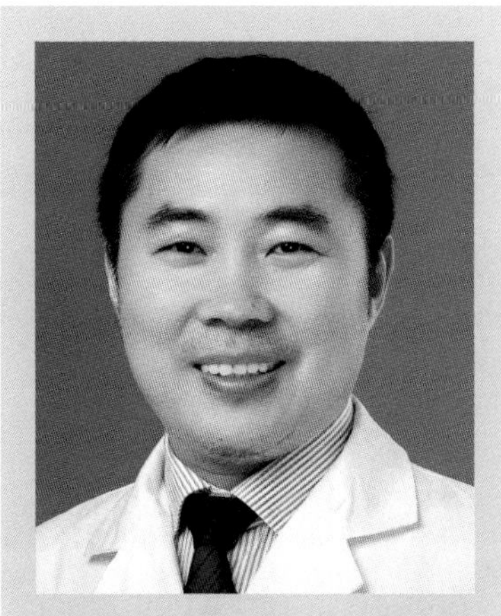

Wang Xiangyang

Chief physician, professor, doctoral supervisor, graduated from Shanghai Jiao Tong University School of Medicine with a doctoral degree, director of the Orthopedic Construction Committee of Yuying Children's Hospital affiliated with Wenzhou Medical University, executive director of Zhejiang Children and Adolescents Spinal Health Guidance Center, leader of national clinical key specialty disciplines, and recipient of the National Top 10 Young and Middle aged Orthopedic Physicians Award. Established the "Yuying Backbone Project" charity fund and the "Jiliang Zhengzi" alliance. Hosted 5 projects funded by the National Natural Science Foundation of China, Zhejiang Provincial Natural Science Outstanding Youth Fund, Zhejiang Provincial "Leading Goose" Key R&D Project, Provincial and Ministerial Joint Construction Project, Zhejiang Qianjiang Talent Project, and other 8 projects. Published over 150 SCI and EI papers as the first and corresponding author, edited "*Anatomy of Spinal Column Fixation*" and co authored 15 books. The person in charge or main researcher has won the second prize of the National Science and Technology Progress Award, the first prize of the Chinese Medical Science and Technology Award, the first prize of the Zhejiang Provincial Science and Technology Progress Award, and the first prize of the Shanghai Municipal Science and Technology Progress Award.

副主编简介

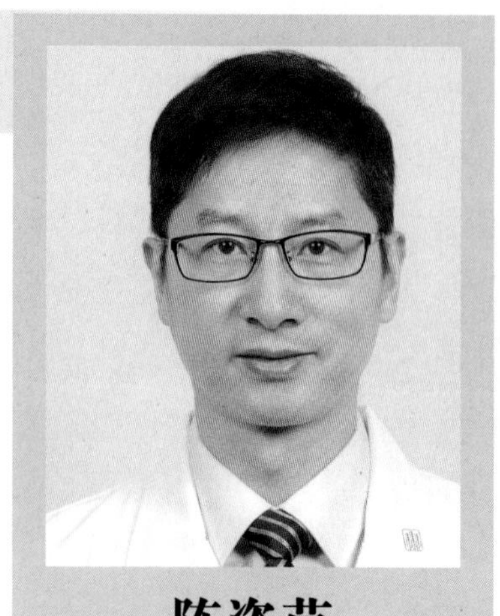

陈迩苗

中共党员，主任医师，副教授，硕士研究生导师，博士，温州医科大学附属第一医院党委委员、副院长，温州医科大学附属第一医院创面修复与再生医学中心副主任。现任浙江省医院协会患者安全管理专业委员会副主任委员，浙江省医学会营养与代谢分会常务委员，中国老年医学学会运动健康分会常务委员，浙江省医师协会内科医师分会委员，浙江省医疗质量管理委员会委员，浙江省医学会临床试验与伦理分会委员，浙江省医学会人文医学分会委员，温州市中西医结合学会常务理事。《糖尿病新世界》杂志社编委会委员。获评医院管理论坛一等奖，校级教学软件比赛二、三等奖。主持参与国家自然科学基金项目、浙江省自然科学基金项目、温州市科技局课题项目多项。

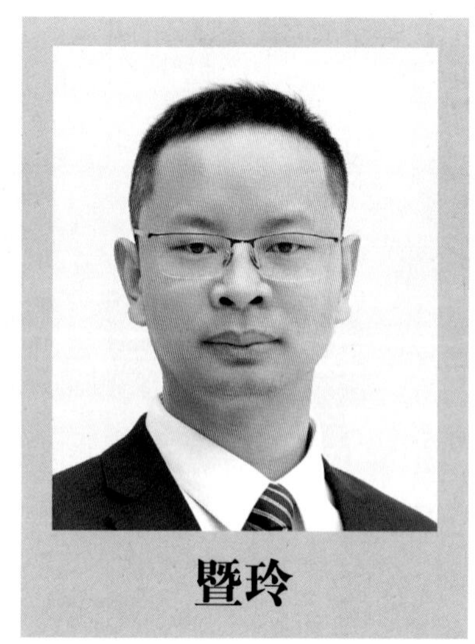

暨玲

温州医科大学附属第一医院医务部主任，大肠外科副主任医师，“肤生工程”国际合作中心主任，浙南紧急医学救援队队长，德国佐林根圣卢卡斯医院访问学者，中国抗癌协会肿瘤与肠道微生物专业委员会青年委员，浙江省医院协会医疗联合体管理专业委员会委员，浙江省医学研究伦理质量控制中心质控专家，浙江省医学会器官移植学分会委员，温州市康复医学会结直肠疾病康复专业委员会委员，第17批援中非共和国医疗队外科主任，中非共和国国家荣誉勋章获得者。

Introduction to the Deputy Editor in Chief

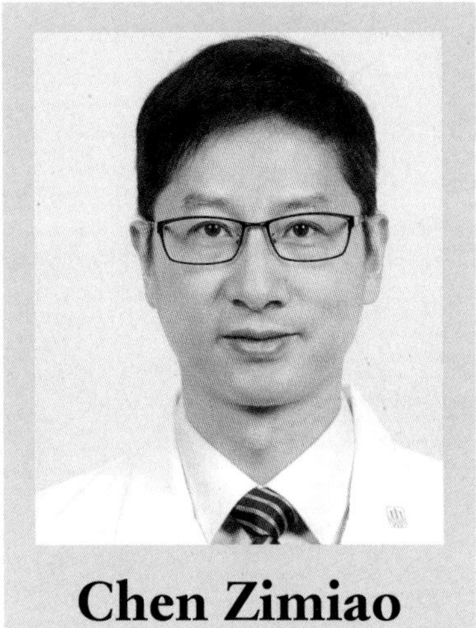

Chen Zimiao

Currently serving as the Vice Chairman of the Patient Safety Management Professional Committee of the Zhejiang Hospital Association, Executive Member of the Nutrition and Metabolism Branch of the Zhejiang Medical Association, Executive Member of the Sports and Health Branch of the Chinese Geriatric Society, Member of the Internal Medicine Branch of the Zhejiang Medical Association, Member of the Zhejiang Medical Quality Management Committee, Member of the Clinical Trial and Ethics Branch of the Zhejiang Medical Association, Member of the Humanities Branch of the Zhejiang Medical Association, and Executive Director of the Wenzhou Association of Traditional Chinese and Western Medicine. Member of the editorial board of *Diabetes New World Magazine*. Won the first prize in the Hospital Management Forum and the second and third prizes in the school level teaching software competition. Hosted and participated in multiple projects funded by the National Natural Science Foundation of China, Zhejiang Provincial Natural Science Foundation, and Wenzhou Science and Technology Bureau.

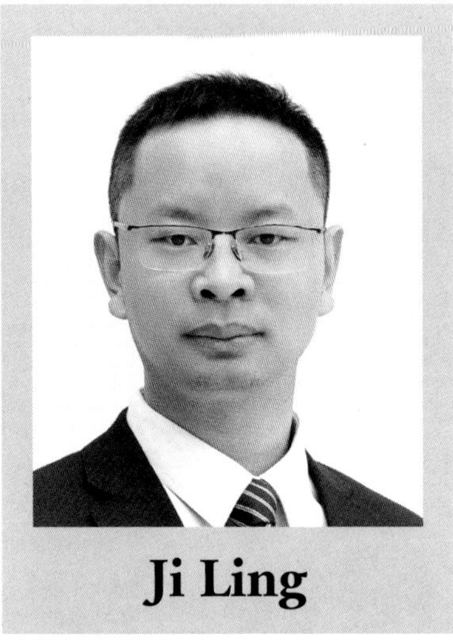

Ji Ling

Director of the Medical Department of the First Affiliated Hospital of Wenzhou Medical University, Deputy Chief Physician of the Department of Colorectal Surgery, Director of the International Cooperation Center for "F&S CHARITY", Captain of the Zhejiang Southern Emergency Medical Rescue Team, Visiting Scholar at St. Lucas Hospital in Solingen, Germany, Youth Member of the Tumor and Gut Microbiota Professional Committee of the China Anti Cancer Association, Member of the Medical Consortium Management Professional Committee of the Zhejiang Hospital Association, Quality Control Expert of the Zhejiang Medical Research Ethics Quality Control Center, Member of the Organ Transplantation Branch of the Zhejiang Medical Association, Member of the Colorectal Disease Rehabilitation Professional Committee of the Wenzhou Rehabilitation Medicine Association, Director of the Surgery Department of the 17th Batch of Aid to the Central African Republic Medical Team, and Recipient of the National Medal of Honor of the Central African Republic.

副主编简介

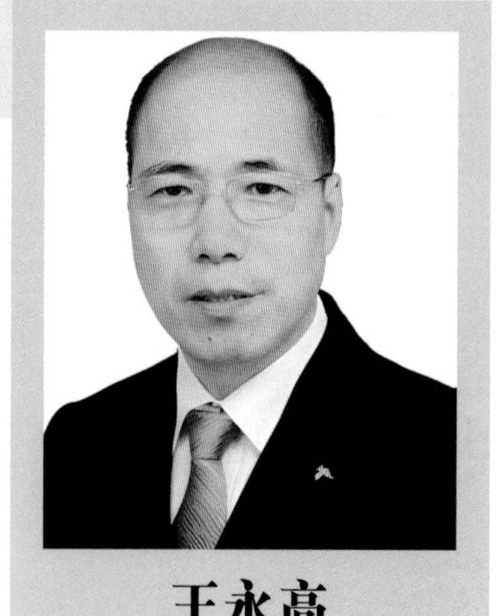

王永高

浙江省中医院副主任医师兼副教授，血管外科学科带头人，创面修复多学科诊疗（MDT）专家组组长，糖尿病足中西医结合诊治获得医院高质量发展助推计划学科建设项目。从事血管外科、普外科临床工作30余年，对血管外科疾病、糖尿病足、创面修复、毒蛇咬伤诊治具有丰富的临床经验。担任中国微循环学会周围血管疾病专业委员会静脉曲张学组副组长，长三角脉管病联盟副理事长，中华医学会急诊医学分会蛇伤专家委员会委员，世界中医药学会联合会痘证专业委员会常务委员，中国医药教育协会蛇伤防治专业委员会常务委员，浙江省中西医结合学会周围血管疾病专业委员会常务委员，中国医药教育协会创面修复学专业委员会常务委员，中华慢病学院伤口分院常务委员，浙江糖尿病足联盟委员。

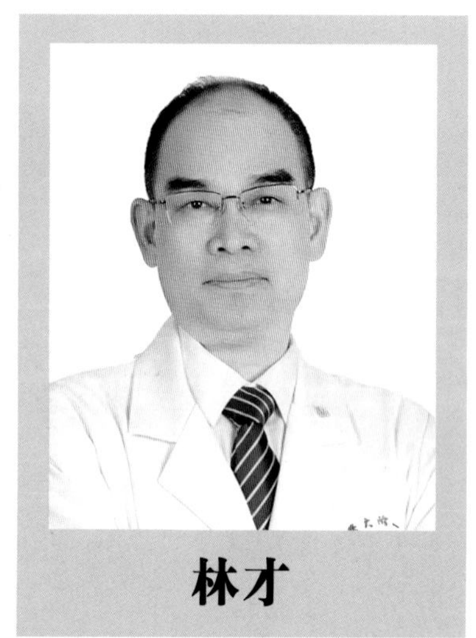

林才

主任医师，生物医学工程博士，博士研究生导师，温州医科大学附属第一医院烧伤•伤口中心主任，温州医科大学组织工程皮肤临床研究中心主任，温州医科大学创面修复与再生医学中心核心成员。学术任职：中华医学会烧伤外科学分会第六届委员会委员，中国生物材料学会生物陶瓷分会委员等。长期从事烧伤与创面修复临床实践及相关研究，主持包括中国科学技术协会“智惠行动”、浙江省自然科学基金项目重点专项等课题20余项，探索性研究人工智能创面识别技术获2023年度省“尖兵领雁”重大专项。连续两年带领烧伤外科进入中国医院科技量值STEM专科排名百强前十，同时作为创面修复科核心成员获国内第一个国家重点临床专科建设项目，实现创面修复学科建设重大突破！

Introduction to the Deputy Editor in Chief

Wang Yonggao

Associate chief physician and associate professor of Zhejiang Provincial Hospital of Traditional Chinese Medicine, leader of vascular surgery discipline, leader of multi-disciplinary diagnosis and treatment (MDT) expert group for wound repair, and obtained the discipline construction project of high-quality development boosting plan of the hospital by combining the diagnosis and treatment of Chinese and western medicine for diabetes foot. He has been engaged in clinical work in vascular surgery and general surgery for more than 30 years, and has rich clinical experience in diagnosis and treatment of vascular surgery diseases, diabetes foot, wound repair, and snake bite. Served as the deputy leader of the varicose vein group of the Specialized Committee of Peripheral Vascular Diseases of the Chinese Microcirculation Society, the vice chairman of the Yangtze River Delta Vascular Disease Alliance, the member of the Snake Wound Expert Committee of the Emergency Medicine Branch of the Chinese Medical Association, the standing member of the Gangrene Professional Committee of the World Federation of Chinese Medical Societies, the standing member of the Snake Wound Prevention Professional Committee of the Chinese Medical Education Association, the standing member of the Specialized Committee of Peripheral Vascular Diseases of the Zhejiang Association of Integrated Traditional and Western Medicine, the standing member of the Wound Repair Professional Committee of the Chinese Medical Education Association, the standing member of the Wound Branch of the Chinese Academy of Chronic Diseases, and the member of the Diabetes.

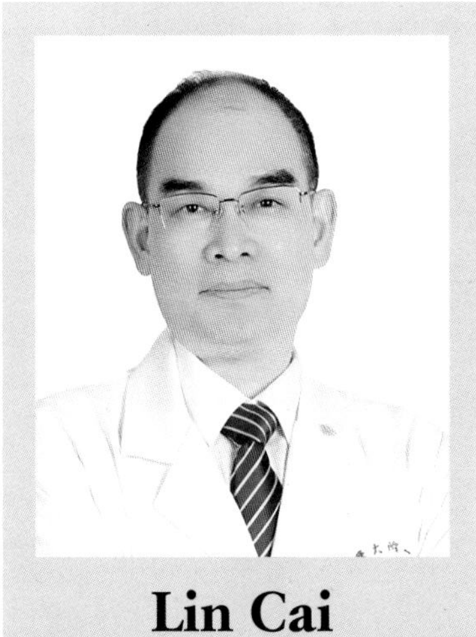

Lin Cai

Chief Physician, Doctor of Biomedical Engineering, Doctoral Supervisor, Director of Burn and Wound Center at the First Affiliated Hospital of Wenzhou Medical University, Director of Clinical Research Center for Tissue Engineering Skin at Wenzhou Medical University, and a core member of Wenzhou Medical University Wound Repair and Regenerative Medicine Center. Academic positions: Member of the 6th Committee of the Burn Surgery Branch of the Chinese Medical Association, member of the Bioceramic Branch of the Chinese Society for Biomaterials, etc. Engaged in clinical practice and related research on burn and wound repair for a long time, led more than 20 projects including the "Smart Benefit Action" of the China Association for Science and Technology and the key special projects of the Zhejiang Provincial Natural Science Foundation. Exploratory research on artificial intelligence wound recognition technology won the "Leading Goose" major special project of the province in 2023. For two consecutive years, we have led burn surgery to enter the top ten of the top 100 STEM specialties in China's hospital science and technology rankings. At the same time, as a core member of the wound repair department, we have won the first national key clinical specialty construction project in China, achieving a major breakthrough in the construction of the wound repair discipline!

副主编简介

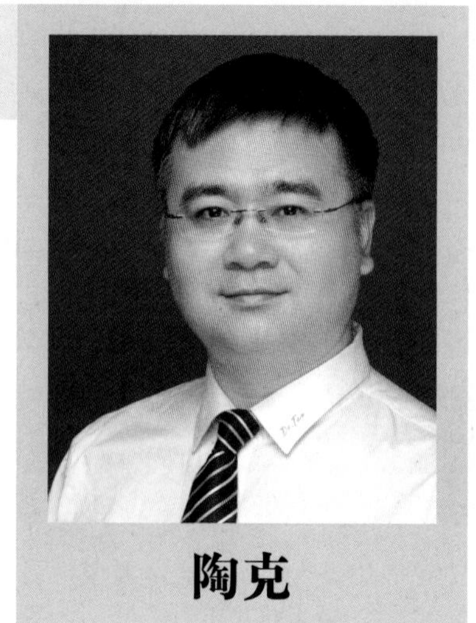

陶克

温州医科大学附属第一医院创面修复科副主任，副主任医师，医学博士、硕士研究生导师。现任中国老年医学学会烧创伤分会副会长，中华医学会烧伤外科学分会瘢痕学组副组长，中国康复医学会再生医学与康复专业委员会常务委员，《中华烧伤杂志》《中华卫生应急电子杂志》编委等。获军队科学技术进步奖一、二等奖各 1 项，中华医学科技奖一等奖 1 项，陕西省科学技术进步奖一等奖 1 项。承担国家自然科学基金项目 4 项，发表论文 80 余篇，获国家发明专利 3 项，主编专著 4 部。

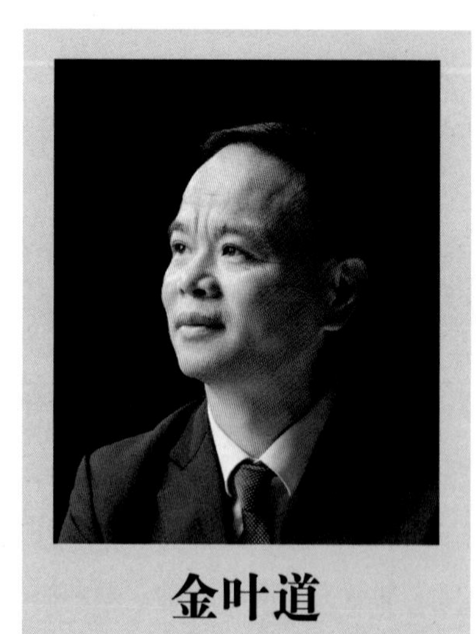

金叶道

温州曙光医院院长，温州市脊椎相关疾病研究所所长，上海惠元医院创始人，毕业于温州医学院、清华大学，香港公开大学 EMBA 硕士、传统医学博士。中华中医药学会整脊分会第三届青年委员，中国医院协会民营医院分会委员，浙江省社会办医协会第一、第二届骨科专业委员会常务委员，温州市社会办医协会副会长，温州市中医药学会骨伤专业委员会常务委员，温州市中医学会常务理事，峨眉正骨术第七代代表性传承人，温州市第八届政协委员，龙湾区第二、第三、第五届政协常务委员。《腰椎整脊学》主编。采用峨眉整脊法从事脊椎及相关疑难杂症临床研究工作30余年，主持多项与脊椎生物力学相关的课题研究，发表与脊椎相关急腹症的手法治疗临床报告等多篇论文。

Introduction to the Deputy Editor in Chief

Tao Ke

Deputy Director of the Department of Wound Repair at the First Affiliated Hospital of Wenzhou Medical University, Deputy Chief Physician, Medical Doctor, and Master's Supervisor. The current Vice President of the Burn and Trauma Branch of the Chinese Geriatric Society, Deputy Leader of the Scar Group of the Burn Surgery Branch of the Chinese Medical Association, Standing Committee Member of the Regenerative Medicine and Rehabilitation Professional Committee of Chinese Rehabilitation Medicine Association, and Editorial Board Member of *Chinese Journal of Burns* and *Chinese Health Emergency Electronic Journal.* Received one first and one second prize of the Military Science and Technology Progress Award, one first prize of the Chinese Medical Science and Technology Award, and one first prize of the Shaanxi Province Science and Technology Progress Award. Undertook 4 National Natural Science Foundation projects, published over 80 papers, obtained 3 national invention patents, and edited 4 monographs.

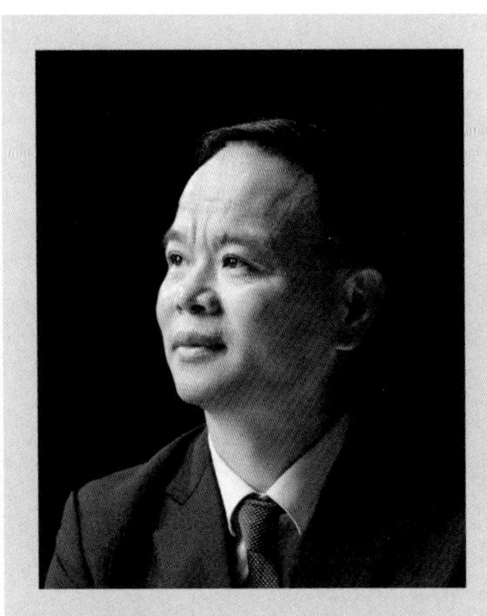

Jin Yedao

Dean of Wenzhou Shuguang Hospital, Director of Wenzhou Institute of Vertebrate Diseases, Founder of Shanghai Huiyuan Hospital, graduated from Wenzhou Medical College, Tsinghua University, EMBA Master's degree from Open University of Hong Kong, and Doctor of Traditional Medicine. The 3rd Youth Member of the Orthopedic Branch of the Chinese Association of Traditional Chinese Medicine, Member of the Private Hospital Branch of the China Hospital Association, Executive Member of the 1st and 2nd Orthopedic Professional Committees of the Zhejiang Provincial Social Medical Association, Vice President of the Wenzhou Social Medical Association, Executive Member of the Orthopedic Professional Committee of the Wenzhou Association of Traditional Chinese Medicine, Executive Director of the Wenzhou Association of Traditional Chinese Medicine, Representative Inheritor of the 7th Generation of Emei Orthopedic Surgery, Member of the 8th Wenzhou Political Consultative Conference, and Standing Committee Member of the 2nd, 3rd, and 5th Longwan District Political Consultative Conference. Editor in Chief of *Lumbar Spine Surgery*. I have been engaged in clinical research on spinal and related difficult and complicated diseases for more than 30 years using the Emei spinal manipulation method. I have led multiple research projects related to spinal biomechanics and published multiple clinical reports on manual therapy for spinal related acute abdomen.

副主编简介

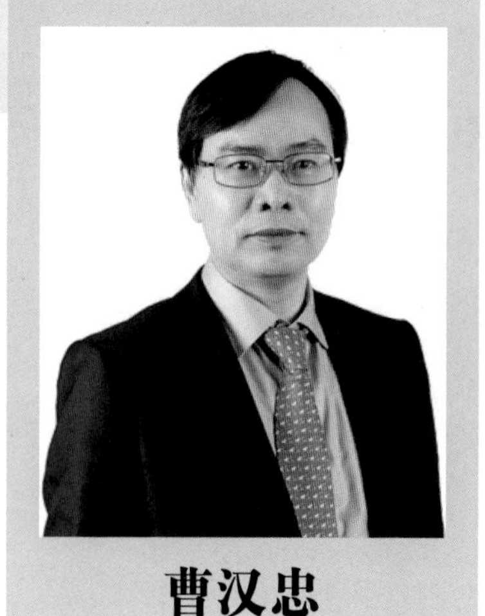
曹汉忠

主任医师，中国抗癌协会肿瘤麻醉与镇痛委员会常务委员，江苏省医院协会麻醉与疼痛管理专业委员会副主任委员，南通大学附属肿瘤医院麻醉科主任，南通市麻醉科质量控制中心主任，专注于急慢性疼痛诊疗与管理研究，主持及参与市级、省级、科技部项目 10 多项。“无线镇痛泵系统研发”于 2011 年获科技部科技型中小企业技术创新基金立项，建立镇痛泵系统产品标准，获国家药品监督管理局Ⅲ类医疗注册，推广至全国上千家大中型医院，2018 年形成了《智能化患者自控镇痛(Ai-PCA)管理专家共识》，2019 年获中国抗癌协会科技奖二等奖；2023 年获华夏医学科技奖二等奖，主编《无痛医院实用技能》，参编专著《智能化病人自控镇痛》及研究生教材《麻醉学》，参与编写《智能化患者自控镇痛管理规范》（T/CATE 0021-2024）。

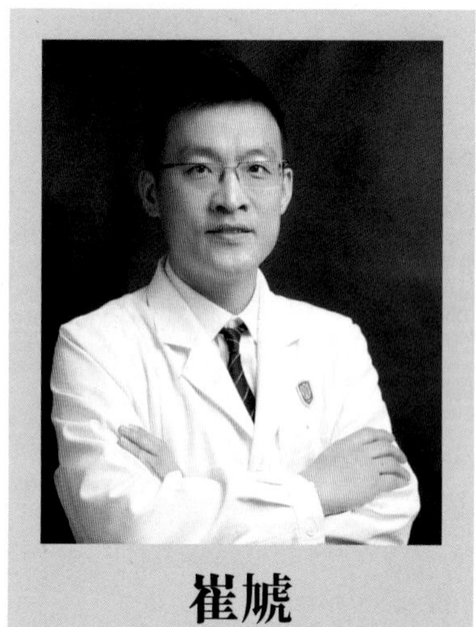
崔旒

现任温州医科大学附属第二医院、育英儿童医院医保物价办公室主任，副主任药师。浙江省医院协会医疗保险管理专业委员会委员、中国优生科学协会基因与药学学组委员、浙江省医师协会临床合理用药专业委员会青年委员、温州市药学会理事、温州市医学会儿童药学学组委员，温州市医保基金监管飞行检查专家组成员。从事医保政策与药物经济学分析、临床药物合理应用和药源性疾病的判断与处理等。主持浙江省基础公益研究计划课题、温州市基础公益研究计划课题。曾获 2018 年浙江省统战理论政策研究优秀成果二等奖、浙江省青年岗位能手、温州医科大学优秀教师等荣誉。带领团队连续荣获第五、第六届中国医影节“金丹奖”。

Introduction to the Deputy Editor in Chief

Cao Hanzhong

Chief physician, standing committee member of the Tumor Anesthesia and Analgesia Committee of the China Anti Cancer Association, vice chairman of the Anesthesia and Pain Management Special Committee of the Jiangsu Hospital Association, director of the Anesthesiology Department of Nantong University Affiliated Cancer Hospital, director of the Nantong Anesthesiology Quality Control Center, specializing in the diagnosis, treatment, and management of acute and chronic pain, leading and participating in more than 10 municipal, provincial, and national science and technology projects. The research and development of wireless analgesia pump system was approved by the Technology Innovation Fund for Science and Technology based Small and Medium sized Enterprises of the Ministry of Science and Technology of China in 2011. It established product standards for analgesia pump system and obtained Class III medical registration from the National Medical Products Administration. It has been promoted to thousands of large and medium-sized hospitals across the country. In 2018, it formed the *Expert Consensus on Intelligent Patient Controlled Analgesia (Ai-PCA) Management* and won the second prize in science and technology from the China Anti Cancer Association in 2019; In 2023, won the second prize of Huaxia Medical Technology, edited *Practical Skills for Painless Hospitals*, participated in the compilation of the monograph *Intelligent Patient Controlled Analgesia* and the graduate textbook *Anesthesiology*, and participated in the compilation of the *Intelligent Patient Controlled Analgesia Management Specification (T/CATE 0021-2024)*.

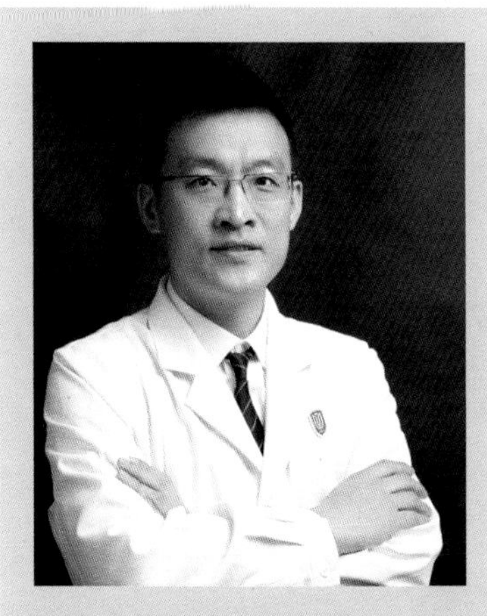

Cui Xiao

Currently serving as the Director of the Medical Insurance Price Office at the Second Affiliated Hospital of Wenzhou Medical University and Yuying Children's Hospital, Deputy Chief Pharmacist. Member of the Medical Insurance Special Committee of Zhejiang Hospital Association, Member of the Genetics and Pharmacy Group of China Eugenics Science Association, Youth Member of the Clinical Rational Drug Use Professional Committee of Zhejiang Physician Association, Director of Wenzhou Pharmaceutical Association, Member of the Children's Pharmacy Group of Wenzhou Medical Association, and Member of the Wenzhou Medical Insurance Fund Supervision Flight Inspection Expert Group. Engaged in medical insurance policy and pharmacoeconomic analysis, rational use of clinical drugs, diagnosis and treatment of drug-induced diseases. He hosted projects under the Zhejiang Province Basic Public Welfare Research Program and the Wenzhou City Basic Public Welfare Research Program. He has won honors such as the Second Prize for Outstanding Achievements in 2018 Zhejiang Province United Front Theory and Policy Research, Zhejiang Province Youth Post Expert, and Wenzhou Medical University Outstanding Teacher. He led the team to win the "Golden Dan Award" at the 5th and 6th China Medical Film Festival consecutively.

副主编简介

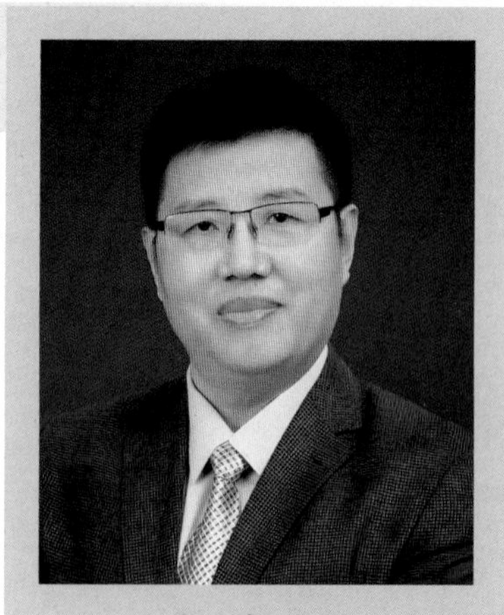

闫合德

医学博士，主任医师，博士研究生导师，温州医科大学附属第二医院手显微外科主任，浙江省医学会显微外科分会现任主任委员，中华医学会显微外科分会委员，*Frontier in Neuroanatomy* 副主编，*Annals of Plastic Surgery* 及 *Microsurgery* 等SCI杂志编委。浙江省卫生创新人才、温州市“551”工程人才。主持国家自然科学基金面上项目2项、浙江省自然科学基金项目3项等10余项课题，以第一作者或通讯作者发表SCI收录论文60余篇，授权专利15项。

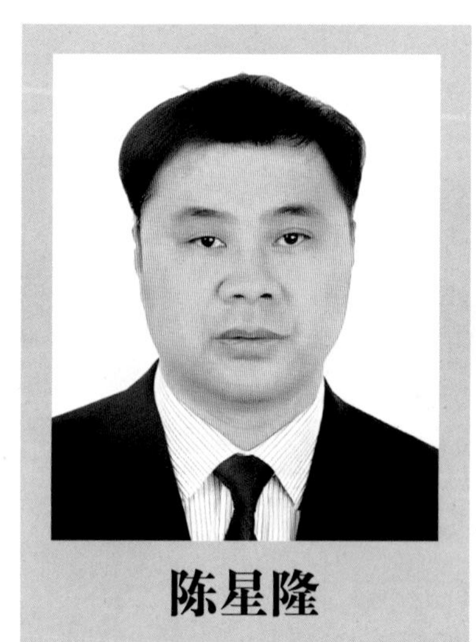

陈星隆

温州医科大学附属第二医院骨科、手显微外科主任医师，科室副主任。现任中华医学会手外科学分会骨与关节学组委员，中国康复医学会修复重建外科专业委员会再造与再植学组委员，中国老年医学会骨与关节分会委员，华东地区手外科学专业委员会委员，浙江省医学会手外科学分会副主任，浙江省医学会显微外科学分会副主任委员，浙江省医师协会手外科医师分会委员，温州市医学会手外科学分会副主任委员，温州市医疗事故鉴定委员会专家库成员，温州市劳动能力鉴定委员会专家。在SCI、中华系列杂志等专业杂志以第一作者或通讯作者发表学术论文近20余篇，主持与参与省部级、厅级课题基金数项，获得2006年度、2011年度浙江省卫生系统应急工作先进个人称号。

Introduction to the Deputy Editor in Chief

Yan Hede

Doctor of Medicine, Chief Physician, Doctoral Supervisor, Director of Hand Microsurgery at the Second Affiliated Hospital of Wenzhou Medical University, Current Chairman of the Microsurgery Branch of the Zhejiang Medical Association, Member of the Microsurgery Branch of the Chinese Medical Association, Deputy Editor in Chief of *Frontier in Neuroanatomy*, and Editorial Board Member of SCI journals such as *Annals of Plastic Surgery* and *Microsurgery*. Zhejiang Province Health Innovation Talents and Wenzhou City "551" Project Talents. I have led over 10 projects, including 2 National Natural Science Foundation of China general projects and 3 Zhejiang Provincial Natural Science Foundation projects. As the first or corresponding author, I have published more than 60 SCI indexed papers and been granted 15 patents.

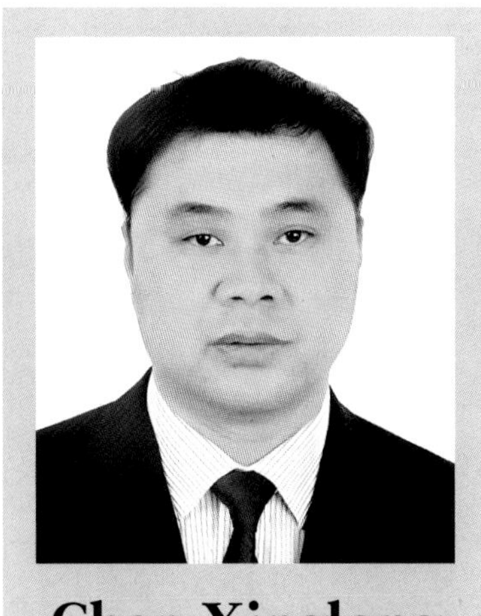

Chen Xinglong

Chief Physician and Deputy Director of Orthopedics and Hand Microsurgery at the Second Affiliated Hospital of Wenzhou Medical University. Currently serving as a member of the Orthopedics and Arthrology Group of the Hand Surgery Credit Association of the Chinese Medical Association, a member of the Reconstruction and Reconstructive Surgery Professional Committee of the Chinese Rehabilitation Medicine Association, a member of the Bone and Joint Branch of the Chinese Geriatrics Association, a member of the Hand Surgery Professional Committee of the East China Region, the Deputy Director of the Hand Surgery Branch of the Zhejiang Medical Association, the Deputy Director of the Microsurgery Branch of the Zhejiang Medical Association, a member of the Hand Surgery Branch of the Zhejiang Medical Association, the Deputy Director of the Hand Surgery Branch of the Wenzhou Medical Association, a member of the Expert Database of the Wenzhou Medical Accident Appraisal Committee, and an expert of the Wenzhou Labor Capacity Appraisal Committee. He has published more than 20 academic papers as the first author or corresponding author in professional journals such as SCI and Chinese series magazines, presided over and participated in several provincial and ministerial level and department level project funds, and won the title of exemplary individual in Zhejiang Health System Emergency Work in 2006 and 2011.

副主编简介

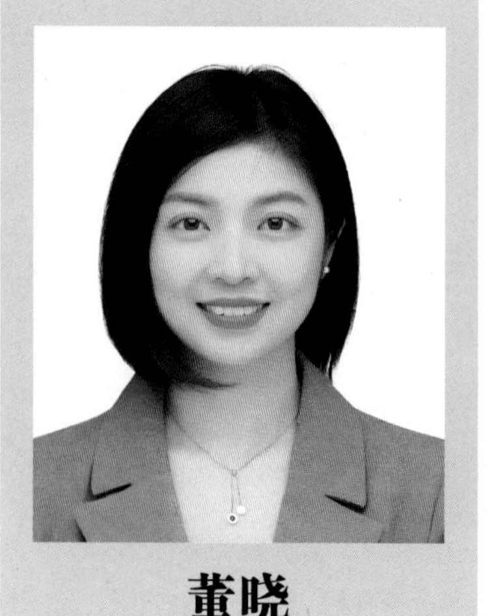

董晓

浙江财经大学管理学硕士研究生，经济师，温州医科大学附属第一医院组织人事部主任、人才办主任，党支部副书记，兼任浙江省医院协会人力资源专业副主任委员。长期在医院组织人事部门工作，熟悉医院组织干部管理、人力资源管理、经济管理等业务，具体涵盖中层干部选拔、中层干部培养、人力资源配置、薪酬管理、人才队伍建设、人才培养、人员绩效管理等。目前已发表中文论文 10 余篇，主持厅局级课题 2 项，曾获医院先进职工、医院先进职能科室负责人、医院优秀党员、温州医科大学优秀党务工作者等荣誉，2022 年度主持案例《引育并重，打造人才集聚“强磁场”》入选国家卫生健康委员会中国现代医院管理典型案例，带领科室多次获批温州市政府人才工作成绩突出集体。

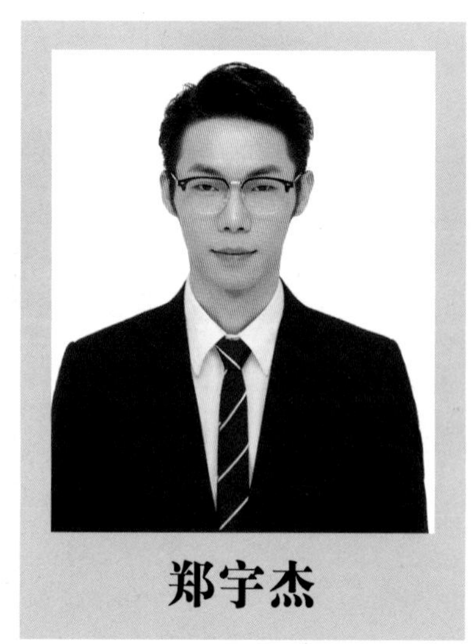

郑宇杰

现任“肤生工程”办公室主任，华奥医学研究（温州）有限公司董事长。具备丰富的商业运营经验，曾成功主导地产、金融、贸易等多个领域的项目投资与运营。近年来，致力于创面修复学科推广，并全身心投入“肤生工程”公益慈善项目。加入“肤生工程”团队后，积极参与策划并筹备了泰顺、永嘉、青藏以及中非共和国等地的慈善公益活动。不仅以企业家的身份身体力行地参与慈善活动，更积极倡导更多企业为慈善事业贡献力量，如慈善捐款、物资捐赠、慈善公益论坛等，共同推动社会公益的发展。

Introduction to the Deputy Editor in Chief

Dong Xiao

A master's student in management at Zhejiang University of Finance and Economics, economist, director of the Organization and Personnel Department and Talent Office of the First Affiliated Hospital of Wenzhou Medical University, deputy secretary of the Party branch, and also serves as the vice chairman of the Human Resources Professional Committee of the Zhejiang Hospital Association. I have been working in the human resources department of the hospital for a long time and am familiar with the management of hospital organizational cadres, human resources, and economic management. This includes the selection and training of middle-level cadres, human resource allocation, salary management, talent team building, talent cultivation, and personnel performance management. At present, more than 10 Chinese papers have been published, and 2 departmental level projects have been presided over. The department has been honored as an advanced employee of the hospital, an advanced functional department head of the hospital, an outstanding party member of the hospital, and an outstanding party worker of Wenzhou Medical University. In 2022, the case study *Emphasizing Education and Talent Agglomeration, Creating a Strong Magnetic Field* was selected as a typical case of modern hospital management in China by the National Health Commission, and the department has been repeatedly approved as an outstanding collective in talent work by the Wenzhou Municipal Government.

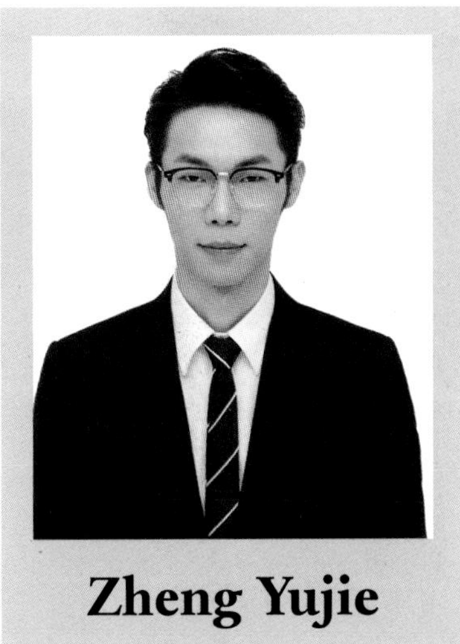

Zheng Yujie

Current Director of the "F&S CHARITY" Office and Chairman of Huaao Medical Research (Wenzhou) Limited Company. With rich experience in business operations, Zheng Yujie has successfully led project investments and operations in multiple fields such as real estate, finance, and trade. In recent years, he has shifted his focus to promoting the discipline of wound repair and devoted himself to the "F&S CHARITY" charity project. After joining the F&S CHARITY team, he actively participated in planning and preparing charity and public welfare activities in Taishun, Yongjia, Qinghai Tibet, and the Central African Republic. Not only does he actively participate in charitable activities as entrepreneurs, but he also advocates for more companies to contribute to charitable causes, such as charitable donations, material donations, charity forums, to jointly promote the development of social welfare.

序

《生长因子与创面修复图鉴》是“肤生工程”团队在开展难愈合创面患者救助公益活动中积累的临床案例集，也是生长因子治疗溃疡和加速损伤组织再生在临床治疗中的一些实践收录。

本书主要分为三部分，即概述、典型个案介绍、附录。第一部分从生长因子讲起。我从事生长因子研究已有三十几年时间，最初是从壁虎断尾再生引发的思考开始，发现生长因子在再生过程中的生理和病理机制，而正是人体内一种神奇的细胞因子——成纤维细胞生长因子，促进了损伤组织再生和创面修复。成纤维细胞生长因子作为从低等动物到哺乳类动物都存在的一类多功能保守蛋白，最早由美国科学家发现，但要将其开发为药物却存在很多的技术瓶颈，中途很多人看不到希望都选择了放弃。但我和团队成员一直坚持不懈，最终取得了成功，使我国成为世界上第一个把成纤维细胞生长因子开发为新药的国家。到目前为止，我们已经有 3 个生长因子自主创新药及 1 个含生长因子的医疗器械生物蛋白海绵“创必复”获批上市并应用于临床。近年来，我们还发现了生长因子的糖脂代谢的调控机制，可用于治疗糖尿病多种并发症，如糖尿病溃疡、糖尿病肾病、糖尿病周围神经病变。围绕以生长因子为代表的蛋白质药物基础理论研究与新药研发，尤其是成纤维细胞生长因子（FGF）家族蛋白的功能、系统理论与新药研究，我们发现了生长因子与一系列疾病的相关机制和大分子药物研发的相关规律，为临床诊治提供了全新的思路，为生长因子系列新药研发奠定了重要基础。这些发现不仅助力药物研发，还将对生命的进化和发育产生新的启示、思考与认识。研发的药物主要用于战创伤、烧烫伤和糖

Foreword

The *Atlas of Growth Factors and Wound Repair* is a collection of clinical cases accumulated by the "F&S CHARITY" team in carrying out public welfare activities to rescue patients with difficult to heal wounds. It is also a practical collection of growth factor therapy for ulcers and accelerated tissue regeneration in clinical treatment.

This book is mainly divided into three parts: an overview of growth factors, introduction of typical cases, and public welfare and wound repair. The first part starts with growth factors. I have been engaged in the research of growth factors for more than 30 years. Initially, I started thinking about the regeneration of geckos' severed tails and discovered the physiological and pathological mechanisms of growth factors in the regeneration process. It is a magical cytokine in the human body – fibroblast growth factor, which promotes the regeneration of damaged tissues and wound repair. Fibroblast growth factor, as a multifunctional conserved protein that exists in both lower animals and mammals, was first discovered by American scientists. However, there were many technical bottlenecks in developing it into a drug, and many people chose to give up halfway because they did not see hope. But my team and I persevered and ultimately achieved success, making our country the first in the world to develop fibroblast growth factor as a new drug. So far, we have obtainod approval for thc marlceting and clinical application of three growth factor independent innovative drugs and one growth factor containing medical device, the biological protein sponge "Chuangbifu". In recent years, we also found the regulation mechanism of glucose and lipid metabolism of growth factors, which can be used to treat various complications of diabetes, such as diabetes ulcer, diabetes nephropathy, and diabetes peripheral neuropathy. Based on the basic theoretical research and new drug development of protein drugs represented by growth factors, especially the function, systematic theory, and new drug research of fibroblast growth factor (FGF) family proteins, we have discovered the relevant mechanisms of growth factors and a series of diseases, as well as the relevant laws of macromolecular drug development. This provides a new approach for clinical diagnosis and treatment and lays an important foundation for the development of growth factor series new drugs. These discoveries will not only aid in drug development, but also provide new insights, thinking, and understanding for the evolution and development of life. The drugs developed are mainly used for the treatment of war wounds, burns, diabetes feet and other refractory ulcers. More than 80 million patients have benefited clinically. They went to the Central African Republic with the Chinese medical team to carry out wound

尿病足等难愈性溃疡的治疗，临床受益患者超 8000 万人，并随中国医疗队远赴中非共和国开展援非创面救治，为国际创伤救治提供了“中国方案”。荣获国家科学技术进步奖一等奖、国家技术发明奖二等奖、国家自然科学二等奖、何梁何利基金科学与技术进步奖、谈家桢生命科学奖、光华工程科技奖、转化医学突出贡献奖等各类奖项。这本《生长因子与创面修复图鉴》中列举的案例，在临床实践上，较为全面地生动佐证了生长因子促进创面修复的良好效果。

第二部分的典型个案介绍以图文形式，展示了生长因子在临床的应用情况，对患者症状、诊治过程、注意事项等治疗信息进行了详细阐述，覆盖急性创面、压力性创面、感染性创面、动脉性创面、糖尿病足创面、癌性创面、烧伤烫伤创面、静脉性创面等各类典型急慢性创面，对生长因子在创面修复临床救治实践有一定的指导意义。图书中难愈合创面案例患病时间最长达 54 年之久，严重影响着患者的生命健康和生活质量，同时也困扰着患者整个家庭。所幸经过生长因子临床科研团队的救治，最终使其创面得到愈合。对此书中每一例患者创面的愈合，我认为愈合的不仅仅是伤口，更是患者心灵的创伤。

第三部分是附录，主要介绍“肤生工程”救助创面患者的公益实践。2020 年 5 月，温州医科大学、温州市慈善总会、温州都市报以及温州曙光医院等单位联合发起“肤生工程”公益慈善项目。团队坚持科技为民、服务社会，以生长因子团队长期从事创面修复与组织再生相关药物研究成果为基础，为全国各地深受创面问题困扰的弱势人群提供慈善救助服务。团队先后在浙、闽、陕、藏等地建立了 68 个创面救助点，开展精准医疗走访 560 人次、手术及住院治疗 213 人次，累计捐款捐物 780 万元，总公益行程超 153 000 公里，足迹遍布温州各地以及我国中西部偏远地区，受益者达 5 万余人。此书收录的大部分案例是在公益实践过程中发现并在“肤生工程”爱心医院——温州曙光医院进行救治的真实案例，对于生长因子在创面修复临床救治实践有实际的指导意义。

rescue in Africa, providing a "Chinese plan" for international trauma treatment. Has won various awards such as the National Science and Technology Progress First Prize, National Technology Invention Second Prize, National Natural Science Second Prize, He Liang He Li Science and Technology Progress Award, Tan Jiazhen Life Science Award, Guanghua Engineering Science and Technology Award, and Outstanding Contribution Award for Translational Medicine. The cases listed in this *Atlas of Growth Factors and Wound Repair* vividly demonstrate the good effect of growth factors in promoting wound repair in clinical practice.

The second part of the typical case introduction shows the clinical application of growth factors in the form of pictures and texts, and elaborates the treatment information of patients such as symptoms, diagnosis and treatment process, and precautions, covering various typical acute and chronic wounds such as acute wounds, pressure wounds, infectious wounds, arterial wounds, diabetes foot wounds, cancerous wounds, burn and scald wounds, venous wounds, which has certain guiding significance for the clinical treatment practice of growth factors in wound repair. The case of difficult to heal wounds in the book has been affected for up to 54 years, seriously affecting the patient's life, health, and quality of life, while also troubling the patient's entire family. Fortunately, with the treatment of the growth factor clinical research team, the wound was finally healed. I believe that the healing of each patient's wound in this book is not only about the wound, but also about the emotional trauma of the patient.

The third part of this book is about public welfare and wound healing, mainly introducing the public welfare practice of the "F&S CHARITY" in rescuing wound patients. In May 2020, Wenzhou Medical University, Wenzhou Charity Federation, Wenzhou Urban Daily, and Wenzhou Shuguang Hospital jointly launched the "F&S CHARITY" public welfare charity project. The team adheres to the principle of technology for the people and serving society. Based on the long-term research achievements of the growth factor team in wound repair and tissue regeneration related drugs, we provide charitable assistance services to vulnerable groups across the country who are deeply troubled by wound problems. The team has established 68 wound relief points in Zhejiang, Fujian, Shaanxi, Tibet and other places, carried out precision medical visits to 560 people, surgeries and hospitalizations to 213 people, donated a total of 7.8 million yuan in donations and goods, and traveled a total of over 153 000 kilometers for public welfare, covering various parts of Wenzhou and remote areas in central and western China, benefiting more than 50 000 people. Most of the cases included in this book are real cases discovered in the process of public welfare practice and treated at Wenzhou Shuguang Hospital, a caring hospital of "F&S CHARITY". They have practical guiding significance for the clinical treatment of growth factors in wound repair.

“肤生工程”团队成员既有科技工作者、医疗工作者、教育工作者，也有对公益事业充满热情的媒体记者、爱心人士。此书的出版得到了出版社的高度重视与大力支持，由“肤生工程”科技、医疗、公益团队主要骨干组成的编委会付出了辛勤的努力，加拿大阿尔伯塔大学医学与牙学院参与英文翻译与校对，此外还有关注难愈合创面患者的社会各界爱心人士们对此书出版的默默支持，在此一并表示感谢。

我们致力于打造结合“医疗、教育、科技、慈善”于一体的新时代慈善公益品牌，因此公益活动每到一处都致力为当地培养医疗力量，以远程帮扶与来温培训相结合的方式，提升当地学科建设水平，变“输血”为“造血”，用优质的创面修复技术为各地培养“带不走的医生”。用科技攻关来提升医疗诊治水平，用教育帮扶来推进创面修复学科发展，用公益慈善来救助创面患者，这是我们的初心和使命，也是我们编撰这本图鉴的缘起，希望此书能够为创面修复领域一线医护人员提供参考和借鉴。

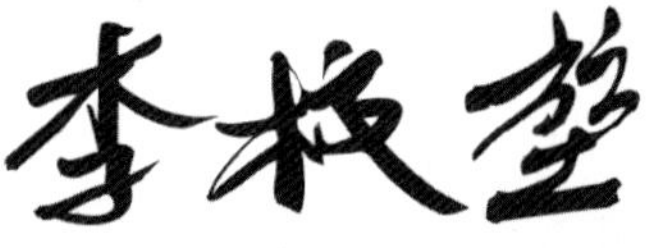

2024 年 10 月

The members of the "F&S CHARITY" team include technology workers, medical workers, educators, as well as media reporters and caring individuals who are passionate about public welfare. The compilation of this book has received high attention and strong support from the publishing house. The editorial committee, composed of key members from the "F&S CHARITY" technology, medical, and public welfare teams, has put in hard work. The School of Medicine and Dentistry at the University of Alberta in Canada has participated in the English translation and proofreading. In addition, caring individuals from all walks of life who focus on patients with difficult to heal wounds have silently supported the publication of this book. We would like to express our gratitude for this.

We are committed to building a new era charity and public welfare brand that combines "medical care, education, technology, and charity". Therefore, every public welfare activity is dedicated to cultivating medical forces for the local area. By combining remote assistance with on-site training, we aim to improve the level of local discipline construction, transform "blood transfusion" into "blood making", and use high-quality wound repair technology to cultivate "doctors who cannot be taken away" for various regions. Our original intention and mission are to improve the level of medical diagnosis and treatment through technological breakthroughs, promote the development of wound repair discipline through educational assistance, and rescue wound patients through public welfare and charity. This is also the origin of our compilation of this guidebook, hoping that this book can provide reference and inspiration for frontline medical staff in the field of wound repair.

Li Xiaokun

October 2024

前　言

随着人口老龄化和疾病谱的改变，除创伤、烧伤等引起的急性创面外，各种疾病导致的体表慢性难愈合创面患者数量逐年增加。这些难愈合慢性创面修复时间长、经济负担重，严重影响人民群众的身心健康和生活质量。

在创面修复领域中，当前已涌现出多种前沿材料和技术，其中，“生长因子”因其对机体生长和发育的显著调节作用而备受瞩目。在李校堃院士的卓越领导下，中国开创性地成为世界上首个将成纤维细胞生长因子成功转化为临床药物的国家。研究团队历经三十余载的不懈探索，将生长因子的科研成果与皮瓣移植、植皮、负压封闭引流、骨搬运等先进技术深度融合，为创面患者的康复赢得了宝贵的时间和空间，极大地推动了创面修复学科的发展。

鉴于难愈合创面患者广泛分布于基层医疗机构和偏远山区的现实挑战，李校堃院士发起“肤生工程”慈善项目，通过科技力量赋能公益慈善，不仅为难愈合创面患者带来了身体上的康复，更在心灵上给予了他们温暖与力量。“肤生工程”团队构建了“千点千点”救助网络，积极收集并整理难愈合创面的临床案例，为临床教学提供了宝贵的实践数据和经验，有力地推动了创面修复学科的持续进步与发展。

本图鉴独具匠心，具备以下显著特点：

1. 真实案例直击人心。例如，文章中第 8 章案例二，独居老人左下肢溃烂，甚至需要用水果刀自行清除坏死腐肉，长段胫骨腓骨外露，全身感染生命垂危。在“肤生工程”公益团队的精准走访下，将老人接到医院救治，及时缓解疼痛，给老人一个体面、干净的临终关怀，这也是科研成果转化成公益慈善的温暖与力量。

Preface

With the aging population and changes in the disease spectrum, in addition to acute wounds caused by trauma, burns, etc., the number of patients with chronic and difficult to heal surface wounds caused by various diseases is increasing year by year. These difficult to heal chronic wounds have a long repair time and heavy economic burden, seriously affecting the physical and mental health and quality of life of the people.

In the field of wound repair, various cutting–edge materials and technologies have emerged, among which "growth factors" have attracted much attention due to their significant regulatory effects on the growth and development of the body. Under the outstanding leadership of Academician Li Xiaokun, China has become the world's first country to successfully convert fibroblast growth factor into clinical drugs. After more than 30 years of unremitting exploration, the research team has deeply integrated the scientific research achievements of growth factors with advanced technologies such as skin flap transplantation, skin grafting, negative pressure closed drainage, and bone transport, winning valuable time and space for the rehabilitation of wound patients and greatly promoting the development of wound repair discipline.

Given the widespread distribution of patients with difficult to heal wounds in grassroots medical institutions and remote mountainous areas, Academician Li Xiaokun initiated the "F&S CHARITY" charity project, empowering public welfare and charity through technological power. This not only brings physical recovery to patients with difficult to heal wounds, but also provides them with warmth and strength in their hearts and spirits. The "F&S CHARITY" team has built a "thousand point" rescue network, actively collecting and organizing clinical cases of difficult to heal wounds, providing valuable practical data and experience for clinical teaching, and effectively promoting the continuous progress and development of wound repair discipline.

This guidebook is unique and has the following notable features:

1. Real cases strike people's hearts. For example, in Case 2 of Chapter 8 of the article, an elderly person living alone has left lower limb ulceration and even needs to use a fruit knife to remove the necrotic flesh on their own. The long tibia and fibula are exposed, and the whole body is infected and in critical condition. Under the precise visits of the "F&S CHARITY" public welfare team, the elderly were taken to the hospital for treatment, and their pain was promptly relieved, providing them with dignified and clean terminal care. This is also the warmth and strength of transforming scientific research achievements into public welfare and charity.

2. 生长因子加速创面新生。图鉴通过实际案例证实了生长因子在促进受损组织重生、加速创面愈合中的显著作用。这种多手段协同合作的策略，为医疗领域带来了新的希望和可能性。

3. 图文并茂，信息丰富。本图鉴以图片案例为核心，力求用直观、真实的方式展示难愈合慢性创面修复医治的全过程。尽管篇幅有限，但我们力求减少文字赘述，使读者能够通过图片直观理解手术步骤与效果。

最后，我们希望《生长因子与创面修复图鉴》能够成为创面修复领域的一本重要参考书，为广大医学工作者和学者提供有益的指导和启示。同时，我们也期待通过本书的传播，能够激发更多人对生长因子与创面修复研究的兴趣和热情，在使用本书时能够不断发现新问题、提出新观点，为实现体表难愈性创面（溃疡）治疗的温州模式、浙江经验、中国标准赓续前行，为我省高质量发展建设共同富裕示范区、推进卫生健康现代化建设做出新的更大的贡献。

本书编委会

2024 年 6 月

2. Growth factors accelerate wound regeneration. The illustrated book confirms the significant role of growth factors in promoting the regeneration of damaged tissues and accelerating wound healing through practical cases. This multi pronged collaborative strategy has brought new hope and possibilities to the medical field.

3. Rich in graphics and text, with abundant information. This guidebook focuses on image cases and strives to present the entire process of repairing and treating difficult to heal chronic wounds in an intuitive and realistic way. Although space is limited, we strive to reduce textual redundancy and enable readers to intuitively understand the surgical steps and effects through images.

Finally, we hope that the *Atlas of Growth Factors and Wound Repair* can become an important reference book in the field of wound repair, providing useful guidance and inspiration for medical workers and scholars. At the same time, we also hope that through the dissemination of this book, it can stimulate more people's interest and enthusiasm in the research of growth factors and wound repair. When using this book, we can constantly discover new problems and propose new perspectives, and continue to advance the Wenzhou model, Zhejiang experience, and Chinese standards for the treatment of difficult to heal wounds (ulcers) on the surface of the body, making new and greater contributions to the high–quality development and construction of a demonstration zone for common prosperity in our province, and promoting the modernization of health and hygiene.

The editorial board of this book

June 2024

目 录

第一部分 概述

第二部分 典型个案介绍

Catalogue

Part 1 Overview

Part 2 Introduction to Typical Cases

第一部分
Part 1

概述
Overview

第 1 章

Chapter 1

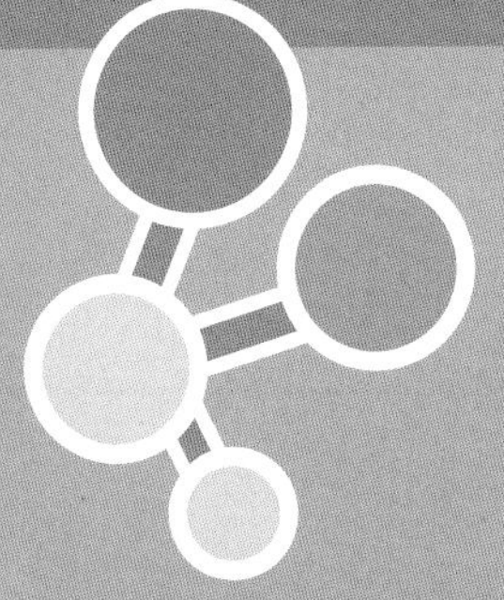

生长因子与创面修复

Growth Factors and Wound Repair

皮肤是人体直接与外界环境接触的最大器官，常易受到多种理化和机械因素的影响从而造成不同程度的损伤，轻度浅表皮肤损伤容易自愈，而基底层的损伤则难以修复，常会伴有皮肤坏死、感染、增生性瘢痕等并发症，严重影响患者的生活质量，所以皮肤创面治疗和修复是亟待解决的临床问题。生长因子是一类能与细胞膜特异受体结合的活性蛋白多肽，广泛存在于生物体内，对机体的生长和发育具有调节作用。生长因子对人体的免疫、造血调控、肿瘤发生、炎症与感染、创伤愈合、血管形成、细胞分化、细胞凋亡、形态发生、胚胎形成等方面也有着重要的调控作用。

第一节　创面分类和修复过程

皮肤是人体最大的器官，它给机体提供了一个保护屏障，以抵御恶劣的外部环境。因此，保持这一屏障的完整性以阻止病原体和毒素的进入对生存至关重要。大多数皮肤损伤会在一两周内愈合。然而，随着年龄的增长，皮肤的愈合能力会下降，即使是轻伤也会导致伤口延迟愈合，甚至无法愈合。这些难以愈合的伤口长期影响患者的生活质量和身心健康，严重者会诱发致死性并发症，如感染性休克、脓毒血症等。随着全球人口老龄化的加速，慢性难愈合性创面的发病率在逐年上升，迫切需要有效的治疗手段来改善这一问题。

创面分类和定义

在创面修复治疗中，首要任务是确定创面形成的原因，然后根据不同的原因制订治疗方案。

根据创面的性质，创面分为开放性创面和闭合性创面。开放性创面是指直接暴露在空气中的创面，是日常生活中最常见的创面，包括刀伤、烧伤、擦伤等；闭合性创面的受伤部位皮肤或体表黏膜仍保持完整，不伴皮肤破裂及外出血，可有皮肤青紫、皮下出血等。

根据创面愈合时间的不同，临床上可以分为急性创面和慢性创面。急性创面主要是指突然性的损伤如擦伤、磨伤、划伤、刺伤等造成的创面，该种创面通常可以在 8 周内恢复。慢性创面主要指无法通过正常、有序、及时地修复而达到解剖和功能上完整状态的创面，这些创面常常延迟愈合甚至不愈合。对于慢性创面的持续时间尚无确切的共识，临床上一般将治疗 1 个月后仍无明显愈合指征的创面称作慢性创面。

创面愈合过程

创面愈合是指由于在致伤因素作用下造成组织缺失后，局部组织通过再生、修复、重建进行修补的一系列病理生理过程。本质上，创面愈合是机体对各种有害因素所致的组织细胞损伤的一种固有的防御性适应性反应。这种再生修复表现于丧失组织结构的恢复上，也能不同程度地恢复其功能。

The skin is the largest organ in direct contact with the external environment in the human body, and is often susceptible to various physical, chemical, and mechanical factors that can cause varying degrees of damage. Mild superficial skin injuries are easy to self heal, while damage to the basal layer is difficult to repair, often accompanied by complications such as skin necrosis, infection, and hypertrophic scars, which seriously affect the quality of life of patients. Therefore, the treatment and repair of skin wounds are urgent clinical problems that need to be solved. Growth factors are a class of active protein peptides that can bind to specific receptors on the cell membrane, widely present in organisms, and have regulatory effects on the growth and development of the body. Growth factors also play important regulatory roles in human immunity, hematopoietic regulation, tumorigenesis, inflammation and infection, wound healing, angiogenesis, cell differentiation, apoptosis, morphogenesis, embryo formation, and other aspects.

Section 1 Classification and repair process of wounds

The skin is the largest organ in the human body, providing a protective barrier to resist harsh external environments. Therefore, maintaining the integrity of this barrier to prevent the entry of pathogens and toxins is crucial for survival. Most skin injuries will heal within one or two weeks. However, as age increases, the healing ability of the skin decreases, and even minor injuries can lead to delayed or even non healing of the wound. These difficult to heal wounds have a long-term impact on the quality of life and physical and mental health of patients, and in severe cases, can lead to fatal complications such as infectious rest and sepsis. With the accelerated aging of the global population, the incidence rate of chronic refractory wounds is increasing year by year. Effective treatment is urgently needed to improve this problem.

Classification and definition of wounds

In wound repair treatment, the primary task is to determine the cause of wound formation and then develop treatment plans based on different reasons.

According to the nature of the wound, it is divided into open wounds and closed wounds. Open wounds refer to wounds that are directly exposed to the air and are the most common types of wounds in daily life, including knife wounds, burns, abrasions, etc; The injured skin or surface mucosa of a closed wound remains intact, without skin rupture or external bleeding, and may have skin bruising, subcutaneous bleeding, etc.

According to the different healing times of wounds, they can be clinically divided into acute wounds and chronic wounds. Acute wounds mainly refer to wounds caused by sudden injuries such as abrasions, abrasions, cuts, stabs, etc., which can usually be fully healed within 8 weeks. Chronic wounds mainly refer to wounds that cannot be repaired in a normal, orderly, and timely manner to achieve anatomical and functional integrity. These wounds often delay healing or even do not heal. There is no definite consensus on the duration of chronic wounds, and in clinical practice, wounds that do not show obvious signs of healing after one month of treatment are generally referred to as chronic wounds.

The process of wound healing

Wound healing refers to a series of pathological and physiological processes in which local tissue is repaired through regeneration, repair, and reconstruction after tissue loss caused by injury factors. Essentially, wound healing is an inherent defensive adaptive response of the body to tissue cell damage caused by various harmful factors. This regenerative repair is manifested in the recovery of lost tissue structure and can also restore its function to varying degrees.

1. 凝血期 从创面形成的一瞬间开始，机体首先出现的生理反应是自身的止血过程。创面产生后周围的小血管、毛细血管等反应性收缩使局部血流量减少，随之而来的是暴露的胶原纤维招募血小板聚集形成血凝块；随后血小板释放血管活性物质如 5- 羟色胺及前列腺素等，使血管进一步收缩，血流减慢，同时释放的磷脂将吸引更多的血小板聚集。最后，内源性及外源性凝血过程也将被启动。凝血过程结束后，机体即开始进行创面的愈合。

2. 炎症期 这一时期自创面形成开始后的 2 ～ 3 天。由于局部血管收缩而导致组织缺血，引起组胺和其他血管活性物质的释放，使创面局部的血管扩张。由坏死组织以及可能存在的致病微生物会引发机体的防御反应，导致粒细胞、巨噬细胞、单核细胞等免疫细胞向创面移动和集中。在这些免疫细胞和自身释放的蛋白溶酶的共同作用下，对坏死组织进行吞噬、消化、清除，以此清洁创面，从而启动组织的修复过程。巨噬细胞除吞噬、消化组织细胞碎片外，还刺激成纤维细胞增殖和分化，合成胶原蛋白，这一过程也被称为清创阶段。临床上，这一时期的创面大多会被黑色的坏死组织所覆盖，因此也被称为黑色期。当这一层坏死组织被清除后，创面仍会被一层薄薄的腐烂失活组织所覆盖，使创面外观呈黄色，此阶段的创面在临床上被称为黄色期。

3. 增殖重塑期 这一时期又可以分为上皮细胞再生和肉芽组织形成两个阶段，从创面形成后的 2 ～ 24 天。①上皮细胞再生阶段：首先是创面周缘的基底细胞开始增生，并向中心部位移行；与此同时，基底细胞的增殖刺激创面基底部毛细血管和结缔组织的反应性增生。②肉芽组织形成阶段：上皮细胞再生后基底细胞的增生刺激肉芽组织的生长。同时巨噬细胞释放的生长因子如血小板源性生长因子（PDGF）、转化生长因子 β（TGF-β）和表皮细胞生长因子（EGF）等，加速肉芽组织的形成。肉芽组织的形成有着重要的生理学意义，主要表现为填补组织的缺损、保护创面、阻止细菌感染、减少出血。

随着肉芽组织的不断形成，创面组织的缺失被填充，上皮细胞便从创面周缘向中心移行，最终使得创面得以完全被再生的上皮细胞覆盖。当创面被再生的上皮细胞完全覆盖后，创面的愈合过程并没有完全结束，新生的肉芽组织和上皮细胞还需要进一步分裂分化、转型，使其力量增强，最后才使创面得以完全愈合。这一过程主要表现为：①新形成的上皮细胞不断分裂，使表皮层增厚。②肉芽组织内部转型，形成的胶原纤维排列发生改变，使新生的结缔组织力量增加；同时，毛细血管数目减少，使创面局部颜色减退，接近于正常色。这一过程需要长达 1 年的时间。

1.The coagulation period begins from the moment the wound is formed, and the first physiological response that the body experiences is its own process of stopping bleeding. After the formation of the wound, the reactive contraction of small blood vessels, capillaries, etc. around the wound reduces local blood flow, followed by the recruitment of platelets by exposed collagen fibers to form blood clots; Subsequently, platelets release vasoactive substances such as serotonin and prostaglandins, which further constrict blood vessels and slow down blood flow. At the same time, the released phospholipids will attract more platelets to aggregate. Finally, both endogenous and exogenous coagulation processes will be initiated. After the coagulation process is completed, the body begins to heal the wound.

2. The inflammatory period is 2-3 days after the formation of the wound. Due to local vascular constriction, tissue ischemia occurs, leading to the release of histamine and other vasoactive substances, causing local vascular dilation in the wound area. Necrotic tissue and potential pathogenic microorganisms can trigger the body's defense response, causing immune cells such as granulocytes, macrophages, and monocytes to move and concentrate towards the wound. Under the joint action of these immune cells and self released proteolytic enzymes, necrotic tissue is engulfed, digested, and cleared to clean the wound and initiate the tissue repair process. Macrophages not only engulf and digest tissue cell debris, but also stimulate fibroblast proliferation and differentiation, synthesize collagen, and this process is also known as the debridement stage. In clinical practice, this period is also known as the black phase because most wounds are covered by black necrotic tissue. After this layer of necrotic tissue is removed, the wound will still be covered by a thin layer of decaying and inactive tissue, making the appearance of the wound yellow. This stage of the wound is clinically known as the yellow phase.

3. The proliferation and remodeling period can be divided into two stages: epithelial cell regeneration and granulation tissue formation, starting from 2-24 days after wound formation Epithelial cell regeneration stage: Firstly, the basal cells around the wound begin to proliferate and migrate towards the central area; At the same time, the proliferation of basal cells stimulates reactive proliferation of capillaries and connective tissue at the base of the wound Granulation tissue formation stage: The proliferation of basal cells after epithelial cell regeneration stimulates the growth of granulation tissue. At the same time, growth factors released by macrophages, such as platelet-derived growth factor (PDGF), transforming growth factor beta (TGF-β), and epidermal growth factor (EGF), accelerate the formation of granulation tissue. The formation of granulation tissue has important physiological significance, mainly manifested as filling tissue defects, protecting wounds, preventing bacterial infections, and reducing bleeding.

With the continuous formation of granulation tissue, the missing wound tissue is filled, and epithelial cells migrate from the periphery of the wound to the center, ultimately allowing the wound to be completely covered by regenerated epithelial cells. After the wound is completely covered by regenerated epithelial cells, the healing process of the wound is not completely completed. The newly formed granulation tissue and epithelial cells need to further divide, differentiate, and transform to enhance their strength, in order to finally achieve complete wound healing. This process is mainly manifested as: ① Newly formed epithelial cells continuously divide, causing thickening of the epidermal layer. ② The internal transformation of granulation tissue results in changes in the arrangement of collagen fibers, leading to an increase in the strength of newly formed connective tissue; At the same time, the number of capillaries decreases, causing the local color of the wound to decrease and approach normal color. This process takes up to one year.

第二节　参与创面修复的生长因子

近年来，随着对创面愈合过程的深入研究，发现生长因子与修复细胞有密切关系，在创面修复中起关键作用。当细胞受到损伤因素刺激后，可释放多种生长因子，刺激同类细胞或同一胚层发育的细胞增生，参与损伤组织重建，促进修复过程。

创面愈合过程中主要涉及的生长因子包括成纤维细胞生长因子 (FGF)、血小板源性生长因子 (PDGF)、转化生长因子 (TGF-α 、TGF-β)、表皮细胞生长因子 (EGF)、血管内皮细胞生长因子 (VEGF) 等，这些生长因子通过协同作用，在促进机体内多种类型组织细胞的分裂和增殖、基质合成和沉积、纤维组织和肉芽组织的形成，以及在增加胶原蛋白合成能力与促进创伤后上皮细胞再生、角质形成细胞增生和新生血管形成等过程中发挥重要作用。

成纤维细胞生长因子 (FGF)

FGF 通过旁分泌或内分泌的方式参与多种生理活动的调节，维护成体组织的正常结构、功能并参与代谢调控。FGF 分泌蛋白配体可分为旁分泌型和内分泌型，FGF1 ~ FGF18、FGF20、FGF22 属于旁分泌型，FGF19、FGF21、FGF23 属于内分泌型。旁分泌型 FGF 需要硫酸乙酰肝素作为受体激活的辅因子，而内分泌型 FGF 依赖 Klotho 协同受体激活受体。成纤维细胞生长因子受体 (FGFR) 是一类跨膜的酪氨酸激酶受体，为单链的糖蛋白分子，包括细胞外区、跨膜区和细胞内激酶区，已知哺乳动物有 FGFR1、FGFR2、FGFR3 和 FGFR4 四种。FGF 通过结合细胞表面酪氨酸激酶受体 FGFR，从而发挥其生物学功能。FGF 与相应的 FGFR 结合后，引发受体二聚化，活化受体酪氨酸激酶，进而激活细胞内信号通路。目前，已知 FGFR 激酶可以引发三条信号通路，包括 MAPKK/MAPK 激酶途径、BAX/BCL-2 相关蛋白途径和 PDK/ 磷酸肌醇 - 依赖蛋白激酶途径。FGF 具有很强的促细胞生长作用和广泛的生物学作用，能影响多种细胞的生长、分化及功能，如血管内皮细胞、成纤维细胞、神经元、星形胶质细胞、卵泡粒层细胞等，同时也是重要的有丝分裂促进因子，是形态发生和分化的诱导因子，在正常生理和病理过程中参与生长发育和组织损伤的修复过程。

FGF1 亚家族由 FGF1 和 FGF2 组成，FGF1 和 FGF2 是最先被发现的 FGF 家族成员，因其各自的等电点分别为酸性和碱性而被称为酸性成纤维细胞生长因子 (aFGF，即 FGF1) 和碱性成纤维细胞生长因子 (bFGF，即 FGF2)。两者氨基酸同源性达 55%，具有促进组织器官的形态发生、损伤修复、血管生成和神经细胞再生等作用。

2005 年，我国研究人员开发的外用重组人酸性成纤维细胞生长因子冻干粉剂就获得国家食品药品监督管理局（SFDA）的批准，并成为世界上第一个上市的 FGF1 产品，批准的适应证为烧伤及慢性溃疡创面的治疗。FGF1 与受体结合后，通过促进创面炎症因子聚集，激活创面修复相关细胞因子，从而调控创面表皮、真皮及皮下组织的全层修复。FGF1 不仅具备分裂原活性，还具有舒张血管、神经调节、降低血糖等内分泌

Section 2 Growth factors involved in wound repair

In recent years, with in-depth research on the wound healing process, it has been found that growth factors are closely related to repair cells and play a key role in wound repair. When cells are stimulated by damaging factors, they can release various growth factors, stimulate the proliferation of cells of the same type or development of the same germ layer, participate in the reconstruction of damaged tissues, and promote the repair process.

The main growth factors involved in wound healing process include fibroblast growth factor (FGF), platelet-derived growth factor (PDGF), transforming growth factor (TGF-α ,TGF-β), epidermal growth factor (EGF), vascular endothelial growth factor (VEGF), etc. These growth factors play an important role in promoting the division and proliferation of various types of tissue cells, matrix synthesis and deposition, formation of fibrous tissue and granulation tissue in the body, as well as increasing collagen synthesis ability and promoting epithelial cell regeneration, keratinocyte proliferation, and neovascularization after trauma.

Fibroblast growth factor (FGF)

FGF participates in the regulation of various physiological activities through paracrine or endocrine pathways, maintaining the normal structure and function of adult tissues and participating in metabolic regulation. FGF secreted protein ligands can be divided into paracrine and endocrine types. FGF1-FGF18, FGF20, and FGF22 belong to paracrine types, while endocrine types include FGF19, FGF21, and FGF23. paracrine FGFs require heparan sulfate as a co factor for receptor activation, while endocrine FGFs rely on Klotho co receptor activation to activate receptors. Fibroblast growth factor receptor (FGFR) is a type of transmembrane tyrosine kinase receptor, which is a single chain glycoprotein molecule consisting of extracellular, transmembrane, and intracellular kinase regions. There are four known mammalian FGFR1, FGFR2, FGFR3, and FGFR4. FGF exerts its biological functions by binding to the cell surface tyrosine kinase receptor FGFR. After binding to the corresponding FGFR, FGF triggers receptor dimerization, activates receptor tyrosine kinase, and subsequently activates intracellular signaling pathways. At present, it is known that FGFR kinase can trigger three signaling pathways, including MAPKK/MAPK kinase pathway, BAX/BCL-2 related protein pathway, and PDK/phosphoinositol dependent protein kinase pathway. FGF has a strong promoting effect on cell growth and a wide range of biological functions, which can affect the growth, differentiation, and function of various cells, such as vascular endothelial cells, fibroblasts, neurons, astrocytes, follicular granulosa cells, etc. It is also an important mitogenic factor, an inducer of morphogenesis and differentiation, and participates in the growth, development, and tissue damage repair process in normal physiological and pathological processes.

The FGF1 subfamily consists of FGF1 and FGF2, with FGF1 and FGF2 being the first members of the FGF family to be discovered. They are referred to as acidic fibroblast growth factor (aFGF, FGF1) and alkaline fibroblast growth factor (bFGF, FGF2) due to their respective isoelectric points being acidic and alkaline, respectively. The amino acid homology between the two is 55%, and they have the ability to promote tissue and organ morphogenesis, injury repair, angiogenesis, and nerve cell regeneration.

In 2005, the externally applied recombinant human acidic fibroblast growth factor freeze-dried powder developed by Chinese researchers was approved by the State Food and Drug Administration (SFDA) and became the world's first FGF1 product to be marketed, with approved indications for the treatment of burns and chronic ulcer wounds. After binding to the receptor, FGF1 promotes the aggregation of inflammatory factors in the wound and activates cytokines related to wound repair, thereby regulating the full layer repair of the wound epidermis, dermis, and subcutaneous tissue. FGF1 not only possesses mitogenic activity, but also has endocrine hormone like activities such as vasodilation, neural regulation, and blood glucose lowering. FGF1 is a highly potent angiogenic factor and

激素样活性。FGF1 是一种作用极强的血管生成因子和促分裂原，它能刺激血管内皮细胞和平滑肌细胞的增生和迁移，刺激内皮细胞分泌胶原酶和蛋白水解酶，抑制成纤维细胞的胶原合成，减少成纤维细胞的胶原蛋白过量沉积。

FGF2 是在一种在牛脑垂体中发现等电点为 9.6 的碱性多肽，由肿瘤细胞和巨噬细胞产生，广泛分布于中胚层和中性胚层来源的组织中。因为缺少信号肽序列，所以它只能通过自分泌或者旁分泌的形式渗透至细胞外，而外源性 FGF2 则可以易位至机体细胞内与靶蛋白或基因发生相互作用。研究发现，FGF2 对成纤维细胞和内皮细胞具有高度的血管生成和趋化作用。因其具有较强的有丝分裂特性，故能促进伤口创面中内皮细胞、真皮成纤维细胞和角化细胞的分裂和增殖，其趋化特性表现为通过影响这些细胞在伤口愈合过程中的迁移、上皮细胞的生长和血管平滑肌细胞的增殖从而形成毛细血管腔。此外，FGF2 能够提高机体白细胞的吞噬功能，加强伤口愈合的炎症反应。

在临床治疗中，FGF 有利于促进血管生成，促进骨、软骨的生长，促进创伤愈合和组织损伤修复以及神经再生，是一种多效能的细胞生长因子。

血小板源性生长因子 (PDGF)

PDGF 主要来源于血小板，是血小板 α 颗粒合成的一种大型糖蛋白多肽生长因子，通过与靶细胞膜上 PDGF 受体接触后促进细胞增殖、分裂和细胞外基质的生成。PDGF 家族有 5 个成员，PDGF-AA、PDGF-BB、PDGF-AB、PDGF-CC 和 PDGF-DD。此外，巨噬细胞、成纤维细胞、血管内皮细胞和角质形成细胞均能产生 PDGF 各亚型，而在创面愈合中 PDGF-BB 被认为是最有效的亚型。PDGF 贯穿伤口愈合的炎症期、增生期和重塑期，PDGF 在炎症期对中性粒细胞、巨噬细胞具有趋化作用，减轻氧化应激及炎症反应。炎症反应后，增生期成纤维细胞、血管内皮细胞等开始增殖分化，恢复受损组织的完整性。

PDGF 不仅可趋化巨噬细胞，还能趋化成纤维细胞及平滑肌细胞迁移至受伤部位，作为有丝分裂原促进成纤维细胞增殖，合成糖胺聚糖、蛋白聚糖和胶原蛋白等细胞外基质，为创面其余细胞的增殖、迁移提供良好的支架，有助于创面肉芽组织的生成，同时活化胶原酶调节细胞外基质的更新。在血管新生过程中 PDGF 起重要作用，PDGF 可促进血管内皮细胞、外膜细胞及血管平滑肌细胞的迁移和增殖，为血管新生提供较好条件。重组人 PDGF 凝胶治疗糖尿病溃疡大鼠创面的研究也表明，重组人 PDGF 凝胶具有促血管新生的作用。PDGF 促进成纤维细胞产生蛋白水解酶和胶原酶去除多余的胶原和细胞外基质成分，并通过上调基质金属蛋白酶调节细胞外基质的降解促进组织重构。

转化生长因子 β (TGF–β)

TGF-β 是一个多功能的细胞因子，可调节细胞增殖、分化、迁移、侵袭，广泛存在于各种组织细胞中，不仅可促进脊椎动物多种组织再生，在伤口愈合中亦起到关键作用。目前在哺乳动物体内被证实存在 TGF-β1、TGF-β2、TGF-β3 三种异构体，在创面愈合的不同阶段，各亚型表达水平有所不同。

mitogen that can stimulate the proliferation and migration of endothelial cells and smooth muscle cells, stimulate the secretion of collagenase and proteolytic enzymes by endothelial cells, inhibit collagen synthesis in fibroblasts, and reduce excessive deposition of collagen proteins in fibroblasts.

FGF2 is an alkaline peptide with an isoelectric point of 9.6 found in the bovine pituitary gland, produced by tumor cells and macrophages, and widely distributed in tissues derived from the mesoderm and mesoderm. Due to the lack of signal peptide sequences, it can only penetrate into the extracellular space through autocrine or paracrine forms, while exogenous FGF2 can translocate into the body's cells and interact with target proteins or genes. Research has found that FGF2 has a high degree of angiogenesis and chemotactic effects on fibroblasts and endothelial cells. Due to its strong mitotic properties, it can promote the division and proliferation of endothelial cells, dermal fibroblasts, and keratinocytes in wound wounds. Its chemotaxis is manifested by affecting the migration of these cells during wound healing, the growth of epithelial cells, and the proliferation of vascular smooth muscle cells, thereby forming capillary lumens. In addition, FGF2 can enhance the phagocytic function of white blood cells in the body and strengthen the inflammatory response of wound healing.

In clinical treatment, FGF is beneficial for promoting angiogenesis, bone and cartilage growth, wound healing, tissue damage repair, and nerve regeneration. It is a multifunctional cell growth factor.

Platelet derived growth factor (PDGF)

PDGF is mainly derived from platelets and is a large glycoprotein peptide growth factor synthesized by platelet alpha granules. It promotes cell proliferation, division, and extracellular matrix production by contacting PDGF receptors on the target cell membrane. The PDGF family consists of five members: PDGF-AA, PDGF-BB, PDGF-AB, PDGF-CC, and PDGF-DD. In addition, macrophages, fibroblasts, endothelial cells, and keratinocytes can all produce various subtypes of PDGF, and PDGF-BB is considered the most effective subtype in wound healing. PDGF runs through the inflammatory, proliferative, and remodeling phases of wound healing. During the inflammatory phase, PDGF has a chemotactic effect on neutrophils and macrophages, reducing oxidative stress and inflammatory response. After the inflammatory response, fibroblasts and endothelial cells in the proliferative phase begin to proliferate and differentiate, restoring the integrity of damaged tissues.

PDGF not only chemotaxis macrophages, but also chemotaxis fibroblasts and smooth muscle cells to migrate to the injured site. As a mitogen, it promotes fibroblast proliferation, synthesizes extracellular matrix such as glycosaminoglycans, proteoglycans, and collagen, and provides a good scaffold for the proliferation and migration of other cells in the wound. It helps to generate granulation tissue in the wound and activates collagenase to regulate the renewal of extracellular matrix. PDGF plays an important role in the process of angiogenesis, as it can promote the migration and proliferation of endothelial cells, outer membrane cells, and vascular smooth muscle cells, providing favorable conditions for angiogenesis. The study of recombinant human PDGF gel in treating diabetes ulcer wounds in rats also showed that recombinant human PDGF gel had the effect of promoting angiogenesis. PDGF promotes the production of proteolytic enzymes and collagenase by fibroblasts to remove excess collagen and extracellular matrix components, and regulates the degradation of extracellular matrix by upregulating matrix metalloproteinases to promote tissue remodeling.

Transforming growth factor beta (TGF-β)

TGF-β is a multifunctional cytokine that can regulate cell proliferation, differentiation, migration, and invasion. It is widely present in various tissue cells and not only promotes the regeneration of various tissues in vertebrates, but also plays a key role in wound healing. At present, it has been confirmed that there are three isoforms of TGF-β1, TGF-β2, and TGF-β3 in mammals, and the expression levels of each subtype vary at different stages of wound healing.

在创面愈合过程的早期阶段，TGF-β1 的释放促使炎症细胞重新聚集到损伤部位，随后通过巨噬细胞释放超氧化物参与负反馈调节。在此过渡阶段，肉芽组织逐渐形成，TGF-β1 促进细胞外基质关键成分的表达，如纤维连接蛋白、Ⅰ型和Ⅲ型胶原蛋白以及血管内皮生长因子。此外，TGF-β1 还通过调节细胞迁移相关的整合素促进角质形成细胞迁移。TGF-β1 是主要的胶原刺激因子之一，尤其是在成纤维细胞中 TGF-β1 是主要的胶原刺激因子之一。TGF-β1 还抑制不同的基质金属蛋白酶，促进胶原纤维的积累。

TGF-β2 和 TGF-β3 在创面愈合过程中的作用与 TGF-β1 类似，TGF-β2 参与了成纤维细胞和免疫细胞从循环和伤口边缘向创面的募集，进而导致颗粒组织的形成、血管生成和胶原的合成和产生。研究人员用 TGF-β1 和 TGF-β2 的抗体治疗动物模型的伤口，发现浸润性免疫细胞特别是单核细胞和巨噬细胞的数量明显减少，Ⅰ型和Ⅲ型胶原蛋白以及纤维连接蛋白的沉积也明显减少，从而抑制瘢痕形成。但进一步的研究表明，这两种抗体不是独立有效地减少瘢痕形成，而是只有这两种抗体结合起来才能看到抑制瘢痕效果。TGF-β3 与 TGF-β1 和 TGF-β2 相比，TGF-β3 在瘢痕形成中具有拮抗 TGF-β1 的作用。在瘢痕形成很少或没有形成瘢痕的伤口中，如口腔黏膜修复过程中 TGF-β1 的水平降低，TGF-β3/TGF-β1 的比率升高。

表皮生长因子 (EGF)

人体中几乎所有的体液、分泌液及大多数组织中都有 EGF。表皮生长因子受体 (EGFR) 主要表达于角质形成细胞，也可表达于其他多种细胞，如成纤维细胞、神经胶质细胞、平滑肌细胞和软骨细胞等。EGF 具有趋化和促进细胞分裂作用，主要通过与细胞膜受体结合，在细胞内递送过程中构成复杂的代谢网络，从而控制细胞的代谢、分化等生物学活动。EGFR 主要存在于上皮细胞，但因为成纤维细胞及血管内皮细胞的胞膜上有表达，所以在创面修复中也发挥重要作用。机体中 EGF 的合成与分泌受神经因素和多种激素调节，如雄激素、孕激素等，但 EGF 在组织中的含量普遍较低，难以满足创面修复的最大需要，外周血中仅含有少量 EGF，血小板颗粒内含量较多。

EGF 的临床作用主要表现为在体内刺激皮肤组织、角膜和气管上皮组织的生长繁殖，促进细胞再生和组织修复。EGF 促进皮肤和黏膜创伤面的愈合作用，减少瘢痕挛缩和皮肤畸形增生，加速角膜、皮肤等表皮创伤的修复，特别用于治疗痤疮后留下的瘢痕疙瘩。EGF 能促进皮肤细胞对营养物质的吸收，加速细胞的新陈代谢，促进皮肤细胞的分裂和增殖，促进透明质酸和糖蛋白的合成，增强表皮细胞的蛋白质、DNA、RNA 的合成和细胞代谢等。EGF 能促进新生细胞生长，替代受紫外线照射损伤的细胞，以降低皮肤中黑色素细胞的数量。EGF 广泛应用于治疗烧伤、烫伤、手术伤、机械伤、皮肤溃疡、激光美容等。

血管内皮生长因子 (VEGF)

VEGF 不仅是一种强烈的内皮细胞有丝分裂原，最近的研究表明 VEGF 在诱导角质形成细胞再生和迁移方面也具有显著的作用。VEGF 的基因位于第 6 号染色体 (6p21.3)，其表达一种同源二聚体糖蛋白，属于 PDGF 家族，同源性约为 20%。目前已鉴定出 VEGF 至少有 7 个成员，即 VEGF-A、VEGF-B、VEGF-C、

In the early stages of wound healing, the release of TGF- β1 promotes the re aggregation of inflammatory cells to the site of injury, followed by the release of superoxide by macrophages to participate in negative feedback regulation. During this transitional stage, granulation tissue gradually forms, and TGF- β1 promotes the expression of key components of the extracellular matrix, such as fibronectin, type I and III collagen, and vascular endothelial growth factor. In addition, TGF- β1 promotes keratinocyte migration by regulating integrins related to cell migration.TGF- β1 is one of the main collagen stimulating factors, especially in fibroblasts. TGF- β1 also inhibits different matrix metalloproteinases and promotes the accumulation of collagen fibers.

The role of TGF- β 2 and TGF- β3 in wound healing is similar to that of TGF- β1. TGF- β 2 is involved in the recruitment of fibroblasts and immune cells from circulation and wound edges to the wound, leading to the formation of granular tissue, angiogenesis, and synthesis and production of collagen. Researchers used antibodies against TGF- β1 and TGF- β 2 to treat wounds in animal models and found a significant decrease in the number of infiltrating immune cells, especially monocytes and macrophages. The deposition of type I and III collagen and fibronectin also decreased significantly, thereby inhibiting scar formation. However, further research has shown that these two antibodies are not independently effective in reducing scar formation, but only when combined can the inhibitory effect on scars be observed. Compared with TGF- β1 and TGF- β 2, TGF- β3 has an antagonistic effect on TGF- β1 in scar formation. In wounds with little or no scar formation, such as during oral mucosal repair, the level of TGF- β 1 decreases and the ratio of TGF- β3/TGF- β1 increases.

第一部分 概述

Epidermal growth factor (EGF)

EGF is present in almost all bodily fluids, secretions, and most tissues in the human body. The epidermal growth factor receptor (EGFR) is mainly expressed in keratinocytes, but can also be expressed in various other cells such as fibroblasts, glial cells, smooth muscle cells, and chondrocytes. EGF has chemotactic and cell division promoting effects, mainly by binding to cell membrane receptors and forming a complex metabolic network during intracellular delivery, thereby controlling biological activities such as cell metabolism and differentiation. EGFR mainly exists in epithelial cells, but is expressed on the membranes of fibroblasts and endothelial cells, so it also plays an important role in wound repair. The synthesis and secretion of EGF in the body are regulated by neural factors and various hormones, such as androgens, progestogens, etc. However, the content of EGF in tissues is generally low, which is difficult to meet the maximum needs of wound repair. Peripheral blood only contains a small amount of EGF but contains a large amount of platelet particles.

The clinical effects of EGF mainly manifest as stimulating the growth and reproduction of skin tissue, corneal and tracheal epithelial tissue in vivo, promoting cell regeneration and tissue repair. EGF promotes the healing of skin and mucosal wounds, reduces scar contractures and skin deformities, accelerates the repair of epidermal wounds such as the cornea and skin, and is particularly used to treat scars left behind after acne. EGF can promote the absorption of nutrients by skin cells, accelerate cell metabolism, promote skin cell division and proliferation, and promote the synthesis of hyaluronic acid and glycoproteins; Enhance the synthesis of proteins, DNA, RNA, and cellular metabolism in epidermal cells. EGF can promote the growth of new cells, replace cells damaged by ultraviolet radiation, and reduce the number of melanocytes in the skin. EGF is widely used in the treatment of burns, scalds, surgical injuries, mechanical injuries, skin ulcers, laser beauty, etc.

Vascular endothelial growth factor (VEGF)

VEGF is not only a strong endothelial cell mitogen, but recent studies have shown that VEGF also plays a significant role in inducing keratinocyte regeneration and migration. The VEGF gene is located on chromosome 6 (6p21.3) and expresses a homodimeric glycoprotein belonging to the PDGF family, with a homology of approximately 20%. At present, at least 7 members of VEGF have been identified, namely VEGF-A, VEGF-B,

VEGF-D、VEGF-E、VEGF-F 和胎盘生长因子，其中以 VEGF-A 活性最强，分布广泛。VEGF-A 蛋白具有至少 7 个同源二聚体的糖蛋白，分别具有 121、145、148、165、183、189 和 206 个氨基酸长度。链长决定了它在细胞外基质中的溶解度。$VEGF\text{-}A_{121}$ 是可溶的且具有活性，而 $VEGF\text{-}A_{189}$、$VEGF\text{-}A_{206}$ 则通过硫酸乙酰肝素分子与细胞外基质紧密结合。$VEGF\text{-}A_{145}$、$VEGF\text{-}A_{165}$ 具有中介亲和力，并且在两种形式之间保持平均分布。

VEGF 的血管生成作用是通过其细胞表面受体 (VEGFR-1 和 VEGFR-2) 介导的。VEGFR-3 与 VEGF-C、VEGF-D 结合，并负责诱导淋巴管生成。

第三节　生长因子递送载体和策略

生长因子在体内的短暂半衰期和在再生的特定阶段的需求是制约它们在临床广泛使用的瓶颈。因此，生物材料对生长因子的递送很重要，使用生物材料作为载体的主要优点是生长因子可以被包裹在生物材料中，避免它们在伤口环境中不被降解。此外，生物材料还可以实现局部和持续的生长因子递送，确保组织再生所需的局部高浓度生长因子的供应，确保生长因子滞留在损伤部位，并提供宿主细胞可以在其上迁移的支架或结构支撑，以促进组织再生。例如，在治疗临界大小的骨缺损时，局部应用生长因子是较难实现的，而胶原海绵或磷酸三钙水泥等生物材料被用作骨再生中生长因子递送的载体。

生物材料分类

1. 天然材料 天然材料如蚕丝、胶原蛋白、明胶、壳聚糖、海藻酸盐、琼脂糖、透明质酸、纤维蛋白、弹性蛋白、淀粉、卡拉胶是常用的生长因子载体。这些材料可能具有一些固有的生物活性，可能有助于再生。这些材料通常溶于水，允许加载对生长因子的生物活性无害的温和制造条件。在大多数天然材料中，生长因子可浸润在材料支架中，或分散在材料支架中，通过扩散或支架的降解释放，对天然材料进行修饰则以实现生长因子控释。

2. 合成材料 通常用于生长因子载体的合成材料包括聚赖氨酸、聚乳酸、聚乙醇酸及其共聚物聚乳酸-乙醇酸、聚乙烯亚胺、聚乙二醇、聚 N-异丙基丙烯酰胺、聚甲基丙烯酸羟乙酯、聚己内酯和聚氨酯。使用合成材料的主要优点，是它们可以基于有利于临床结果的所需性质来合成。此外，有时还会使用不同材料的复合材料来优化每种材料的个体效益，提高生长因子的递送效率。例如，聚赖氨酸和聚己内酯的混合物已被用于递送神经生长因子（NGF），并有效地促进坐骨神经再生。这些聚合物可以配制成与生长因子释放相关的各种物理结构，如锥形支架、水凝胶、纳米颗粒和纳米纤维。此外，与天然材料类似，合成材料也可用不同的材料(如肝素)进行功能化以增强生长因子的包载。虽然这些材料可用作生长因子载体，但需要注意，这些材料不是天然的，其降解产物可能有毒或难以从体内清除。

VEGF-C, VEGF-D, VEGF-E, VEGF-F, and placental growth factor. Among them, VEGF-A has the strongest activity and is widely distributed. VEGF-A protein has at least 7 homologous dimeric glycoproteins, each with a length of 121, 145, 148, 165, 183, 189, and 206 amino acids. The chain length determines its solubility in the extracellular matrix. VEGF-A_{121} is soluble and active, while VEGF-A_{189} and VEGF-A_{206} tightly bind to the extracellular matrix through heparan sulfate molecules. VEGF-A_{145} and VEGF-A_{165} have intermediate affinity and maintain an average distribution between the two forms.

The angiogenic effect of VEGF is mediated by its cell surface receptors (VEGFR-1 and VEGFR-2). VEGFR-3 binds to VEGF-C and D and is responsible for inducing lymphangiogenesis.

Section 3 Growth factor delivery vehicles and strategies

The short half-life of growth factors in the body and the specific requirements during regeneration are the bottlenecks that limit their widespread clinical use. Therefore, the delivery of growth factors by biomaterials is crucial, and the main advantage of using biomaterials as carriers is that growth factors can be encapsulated within the biomaterials, avoiding their degradation in the wound environment. In addition, biomaterials can achieve local and sustained delivery of growth factors, ensuring the supply of locally high concentrations of growth factors required for tissue regeneration, ensuring that growth factors remain at the site of injury, and providing a scaffold or structural support on which host cells can migrate to promote tissue regeneration. For example, local application of growth factors is difficult to achieve in the treatment of critical sized bone defects, and biomaterials such as collagen sponge or tricalcium phosphate cement are used as carriers for growth factor delivery in bone regeneration.

Classification of Biomaterials

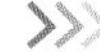

1. Natural materials such as silk, collagen, gelatin, chitosan, alginate, agarose, hyaluronic acid, fibrin, elastin, starch, and carrageenan are commonly used growth factor carriers. These materials may have some inherent biological activity and may contribute to regeneration. These materials are typically soluble in water, allowing for mild manufacturing conditions that are harmless to the biological activity of growth factors. In most natural materials, growth factors can infiltrate or disperse within the material scaffold, and can be modified through diffusion or scaffold degradation to achieve controlled release of growth factors.

2. Synthetic materials commonly used as growth factor carriers include polylysine, polylactic acid, polyglycolic acid and its copolymers polylactic acid glycolic acid, polyethyleneimine, polyethylene glycol, poly (N-isopropylacrylamide), hydroxyethyl methacrylate, polycaprolactone, and polyurethane. The main advantage of using synthetic materials is that they can be synthesized based on desired properties that are beneficial for clinical outcomes. In addition, sometimes composite materials of different materials are used to optimize the individual benefits of each material and improve the delivery efficiency of growth factors. For example, a mixture of polylysine and polycaprolactone has been used to deliver nerve growth factor (NGF) and effectively promote sciatic nerve regeneration. These polymers can be formulated into various physical structures related to the release of growth factors, such as conical scaffolds, hydrogels, nanoparticles and nanofibers. In addition, similar to natural materials, synthetic materials can also be functionalized with different materials (such as heparin) to enhance the loading of growth factors. Although these materials can be used as growth factor carriers, it should be noted that they are not natural and their degradation products may be toxic or difficult to remove from the body.

载体结构和形式与递送策略

生物材料载体可用作不同的物理结构和形式，包括支架、可注射水凝胶、纳米颗粒和纳米纤维。此外，这些结构的组合也可用于生长因子的双重释放。这种灵活性较强的生物材料载体对生长因子的递送极具吸引力。

1. 支架 组织工程和再生医学中的支架有两个关键功能，一是作为细胞附着和支撑结构，二是作为递送多种生长因子的平台。通常生长因子通过物理吸附加载到支架上，然后将这种含有生长因子的支架植入组织缺损处，不仅覆盖了缺损处，而且通过递送生长因子促进再生。支架可以通过各种不同的技术来制备，如颗粒浸出和溶剂浇注、冷冻干燥、相分离、熔融成型、原位聚合、气体发泡和乳化。

在支架上包载生长因子的主要问题之一是可能导致生长因子的突释。在某些情况下，生长因子的缓慢释放有利于创面修复。研究人员还设计了一种由生长因子和与支架结合的结合域组成的融合蛋白，如将脑源性神经生长因子（BDNF）和胶原结合结构域的融合蛋白负载到线性有序的胶原支架上，显著地促进了脊髓损伤的恢复。对 FGF 和 NGF 也采用了类似的策略，将它们与胶原结合结构域融合，并加载到胶原膜上，分别用于治疗腹壁缺损和皮肤溃疡的愈合。还有策略将生长因子结合位点连接到支架中以增强生长因子与支架的结合。例如，改造藻酸盐硫酸盐结构模拟肝素，从而与 VEGF、TGF-β1、EGF 和 PDGF 结合。肝素共价连接到大孔聚乳酸 - 乙醇酸支架的表面，将肝素结合的生长因子 FGF 负载到支架上，显著促进血管的形成。

2. 水凝胶 水凝胶有较高的水分含量，可以注射并填充到缺损的部位。此外，通过水凝胶递送生长因子的策略类似于上述支架的策略。目前美国食品药品监督管理局（FDA）批准了以羟乙基纤维素 (HEC) 包载 PDGF 用于治疗糖尿病下肢溃疡。有临床试验表明，使用包载 FGF2 的可生物降解的水凝胶治疗截骨手术患者是安全有效的。使用水凝胶作为粒细胞 - 巨噬细胞集落刺激因子 (GM-CSF) 递送载体治疗Ⅱ度烧伤也是安全有效的，还有报道在纤维蛋白凝胶中使用 FGF1 治疗脊髓损伤，在凝胶载体中包载 PDGF 和胰岛素样生长因子 1(IGF-1) 促进牙周骨缺损患者的骨再生。纤维蛋白 / 透明质酸水凝胶包载骨形态发生蛋白（BMP）-2 涂覆在固体自由支架上以促进骨再生。聚丙交酯 - 己内酯支架上涂覆肝素水凝胶用于骨再生中 BMP-2 的递送可促进骨形成和矿化；聚 -L- 乳酸支架和含有 FGF 的水凝胶用于前十字韧带再生，钛植入物和含有 FGF 的水凝胶用于骨再生，磷酸三钙多孔支架填充含 VEGF 的纤维蛋白凝胶密封剂用于严重骨缺损。为了防止生长因子从水凝胶中突释效应，可以利用生长因子与水凝胶的共价结合，如制备高肝素含量的水凝胶，以便肝素更容易地结合生长因子；调整水凝胶的电荷以增强生长因子的结合；制备能够共价连接生长因子的多肽纤维蛋白水凝胶，等等。

3. 颗粒系统 微粒系统与其他递送系统的不同之处在于其尺寸较小，微粒的范围为 1 ~ 1000 μm，纳米颗粒的范围 <1 μm，并已被用作生长因子递送载体，用于不同组织的再生。由于其尺寸小，纳米颗粒可以系统地给药，并可能改善传输特性和体内的药代动力学特征，因为它们可以通过细小的毛细血管和衬里

Carrier structure and form and delivery strategy

Biomaterial carriers can be used as different physical structures and forms, including scaffolds, injectable hydrogels, nanoparticles and nanofibers. In addition, the combination of these structures can also be used for dual release of growth factors. This flexible biomaterial carrier is highly attractive for the delivery of growth factors.

1.Scaffolds in tissue engineering and regenerative medicine have two key functions: serving as cell attachment and support structures, and as platforms for delivering various growth factors. Usually, growth factors are loaded onto scaffolds through physical adsorption, and then the scaffolds containing growth factors are implanted into tissue defects, not only covering the defects but also promoting regeneration by delivering growth factors. Brackets can be prepared using various techniques, such as particle leaching and solvent casting, freeze-drying, phase separation, melt forming, in-situ polymerization, gas foaming, and emulsification.

One of the main issues with encapsulating growth factors on scaffolds is the potential for burst release of growth factors. In some cases, slow release of growth factors is beneficial for wound repair. The researchers also designed a fusion protein consisting of growth factors and a binding domain that binds to the scaffold, such as loading the fusion protein of brain-derived neurotrophic factor (BDNF) and collagen binding domain onto a linearly ordered collagen scaffold, significantly promoting the recovery of spinal cord injury. A similar strategy was adopted for FGF and NGF, which were fused with collagen binding domains and loaded onto collagen membranes for the treatment of abdominal wall defects and skin ulcer healing, respectively. There are also strategies to connect growth factor binding sites to the scaffold to enhance the binding of growth factors to the scaffold. For example, modifying the structure of alginate sulfate to mimic heparin, thereby binding to VEGF, TGF-β1, EGF, and PDGF. Heparin is covalently attached to the surface of a macroporous polylactic acid glycolic acid scaffold, loading heparin bound growth factor FGF onto the scaffold and significantly promoting vascular formation.

2. The hydrogel gel has a high moisture content and can be injected and filled to the defect site. In addition, the strategy of delivering growth factors through hydrogels is similar to the strategy of the scaffold described above. At present, the US Food and Drug Administration (FDA) has approved the use of hydroxyethyl cellulose (HEC) encapsulated PDGF for the treatment of diabetes leg ulcers. Clinical trials have shown that FGF2 loaded biodegradable hydrogel is safe and effective for osteotomy patients. It is also safe and effective to use hydrogel as a delivery carrier of granulocyte macrophage colony stimulating factor (GM-CSF) to treat second degree burns. It is also reported that FGF1 is used in fibrin gel to treat spinal cord injury, and PDGF and insulin-like growth factor-1 (IGF-1) are encapsulated in gel carrier to promote bone regeneration in patients with periodontal bone defects. Fibrin/hyaluronic acid hydrogel encapsulated bone morphogenetic protein (BMP) -2 was coated on solid free scaffolds to promote bone regeneration. Heparin hydrogel coated on poly (lactide caprolactone) scaffold for BMP-2 delivery in bone regeneration can promote bone formation and mineralization; Poly-L-lactic acid scaffold and FGF containing hydrogel are used for anterior cruciate ligament regeneration, titanium implants and FGF containing hydrogel are used for bone regeneration, and tricalcium phosphate porous scaffold filled with fibrin gel sealant containing VEGF is used for severe bone defects. In order to prevent the sudden release of growth factors from hydrogels, covalent binding of growth factors and hydrogels can be used, such as preparing hydrogels with high heparin content, so that heparin can bind growth factors more easily; Adjust the charge of hydrogel to enhance the combination of growth factors; Preparation of polypeptide fibrin hydrogel capable of covalently linking growth factors, etc.

3. Particle systems. The difference between particle systems and other delivery systems lies in their smaller size, with particles ranging from 1-1000 μm and nanoparticles ranging from<1 μm. They have been used as growth factor delivery carriers for regeneration of different tissues. Due to their small size, nanoparticles can be systematically administered and may improve transport properties and pharmacokinetic characteristics in vivo, as

上皮更深入地渗透到组织中，从而允许更有效地递送生长因子。此外，纳米尺度赋予纳米颗粒系统独特的物理化学性质，如溶解性、生物分布、免疫原性和释放特性，最重要的是能够以最小限度分布到正常组织来靶向特定组织的能力。

目前有多项这方面的研究报道。例如，将 FGF 包裹在多孔二氧化硅纳米颗粒中，或者将 FGF 物理和化学结合到磁性氧化铁纳米颗粒中，把 BMP-2 固定在甲基丙烯酸缩水甘油酯葡聚糖 / 明胶纳米颗粒中用于牙周再生，PDGF 负载到透明质酸多孔纳米颗粒用于治疗皮肤溃疡，肝细胞生长因子（HGF）包埋在壳聚糖纳米颗粒中用于治疗肝硬化，PDGF 和 FGF 包裹在聚乳酸 - 乙醇酸 -Poloxamer 纳米颗粒中用于血管生成，聚乳酸 - 乙醇酸颗粒负载 EGF 用于糖尿病伤口的愈合。此外，为了提高生长因子对纳米颗粒的负载效率，通常在纳米颗粒配方中包括生长因子结合分子，如肝素等。

生长因子在创面修复临床应用上已经显示出巨大潜力，但为了充分发挥其潜力，还需要多学科的研究人员和临床医生共同开发新的生长因子递送方法用于组织再生和复杂创面的治疗。

第四节　生长因子调控创面修复的进展和思考

生长因子系列药物的研发，离不开以创伤和药学领域两位中国科学家为代表的本土科研团队所做出的杰出贡献。1991 年，付小兵院士出版了国际上第一部论述生长因子与创伤修复问题的学术专著《生长因子与创伤修复》；1996 年，李校堃院士团队经过艰苦的自主创新，将生长因子首次开发为烧创伤患者可用的新药，获得世界上第一个 FGF 新药证书；1998 年，付小兵院士团队在 *The Lancet* 杂志最早报道了 600 例多中心不同程度烧伤创面患者应用 bFGF 的临床试验结果，表明 bFGF 显著加速烧伤创面肉芽组织形成和再上皮化，促进创面愈合。2002 年和 2006 年，李校堃院士团队又先后开发了重组人碱性成纤维细胞生长因子和重组人酸性成纤维细胞生长因子系列新药。这些原创性的工作被国际创伤领域的专家评述为“了解中国创面治疗的窗口”“向东方看”，FGF 系列新药为创伤修复和组织再生提供了安全有效的主动修复和功能修复治疗新手段，创建了以生长因子为代表的创烧伤治疗特色体系，“中国方案”获得了国际同行的高度认可，是我国科技自主创新的一个颇具典型的案例。

从中国科学家研发生长因子新药至今已 30 多年，尽管生长因子系列新药已经广泛应用于创面修复领域，国内外的科学家在基础和临床研究上对生长因子不断有新的认识，特别是李校堃院士团队几十年如一日对 FGF 的研究，提出了生长因子代谢轴的概念，正在逐步拓宽 FGF 的临床适应证，挖掘生长因子新的潜在应用价值如治疗糖尿病、脂肪肝等。前沿交叉学科的进展，也使得我们从免疫、神经、脂肪等多个新的角度

they can penetrate deeper into tissues through small capillaries and lining epithelium, allowing for more effective delivery of growth factors. In addition, the nanoscale endows nanoparticle systems with unique physicochemical properties such as solubility, biological distribution, immunogenicity, and release characteristics, and most importantly, the ability to target specific tissues with minimal distribution to normal tissues.

There are currently multiple research reports in this area. For example, FGF is wrapped in porous silica nanoparticles, or FGF is physically and chemically combined into magnetic iron oxide nanoparticles, BMP-2 is fixed in glycidyl methacrylate dextran/gelatin nanoparticles for periodontal regeneration, PDGF is loaded into hyaluronic acid porous nanoparticles for treatment of skin ulcers, hepatocyte growth factor (HGF) is embedded in chitosan nanoparticles for treatment of liver cirrhosis, PDGF and FGF are wrapped in polylactic acid glycolic acid polyoxamer nanoparticles for angiogenesis, and polylactic acid glycolic acid particles loaded with EGF are used for healing of diabetes wounds. In addition, in order to improve the loading efficiency of growth factors on nanoparticles, growth factor binding molecules such as heparin are usually included in the nanoparticle formulation.

Growth factors have shown great potential in clinical applications of wound repair, but in order to fully unleash their potential, multidisciplinary researchers and clinical doctors need to jointly develop new growth factor delivery methods for tissue regeneration and treatment of complex wounds.

Section 4 Progress and reflection on the regulation of growth factors in wound repair

The development of growth factor series drugs cannot be separated from the outstanding contributions made by local research teams represented by two Chinese scientists in the fields of trauma and pharmacy. In 1991, Academician Fu Xiaobing published the first international academic monograph on the relationship between growth factors and trauma repair, titled *Growth Factors and Trauma Repair*; In 1996, the team led by Academician Li Xiaokun, after arduous independent innovation, developed growth factors into a new drug that could be used for burn trauma patients for the first time, and obtained the world's first FGF new drug certificate; In 1998, Academician Fu Xiaobing's team first reported the clinical trial results of using bFGF in 600 patients with different degrees of burn wounds from multiple centers in *The Lancet*. The results showed that bFGF significantly accelerated granulation tissue formation and re epithelialization of burn wounds, promoting wound healing. In 2002 and 2006, the team led by Academician Li Xiaokun developed a series of new drugs, recombinant human basic fibroblast growth factor and recombinant human acidic fibroblast growth factor. These original works have been praised by experts in the international trauma field as a "window to understand wound treatment in China" and a "look to the east". The FGF series of new drugs provide a safe and effective new means of active repair and functional repair for trauma repair and tissue regeneration, creating a unique system for burn treatment represented by growth factors. The "Chinese solution" has been highly recognized by international peers and is a typical case of China's independent scientific and technological innovation.

It has been more than 30 years since Chinese scientists developed new growth factor drugs. Although new growth factor series drugs have been widely used in the field of wound repair, scientists at home and abroad continue to have new understanding of growth factors in basic and clinical research. In particular, Academician Li Xiaokun's team has been studying FGF for decades, putting forward the concept of growth factor metabolic axis, gradually broadening the clinical indications of FGF, and tapping new potential application values of growth factors, such as treating diabetes, fatty liver, etc. The progress of cutting-edge interdisciplinary fields has also led us to rethink the

来重新思考生长因子对创面修复的调控及其对创面愈合的影响。

生长因子在创面治疗的临床研究

生长因子的临床研究在我国有很好的优势，2017 年中华医学会烧伤外科学分会多位专家联合起草和发布了《皮肤创面外用生长因子的临床指南》，全面总结和梳理了多种外用生长因子促进不同类型创面愈合的推荐分级的评估、制订与评价（GRADE）证据等级并做了专家推荐，对生长因子的剂型、浓度、常用剂量、频次，以及不良反应和注意事项都有了详细的说明。2020 年又发布该指南的英文版，也是国际上第一份生长因子药物在创面修复的临床指南。中外学者两篇最新的荟萃分析论文也表明，生长因子药物促进患者各类创面的愈合，但也都提到需要更多高质量的生长因子创面治疗临床试验。

生长因子和瘢痕形成密切联系，尽管已有不少动物实验证实生长因子减少创面愈合过程中瘢痕形成，但临床报道非常少。仅有的中国和日本的一些临床案例显示，bFGF 可缩短创面愈合同时减少病理性瘢痕产生。值得注意的是，一项关于 TGF-β3 的Ⅰ/Ⅱ期临床试验表明，重组 TGF-β3 蛋白显著改善志愿者皮肤瘢痕形成，然而Ⅲ期临床试验未能显示其对瘢痕的疗效，Ⅲ期使用的剂量是Ⅰ/Ⅱ期的 50%，因此研究人员推测可能是 TGF-β3 剂量不足导致对瘢痕的疗效不显著。结缔组织生长因子（CTGF）和 TGF-β1 被认为是治疗瘢痕的有效靶点，国外企业研发的 2 个 CTGF 的抑制剂 RXI-109 和 FS2 均显示了对临床患者皮肤瘢痕有较好治疗效果，但目前都还没有Ⅲ期临床试验结果；抗过敏药物曲尼司特是一种 TGF-β1 抑制剂，临床研究显示曲尼司特可显著改善剖宫产术后瘢痕形成，或有可能成为皮肤瘢痕治疗药物。

尽管生长因子在烧创伤和创面修复领域已经是一个“老药”，但对其深入研究很有可能拓展生长因子的临床适应证。已有不少的国内临床研究报道了生长因子可以用于气道插管所致的损伤、放射性皮炎、口腔扁平苔藓、咽瘘甚至白癜风的临床治疗，但高质量的临床研究或临床试验仍然不足，有必要进一步开展生长因子的临床研究，特别是生长因子和其他创面治疗手段如何协作也需要更多的临床探索。

生长因子对创面修复机制的研究

尽管生长因子在国内已经有 20 多年的临床应用，但进一步深入探讨已上市的生长因子对创面修复的作用机制仍然是研究方向。

李校堃院士带领团队进一步解析了 aFGF 和 bFGF 对糖尿病溃疡的机制。研究表明，bFGF 通过调控高糖环境下蛋白质 S-亚硝基化稳态化，从而缓解糖尿病诱导的血管内皮细胞功能障碍，促进血管新生。人脐静脉内皮细胞（HUVEC）在高血糖条件下显著降低内源性 IκB 激酶 β^{C179}（$IKK\beta^{C179}$）和转录因子 $p65^{C38}$ 的 S-亚硝基化，促进血管内皮功能慢性炎症导致功能障碍；抗亚硝基化的 $IKK\beta^{C179S}$ 和 $p65^{C38S}$ 突变体加重 db/db 小鼠和高血糖、高脂血症培养的 HUVEC 的内皮功能障碍，而 bFGF 可激活 AMPK/Akt-eNOS 通路促

regulation of growth factors on wound repair and their impact on wound healing from multiple new perspectives such as immunity, neurology, and adipose tissue.

Clinical study on growth factors in wound treatment >>>

The clinical research of growth factors has great advantages in China. In 2017, several experts from the Burn Surgery Branch of the Chinese Medical Association jointly drafted and released the *Clinical Guidelines for External Application of Growth Factors to Skin Wounds*, which comprehensively summarized and sorted out the recommended grading evaluation, formulation, and assessment (GRADE) evidence levels for various external growth factors to promote wound healing of different types, and made expert recommendations. Detailed explanations were provided on the dosage form, concentration, commonly used dosage, frequency, adverse reactions, and precautions of growth factors. The English version of the guideline was released in 2020, which is also the first clinical guideline for growth factor drugs in wound repair internationally. Two latest meta-analysis papers by Chinese and foreign scholars also indicate that growth factor drugs promote the healing of various types of wounds in patients, but both also mention the need for more high-quality clinical trials of growth factor wound treatment.

There is a close relationship between growth factors and scar formation. Although many animal experiments have shown that growth factors reduce scar formation during wound healing, there are very few clinical reports. The only clinical cases in China and Japan have shown that bFGF can shorten wound healing time and reduce pathological scar formation. It is worth noting that a phase I/II clinical trial on TGF - β3 showed that the recombinant TGF - β3 protein significantly improved scar formation in volunteers' skin. However, the phase III clinical trial did not demonstrate its therapeutic effect on scars, and the dosage used in phase III was 50% of that in phase I/II. Therefore, researchers speculate that insufficient TGF- β3 dosage may have led to insignificant therapeutic effects on scars. Connective tissue growth factor (CTGF) and TGF- β1 are considered effective targets for treating scars. Two CTGF inhibitors, RXI-109 and FS2, developed by foreign companies, have shown good therapeutic effects on skin scars in clinical patients, but there are currently no phase III clinical trial results; The anti allergic drug tranilast is a TGF- β1 inhibitor. Clinical studies have shown that tranilast can significantly improve scar formation after cesarean section and may become a skin scar treatment drug.

Although growth factors are already an "old medicine" in the fields of burn injury and wound repair, in-depth research on them is likely to expand the clinical indications of growth factors. Many domestic clinical studies have reported that growth factors can be used for the clinical treatment of injuries caused by airway intubation, radiation dermatitis, oral lichen planus, pharyngeal fistula, and even vitiligo. However, high-quality clinical research or trials are still insufficient, and it is necessary to further carry out clinical research on growth factors, especially how to cooperate with other wound treatment methods, which also requires more clinical exploration.

Research on the mechanism of growth factors in wound repair >>>

Although growth factors have been clinically applied in China for over 20 years, further exploration of the mechanism of action of already marketed growth factors on wound repair is still a research direction.

Academician Li Xiaokun led the team to further analyze the mechanism of aFGF and bFGF on diabetes ulcer. Research shows that bFGF can alleviate the dysfunction of vascular endothelial cells induced by diabetes and promote angiogenesis by regulating the protein S-nitrosation homeostasis in high glucose environment. Under hyperglycemic conditions, human umbilical vein endothelial cells (HUVECs) significantly reduce the S-nitrosylation of endogenous I κ B kinase β^{C179} (IKK β^{C179}) and transcription factor $p65^{C38}$, promoting chronic inflammation and dysfunction of vascular endothelial function; The IKK β^{C179S} and $p65^{C38S}$ mutants that resist nitrosylation exacerbate endothelial dysfunction in db/db mice and HUVECs cultured with hyperglycemia and hyperlipidemia, while bFGF

进 IKKβ 及 p65 的亚硝基化修饰，显著逆转高糖导致的血管内皮细胞功能障碍，促进血管新生及皮肤创面愈合。因此，研究人员首次从 S- 亚硝基化途径解释了 bFGF 对糖尿病患者血管功能保护作用，为 bFGF 临床应用于慢性难愈合患者提供了全新的理论支持。研究人员还发现，aFGF 可显著降低 db/db 小鼠和高糖环境下血管内皮细胞线粒体超氧化物的产生，并激活 Wnt/β-catenin 信号通路保护血管内皮细胞功能，*c-Myc* 基因敲除和抑制己糖激酶 2（HXK-2）可部分抵消 aFGF 对血管内皮细胞的保护，因此 Wnt/β-catenin/c-Myc/HXK-2 信号通路介导了 aFGF 的促愈合作用。该研究首次报道了 aFGF 通过 HXK-2 抑制线粒体超氧化物生成来促进糖尿病创面愈合。

针对 FGF 家族的其他成员，本团队的研究人员发现，FGF21 通过 SIRT1 介导的自噬信号通路促进角质细胞的迁移和分化，进而促进皮肤创面愈合，在角质细胞特异性敲除 *SIRT1* 基因以及 *Atg7* 基因敲除小鼠中，FGF21 的促创面愈合作用均显著下降。另外，FGF21 能够通过上调自噬，激活 AMPK-FoxO3a-SPK2-CARM1 和 AMPK-mTOR 信号通路，抑制血管内皮细胞凋亡、减少氧化应激促进血管新生，从而增强皮瓣存活。本团队的研究显示，FGF10 对创伤愈合后瘢痕形成起重要的调控作用，通过转录组学分析发现，FGF10 促进创面愈合的同时，抑制 *STAP2* 基因表达和信号转导及转录激活蛋白 3（STAT3）的激活，降低Ⅰ型胶原和Ⅲ型胶原蛋白水平，减少机械应力诱导的瘢痕形成。

本团队的这些系列研究工作不仅加深了生长因子对创面修复的调控机制的理解，而且也更好的指导了生长因子在临床的应用。笔者认为可从以下几个方面开展工作：①创面修复过程中生长因子表达时空的图谱、应用前沿的时空组学技术有可能给人们更多的启示。②生长因子对创面修复过程中毛囊、汗腺、末梢神经的作用及机制研究还有待于进一步阐明。③机体内生长因子是一个复杂的调控网络，给予的外源性生长因子也可促进内源性生长因子表达。外源性生长因子对创面愈合过程中内源性生长因子表达图谱需要进一步解析，有望更好地指导生长因子药物的精准治疗。

生长因子与免疫系统相互作用影响创面愈合的研究

随着条件性敲除动物、各类组学技术、单细胞分析技术等在慢性创面研究的广泛应用，从免疫系统的角度来探讨创面愈合取得了一系列重要的进展，值得注意的是，生长因子在免疫系统调控创面修复过程中充当了不可或缺的角色。

一项研究表明，TGF-β 是促使创面愈合过程瘙痒发生重要调控因素。创面愈合过程中局部的免疫调节细胞 TGF-β 的增高可促使真皮层内的 2 型经典树突状细胞（cDC2）分泌白介素 -31（IL-31），使得具有 IL-31 受体的瘙痒相关神经元敏感并兴奋，造成创面愈合过程中产生局部瘙痒。*IL31* 基因敲除小鼠在皮肤愈合过程的搔抓行为大幅减少，证明 IL-31 是引起创面愈合过程中产生瘙痒的主要原因。将 TGF-β 处理后的 cDC2 注射回小鼠皮内，也可使其出现抓搔行为，而特异性敲除树突样细胞的 TGF-β 受体小鼠，在皮肤愈

can activate the AMPK/Akt eNOS pathway to promote nitrosylation modification of IKK β and p65, significantly reversing the dysfunction of vascular endothelial cells caused by high glucose, promoting angiogenesis and skin wound healing. Therefore, researchers explained the protective effect of bFGF on vascular function of diabetes patients from the S-nitroso pathway for the first time, providing a new theoretical support for the clinical application of bFGF in chronic refractory patients. Researchers also found that aFGF can significantly reduce the production of mitochondrial superoxide in db/db mice and vascular endothelial cells under high glucose conditions, and activate the Wnt/ β-catenin signaling pathway to protect the function of vascular endothelial cells. *c-Myc* gene knockout and inhibition of hexokinase 2 (HXK-2) can partially offset the protective effect of aFGF on vascular endothelial cells. Therefore, the Wnt/ β-catenin/c-Myc/HXK-2 signaling pathway mediates the pro healing effect of aFGF. This study is the first report that aFGF promotes wound healing in diabetes by inhibiting mitochondrial superoxide generation through HXK-2.

For other members of the FGF family, our team's researchers found that FGF21 promotes the migration and differentiation of keratinocytes through the SIRT1 mediated autophagy signaling pathway, thereby promoting skin wound healing. In keratinocyte specific knockout of *SIRT1* gene and *Atg7* gene knockout mice, the wound healing promoting effect of FGF21 was significantly reduced. In addition, FGF21 can upregulate autophagy, activate the AMPK-FoxO3a-SPK2-CARM1 and AMPK mTOR signaling pathways, inhibit endothelial cell apoptosis, reduce oxidative stress, promote angiogenesis, and enhance flap survival. Our team's research shows that FGF10 plays an important regulatory role in scar formation after wound healing. Through transcriptomic analysis, it was found that FGF10 promotes wound healing while inhibiting the expression of *STAP2* gene and the activation of signal transduction and transcriptional activator protein 3 (STAT3), reducing the levels of type I collagen and type III collagen, and reducing mechanical stress-induced scar formation.

Our team's series of research works not only deepen our understanding of the regulatory mechanism of growth factors on wound repair, but also better guide the clinical application of growth factors. The author believes that work can be carried out from the following aspects: ① Spatiotemporal mapping of growth factor expression during wound repair process, and the application of cutting-edge spatiotemporal omics technology may provide more insights for people. ② The role and mechanism of growth factors in hair follicles, sweat glands, and peripheral nerves during wound repair process still need further clarification The growth factors in the body are a complex regulatory network, and exogenous growth factors administered can also promote the expression of endogenous growth factors. The expression profile of endogenous growth factors during wound healing process by exogenous growth factors needs further analysis, which is expected to better guide the precise treatment of growth factor drugs.

Study on the interaction between growth factors and immune system affecting wound healing

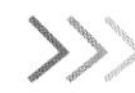

With the widespread application of conditional knockout animals, various omics techniques, single-cell analysis techniques, etc. in the study of chronic wounds, a series of important advances have been made in exploring wound healing from the perspective of the immune system. It is worth noting that growth factors play an indispensable role in regulating the process of wound repair by the immune system.

A study suggests that TGF- β is an important regulatory factor that promotes itching during wound healing. The increase of local immune regulatory cells TGF- β during wound healing can promote the secretion of interleukin-31 (IL-31) by type 2 classical dendritic cells (cDC2) in the dermis, making itch related neurons with IL-31 receptors sensitive and excited, resulting in local itching during wound healing. *IL31* gene knockout mice showed a significant reduction in scratching behavior during skin healing, indicating that IL-31 is the main cause of itching during wound healing. Injecting cDC2 treated with TGF- β back into the skin of mice can also induce scratching behavior, while TGF- β receptor mice specifically knocking out dendritic like cells significantly reduce scratching behavior during

合过程中的抓搔行为显著减少，表明 TGF-β 促进 cDC2 分泌 IL-31 是创面愈合过程中产生瘙痒的主要原因。

另一项研究表明，GM-CSF 也可通过免疫系统介导创面愈合进程。在皮肤损伤期间必须协调免疫反应和修复机制以实现快速皮肤再生和预防微生物感染，研究证实自然杀伤（NK）细胞中缺乏缺氧诱导因子 -1α（HIF-1α）的小鼠表现出干扰素 γ（IFN-γ）和 GM-CSF 的释放受损，使得免疫（炎症）反应减弱，从而加速皮肤血管生成和创面愈合。尽管创面迅速闭合，皮肤免疫系统的杀菌作用和限制全身细菌感染的能力仍受到损害；相反，HIF-1α 信号通路的激活增强 NK 细胞介导的抗菌防御，NK 细胞可直接杀死细菌，同时释放 IFN-γ 和 GM-CSF，促进免疫（炎症）反应增强。因此，生长因子的释放对于 NK 细胞发挥皮肤抗菌防御和促进修复也是重要的环节。

众所周知，免疫细胞分泌大量的细胞因子和生长因子可调控创面愈合全过程。事实上，在生理状态下，皮肤免疫系统内的树突状表皮 T 细胞也分泌少量的生长因子和炎症因子来维持皮肤的稳态。笔者认为有必要从以下三个方面考虑：①探讨皮肤免疫系统重要的免疫细胞分泌各类生长因子对免疫系统自身的影响，对创面微环境的表皮细胞、成纤维细胞、角质细胞等的作用和再上皮化机制。②巨噬细胞通过释放多种生长因子影响创面愈合进程，有必要通过组学技术探讨各种常见慢性皮肤溃疡巨噬细胞来源的生长因子图谱，鉴别不同阶段生长因子对创面微环境的影响。③创面愈合过程中，外源性生长因子如何作用于皮肤免疫系统，如何调控免疫系统分泌细胞因子和内源性生长因子，也有待进一步研究。

生长因子与神经系统相互作用影响创面愈合的研究

皮肤是一种极其敏感的神经依赖器官，人体皮肤真皮层含有神经末梢，属于周围神经系统的一部分，其中感觉神经纤维末梢使皮肤能感受触觉、温觉、冷觉、痛觉和压觉，运动神经末梢主要分布于皮肤附属器周围，支配肌肉活动。

已有临床研究表明，脊髓损伤、周围神经损伤、糖尿病神经病变等都会导致皮肤神经末梢损害，导致创面难愈合。动物模型试验也证实，神经源性刺激能够影响创面愈合，通过手术切断支配神经（去神经支配）能够延迟创面修复，神经支配和神经介质对创面修复起主要作用。神经支配主要通过神经元的轴突出芽以及分泌的各种生长因子调控创面愈合；而神经介质主要是生长因子如 BDNF、NGF、神经营养素 3（NT-3）神经元及其他皮肤细胞分泌的多种神经肽，包括降钙素基因相关肽（CGRP）、P 物质（SP）、促肾上腺皮质激素释放激素（CRH）、血管活性肠肽（VIP）等，这些神经肽对多种皮肤细胞具有调控增殖、迁移作用，还参与创伤后免疫、内分泌的调控。因此，神经创伤导致的周围神经损伤能够延迟创面愈合导致的慢性创面，但神经损伤对创面难愈合的分子机制还有待于进一步阐明。

另外，烧创伤、慢性溃疡也伴随皮肤神经纤维的破坏，进一步影响了创面愈合。临床研究发现，Ⅱ度烧伤患者新生的肉芽组织中有大量不依赖于血管的神经纤维，这些神经纤维被施万细胞包绕，说明表皮神

skin healing, indicating that TGF-βpromotes the secretion of IL-31 by cDC2 and is the main cause of itching during wound healing.

Another study suggests that GM-CSF can also mediate the wound healing process through the immune system. During skin injury, it is necessary to coordinate immune response and repair mechanisms to achieve rapid skin regeneration and prevent microbial infections. Studies have shown that mice lacking hypoxia inducible factor-1 alpha (HIF-1 alpha) in natural killer (NK) cells exhibit impaired release of interferon gamma (IFN-γ) and GM-CSF, leading to weakened immune (inflammatory) response and accelerated skin angiogenesis and wound healing. However, despite the rapid closure of the wound, the bactericidal effect of the skin's immune system and its ability to limit systemic bacterial infections are still compromised; On the contrary, activation of the HIF-1α signaling pathway enhances the antibacterial defense mediated by NK cells, which can directly kill bacteria while releasing IFN-γ and GM-CSF, promoting an enhanced immune (inflammatory) response. Therefore, the release of growth factors is also an important link for NK cells to exert skin antibacterial defense and promote repair.

As is well known, immune cells secrete a large amount of cytokines and growth factors that can regulate the entire process of wound healing. In fact, under physiological conditions, dendritic epidermal T cells within the skin's immune system also secrete small amounts of growth factors and inflammatory factors to maintain skin homeostasis. The author believes that it is necessary to consider the following three aspects: ① Exploring the effects of various growth factors secreted by important immune cells in the skin immune system on the immune system itself, the role of epidermal cells, fibroblasts, keratinocytes, etc. in the wound microenvironment, and the re epithelialization mechanism. ② Macrophages affect the wound healing process by releasing multiple growth factors. It is necessary to explore the growth factor profiles of macrophages from various common chronic skin ulcers through omics techniques to identify the effects of growth factors on the wound microenvironment at different stages. ③ Further research is needed on how exogenous growth factors act on the skin immune system during wound healing, and how they regulate the secretion of cytokines and endogenous growth factors by the immune system.

Study on the interaction between growth factors and the nervous system affecting wound healing

The skin is an extremely sensitive nerve dependent organ, and the dermis layer of human skin contains nerve endings, which are part of the peripheral nervous system. Among them, sensory nerve fiber endings enable the skin to sense touch, temperature, cold, pain, and pressure, while motor nerve endings are mainly distributed around the skin appendages, controlling muscle activity.

Clinical studies have shown that spinal cord injury, peripheral nerve injury, diabetes neuropathy, etc. can lead to skin nerve endings damage, resulting in difficult wound healing. Animal model experiments have also confirmed that neurogenic stimulation can affect wound healing. Surgical cutting of innervated nerves (denervation) can delay wound repair, and innervation and neural mediators play a major role in wound repair. Neural innervation mainly regulates wound healing through axonal sprouting and secretion of various growth factors by neurons; And the main neurotransmitters are growth factors such as BDNF, NGF, neurotrophin-3 (NT-3) neurons, and various neuropeptides secreted by other skin cells, including calcitonin gene-related peptide (CGRP), substance P (SP), corticotropin releasing hormone (CRH), vasoactive intestinal peptide (VIP), etc. These neuropeptides have regulatory effects on the proliferation and migration of various skin cells, and also participate in the regulation of immune and endocrine functions after trauma. Therefore, peripheral nerve injury caused by nerve trauma can delay chronic wound healing, but the molecular mechanism of nerve injury on difficult wound healing still needs further clarification.

In addition, burn wounds and chronic ulcers are also accompanied by the destruction of skin nerve fibers, further affecting wound healing. Clinical studies have found that there are a large number of nerve fibers in the newly formed granulation tissue of patients with second degree burns that do not rely on blood vessels. These nerve

经与创面愈合早期的调控密切相关。烧伤后愈合过程中，伴随肉芽组织增生，神经末梢也呈现持续再生，瘢痕增生期神经纤维容积分数达到最高，但存在扭曲变形、崩解断裂现象，到成熟期神经纤维趋于正常，容积分数则低于正常。愈合过程中胶原蛋白的沉积，一方面为神经再生提供支架，另一方面胶原蛋白会对神经纤维进行缠绕，阻止其分泌神经肽，不利于创面重塑调控。糖尿病大鼠皮肤损伤模型也出现周围神经末梢缺损，SP 释放减少。此外，创面修复时角质形成细胞表达的 NGF 上调，NGF 作用于人真皮微血管内皮细胞（HDMEC）使其增殖，增加 HDMEC 中细胞间黏附分子（ICAM）的表达；NGF 还参与募集炎症细胞和 T 细胞浸润、诱导巨噬细胞聚集，也可能是炎症的重要介导因素。因此，在创面修复过程中，皮肤神经也对创面愈合起到重要的调控作用，但神经因素如 NGF 等对创面修复的分子机理仍然研究不多，也有待于进一步阐明。

生长因子在脂肪调控创面愈合中的重要作用

多项研究表明，脂肪组织在创面修复过程中起重要的作用，特别是脂肪细胞脂解在调节炎症和皮肤损伤后修复中有重要作用。在小鼠中进行的遗传研究表明，皮肤脂肪细胞对于损伤后引发炎症并促进后续修复是必不可少的。

厦门大学张凌娟教授团队对不同年龄段的小鼠和人的皮肤做了系统的分析，发现婴儿皮肤里有大量的不成熟脂肪，这些脂肪表达大量抗菌肽，但随着年龄增长，这些皮下脂肪慢慢消失，在老龄鼠的人的皮肤里皮下脂肪完全被纤维化细胞取而代之。该团队发现，老化过程中皮肤脂肪丢失是和真皮成纤维细胞失去脂肪分化能力密切相关的。进一步对不同年龄段提取的真皮成纤维细胞做转录组基因测序分析发现，TGF-β 信号通路在成纤维细胞的成长过程中被激活，TGF-β2 通过激活下游 TGFβR 和 SMAD2/3 信号通路，直接导致真皮成纤维细胞丧失脂肪分化的功能，取而代之的是纤维化功能增加。在成年或老化小鼠中使用 TGF-β 受体小分子抑制剂阻断 TGF-β 信号通路，可促进真皮成纤维细胞恢复脂肪分化功能，从而增加皮肤对金黄色葡萄球菌的天然免疫抵抗力。因此，TGF-β 抑制剂有可能用于老年患者的创面修复。张凌娟教授等进一步的研究发现，高脂饮食喂养的小鼠皮肤有大量成熟脂肪细胞增生，这类成熟脂肪细胞释放 TGF-β，反而降低了脂肪干细胞分化及表达抗菌肽的能力，使肥胖小鼠容易受到金黄色葡萄球菌的感染，而过氧化物酶体增殖物激活受体（PPARγ）激动剂罗格列酮或 TGF-β 受体阻滞剂可恢复肥胖小鼠的皮肤防御金葡菌感染的能力。这两项研究都证实了 TGF-β 在脂肪调控创面愈合中起重要作用。

在另一项研究中，科研人员对成纤维细胞的遗传特性进行了分析。结果发现，皮肤出现损伤后，一类在正常情况下能分化为脂肪前体细胞的成纤维细胞亚群，能形成瘢痕组织并促进皮肤创面愈合。进一步研究发现，表达 CD301b 的巨噬细胞是通过两种重要的生长因子，即 IGF-1 和 PDGF-CC 来促进这类特殊的成纤维细胞亚群的增殖；相比小鼠皮肤组织，这类能分化为脂肪前体细胞的成纤维细胞亚群在人类皮肤组织

fibers are surrounded by Schwann cells, indicating that the epidermal nerve is closely related to the regulation of early wound healing. During the healing process after burn injury, granulation tissue proliferation is accompanied by continuous regeneration of nerve endings. The nerve fiber volume fraction reaches its highest point during scar hyperplasia, but there is distortion, deformation, disintegration, and fracture. In the mature stage, the nerve fibers tend to be normal, and the volume fraction is lower than normal. The deposition of collagen during the healing process provides a scaffold for nerve regeneration on one hand, and on the other hand, collagen wraps around nerve fibers, preventing their secretion of neuropeptides, which is not conducive to wound remodeling regulation. The skin injury model of diabetes rats also showed peripheral nerve endings defect, and SP release was reduced. In addition, during wound repair, the expression of NGF in keratinocytes is upregulated. NGF acts on human dermal microvascular endothelial cells (HDMEC) to promote their proliferation and increase the expression of intercellular adhesion molecules (ICAM) in HDMEC; NGF also participates in recruiting inflammatory cells and T cell infiltration, inducing macrophage aggregation, and may be an important mediator of inflammation. Therefore, in the process of wound repair, skin nerves also play an important regulatory role in wound healing, but the molecular mechanism of nerve factors such as NGF on wound repair is still not well studied and needs further clarification.

The important role of growth factors in fat regulation of wound healing

Multiple studies have shown that adipose tissue plays an important role in wound repair, particularly in regulating inflammation and repairing skin injuries through adipocyte lipolysis. Genetic studies conducted in mice have shown that skin adipocytes are essential for triggering inflammation and promoting subsequent repair after injury.

Professor Zhang Lingjuan's team from Xiamen University conducted a systematic analysis of the skin of mice and humans of different age groups and found that there is a large amount of immature fat in infant skin, which expresses a large amount of antimicrobial peptides. However, as age increases, this subcutaneous fat gradually disappears, and in the skin of elderly mice, subcutaneous fat is completely replaced by fibrotic cells. The team found that the loss of skin fat during aging is closely related to the loss of fat differentiation ability of dermal fibroblasts. Further transcriptome gene sequencing analysis of dermal fibroblasts extracted from different age groups revealed that the TGF-β signaling pathway is activated during fibroblast growth. TGF-β2 activates downstream TGF βR and SMAD2/3 signaling pathways, directly leading to the loss of adipogenic differentiation function in dermal fibroblasts and an increase in fibrotic function. Blocking the TGF-β signaling pathway with TGF-β receptor small molecule inhibitors in adult or aging mice can promote the restoration of adipogenic differentiation function in dermal fibroblasts, thereby increasing the skin's natural immune resistance to Staphylococcus aureus. Therefore, TGF-β inhibitors may be used for wound repair in elderly patients. Further research by Professor Zhang Lingjuan and others has found that mice fed a high-fat diet have a significant increase in mature adipocytes in their skin. These mature adipocytes release TGF-β, which in turn reduces the ability of adipose stem cells to differentiate and express antimicrobial peptides, making obese mice more susceptible to Staphylococcus aureus infection. However, peroxisome proliferator activated receptor (PPAR γ) agonists such as Rosiglitazone or TGF-β receptor blockers can restore the skin's ability to defend against Staphylococcus aureus infection in obese mice. Both studies have confirmed the important role of TGF-β in regulating fat induced wound healing.

In another study, researchers analyzed the genetic characteristics of fibroblasts. It was found that after skin damage, a subpopulation of fibroblasts that can normally differentiate into adipocyte precursor cells can form scar tissue and promote skin wound healing. Further research has found that macrophages expressing CD301b promote the proliferation of this particular fibroblast subpopulation through two important growth factors, IGF-1 and PDGF-CC; Compared to mouse skin tissue, the level of fibroblast subpopulations that can differentiate into adipocyte precursor cells is significantly reduced in human skin tissue, indicating that human skin scars are much more

中的水平显著下降，也表明人类的皮肤瘢痕要远多于小鼠的原因。该研究也证实，巨噬细胞可通过分泌生长因子，来调控特殊成纤维细胞亚群，从而影响创面愈合。

脂肪与创面修复是创面研究的热点，已有很多临床报道脂肪组织用于创面治疗，生长因子和脂肪如何相互作用并影响创面愈合进程，是值得研究人员去挖掘的重要研究方向。

改造生长因子扩展其应用的研究

生长因子药物尽管已经广泛应用于临床，但如何获得功能更加强大的生长因子也一直是科研工作者的目标。澳大利亚莫纳什大学 Mikal M. Martino 教授等报道了一种基于蛋白质工程的技术，对生长因子进行改造，引入层粘连蛋白亚基 - α 1 的方法，从而增强生长因子与细胞表面的受体的结合，可触发一种可控持久的生长因子信号传递通路，显著促进皮肤创面修复。加强型生长因子与受体结合启动一种相对较低但持续的信号，与野生型生长因子（磷酸化强烈且迅速降低）相比，在前 30 分钟内可诱导较低的磷酸化水平，显示出非常不同的信号动力学，避免了因快速磷酸化导致的生长因子受体内化和降解，对糖尿病创面等有持续显著的修复作用。因此，通过控制生长因子与多配体蛋白聚糖的结合来控制生长因子信号，可能是促进难愈合创面修复有效的策略。

瑞士洛桑联邦理工学院的 Jeffrey A. Hubbell 教授等对 25 种生长因子与 6 种重要细胞外基质蛋白之间的作用进行了筛查研究，挑选出了与所有 6 种蛋白显示最强力结合的胎盘胰岛素样生长因子 2（PIGF-2）。进一步分析 PIGF-2 的序列，鉴定出导致 PIGF-2 与细胞外基质蛋白强有力结合的原因是含有一个 22 个氨基酸的区域。通过将这段 22 个氨基酸序列与另外 3 种生长因子融合，能够将生长因子的结合亲和力提高 2 ~ 100 倍，且显著促进创面修复。该团队还发现，小鼠血管血友病因子（vWF）缺陷可导致创面愈合延迟，同时伴随创面中的血管形成减少、促血管形成的生长因子减少；vWF 主要通过 vWF A1 结构域中的肝素结合结构域（HBD）与多种生长因子结合，如 VEGF-A 和 PDGF-BB。在 vWF A1 HBD 功能化纤维蛋白基质中加入 $VEGF\text{-}A_{165}$ 和 PDGF-BB 可以缓释生长因子，显著促进糖尿病溃疡小鼠的创面愈合，促进血管新生和平滑肌细胞增殖。

总之，生长因子作为在临床创面治疗的常用药物，在创面修复领域依然是一个热点研究方向，需要研究人员进一步继承和发扬为生长因子研究做出卓越贡献的中国科学家的首创精神，努力在生长因子和创面修复领域做出新的贡献。

common than in mice. This study also confirms that macrophages can regulate specific subpopulations of fibroblasts by secreting growth factors, thereby affecting wound healing.

Fat and wound repair are hot topics in wound research, and there have been many clinical reports on the use of adipose tissue for wound treatment. How growth factors and fat interact and affect the wound healing process is an important research direction worth exploring by researchers.

Research on expanding the application of modified growth factors

Although growth factor drugs have been widely used in clinical practice, how to obtain more powerful growth factors has always been the goal of researchers. Professor Mikal M. Martino from Monash University in Australia reported a protein engineering based technique to modify growth factors by introducing the laminin subunit-α 1, thereby enhancing the binding of growth factors to cell surface receptors. This can trigger a controllable and persistent growth factor signaling pathway, significantly promoting skin wound repair. The combination of enhanced growth factor and receptor initiates a relatively low but persistent signal. Compared with wild growth factor (phosphorylation is intense and rapidly reduced), it can induce a lower phosphorylation level in the first 30 minutes, showing very different signal dynamics, avoiding the internalization and degradation of growth factor receptor caused by rapid phosphorylation, and has a sustained and significant repair effect on diabetes wounds. Therefore, controlling the binding of growth factors to multi ligand proteoglycans to regulate growth factor signaling may be an effective strategy for promoting the repair of difficult to heal wounds.

Professor Jeffrey A. Hubbell and colleagues from the Swiss Federal Institute of Technology in Lausanne conducted a screening study on the interactions between 25 growth factors and 6 important extracellular matrix proteins, and selected placental insulin-like growth factor 2 (PIGF-2), which showed the strongest binding to all 6 proteins. Further analysis of the sequence of PIGF-2 identified that the strong binding of PIGF-2 to extracellular matrix proteins is due to a region containing 22 amino acids. By fusing this 22 amino acid sequence with three other growth factors, the binding affinity of the growth factors can be increased by 2-100 times, and wound repair can be significantly promoted. The team also found that defects in von Willebrand factor (vWF) in mice can lead to delayed wound healing, accompanied by reduced angiogenesis and growth factors that promote angiogenesis in the wound; VWF mainly binds to various growth factors such as VEGF-A and PDGF-BB through the heparin binding domain (HBD) in the vWF A1 domain. Adding VEGF-A_{165} and PDGF-BB to vWF A1 HBD functionalized fibrin matrix can release growth factors, significantly promote wound healing in diabetes ulcer mice, and promote angiogenesis and smooth muscle cell proliferation.

In summary, growth factors, as commonly used drugs in clinical wound treatment, remain a hot research direction in the field of wound repair. Researchers need to further inherit and carry forward the pioneering spirit of Chinese scientists who have made outstanding contributions to growth factor research, and strive to make new contributions in the field of growth factors and wound repair.

第一部分 概述

第 2 章
Chapter 2

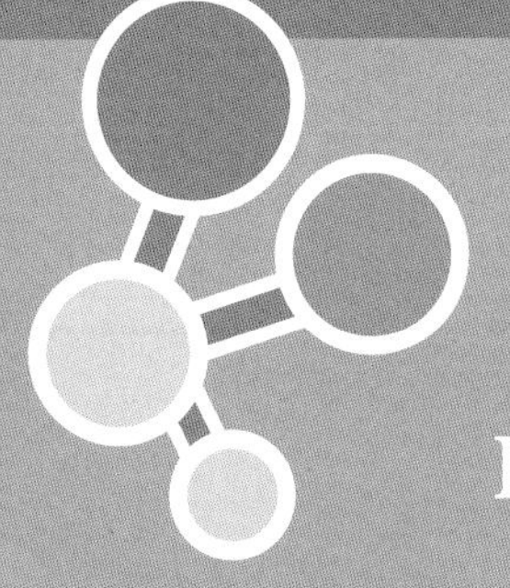

生长因子的研发与新理论
Development and New Theory of Growth Factors

第一节　生长因子自主研发之路

20 世纪 30 年代末 40 年代初，Trowell 和 Hoffman 等在研究垂体激素时发现，垂体提取液能够刺激小鼠成纤维细胞分裂增殖，经已知的各种垂体激素实验证实均无此作用，说明垂体提取液中存在着一种新的物质。由于这种新物质能够刺激成纤维细胞增殖，故称为成纤维细胞生长因子（FGF）。随后的研究表明，FGF 也可以刺激中胚层和神经外胚层来源细胞如角膜内皮细胞、血管内皮细胞、上皮细胞等生长，因而对血管生成、肢体发育、伤口愈合起促进作用。近来发现其对神经系统、代谢系统、骨骼系统等都有重要调控作用，实际上是一种对多种细胞具有增殖和分化调控的活性多肽，目前已陆续发现具有类似结构和功能的 23 个成员，组成了 FGF 家族。

FGF 药物的发现

20 世纪 80 年代以来，生物技术特别是基因工程技术迅猛发展，不仅给生物制药业本身带来了革命性的突破，也给相关或相邻学科与产业带来了变革的契机。1989 年，暨南大学林剑教授从美国留学归来率先进行了 FGF 的研制开发。1992 年，李校堃加入导师林剑教授科研团队，并很快成为项目的核心骨干。从 FGF 被发现，在长达 50 多年的时间没有成药，主要是因为 FGF 结构与功能十分复杂，成药研发遇到重大技术瓶颈，表达量低、活性低、稳定性差，是 FGF 成药需翻越的三座大山。早期获得 FGF 是通过动物组织提取，大约上万头牛才能提取 1g，高昂的成本无法用于临床应用，而本团队的研究人员通过基因工程与分子修饰技术实现了突破，通过分子伴侣技术实现了从活性低的包涵体表达到高活性的可溶性表达。蛋白生产周期从 14 天缩短为 2 天，产率提高了 6 倍。通过对 FGF 结构的研究，发现其可与长链肝素修饰物特异性结合的特性，由此开发了新型亲和层析系统，蛋白纯度超过 99%，完全满足了产业化的需求。基于其亲疏水基团分布的特征，通过高通量筛选获得了 FGF 蛋白稳态体系，为后续多种制剂开发奠定了基础。1996 年 1 月，团队获得了卫生部颁发的重组牛源 FGF2 一类新药证书。这是世界上第一个上市的 FGF 新药，主要适应证为烧伤、创伤。

由于牛源的 FGF2 和人源在氨基酸序列方面存在差异，本团队又进一步开发了全人源化的 FGF2 新药，适应证为各类复杂创面。其间，付小兵教授领导的解放军总医院 304 医院创伤修复重点实验室作为牵头单位，在 34 家医院开展了 FGF2 药物的多中心临床应用研究，试验结果先后发表于国内专业杂志和 *The Lancet* 杂志。试验涉及的 1000 余例患者包括不同深度烧伤和手术供皮区等急性创面，采用 FGF2[150AU/(cm^2·d)] 处理，另有 800 余例创面作为对照。结果显示，FGF2 能显著加速肉芽组织的形成和创面再上皮化，即重组 FGF2 加速烧伤供皮区创面的愈合，与对照组相比，浅Ⅱ度和深Ⅱ度烧伤创面的愈合时间较对照组的明显缩短；

Section 1 The path of independent research and development of growth factors

In the late 1930s and early 1940s, Trowell and Hoffman found that pituitary extract could stimulate the division and proliferation of mouse fibroblasts while studying pituitary hormones. However, various known pituitary hormone experiments confirmed that there was no such effect, indicating the presence of a new substance in pituitary extract. Due to its ability to stimulate fibroblast proliferation, this new substance is called fibroblast growth factor (FGF). Subsequent studies have shown that FGF can also stimulate the growth of cells derived from the mesoderm and neuroectoderm, such as corneal endothelial cells, vascular endothelial cells, epithelial cells, etc., thus promoting angiogenesis, limb development, and wound healing. Recently, it has been discovered that FGF plays an important regulatory role in the nervous system, metabolic system, skeletal system, etc. It is actually an active peptide that has proliferation and differentiation regulation on various cells. Currently, 23 members with similar structures and functions have been discovered, forming the FGF family.

Discovery of FGF drugs

Since the 1980s, the rapid development of biotechnology, especially genetic engineering technology, has not only brought revolutionary breakthroughs to the biopharmaceutical industry itself, but also provided opportunities for transformation in related or adjacent disciplines and industries. In 1989, Professor Lin Jian from Jinan University returned from studying in the United States and was the first to develop FGF. In 1992, Li Xiaokun joined the research team led by his mentor Professor Lin Jian and quickly became a core member of the project. From the discovery of FGF, it has not been developed into a drug for more than 50 years, mainly due to the complex structure and function of FGF, major technical bottlenecks in drug development, low expression levels, low activity, and poor stability, which are the three major obstacles that FGF drugs need to overcome. Early acquisition of FGF was achieved through animal tissue extraction, which required approximately 10 000 cows to extract 1g. The high cost made it impossible to use it for clinical applications. However, our team's researchers achieved a breakthrough through genetic engineering and molecular modification techniques, using molecular chaperone technology to achieve expression from low activity inclusion bodies to high activity soluble expression. The protein production cycle has been shortened from 14 days to 2 days, resulting in a 6-fold increase in yield. Through the study of FGF structure, it was found that it can specifically bind to long-chain heparin modifications. As a result, a new affinity chromatography system was developed, with protein purity exceeding 99%, fully meeting the needs of industrialization. Based on the distribution characteristics of its hydrophilic and hydrophobic groups, a stable FGF protein system was obtained through high-throughput screening, laying the foundation for the development of various formulations in the future. In January 1996, the team obtained the Class I new drug certificate for recombinant bovine FGF2 issued by the Ministry of Health. This is the world's first FGF new drug to be launched, with main indications for fever and trauma.

Due to the differences in amino acid sequences between bovine FGF2 and human FGF2, our team has further developed a fully humanized FGF2 new drug, which is suitable for various complex wounds. During this period, Professor Fu Xiaobing led the Key Laboratory of Trauma Repair at 304 Hospital of the People's Liberation Army General Hospital as the leading unit to conduct multi center clinical application studies of FGF2 drugs in 34 hospitals. The experimental results have been published in domestic professional journals and *The Lancet*. More than 1000 patients involved in the experiment, including acute wounds with different depths of burns and surgical skin supply areas, were treated with FGF2 [150AU/(cm^2 · d)], and over 800 wounds were used as controls. The results

供皮区的愈合时间同样较安慰剂组为短。病理结果证实，FGF2 促进愈合，一方面是显著增加了肉芽组织中毛细血管数量，另一方面提高了上皮化的表皮细胞的增殖速率。2002 年，重组人碱性成纤维细胞生长因子获得上市批准，成为国际上第一个人源化的 FGF 新药，适应证为各类复杂创面。

临床应用表明，FGF 新药改变了在创伤修复过程中以抗感染为主的传统治疗方式，为创伤修复和组织再生提供了安全有效的主动修复和功能修复新治疗手段。FGF2 药物的临床应用已写入《外科学》等临床医学本科教材，Springer 出版的 *Wound Healing and Ulcers of the Skin Diagnosis and Therapy - The Practical Approach* 和 Wiley 出版的 *The Foot in Diabetes* 将 FGF 列为临床医生指导用药。外用重组人碱性成纤维细胞生长因子被国际创伤愈合学会写入“急性创伤愈合治疗指南”，并列入国防战备用药及国家医保药品目录。

FGF 的基础研究 >>>

随着经济社会的发展，创伤谱也发生了相应的变化，糖尿病发病率越来越高，引起的糖尿病足也越来越多，社会老龄化引起的各类老年创伤如脉管炎等也日益剧增。通过研究发现，FGF 家族的 FGF1 具有一定的抗氧化作用。本团队又开发了 FGF1 国家一类新药，主要适应证为糖尿病足等慢性难愈性溃疡。2006 年的最后一天，“重组人酸性成纤维细胞生长因子”基因工程一类新药获得 SFDA 新药证书，主要用于糖尿病足等慢性溃疡，成为国际上第一个 aFGF 药物。

接下来的几年，FGF 的发展遇到了瓶颈。因为基础研究的落后，FGF 结构和功能机制尚不够清楚。作为促成纤维细胞增殖的生长因子，它在临床应用中潜在的致肿瘤安全风险也受到质疑。几个上市药物的应用推广受到限制，甚至团队内部也有一部分人对 FGF 未来前景充满悲观，有的选择放弃和离开。在这种情况下，本团队决定进一步加强 FGF 基础研究，主要在 FGF 的结构与功能、细胞效应与分子调控机制、临床应用适用证与安全性及相关材料制剂等方面进行深入探索。在国内，本团队在吉林农业大学、吉林大学开展了 FGF 在植物表达系统、动物表达系统等生物反应器蛋白表达，以及 FGF 在病理和生理学机制的研究；国际上，与哈佛大学、纽约大学、得克萨斯农工大学和路易斯维尔大学的 FGF 研究小组合作，共同对 FGF 及其受体（FGFR）的作用方式结构解析、FGF 与糖尿病心肌病损伤修复的作用机制、FGF 与肿瘤、FGF 与代谢和 FGF 与信号传导等研究方向展开了全面深入的探索。经过近十年的不懈努力，FGF 基础研究工作得到夯实，主要功能特征和机制也越来越清晰，进一步促进了 FGF 在创新药物开发和应用方面的长足进展。

本团队研究发现，FGF2 可显著抑制瘢痕形成；可改善局部微环境，促进成纤维细胞的迁移有利于创

showed that FGF2 significantly accelerated the formation of granulation tissue and wound re epithelialization, i.e. recombinant FGF2 accelerated the healing of burn donor skin wounds. Compared with the control group, the healing time of shallow and deep second degree burn wounds was significantly shortened; The healing time of the donor skin area was also shorter than that of the placebo group. Pathological results confirm that FGF2 promotes healing by significantly increasing the number of capillaries in granulation tissue and increasing the proliferation rate of epithelialized epidermal cells. In 2002, recombinant human basic fibroblast growth factor obtained market approval, becoming the first humanized FGF new drug internationally, with indications for various complex wounds.

Clinical applications have shown that FGF new drugs have changed the traditional treatment approach of mainly anti infection during trauma repair, providing a safe and effective new treatment method for active repair and functional repair of trauma and tissue regeneration. The clinical application of FGF2 drugs has been included in clinical undergraduate textbooks such as *"Surgery"*. Springer's *"Wow Healing and Ulcers of the Skin Diagnosis and Therapy - The Practical Approach"* and Wiley's "The Foot in Diabetes" list FGF as a clinical guidance medication. The topical recombinant human basic fibroblast growth factor has been included in the "Guidelines for the Treatment of Acute Trauma Healing" by the International Society for Trauma Healing, and has been listed in the National Defense and Medical Insurance Drug Catalogue.

Basic research on FGF

With the development of economy and society, the trauma spectrum has also undergone corresponding changes. The incidence rate of diabetes is getting higher and higher, resulting in more and more diabetes feet. Various elderly injuries such as vasculitis caused by social aging are also increasing dramatically. Through research, it has been found that FGF1 in the FGF family has certain antioxidant effects. The team has also developed FGF1 national class I new drug, whose main indications are chronic refractory ulcers such as diabetes foot. On the last day of 2006, "recombinant human acidic fibroblast growth factor" genetic engineering class I new drug obtained the SFDA new drug certificate, mainly used for chronic ulcers such as diabetes foot, and became the first aFGF drug in the world.

In the following years, the development of FGF encountered bottlenecks. Due to the backwardness of basic research, the structure and functional mechanism of FGF are not yet clear enough. As a growth factor that promotes fibroblast proliferation, its potential tumorigenic safety risks in clinical applications have also been questioned. The application and promotion of several marketed drugs have been restricted, and even some members of the team are pessimistic about the future prospects of FGF, with some choosing to give up or leave. In this situation, our team has decided to further strengthen basic research on FGF, mainly exploring the structure and function of FGF, cellular effects and molecular regulatory mechanisms, clinical applicability and safety, and related material formulations. In China, our team has conducted research on the expression of FGF in plant expression systems, animal expression systems, and other bioreactor proteins, as well as the pathological and physiological mechanisms of FGF, at Jilin Agricultural University and Jilin University; Internationally, in cooperation with the FGF research group of Harvard University, New York University, Texas A&M University and the University of Louisville, we have carried out a comprehensive and in-depth exploration on the research direction of the structural analysis of the mode of action of FGF and its receptor (FGFR), the mechanism of FGF and the damage repair of diabetes cardiomyopathy, FGF and tumor, FGF and metabolism, FGF and signal transduction. After nearly a decade of unremitting efforts, the basic research work of FGF has been consolidated, and the main functional characteristics and mechanisms have become increasingly clear, further promoting the significant progress of FGF in innovative drug development and application.

Our team's research found that FGF2 can significantly inhibit scar formation; Improving the local microenvironment and promoting the migration of fibroblasts are beneficial for wound closure, while promoting the migration of melanocytes is beneficial for reducing pigment deposition; Multiple FGFs can significantly promote

面闭合，促进黑色素细胞迁移有利于减少色素沉积；多种 FGF 能显著促进毛囊增生，可用于脱发的治疗；证实 FGF2 可促进创面微血管新生，上调内源性 VEGF 表达，促进创面修复。由此，本团队较系统地阐明了生长因子对于创面皮肤的“功能”愈合机制，为 FGF 的进一步临床应用提供了重要的理论指导。

FGF 载体的研发

由于生长因子半衰期较短，如何延长 FGF 的半衰期、保持其活性是重要的科学问题。通过对多种载药材料进行筛选，在国际上首次成功研制适用于如瘘管、褥疮和子宫糜烂等的重组人 FGF2 与胶原复合活性材料，该材料成为我国第一个上市的载药医疗器械。率先建立了该生物材料的生产工艺及活性标准，建立了特殊冻干曲线下的海绵状成型技术。该材料入选商务部对外国际援助目录和全军战储目录，用于国防及军事救急配备品，成为我国具有自主知识产权的重要战略军需产品。

2008 年，本团队立项了拥有自主知识产权的第二代 FGF 新型温敏凝胶剂，用于糖尿病引起的慢性溃疡的治疗；该药获得科技部国家“重大新药创制”立项的支持，并于 2009 年取得国家发明专利证书。本团队开发的 FGF7 冻干粉注射制剂作为治疗肿瘤化疗引起的黏膜溃疡创新药物也已进入Ⅱ期临床试验，Ⅰ期临床试验（四川大学华西医院完成）报告表明，在 40 ~ 60 μg/(kg·d) 的治疗组，其用药 3 天后在促进右侧颊黏膜溃疡修复的效果显著高于安慰剂治疗组，用药 1 周后就能基本修复损伤的黏膜溃疡，而且在该剂量下患者的耐受性好，安全性强；FGF10 冻干粉外用制剂和角膜溃疡修复制剂已分别进入Ⅲ期临床试验或Ⅰ期研究阶段，Ⅱb 期临床试验结果表明 FGF10 促进烧伤创口愈合的有效、安全。随着 FGF 家族系列新理论的揭示和新成员的应用，FGF 药物进入了一个新的黄金发展期。

新型 FGF 药物的研制

在 FGF 研究方向上坚持不懈多年努力，终于取得了突破性进展。在开展 FGF 对糖尿病足等慢性创面的治疗的同时，本团队对该类患者的血样进行了分析研究，发现 FGF 与糖代谢有关，糖尿病患者 FGF21 水平会明显上调。本团队以 2 型糖尿病为模型，研究 FGF21 调控血糖的网络调控机制，结果发现 FGF21 有很好的降糖效果，进一步研究其调控信号机制，阐明了 FGF21 以脂肪组织为靶标，激活 PLCγ-PPARγ 通路，促进脂联素分泌，进而发挥胰岛素增敏作用。其成果发表于 2013 年的 *Cell Metabolism* 杂志。本团队进一步以动脉粥样硬化为模型，率先发现其对脂代谢也有重要调控作用，同时阐明其调控脂代谢的药理机制，研究结果发表在 *Circulation* 杂志。该项研究不仅明确了 FGF21 对糖脂代谢的调控机制，而且对于开发肥胖、糖尿病的药物有重要的意义。FGF21 通过调控脂联素的表达分泌来发挥其降血糖、调节脂质代谢和增加胰岛素敏感性等生物功能的理论，被 *Cell Metabolism* 杂志评选为十年代谢领域十大新

hair follicle proliferation and can be used for the treatment of hair loss; Confirmed that FGF2 can promote wound microvascular regeneration, upregulate endogenous VEGF expression, and promote wound repair. Thus, our team systematically elucidated the "functional" healing mechanism of growth factors on wound skin, providing important theoretical guidance for the further clinical application of FGF.

Research and development of FGF carrier

Due to the short half-life of growth factors, extending the half-life of FGF and maintaining its activity is an important scientific issue. By screening various drug carrying materials, a recombinant human FGF2 and collagen composite active material suitable for conditions such as fistulas, pressure ulcers, and uterine erosion has been successfully developed for the first time internationally. This material has become the first drug carrying medical device to be launched in China. We were the first to establish the production process and activity standards for this biomaterial, and developed sponge like molding technology under a special freeze-drying curve. This material has been included in the Ministry of Commerce's Catalogue of International Aid to Foreign Countries and the Military Reserve Catalogue, and is used for national defense and military emergency equipment, becoming an important strategic military supply product with independent intellectual property rights in China.

In 2008, the team set up a project of the second generation FGF new temperature sensitive gel with independent intellectual property rights for the treatment of chronic ulcers caused by diabetes; The drug received support from the Ministry of Science and Technology's national "Major New Drug Creation" project and obtained a national invention patent certificate in 2009. The FGF7 freeze-dried powder injection formulation developed by our team as an innovative drug for treating mucosal ulcers caused by tumor chemotherapy has also entered phase II clinical trials. The phase I clinical trial (completed by West China Hospital of Sichuan University) report shows that in the treatment group of 40-60 μg/(kg · d), the effect of promoting the repair of right cheek mucosal ulcers after 3 days of medication is significantly higher than that of the placebo treatment group. After 1 week of medication, the damaged mucosal ulcers can be basically repaired, and patients have good tolerance and strong safety at this dose; FGF10 freeze-dried powder topical preparation and corneal ulcer repair preparation have entered phase III clinical trials or phase I research stages respectively. The results of phase IIb clinical trials show that FGF10 is effective and safe in promoting burn wound healing. With the revelation of new theories and the application of new members in the FGF family, FGF drugs have entered a new golden period of development.

Development of new FGF drugs

After years of persistent efforts in the research direction of FGF, breakthrough progress has finally been made. While carrying out FGF treatment for chronic wounds such as diabetes foot, the team analyzed and studied the blood samples of such patients, and found that FGF was related to glucose metabolism, and the level of FGF21 in diabetes patients would be significantly increased. Our team took type 2 diabetes as a model to study the network regulation mechanism of FGF21 regulating blood glucose. The results showed that FGF21 has a good hypoglycemic effect. Further research on its regulatory signal mechanism has clarified that FGF21 targets adipose tissue, activates PLC γ - PPAR γ pathway, promotes adiponectin secretion, and then plays an insulin sensitizing role. Its results were published in the journal *Cell Metabolism* in 2013. The team further took atherosclerosis as a model, and took the lead in discovering that it also has an important role in regulating lipid metabolism, and clarified its pharmacological mechanism in regulating lipid metabolism. The research results were published in the journal *Circulation*. This study not only clarifies the regulation mechanism of FGF21 on glucose and lipid metabolism, but also has important significance for developing drugs for obesity and diabetes. The theory that FGF21 exerts its biological functions such as lowering blood sugar, regulating lipid metabolism, and increasing insulin sensitivity by regulating the expression and secretion of adiponectin has been selected as one of the top ten new discoveries in the field of

发现之一。*Nature Review* 杂志也对此进行了专题评论，认为有关 FGF21 代谢调控网络的阐明为开发新型糖尿病药物提供了重要的理论依据。

以上研究明晰了 FGF 通过胞内 PPAR γ 和脂联素等分子发挥糖脂代谢调控的功能，但 FGF 如何与细胞膜结合起始信号转导、如何启动膜内信号级联过程，仍是 FGF 蛋白质机器网络的重大科学问题。历时 6 年攻关，本团队最终获得了高纯度单体及复合物，成功获得几种目标结晶。经过结构与功能分析，终于解开 FGF 与受体结合的膜外启动机制，即 FGF、受体、肝素与 Klotho 形成四元复合物形式，研究结果发表在 *Nature* 杂志。四元复合物启动后的信号级联过程也是了解药物机制的重要源头，本团队在 *Molecular Cell* 发表文章第一次揭示了 FGF 受体与下游底物磷酸化的模式，发现并确证了 FGF 二步激活的模式，改变了过去学术界一直认为的同步激活模式的观点。

本团队针对创伤修复组织再生进行大量的实验研究，并研制出一批可产业化的技术产品，与解放军总医院付小兵院士团队联合获得国家科学技术进步奖一等奖。该获奖项目是由我国创伤医学领域与药学医疗器械、材料学等多学科交叉的系列成果，体现了我国在创伤修复、慢性病及老年病领域领先国际的救治及研究水平。

已有研究表明，生长因子参与调控创伤修复的全过程，其中 FGF1 和 FGF2 对创伤修复有促进作用已得到充分证实，尽管 FGF2 较 FGF1 有相对更强的促增殖活性，但生物材料结合不同生长因子对创面愈合效果可能不同。本团队的研究发现，利用肝素泊洛沙姆材料 (HP) 结合 FGF1 与 FGF2，均可促进小鼠皮肤全层切除创面模型的组织修复与再生，但是相比于 HP-FGF2，HP-FGF1 具有更加显著的修复效果。这可能与不同生长因子本身带的电荷不同，导致了生长因子与材料结合的程度不同，进而影响了材料对生长因子的释放和促修复效果。进一步研究发现，HP-FGF1 能够更加高效地控制释放生长因子，从而促进细胞增殖、肉芽组织的形成、胶原沉积和再上皮化的发生，并加速血管生成，减少创面愈合时间；而 HP-FGF2 控释差，其创面愈合效果弱于 HP-FGF1。该项研究对于开发结合生长因子的生物材料或医疗器械有较重要的参考价值。

2018 年，本团队开发的治疗类生物制品一类新药“重组人角质细胞生长因子 -2(FGF10) 滴眼液”获得 SFDA 颁发的“药物临床试验批准文件”，该药物用于角膜手术及糖尿病溃疡性角膜损伤治疗。角膜损伤是眼科临床的常见病和多发病，FGF10 加速角膜损伤愈合，抑制角膜新生血管形成、减少角膜损伤修复后的瘢痕，有效提高角膜透明度。本团队 2014 年转让安徽鑫华坤生物工程有限公司的“重组人酸性成纤维细胞生长因子凝胶”新药，也于 2018 年 6 月获得 SFDA 核发的“药物临床试验批件”。

FGF1 蛋白在凝胶等高水分状态下容易聚集失活，限制了 FGF1 蛋白在临床上的应用。本团队经过大量试验，成功制备出以高分子材料卡波姆 940 和人血清白蛋白等保护剂组成的高稳定性 FGF1 水凝胶，

metabolism in the decade by the journal *Cell Metabolism*. The journal *Nature Review* also made a special comment on this, believing that the clarification of FGF21 metabolic regulation network provides an important theoretical basis for the development of new diabetes drugs.

The above research has clarified the function of FGF in regulating glucose and lipid metabolism through intracellular molecules such as PPAR γ and adiponectin. However, how FGF binds to the cell membrane to initiate signal transduction and how to initiate the membrane signal cascade process remain major scientific issues in the FGF protein machine network. After 6 years of research and development, our team finally obtained high-purity monomers and complexes, and successfully obtained several target crystals. After structural and functional analysis, the extracellular activation mechanism of FGF receptor binding was finally unlocked, namely the formation of a quaternary complex between FGF, receptor, heparin, and Klotho. The research results were published in the journal *Nature*. The signal cascade process after the initiation of quaternary complexes is also an important source for understanding drug mechanisms. Our team published an article in *Molecular Cell*, which for the first time revealed the phosphorylation pattern of FGF receptors and downstream substrates, and discovered and confirmed the two-step activation mode of FGF, changing the previous academic view of synchronous activation mode.

Our team has conducted extensive experimental research on wound repair tissue regeneration and developed a batch of industrializable technological products. Together with the team of Academician Fu Xiaobing from the General Hospital of the People's Liberation Army, we have won the first prize of the National Science and Technology Progress Award. This award-winning project is a series of interdisciplinary achievements in the fields of trauma medicine, pharmaceutical medical devices, materials science, etc. in China, reflecting the country's leading international level of treatment and research in trauma repair, chronic diseases, and geriatric diseases.

Previous studies have shown that growth factors are involved in regulating the entire process of wound repair, among which FGF1 and FGF2 have been fully confirmed to have a promoting effect on wound repair. Although FGF2 has relatively stronger proliferative activity than FGF1, the effect of biomaterials combined with different growth factors on wound healing may vary. Our team's research found that using heparin poloxamer material (HP) combined with FGF1 and FGF2 can promote tissue repair and regeneration in a mouse skin full-thickness excision wound model. However, compared to HP-FG2, HP-FG1 has a more significant repair effect. This may be due to the different charges carried by different growth factors themselves, resulting in varying degrees of binding between growth factors and materials, which in turn affects the release and repair promoting effect of materials on growth factors. Further research has found that HP-FF1 can more efficiently control the release of growth factors, thereby promoting cell proliferation, granulation tissue formation, collagen deposition, and re epithelialization, as well as accelerating angiogenesis and reducing wound healing time; However, HP-FG2 has poor controlled release and weaker wound healing effect than HP-FG1. This study has significant reference value for the development of biomaterials or medical devices that combine growth factors.

In 2018, the first class new drug "Recombinant human keratinocyte growth factor-2 (FGF10) eye drops" developed by the team for therapeutic biological products obtained the Approval Document of Drug Clinical Trial issued by SFDA, which is used for corneal surgery and the treatment of diabetes ulcerative corneal injury. Corneal injury is a common and frequently occurring disease in ophthalmic clinical practice. FGF10 accelerates corneal injury healing, inhibits corneal neovascularization, reduces scarring after corneal injury repair, and effectively improves corneal transparency. In 2014, the team transferred the new drug of "recombinant human acidic fibroblast growth factor gel" from Anhui Xinhuakun Biological Engineering Co., Ltd., and also obtained the "Drug Clinical Trial Approval" issued by SFDA in June 2018.

FGF1 protein is easy to accumulate and inactivate under high water conditions such as gel, which limits the clinical application of FGF1 protein. After a lot of experiments, our team successfully prepared a highly stable FGF1 hydrogel composed of polymer material Carbomer 940 and human serum albumin and other protective agents,

克服 FGF1 水凝胶的稳定性问题。该水凝胶在 4℃可以稳定保存 24 个月。临床上的应用证实，其可以有效降低糖尿病溃疡患者截肢率 35%，降低患者医疗费用 50%，降低治疗时间达 40%，使临床用药更加方便快捷，从而造福广大糖尿病溃疡患者。

FGF 家族是存在于各种细胞和组织系统的多效性信号分子。除四种 FGF 外，根据其独特的功能和生物学效应可分为有丝分裂型和代谢型。有丝分裂型调节细胞增殖，而代谢型调节能量代谢。这两类 FGF 都通过同一类型的跨膜受体酪氨酸激酶 FGFR1、FGFR2、FGFR3、FGFR4 以及它们的异构体发挥生理学作用。在生理学上，这两类由 FGF 驱动的两种调节活动似乎在空间和时间上是分离的。一方面，促进创面愈合的有丝分裂 FGF 在生理水平上似乎不能向包括代谢组织在内的其他组织移动，以促进细胞代谢，因为分泌后的细胞因子是必须通过与细胞外基质硫酸肝素的亲和介导。另一方面，由于缺乏关键的跨膜辅助共受体，代谢性型 FGF 在非代谢性组织或细胞中循环，对那些经常通过细胞增殖和种群增长的新周期进行积极组织重塑的细胞不起作用。从进化的观点来看，尽管这两类 FGF 基本上平行，并通过不同的细胞内机制驱动差异效应，但正如研究人员总结的那样，它们注定要达到一个共同的目标，即调控每个细胞 / 组织系统和整个有机体的生存和内环境平衡。因此，FGF 促进创面愈合的作用机制必定与促进细胞代谢的作用机制通过某种途径联系在一起，达到统一，这将是未来研究探索的方向之一。

第二节 生长因子调节系统

生物，特别是动物与人体的生长发育、衰老、疾病发生等是受体内不同的调节系统所调节的。传统的调节系统，如神经、内分泌、代谢与免疫调节系统等，是机体生长、发育、代谢所必需的。在正常情况下，这些系统保持平衡，精确调节着生命活动的各个环节。但在异常情况下，这些调节系统本身出现障碍或外源性打击导致调节系统发生障碍，就会导致疾病或损伤的发生。例如，经典的神经内分泌调节系统中，库欣综合征就是由于肾上腺皮质长期分泌过多的糖皮质激素产生的一系列异常临床综合征，如出现满月脸、水牛背，累及血液循环、骨代谢、性腺功能等。又如，严重创伤烧伤导致免疫调节系统失衡，产生过度炎症反应，导致脓毒症发生。这些例子说明机体内多个调节系统之间独立或相互之间精确的调控，对机体稳态维持、健康发育、生长十分重要。

近 20 年来，本团队研究和国际上的相关研究越来越倾向于生物体内存在另一个十分重要而又尚未被人们完全认识与阐明的调节系统，即生长因子调节系统（GFRS）。生长因子是一类可促进细胞增殖与分化、分子结构存在差异的多家族蛋白。生长因子主要通过结合和激活靶细胞中含胞质酪氨酸激酶结构域的跨膜受体，引发一系列的胞内信号级联反应，从而发挥多种生物学活性，包括在发育过程中调节组织形态发

which overcame the stability problem of FGF1 hydrogel. The hydrogel can be stored stably for 24 months at 4 ℃. Its clinical application has proved that it can effectively reduce the amputation rate of diabetes ulcer patients by 35%, reduce the medical expenses of patients by 50%, and reduce the treatment time by 40%, making clinical medication more convenient and quick, thus benefiting the majority of diabetes ulcer patients.

The FGF family is a multifunctional signaling molecule that exists in various cellular and tissue systems. Besides the four types of FGFs, they can be classified into mitotic and metabolic types based on their unique functions and biological effects. Mitotic type regulates cell proliferation, while metabolic type regulates energy metabolism. These two types of FGFs exert physiological effects through the same type of transmembrane receptor tyrosine kinases FGFR1, FGFR2, FGFR3, FGFR4, and their isomers. Physiologically, these two types of regulatory activities driven by FGF seem to be separated in space and time. On the one hand, the mitotic FGF that promotes wound healing does not seem to be able to move to other tissues, including metabolic tissues, at the physiological level to promote cellular metabolism, as secreted cytokines must be mediated through affinity with the extracellular matrix heparin sulfate. On the other hand, due to the lack of key transmembrane co receptors, metabolic FGFs circulate in non metabolic tissues or cells and do not work on cells that undergo active tissue remodeling through new cycles of cell proliferation and population growth. From an evolutionary perspective, although these two types of FGFs are essentially parallel and drive differential effects through different intracellular mechanisms, as summarized by researchers, they are destined to achieve a common goal of regulating the survival and internal environment balance of each cell/tissue system and the entire organism. Therefore, the mechanism by which FGF promotes wound healing must be linked to the mechanism by which it promotes cellular metabolism through some pathway, achieving unity. This will be one of the directions for future research exploration.

Section 2 Growth factor regulation system

The growth, development, aging, and disease occurrence of organisms, especially animals and humans, are regulated by different regulatory systems in the body. The traditional regulatory systems, such as the nervous, endocrine, metabolic, and immune regulatory systems, are essential for the growth, development, and metabolism of the body. Under normal circumstances, these systems maintain balance and precisely regulate various aspects of life activities. However, in abnormal situations, if these regulatory systems themselves experience obstacles or external shocks that cause obstacles in the regulatory system, it can lead to the occurrence of diseases or injuries. For example, in the classic neuroendocrine regulation system, Cushing's syndrome is a series of abnormal clinical syndromes caused by long-term excessive secretion of glucocorticoids from the adrenal cortex, such as the appearance of a full moon face, buffalo back, involving blood circulation, bone metabolism, gonadal function, etc. For example, severe traumatic burns can cause an imbalance in the immune regulatory system, leading to excessive inflammatory reactions and the occurrence of sepsis. These examples illustrate the importance of independent or precise regulation among multiple regulatory systems within the body, which is crucial for maintaining homeostasis, healthy development, and growth.

In the past 20 years, our team's research and international studies have increasingly focused on the existence of another important and yet to be fully understood and elucidated regulatory system in organisms, namely the Growth Factor Regulatory System (GFRS). Growth factors are a class of multi family proteins that can promote cell proliferation and differentiation, and have different molecular structures. Growth factors initiate a series of intracellular signal cascades by binding and activating transmembrane receptors containing cytoplasmic tyrosine

生、细胞增殖、细胞分化、血管生成和神经轴突生长；在成人器官中维持组织稳态，参与组织创伤修复和代谢调控等。生长因子信号的持续激活与细胞转化和肿瘤形成密切相关。常见的生长因子包括 FGF 家族、TGF-β 超家族、IGF 家族、EGF 家族和 PDGF 家族等。

生长因子调节系统主要由生长因子、生长因子受体及下游信号传递通路、靶器官或靶细胞组成，分为促分裂生长因子调节系统、类激素类生长因子调节系统和非促分裂生长因子调节系统三大功能部分。不同于有相对独立的实质性器官的机体调控系统，生长因子调节系统没有独立的器官组成，但又几乎调控了机体所有器官的发育及相关生理功能、病理变化，如血压、血糖和血脂等，可以理解为不同于传统神经系统、内分泌系统等的另一纬度的重要机体调节组成部分。

我们之所以把生长因子作为生物体内一个尚未被真正认识的新的调节系统，主要是基于以下的证据与认识。

生长因子调节系统具备经典调节系统的基本要素

基本要素即效应物质，效应物质作用的靶器官、细胞上的受体、信号通路、网络调节以及有序调节等，同时具备全身与局部效应的调节机制。已有的研究表明，生长因子在体内有几十种，如人们熟知的 FGF 系统、EGF 系统、肿瘤坏死因子 (TNF) 系统等，这几十种生长因子有自己独立或相对独立的分泌源，有作用的靶器官及相应受体，有共同或独特的信号调节系统，如 ERK、MAPK 等。因此，生长因子作为新的调节系统的组织学要素已完全具备。

例如，TGF 包括两个成员：TGF-α 和 TGF-β。TGF-α 是由 50 个氨基酸组成的单链多肽，属表皮生长因子相关蛋白家族成员，亦称为类表皮生长因子，其一级序列和三维构象与 EGF 相似，两者的氨基酸序列具有 30% ~ 40% 的同源性。TGF-α 和 EGF 的受体相同，两者具有相似的生物学活性。TGF-α 在诱导上皮发育、肺纤维化发生发展中具有重要作用。

TGF-β 属 TGF-β 超家族成员，通过结合并激活细胞表面的丝氨酸 / 苏氨酸激酶受体，参与多种细胞的增殖、分化、凋亡及免疫调节等。TGF-β 具有相对独立的信号调节系统，该信号调节系统是由其信号转导通路中大量的下游效应因子决定的。目前已发现的下游效应因子主要有四大类（表 2.2.1）。第一类效应因子是细胞增殖周期相关因子，包括细胞周期蛋白、周期蛋白依赖性激酶 (CDK)、CDK 抑制因子（CDI），TGF-β 通过影响上述因子的表达水平高低或活化程度，抑制或促进细胞增殖。第二类是转录因子，如 c-myc、c-fos、E2F 等。第三类效应因子是凋亡相关因子，如 TGF-β 可下调 Bcl-2 的表达。第四类效应因子是包括层粘连蛋白、纤维连接蛋白在内的细胞间质组分及其他因子，TGF-β 诱导间质组分改变可直接影响邻近细胞的生物学行为。由于这些下游效应因子的存在，使 TGF-β 在机体的胚胎发育、炎症修复、骨骼生长、肿瘤发生、表皮生长、神经保护、器官纤维化等过程中起重要调控作用。

kinase domain in target cells, thus exerting various biological activities, including regulating histomorphogenesis, cell proliferation, cell differentiation, angiogenesis and neurite growth during development; Maintaining tissue homeostasis in adult organs, participating in tissue wound repair and metabolic regulation. The sustained activation of growth factor signals is closely related to cell transformation and tumor formation. Common growth factors include FGF family, TGF-β superfamily, IGF family, EGF family, and PDGF family.

The growth factor regulatory system is mainly composed of growth factors, growth factor receptors, downstream signaling pathways, and target organs or cells. It is divided into three functional parts: the mitotic growth factor regulatory system, the hormone like growth factor regulatory system, and the non mitotic growth factor regulatory system. Unlike the body regulatory system with relatively independent substantive organs, the growth factor regulatory system does not have independent organ components, but almost regulates the development and related physiological functions, pathological changes of all organs in the body, such as blood pressure, blood glucose, and blood lipids. It can be understood as an important regulatory component of the body in another dimension different from the traditional nervous system, endocrine system, etc.

The reason why we consider growth factors as a new regulatory system in organisms that has not yet been truly understood is mainly based on the following evidence and understanding.

The growth factor regulatory system has the basic elements of classical regulatory systems

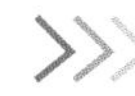

The basic elements are the effector substances, which act on target organs, receptors on cells, signaling pathways, network regulation, and orderly regulation, while possessing regulatory mechanisms for both systemic and local effects. Previous studies have shown that there are dozens of growth factors in the body, such as the well-known FGF system, EGF system, tumor necrosis factor (TNF) system, etc. These dozens of growth factors have their own independent or relatively independent secretion sources, target organs and corresponding receptors, and common or unique signaling regulatory systems, such as ERK, MAPK, etc. Therefore, growth factors as histological elements of a new regulatory system are fully available.

For example, TGF consists of two members: TGF-α and TGF-β. TGF-α is a single chain polypeptide composed of 50 amino acids, belonging to the epidermal growth factor related protein family, also known as epidermal growth factor like. Its primary sequence and three-dimensional conformation are similar to EGF, and their amino acid sequences have 30% to 40% homology. TGF-α and EGF have the same receptors and similar biological activities. TGF-α plays an important role in inducing epithelial development and the occurrence and development of pulmonary fibrosis.

TGF-β belongs to the TGF-β superfamily and participates in various cell proliferation, differentiation, apoptosis, and immune regulation by binding to and activating serine/threonine kinase receptors on the cell surface. TGF-β has a relatively independent signaling regulatory system, which is determined by a large number of downstream effector factors in its signaling pathway. There are four main categories of downstream effect factors that have been identified so far (Table 2.2.1). The first type of effector factor is cell proliferation cycle related factors, including cyclin, cyclin dependent kinase (CDK), CDK inhibitor (CDI). TGF-β inhibits or promotes cell proliferation by affecting the expression level or activation degree of these factors. The second type is transcription factors, such as c-myc, c-fos, E2F, etc. The third type of effector factor is apoptosis related factors, such as TGF-β, which can downregulate the expression of Bcl-2. The fourth type of effector factors includes mesenchymal components such as laminin and fibronectin, as well as other factors. TGF-β - induced changes in mesenchymal components can directly affect the biological behavior of adjacent cells. Due to the presence of these downstream effector factors, TGF-β plays an important regulatory role in embryonic development, inflammation repair, bone growth, tumorigenesis, epidermal growth, neuroprotection, organ fibrosis, and other processes in the body.

表 2.2.1 TGF-β 下游效应因子

下游效应因子		在 TGF-β 作用下发生的变化
细胞增殖周期相关因子	细胞周期蛋白	Cyclin A 表达下降
		Cyclin D1、2 表达下降或不变
	CDK	CDK2 翻译下降 或 160 位点丝氨酸去磷酸化
		CDK4 表达或翻译下降
		CDK4 表达或翻译下降
		CDK1（CDC25A）表达下降
		CDK1 蛋白磷酸化降低
	CDI	p15INK4B 表达增强
		p21/WAF1/CIP1 蛋白水平升高或活化
		P27KIP1 表达增强
转录因子		c-myc 表达下降
		视网膜母细胞瘤蛋白 (RB 蛋白) 磷酸化水平降低
		c-fos(c-jun) 表达升高
		myb 表达下降
		E2F 表达降低
凋亡相关因子		Bcl-2 表达下降
间质成分及其他		层粘连蛋白、纤维连接蛋白表达增强
		谷胱甘肽 S- 转移酶（GST）表达下降
		纤溶酶原激活物抑制物 1(PAI-1) 表达增强
		精脒合成酶表达降低
		鸟氨酸脱羧酶表达降低
		S- 腺苷蛋氨酸脱羧酶表达降低
		甘油醛 -3- 磷酸脱氢酶表达增强

生长因子调节系统具有独特的、传统调节系统不可替代的生物调节作用 >>>

以 FGF 家族为例，它具有促分裂效应与非促分裂激素样活性两大调节作用。生长因子系统通过其非促分裂功能直接参与机体生命活动的调控过程。研究发现，FGF 的非促分裂活性又可以分为旁分泌型和内分泌型两类。其中 FGF11 亚家族由 FGF11、FGF12、FGF13、FGF14 组成。这些因子是细胞内分泌的，不与 FGFRS 相互作用，其主要作用是调节神经元和其他可兴奋细胞（如心肌细胞）的电兴奋性。

旁分泌型 FGF 由 FGF1 亚家族（FGF1、FGF2）、FGF4 亚家族（FGF4、FGF5、FGF6）、FGF7 亚家族（FGF3、FGF7、FGF10、FGF22）、FGF9 亚家族（FGF9、FGF17、FGF18）和 FGF8 亚家族（FGF8、FGF17、FGF18）组成。这些是结合到 FGFRS 并使用肝素 / 硫酸肝素作为辅助因子的分泌蛋白，FGF1、FGF2、FGF3 可以直接转移到细胞核并作为内蛋白发挥作用，通过调节细胞增殖、分化和存活参与胚胎发生和组织修复。

Table 2.2.1 Downstream effector factors of TGF-β

Downstream effect factors		Changes occurring under the action of TGF-β
Cell proliferation cycle related factors Decreased expression or translation of CDK4	cyclin	Decreased expression of Cyclin A
		Decreased or unchanged expression of Cyclin D1, 2
	CDK Decreased expression or translation of CDK4	CDK2 translation decrease or serine dephosphorylation at position 160
		Decreased expression or translation of CDK4
		Decreased expression or translation of CDK4
		Decreased expression of CDK1（CDC25A）
		Reduced phosphorylation of CDK1 protein
	CDI	Enhanced expression of p15INK4B
		Elevated or activated levels of p21/WAF1/CIP1 protein
		Enhanced expression of P27KIP1
transcription factor		Decreased expression of c-myc
		Reduced phosphorylation level of retinoblastoma protein (RB protein)
		Increased expression of c-fos(c-jun)
		Decreased expression of myb
		Decreased expression of E2F
Apoptosis related factors		Decreased expression of Bcl-2
Interstitial components and others		Enhanced expression of laminin and fibronectin
		Decreased expression of GST
		Enhanced expression of plasminogen activator inhibitor-1 (PAI-1)
		Reduced expression of spermidine synthase
		Reduced expression of ornithine decarboxylase
		Reduced expression of S-adenosylmethionine decarboxylase
		Enhanced expression of glyceraldehyde-3-phosphate dehydrogenase

The growth factor regulatory system has unique and irreplaceable biological regulatory effects that traditional regulatory systems cannot replace

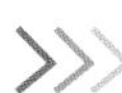

Taking FGF family as an example, it has two major regulatory effects: mitogenic effect and non mitogenic hormone like activity. The growth factor system directly participates in the regulation of biological activities through its non mitotic function. Research has found that the non mitogenic activity of FGF can be divided into two types: paracrine and endocrine. The secreted FGF is composed of the FGF11 subfamily (FGF11, FGF12, FGF13, FGF14). These factors are cellular endocrine and do not interact with FGFRS. Their main function is to regulate the electrical excitability of neurons and other excitable cells, such as cardiomyocytes.

The paracrine FGF is composed of the FGF1 subfamily (FGF1, FGF2), FGF4 subfamily (FGF4, FGF5, FGF6), FGF7 subfamily (FGF3, FGF7, FGF10, FGF22), FGF9 subfamily (FGF9, FGF17, FGF18), and FGF8 subfamily (FGF8, FGF17, FGF18). These are secreted proteins that bind to FGFRS and use heparin/heparin sulfate as cofactors. FGF1, FGF2, and FGF3 can be directly transferred to the nucleus and act as intracellular proteins, participating in embryonic development and tissue repair by regulating cell proliferation, differentiation, and survival.

内分泌型 FGF 由 FGF15/FGF19 亚家族（FGF15/FGF19、FGF21、FGF23）组成。内分泌型 FGF 与肝素 / 硫酸肝素的亲和力较低，并以 Klotho 家族蛋白作为辅因子与 FGFR 结合，调节胆汁酸、脂质和碳水化合物稳态。其信号需要由 FGFR 及其共同受体 Klotho/β-Klotho 形成的复合物共同介导，组成 FGF-FGFR-KL/KLB 信号复合物。该信号复合物的功能获得和功能缺失改变与人体多种代谢性疾病，包括但不限于肥胖、糖尿病、脂肪肝疾病、血脂异常、组织特异性共病，以及与胆汁酸和矿物质代谢紊乱有重要的关系。以 FGF21 为例，FGF21 的信号 FGFR/β-Klotho 介导，并通过脂联素 / 血管紧张素转换酶Ⅱ (ACE2) 等信号因子的介导其下游效应。FGF21- 脂联素信号轴在维持机体代谢健康状态中的作用受到越来越多的认可，在维持糖稳态、脂代谢平衡、心血管健康和能量代偿中发挥着重要的作用。

本团队的研究发现，FGF21 具有降低机体血糖血脂、改善胰岛素抵抗、保护胰岛 β 细胞等多种糖脂代谢调控的功能，在 2 型糖尿病、动脉粥样硬化等多种代谢综合征的临床应用方面极具潜力。FGF21 能够对机体胰岛素产生增敏效应主要是通过胰岛素增敏因子 - 脂联素来发挥作用 (*Cell Metab*, 2013)。FGF21 还可通过调节机体胆固醇代谢和脂联素的表达与分泌直接发挥其抗动脉粥样硬化效应 (Circulation, 2015)。FGF21 缺失（FGF21-KO）引起糖尿病心肌组织的脂肪酸蓄积和糖脂代谢紊乱、加快糖尿病心肌病的发生和发展，给予外源重组 FGF21 能通过激活 MAPK-AMPK 通路预防脂毒性诱导的心肌细胞凋亡和糖尿病心肌病的发生和发展，表明 FGF21 也是治疗糖尿病心肌损伤潜在手段（*Diabetologia*, 2015）。此外，FGF21 通过激活脂肪和肾脏组织细胞中 ACE2/Angiotensin-（1-7）/Mas 信号轴，调节机体血压平稳，发挥其血管、心脏、肾脏等多器官保护效应（*Cell Metabolism*, 2018）。这些结果说明，内分泌型 FGF 成员的非促分裂效应与机体生命活动、疾病病理病变过程存在密切的关系。

相关研究表明，当 FGF 分泌或与受体结合障碍时，机体发育受损，产生骨发育异常，形成疾病。以 FGF23 为例，Klotho 和 FGFR4 是 FGF23 的下游信号。Klotho 缺乏是一个导致慢性肾病和心血管疾病发生发展的致病因素。轻度慢性肾脏病（CKD）患者血清 Klotho 水平下降先于血清 FGF23、甲状旁腺激素和磷的升高，提示 Klotho 可能是肾功能下降的敏感生物标志物。而预防 Klotho 下降、内源性 Klotho 产生的再活化或补充外源性 Klotho，均可减轻肾纤维化、延缓 CKD 进展、改善矿物质代谢、改善心肌病和减轻 CKD 中的血管钙化。FGFR3 的突变可以导致侏儒症和软骨发育不全。*FGFR4* 基因敲除可导致肾钙质沉着症、婴儿高钙血症。而当 FGF 非促分裂激素样活性异常时，机体亦会发生代谢和心血管系统方面的疾病，如 FGF23 的过度表达与心血管疾病和慢性肾病相关。

此外，本团队前期的研究也表明，FGF21 的缺失会加速动脉粥样病变和加重血管紧张素Ⅱ高血压病变。胰腺 FGF21 表达的下降，是肥胖症小鼠胰腺结构和功能损伤的重要原因。

Endocrine FGF is composed of the FGF15/FGF19 subfamily (FGF15/FGF19, FGF21, FGF23). Endocrine FGF has a low affinity for heparin/heparin sulfate and binds to FGFR using Klotho family proteins as co factors to regulate bile acid, lipid, and carbohydrate homeostasis. The signal needs to be mediated by a complex formed by FGFR and its common receptor Klotho/ β -Klotho, forming the FGF-FGFR-KL/KLB signaling complex. The functional acquisition and loss changes of this signal complex have an important relationship with a variety of metabolic diseases in the human body, including but not limited to obesity, diabetes, fatty liver disease, dyslipidemia, tissue-specific comorbidity, and metabolic disorders of bile acids and minerals. Taking FGF21 as an example, its signaling is mediated by FGFR/ β -Klotho and its downstream effects are mediated by signaling factors such as adiponectin/angiotensin-converting enzyme II (ACE2). The role of FGF21 adiponectin signaling axis in maintaining metabolic health in the body is increasingly recognized, playing an important role in maintaining glucose homeostasis, lipid metabolism balance, cardiovascular health, and energy compensation.

The research of our team found that FGF21 has the functions of reducing blood glucose and lipids, improving insulin resistance, protecting islet β cells and other glucose and lipid metabolism regulation, and has great potential in clinical application of type 2 diabetes, atherosclerosis and other metabolic syndromes. FGF21 can enhance insulin sensitivity in the body mainly through the action of insulin sensitizing factor adiponectin (*Cell Metab*, 2013). FGF21 can also exert its anti atherosclerosis effect directly by regulating cholesterol metabolism and adiponectin expression and secretion (*Circulation*, 2015). FGF21 deletion (FGF21-KO) causes fatty acid accumulation and glycolipid metabolism disorder in diabetes myocardium, accelerates the occurrence and development of diabetes cardiomyopathy, and exogenous recombinant FGF21 can prevent lipotoxic induced cardiomyocyte apoptosis and the occurrence and development of diabetes cardiomyopathy by activating MAPK-AMPK pathway, indicating that FGF21 is also a potential means of treating diabetes myocardial injury (*Diabetology*, 2015). In addition, FGF21 activates the ACE2/Angiotensin - (1-7)/Ma signaling axis in adipose and renal tissue cells, regulating blood pressure stability and exerting its protective effects on multiple organs such as blood vessels, heart, and kidneys (*Cell Metabolism*, 2018). These results indicate that the non mitogenic effects of endocrine type FGF members are closely related to biological activities and pathological processes of diseases.

Related studies have shown that when FGF secretion or receptor binding is impaired, the body's development is impaired, leading to abnormal bone development and the formation of diseases. Taking FGF23 as an example, Klotho and FGFR4 are downstream signals of FGF23. Klotho deficiency is a pathogenic factor that leads to the occurrence and development of chronic kidney disease and cardiovascular disease. The decrease in serum Klotho levels in patients with mild chronic kidney disease (CKD) precedes the increase in serum FGF23, parathyroid hormone, and phosphorus, suggesting that Klotho may be a sensitive biomarker for renal dysfunction. Preventing the decline of Klotho, reactivation of endogenous Klotho production, or supplementing exogenous Klotho can all alleviate renal fibrosis, delay CKD progression, improve mineral metabolism, alleviate cardiomyopathy, and reduce vascular calcification in CKD. Mutations in FGFR3 can lead to dwarfism and chondrodysplasia. Knockout of *FGFR4* gene can lead to renal calcium deposition and infantile hypercalcemia. When FGF non mitogenic hormone like activity is abnormal, metabolic and cardiovascular diseases can also occur in the body, such as overexpression of FGF23 being associated with cardiovascular disease and chronic kidney disease.

In addition, the previous research of our team also showed that the absence of FGF21 would accelerate arterial atherosclerosis and aggravate angiotensin II hypertension. The decrease in pancreatic FGF21 expression is an important cause of pancreatic structural and functional damage in obese mice.

生长因子调节系统在保持其独特调节作用的前提下与传统、经典的调节系统具有交叉、双相的调节作用

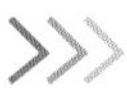

TNF 与 IL、FGF 等既是生长因子调节系统的效应因子，也是免疫、炎症调节系统的效应因子。

以 FGF21 为例，FGF21 可以抑制许多疾病状态下炎症因子的表达，抑制由此引发的单核细胞和巨噬细胞浸润，从而抑制自噬作用这一细胞免疫反应。在血管紧张素Ⅱ诱导的高血压病变过程中，FGF21 除了激活 ACE2/Angiotensin-（1-7）/Mas 信号轴，调节血压平稳之外，对血管紧张素Ⅱ引发的血管炎症因子 (IL-1b、IL-6、TNF-α、MCP-1 和 VCAM-1) 具有显著的抑制效应。相似地，对乙酰氨基酚诱导的急性肝功能衰竭中，FGF21 亦能抑制炎症因子 IL-6 和 TNF-α 的表达。此外，体外成骨样细胞培养的结果也表明，bFGF 可以调节 IL-4、IL-12、IL-15、IL-18 和 IFN-γ 等苗裔调节系统效应因子的表达。相反地，炎症因子亦能刺激生长因子的表达分泌。在分化的成骨细胞 IDG-SW3 培养中，FGF23 的 mRNA 表达水平受 TNF、IL-1β 剂量依赖的上调，并且这种上调作用是核因子 κB 通路依赖的。在 UMR106 成骨细胞样细胞，TGF-β2 亦能刺激 FGF23 通路的表达。

此外，越来越多的证据表明，生长因子的调节系统与经典的信号通路有互作，并组成一个复杂的调控网络，维持着机体的发育、代谢稳态，影响疾病的发生发展。以 FGF21 为例，FGF21 与 PI3K/Akt 信号通路的互作。在离体心肌细胞中治疗外源性 FGF21，直接与 FGFR1 和 β-Klotho 相互作用，进而激活 PI3K/Akt 信号级联和上调抗氧化基因，从而防止细胞死亡和减少活性氧化物质的产生。体外朗根多夫系统也强调了 FGF21 的自分泌作用，在该系统中，FGF21 给药可诱导显著的心肌缺血保护，而其作用在抑制 PI3K/Akt、AMPK、ERK1/2 或视黄酸受体 A 途径上显著减弱。FGF21 通过激活 PI3K/Akt 等经典的信号通路保护小鼠肝脏抵抗果糖引起的氧化应激和细胞凋亡。这些证据提示，生长因子调节系统与机体内的经典信号通路存在密切的关系，并形成负责的调控网络系统，参与机体的生命活动过程。

例如，FGF21 信号与 mTORC 信号通路的交叉调控。FGF21 通过对脂肪细胞的作用改善肥胖动物的代谢状况。FGF21 调控 542 个蛋白质上 821 个磷酸位点的网络。一个主要的 FGF21 调节信号节点就是 mTORC1/S6K，与胰岛素不同，FGF21 通过 MAPK 激活 mTORC1，而不是通过典型的 PI3K/Akt 途径。通过 FGF21 激活 mTORC1/S6K 被认为有助于有害的代谢效应，如肥胖和胰岛素抵抗。相反，mTORC1 介导了 FGF21 在体外的许多有益作用，包括 UCP1 和 FGF21 的诱导、脂联素分泌增加和葡萄糖摄取增加，而对胰岛素作用没有任何不良影响。

生长因子调节系统的异常引发重大疾病

生长因子调节系统异常可能造成人体重大疾病发生发展，例如生长因子受体发生异常可能导致全身各脏器发生功能缺失或结构异常。例如，IGF-1 受体（IGF-1R）与机体多种组织及胚胎的生长密切相关。在新生小鼠中，*IGF1R* 基因敲除小鼠的体重只有野生型的 45%，并且 *IGF1R* 敲除小鼠会在出生后不久死亡。

The growth factor regulatory system has a cross-over and biphasic regulatory effect with traditional and classical regulatory systems while maintaining its unique regulatory function 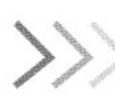

TNF, IL, FGF, and other factors are not only effectors of the growth factor regulatory system, but also effectors of the immune and inflammatory regulatory systems.

Taking FGF21 as an example, FGF21 can inhibit the expression of inflammatory factors in many disease states, suppress the infiltration of monocytes and macrophages caused by it, and thus inhibit autophagy, a cellular immune response. In the process of hypertension induced by angiotensin II, FGF21 not only activates the ACE2/angiotensin -(1-7)/Ma signaling axis and regulates blood pressure stability, but also has a significant inhibitory effect on vascular inflammatory factors (IL-1b, IL-6, TNF - α, MCP-1, and VCAM-1) induced by angiotensin II. Similarly, in acute liver failure induced by acetaminophen, FGF21 can also inhibit the expression of inflammatory factors IL-6 and TNF - α. In addition, the results of in vitro osteogenic cell culture also indicate that bFGF can regulate the expression of effector factors such as IL-4, IL-12, IL-15, IL-18, and IFN-γ in the seedling regulatory system. On the contrary, inflammatory factors can also stimulate the expression and secretion of growth factors. In the culture of differentiated osteoblasts IDG-SW3, the mRNA expression level of FGF23 is upregulated in a dose-dependent manner by TNF and IL-1 β, and this upregulation is dependent on the nuclear factor kappa B pathway. In UMR106 osteoblast like cells, TGF-β2 can also stimulate the expression of the FGF23 pathway.

In addition, increasing evidence suggests that the regulatory system of growth factors interacts with classical signaling pathways and forms a complex regulatory network that maintains the development and metabolic homeostasis of the body, affecting the occurrence and development of diseases. Taking FGF21 as an example, the interaction between FGF21 and the PI3K/Akt signaling pathway. Treating exogenous FGF21 in ex vivo cardiomyocytes directly interacts with FGFR1 and β-Klotho, thereby activating the PI3K/Akt signaling cascade and upregulating antioxidant genes, thereby preventing cell death and reducing the production of reactive oxygen species. The in vitro Langgendorf system also emphasizes the autocrine effect of FGF21. In this system, administration of FGF21 can induce significant myocardial ischemic protection, while its effect is significantly weakened in inhibiting the PI3K/Akt, AMPK, ERK1/2, or retinoic acid receptor A pathways. FGF21 protects mouse liver against fructose induced oxidative stress and cell apoptosis by activating classic signaling pathways such as PI3K/Akt. These pieces of evidence suggest a close relationship between the growth factor regulatory system and classical signaling pathways within the body, forming a responsible regulatory network system that participates in the body's life processes.

For example, the cross regulation of FGF21 signaling and mTORC signaling pathways. FGF21 improves the metabolic status of obese animals by acting on adipocytes. FGF21 regulates a network of 821 phosphate sites on 542 proteins. A major signaling node regulated by FGF21 is mTORC1/S6K. Unlike insulin, FGF21 activates mTORC1 through MAPK instead of the typical PI3K/Akt pathway. Activation of mTORC1/S6K through FGF21 is believed to contribute to harmful metabolic effects such as obesity and insulin resistance. On the contrary, mTORC1 mediates many beneficial effects of FGF21 in vitro, including induction of UCP1 and FGF21, increased adiponectin secretion, and glucose uptake, without any adverse effects on insulin action.

Abnormal growth factor regulatory system triggers major diseases 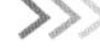

Abnormalities in the growth factor regulatory system may lead to the occurrence and development of major diseases in the human body, such as abnormal growth factor receptors that may cause functional or structural abnormalities in various organs throughout the body. For example, IGF-1 receptor (IGF-1R) is closely related to the growth of various tissues and embryos in the body. In newborn mice, *IGF1R* gene knockout mice weigh only 45%

在肝脏中条件敲除 *IGF1R* 基因会降低肝再生的能力。在小鼠大脑中失活 *IGF1R* 基因使髓鞘再生能力受损。缺失 IGF-1R 的胰脏 B 细胞失去胰岛素分泌能力。脂肪组织中条件失活 *IGF1R* 基因并不影响脂肪的生成，但增加脂肪组织的更替速度。值得注意的是，脂肪组织中 IGF-1R 的缺失会导致循环水平中 IGF-1 浓度的升高，并伴随全身性的机体生长。

疾病如肿瘤往往也会导致生长因子调节系统异常，生长因子调节系统的异常又反馈性地促进肿瘤的发生发展。例如，*FGF2* 与肿瘤关系密切，在神经胶质瘤、黑色素瘤、前列腺瘤、纤维瘤和横纹肌肉瘤等多种肿瘤细胞中存在 *FGF2* 基因的高水平表达，最高可以超出正常值 100 倍以上。FGF2 一方面通过诱导癌基因 *c-Jun*、*c-fos*、*c-Myc*、*c-Myb* 等的表达，促进肿瘤细胞增殖；另一方面通过调控间质胶原酶、纤维蛋白酶原激活物、纤维蛋白酶原受体等分子的表达，促进血管内皮细胞的增殖及迁移，参与血管生成的整个过程，而新生血管不仅为肿瘤细胞提供养分和氧气，促进其生长，还为肿瘤细胞的侵袭、转移和扩散提供了基础。因此，FGF2 被视为肿瘤治疗的靶标之一而备受关注。

事实上，人体的生长因子水平被精确的进行调控，维持相对稳定状态，生长因子调节系统出现异常，导致生长因子组织浓度变化很可能导致严重的功能障碍。例如，*FGF23* 基因主要在骨中表达，并从骨进入血液循环，调节肾脏中维生素 D 和磷酸盐代谢，是体液中维持磷平衡的主要调节蛋白。FGF23 一方面通过降低维生素 D 代谢酶活性；另一方面通过抑制甲状旁腺激素分泌，减少可增强肠道磷酸盐吸收的活化 1,25- 二羟维生素 D 水平，从而降低磷酸盐水平。*FGF23* 基因过表达小鼠，肾脏中磷酸盐重吸收受到抑制。FGF23 敲除小鼠则出现高磷酸盐血症，其 1,25- 二羟维生素 D 水平及血清中甘油三酯水平升高、胸腺萎缩、生殖器官发育不成熟。而 FGF23 枯草杆菌样前蛋白转化酶切割位点突变则使 FGF23 不易被降解，增强 FGF23 的生物学活性，引起低磷酸盐血症佝偻病。编码 M13 家族金属蛋白酶的 *PHEX* 基因的失活突变可增加 FGF23 的水平，引起 X 相关性低磷酸盐血症佝偻病。

综上所述，生长因子系统不仅具有传统的调控系统的功能，同时又具有独特调节特性。虽然不具有相对独立的实质性器官的机体调控系统，但又几乎调控了机体所有器官的发育及相关生理功能、病理变化，如血压、血糖和血脂等，对维护生命健康和生命活动扮演着不可或缺的重要角色，是机体内存在的另外一个新型调控系统。生长因子调节系统作为一类有别于传统器官组织系统的新的调节系统（表 2.2.2），受到体内各因素的精密调节，一旦该调控系统异常，将可能导致严重的病理生理障碍，引发各类疾病。深入研究与阐明机体生长因子调节系统的结构、功能、效应与调节，可能对进一步了解人体生长发育、稳态维持、多种疾病发生、肿瘤预防与治疗以及完美修复与再生具有重要意义。

of wild-type mice, and *IGF1R* knockout mice die shortly after birth. Knocking out the *IGF1R* gene in the liver will reduce the ability of liver regeneration. Inactivation of *IGF1R* gene in mouse brain impairs myelin regeneration ability. Pancreatic B cells lacking IGF-1R lose their insulin secretion ability. Conditional inactivation of IGF1R gene in adipose tissue does not affect fat production, but increases the turnover rate of adipose tissue. It is worth noting that the absence of IGF-1R in adipose tissue leads to an increase in circulating IGF-1 concentration, accompanied by systemic body growth.

Diseases such as tumors often lead to abnormalities in the growth factor regulatory system, which in turn feedback promote the occurrence and development of tumors. For example, FGF2 is closely related to tumors, with high levels of *FGF2* gene expression in various tumor cells such as glioma, melanoma, prostate adenoma, fibroadenoma, and rhabdomyosarcoma, which can exceed normal values by more than 100 times. FGF2 promotes tumor cell proliferation by inducing the expression of oncogenes *c-Jun*, *c-fos*, *c-Myc*, *c-Myb*, etc; On the other hand, by regulating the expression of molecules such as interstitial collagenase, fibrinogen activator, and fibrinogen receptor, it promotes the proliferation and migration of endothelial cells and participates in the entire process of angiogenesis. Neovascularization not only provides nutrients and oxygen for tumor cells, promoting their growth, but also provides a basis for tumor cell invasion, metastasis, and diffusion. Therefore, FGF2 is regarded as one of the targets for tumor therapy and has attracted much attention.

In fact, the levels of growth factors in the human body are precisely regulated to maintain a relatively stable state. Abnormalities in the growth factor regulatory system can lead to changes in tissue concentration of growth factors, which may result in serious functional impairments. For example, the *FGF23* gene is mainly expressed in bones and enters the bloodstream from bones to regulate vitamin D and phosphate metabolism in the kidneys. It is the main regulatory protein that maintains phosphorus balance in body fluids. FGF23 reduces the activity of vitamin D metabolizing enzymes on one hand; On the other hand, by inhibiting parathyroid hormone secretion and reducing activated 1,25-dihydroxyvitamin D levels that can enhance intestinal phosphate absorption, phosphate levels can be lowered. Overexpression of *FGF23* gene in mice results in inhibition of phosphate reabsorption in the kidneys. FGF23 knockout mice exhibit hyperphosphatemia, with elevated levels of 1,25-dihydroxyvitamin D and serum triglycerides, thymic atrophy, and immature reproductive organ development. The mutation of the cleavage site of FGF23 Bacillus subtilis like pre protein convertase makes FGF23 difficult to degrade, enhances its biological activity, and causes hypophosphatemia rickets. The inactivation mutation of *PHEX* gene encoding M13 family metalloproteinases can increase the level of FGF23 and cause X-related hypophosphatemia rickets.

In summary, the growth factor system not only has the functions of traditional regulatory systems, but also has unique regulatory characteristics. Although the body's regulatory system does not have relatively independent substantive organs, it almost regulates the development and related physiological functions, pathological changes of all organs in the body, such as blood pressure, blood glucose, and blood lipids, playing an indispensable and important role in maintaining life, health, and life activities. It is another new type of regulatory system that exists in the body. The growth factor regulatory system, as a new type of regulatory system different from traditional organ and tissue systems (Table 2.2.2), is precisely regulated by various factors in the body. Once the regulatory system is abnormal, it may lead to serious pathological and physiological disorders, causing various diseases. In depth research and elucidation of the structure, function, effects, and regulation of the body's growth factor regulatory system may be of great significance for further understanding human growth and development, homeostasis maintenance, the occurrence of various diseases, tumor prevention and treatment, as well as perfect repair and regeneration.

表 2.2.2　生长因子调节系统与传统调节系统的差异

差异点	生长因子调节系统	传统调节系统	备注
基本类型	促分裂、类激素、非促分裂生长因子调节系统（根据功能分类）	运动、循环、消化、呼吸、泌尿、神经、内分泌、免疫、生殖系统（根据主要器官分类）	主要生长因子包括 FGF、EGF、TGF、IGF、PDGF、NGF、IL、EPO、CSF 等
组成结构	没有独立的器官组成	共同完成某些生理功能的一个或几个器官的组合	GFRS 有独立或相对独立的分泌源，有作用的靶器官及相应受体，有共同或独特的信号调节系统
生理功能	几乎调控机体所有器官的发育及相关生理、病理机能	相对独立，维持正常生理功能	GFRS 从全身各器官组织协调联动维持正常生理功能
病理变化	系统障碍导致复杂疾病，包括遗传性疾病，可影响多器官	系统障碍导致相对独立的疾病，如呼吸系统疾病等	GFRS 从全身影响疾病发生发展
常见症状和体征	系统障碍没有特异的症状和体征，没有明确指标可以检测，但可能影响全身各脏器	系统障碍导致相对特异的症状和体征，有较明确的指标可以检测	GFRS 可能提供研究疾病治疗的新思路

（肖　健）

Table 2.2.2 Differences between growth factor regulation system and traditional regulation system

Difference points	Growth factor regulatory system	Traditional regulation system	Notes
Basic type	Regulation system of mitogenic, steroid like, and non mitogenic growth factors (classified by function)	Exercise, circulation, digestion, respiration, urinary system, nervous system, endocrine system, immune system, reproductive system (classified according to major organs)	The main growth factors include FGF, EGF, TGF, IGF, PDGF, NGF, IL, EPO, CSF, etc
Composition structure	No independent organ composition	A combination of one or several organs that collectively perform certain physiological functions	GFRS has independent or relatively independent secretion sources, effective target organs and corresponding receptors, and a common or unique signaling regulatory system
physiologic function	Almost regulates the development and related physiological and pathological functions of all organs in the body	Relatively independent, maintaining normal physiological functions	GFRS coordinates and links various organs and tissues throughout the body to maintain normal physiological functions
pathological change	Systemic disorders lead to complex diseases, including genetic disorders, which can affect multiple organs	Systemic disorders lead to relatively independent diseases, such as respiratory diseases, etc	GFRS affects the occurrence and development of diseases throughout the body
Common Symptoms and Signs	Systemic disorders have no specific symptoms or signs, and there are no clear indicators to detect, but they may affect various organs throughout the body	Systemic disorders lead to relatively specific symptoms and signs, with clear indicators that can be detected	GFRS may provide new ideas for researching disease treatments

(Xiao Jian)

第二部分
Part 2

典型个案介绍
Introduction to Typical Cases

第 3 章
Chapter 3

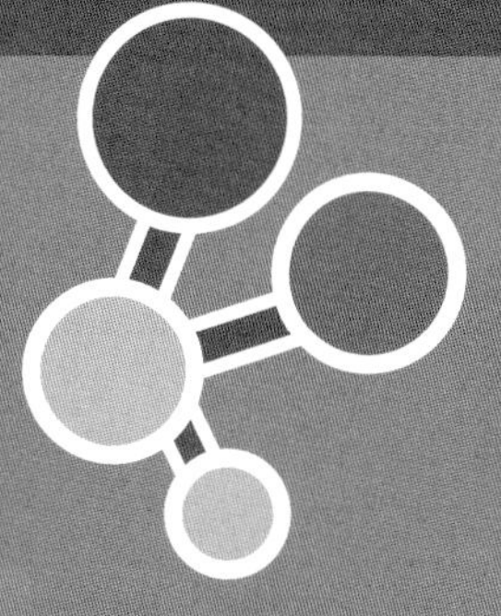

急性创面修复
Acute Wound Repair

案例一　肩部火车压轧性离断

◆ 损伤原因

患者因火车压轧性损伤，致右肩部完全离断。

◆ 症状与体征

剧烈疼痛，表情痛苦，贫血面容，心悸气促，血压下降，肢体完全离断，断面有火车轮压痕，创面出血活跃，血管神经有抽脱，肱骨干部粉碎骨折，远端苍白无血运（图 3.1.1）。

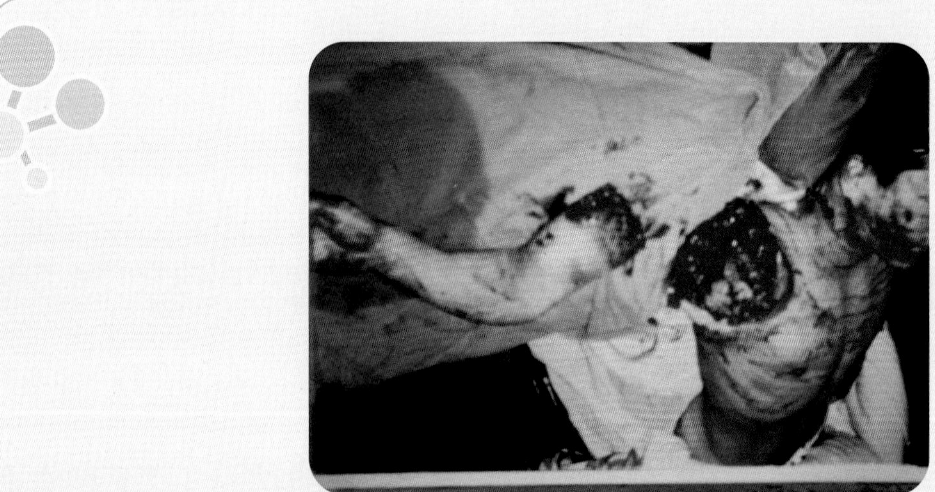

图 3.1.1　手术前，右肩部被火车压断，肢体离体，肩部形成巨大的创面

◆ 治疗方案

1. 立即加压包扎止血，建立静脉通道，输血补液积极抗休克。
2. 纠正休克后，在全麻下进行清创断肢再植术。
3. 生长因子喷洒创面，促进创面愈合，肌肉血管神经再生。
4. 手术后扩容、解痉，继续纠正休克，预防感染。
5. 手术后加强换药，3 天拔出引流条，换药时创口喷洒生长因子。
6. 抬高患肢利于减轻肿胀，保持室温 26℃。
7. 术后断肢再植成活，比健侧短缩 6 cm。术后 1 年随访，可以端水 10 kg（图 3.1.2、图 3.1.3）。

Case 1 Shoulder train crush fracture

◆ Cause of injury

The patient suffered from a rolling injury caused by the train, resulting in complete detachment of the right shoulder.

◆ Signs and symptoms

Severe pain, painful expression, anemic facial features, palpitations and shortness of breath, decreased blood pressure, complete limb separation, train wheel indentation on the cross section, active bleeding on the wound, extraction of blood vessels and nerves, comminuted fracture of the humeral shaft, pale and bloodless distal end (Figure 3.1.1).

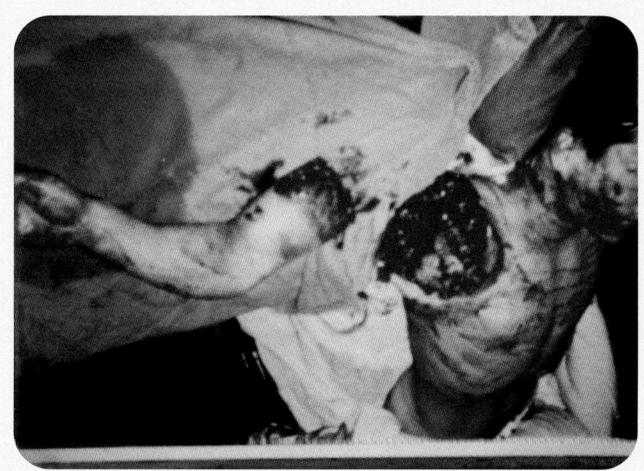

Figure 3.1.1 Before the surgery, the right shoulder was crushed by a train, causing the limb to detach and forming a huge wound on the shoulder

◆ Treatment plan

1. Immediately apply pressure and bandage to stop bleeding, establish a venous channel, and actively administer blood and fluids to combat shock.

2. After correcting shock, perform debridement and limb replantation surgery under general anesthesia.

3. Spraying growth factors on wounds promotes wound healing and muscle vascular and nerve regeneration.

4. Expand and relieve spasms after surgery, continue to correct shock, and prevent infection.

5. Strengthen dressing change after surgery, remove the drainage strip within 3 days, and spray growth factor on the wound during dressing change.

6. Raising the affected limb is beneficial for reducing swelling and maintaining a room temperature of 26 ℃.

7. After the surgery, the severed limb was replanted and survived, shortening by 6 cm compared to the healthy side. One year follow-up after surgery, it is possible to carry 10 kg of water (Figure 3.1.2, Figure 3.1.3).

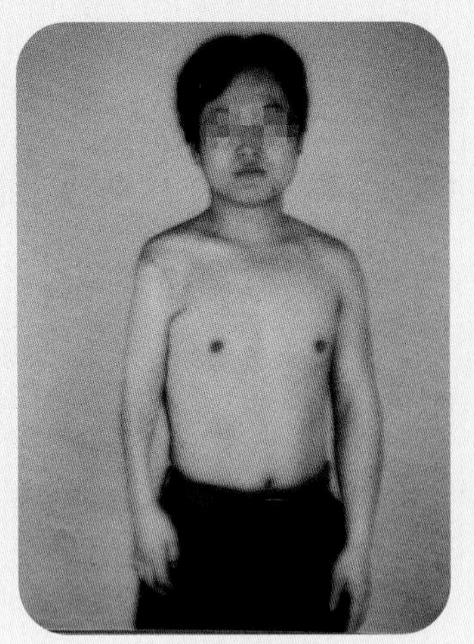

图 3.1.2 术后，断肢再植成活，比健侧短缩 6 cm

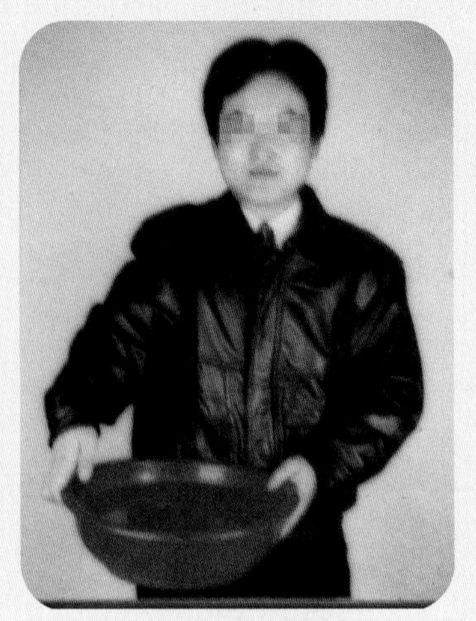

图 3.1.3 术后 1 年随访，可以端水 10 kg

（陈善亮）

案例二 断腕伴组织缺损

◆ 损伤原因

患者因制笔磨具冲压，致左手断腕伴组织缺损。

◆ 症状与体征

急性病容，伤手剧痛，面色苍白，前臂中段有尼龙绳捆扎，出血不多，手掌毁损较重，皮肤有多处压痕，示指在掌指关节处离断，远端缺损，手掌处有 3 cm 横行裂伤，中指、环指、小指指甲脱落，虎口区有 6 cm × 4 cm 皮肤缺损，大鱼际部分缺损，第 2 掌骨中远段缺损；前臂近端纵行劈裂，肌腱血管抽脱伴缺损，离断手背手掌有多处瘀斑（图 3.2.1 ~ 图 3.2.3）。

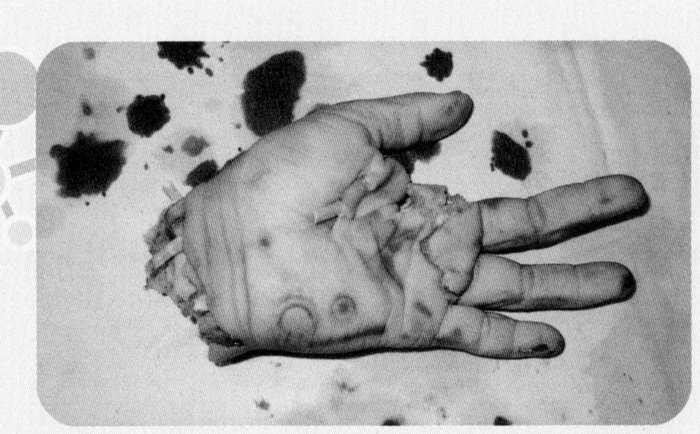

图 3.2.1 手术前，伴有手掌多出裂伤伴压痕，示指缺损

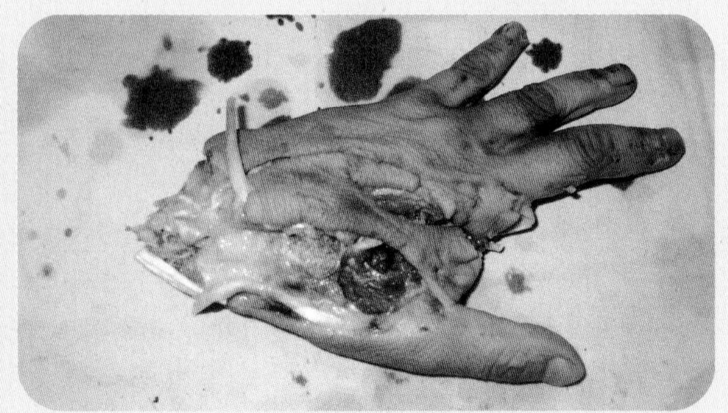

图 3.2.2 手术前，手背瘀斑，指甲缺失，甲床破裂，示指和虎口区有大面积缺损

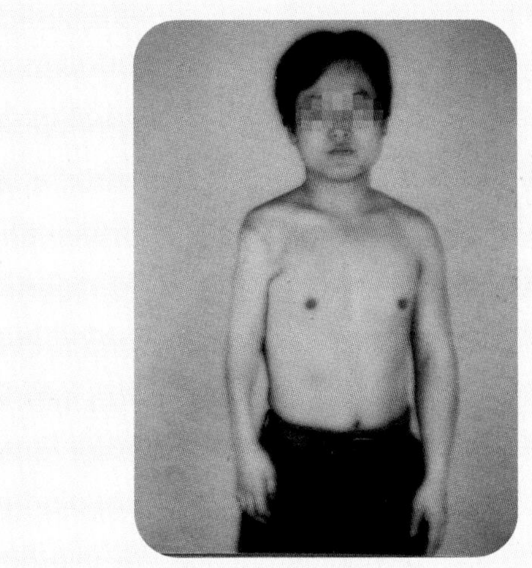
Figure 3.1.2 After surgery, the severed limb was replanted and survived, with a reduction of 6 cm compared to the healthy side

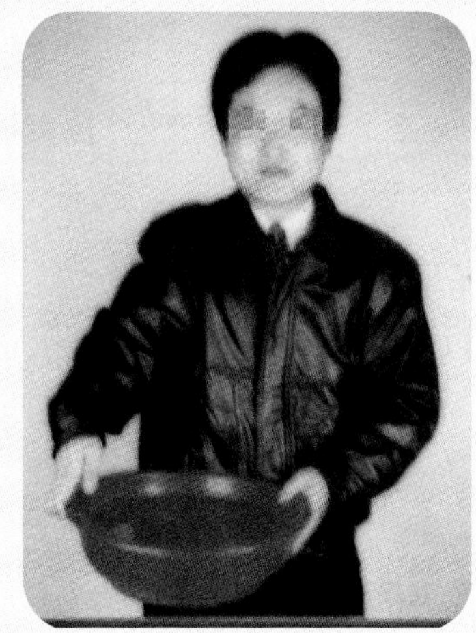
Figure 3.1.3 1-year follow-up after surgery, can carry 10kg of water

(Chen Shanliang)

Case 2 Broken wrist with tissue defect

◆ Cause of injury

The patient suffered a wrist fracture with tissue defects in the left hand due to stamping of the pen and grinding tool.

◆ Signs and symptoms

Acute appearance, severe pain in the injured hand, pale complexion, nylon rope tied in the middle of the forearm, minimal bleeding, severe damage to the palm, multiple pressure marks on the skin, detachment of the index finger at the metacarpophalangeal joint, distal defect, 3 cm transverse laceration on the palm, detachment of nails on the middle finger, ring finger, and little finger, 6 cm × 4 cm skin defect in the tiger's mouth area, defect in the large fish margin, and defect in the middle and distal segments of the second metacarpal bone; The proximal forearm is longitudinally split, with tendon and vascular detachment and defects. There are multiple bruises on the palm of the severed hand (Figure 3.2.1-Figure 3.2.3).

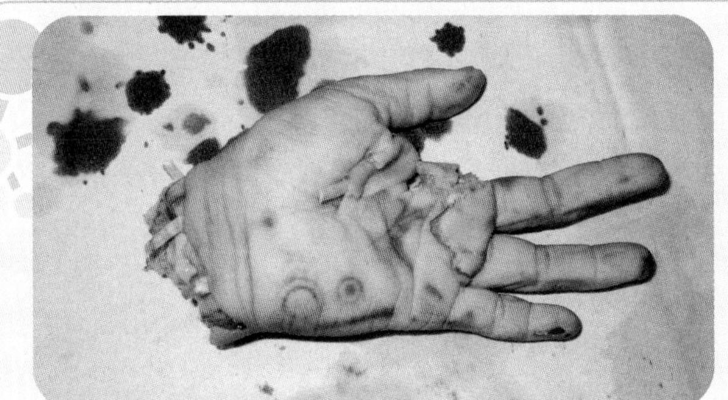
Figure 3.2.1 Prior to surgery, there were multiple lacerations and pressure marks on the palm, as well as a defect in the index finger

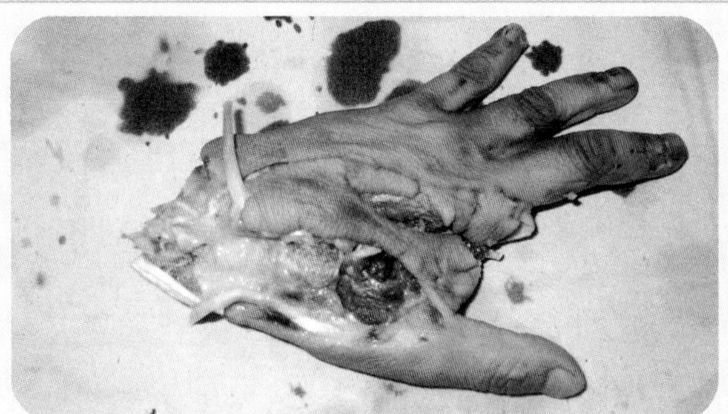
Figure 3.2.2 Before surgery, there were bruises on the back of the hand, missing nails, cracked nail beds, and large areas of defects in the index finger and tiger mouth area

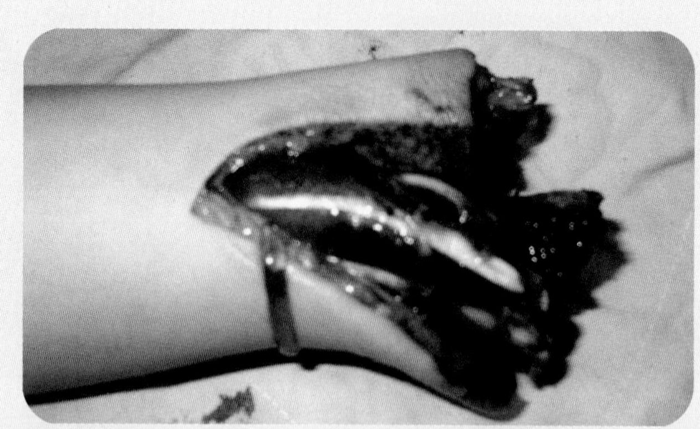

图 3.2.3　手术前，前臂近端纵行裂开，尺桡骨骨折，肌肉肌腱断裂，血管神经抽脱断裂

◆ 治疗方案

此类断腕比较复杂，因为手背有多出皮肤软组织损害，修复起来较为复杂，病程也长。

1. 急诊加压包扎止血，建立静脉通道预防失血性休克。

2. 做好手术前准备，全身检查是否伴有内脏复合伤。

3. 在臂丛麻醉下断肢再植，清创，骨支架建立、肌腱修复，修复尺神经、正中神经及尺神经手背支，吻合桡动脉尺动脉及其伴行静脉，吻合手背静脉。重组人酸性成纤维细胞生长因子喷洒伤口，闭合断腕伤口。

4. 手术后积极解痉预防血管痉挛，预防感染。

5. 由于手部虎口区有大面积皮肤软组织缺损，每天加强局部换药，并喷洒重组人酸性成纤维细胞生长因子，待创面新鲜后，采用腹部带蒂皮瓣移植，3 周后皮瓣断蒂，断腕和皮瓣成活（图 3.2.4、图 3.2.5），并康复出院。

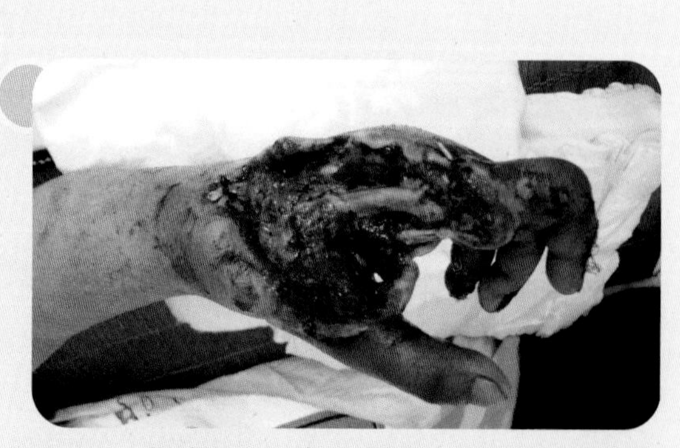

图 3.2.4　断腕再植后虎口区组织坏死伴组织缺损、面积较大，通过清创 + 生长因子喷洒，创面新鲜

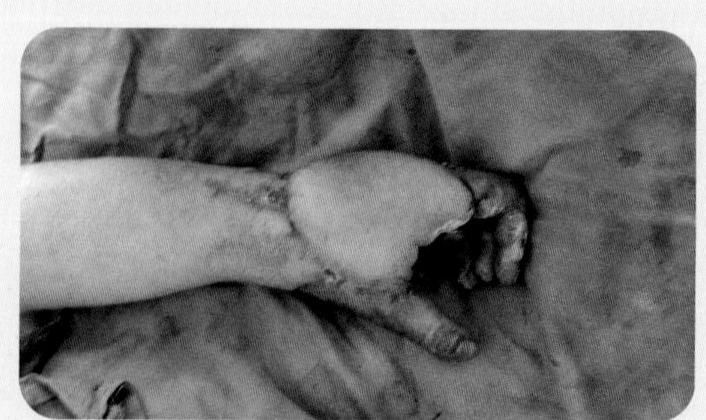

图 3.2.5　手掌背侧创面行腹部皮瓣移植术，皮瓣成活

（陈善亮）

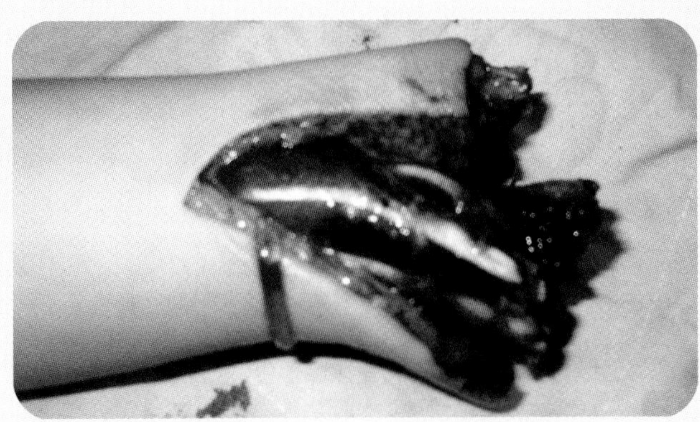

Figure 3.2.3 Prior to surgery, the proximal forearm was longitudinally split, with fractures of the radius and ulna, muscle and tendon ruptures, and vascular and nerve detachment ruptures

◆ Treatment plan

This type of wrist fracture is more complex because there are multiple skin and soft tissue damages on the back of the hand, making repair more complicated and the course of the disease longer.

1. Emergency pressure bandaging to stop bleeding and establish venous access to prevent hemorrhagic shock.

2. Prepare for surgery and conduct a full body examination to check for any accompanying visceral injuries.

3. Limb replantation under brachial plexus anesthesia, debridement, establishment of bone scaffolds, tendon repair, repair of ulnar nerve, median nerve, and dorsal branch of ulnar nerve, anastomosis of radial artery ulnar artery and its accompanying veins, and anastomosis of dorsal vein. Recombinant human acidic fibroblast growth factor was sprayed onto the wound to close the severed wrist wound.

4. Actively relieve spasms after surgery to prevent vascular spasms and infections.

5. Due to the large area of skin and soft tissue defects in the tiger mouth area of the hand, local dressing changes were strengthened daily, and recombinant human acidic fibroblast growth factor was sprayed. After the wound was fresh, abdominal pedicled skin flap transplantation was used. Three weeks later, the flap pedicle was severed, the wrist was severed, and the skin flap survived (Figure 3.2.4, Figure 3.2.5), and the patient recovered and was discharged from the hospital.

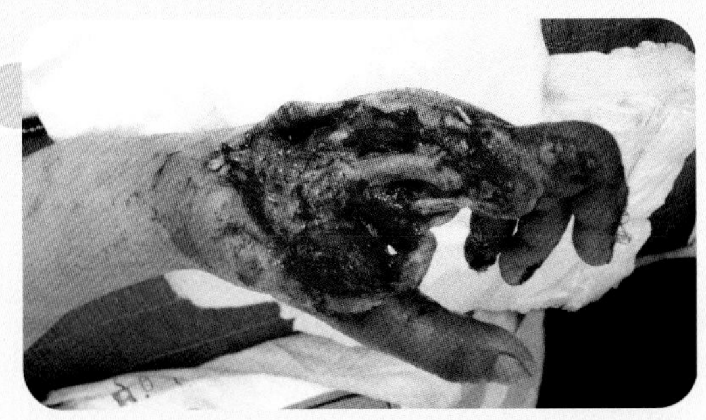

Figure 3.2.4 After wrist replantation, there is tissue necrosis and tissue defect in the tiger's mouth area, with a large area. Through debridement and growth factor spraying, the wound is fresh

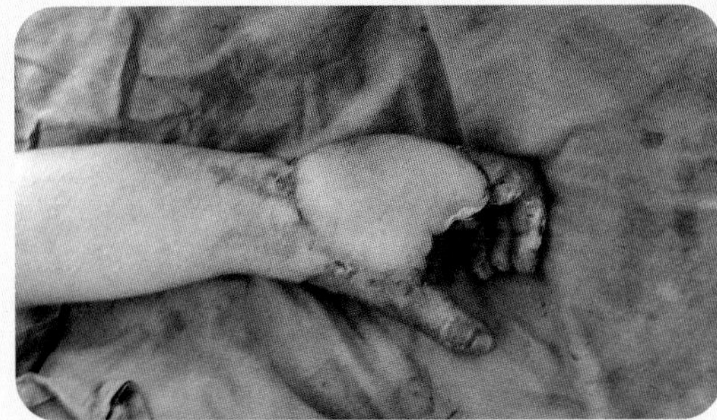

Figure 3.2.5 Abdominal skin flap transplantation surgery performed on the dorsal wound of the palm, and the skin flap survived

(Chen Shanliang)

案例三　腕部抽脱性离断伤

◆ 损伤原因

患者左手因打包机压伤、机器带缠绞手臂，致旋转撕脱离断。

◆ 症状与体征

面色苍白，急性病容，抬入病房，血压 90/50 mmHg，脉搏纤细，心率 110 次 / 分，左手从腕关节处完全离断，伸指、伸腕和屈指、屈腕肌腱从肌腹处抽脱，尺动脉和桡动脉及其伴行静脉长段抽脱断离，尺神经和正中神经游离抽脱 11 cm，手背皮肤撕脱并缺损 4 cm × 3 cm（图 3.3.1、图 3.3.2）。

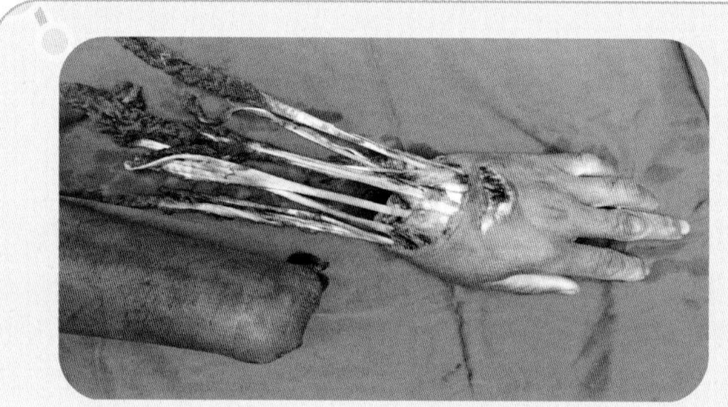

图 3.3.1　手背撕脱情况

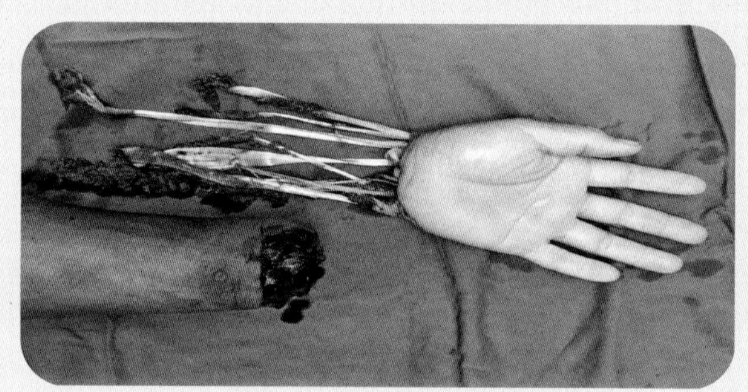

图 3.3.2　手掌面情况

◆ 治疗方案

此类案例手术往往很难一期愈合，都会有不同的创面需要择期修复。因离断伤肌腱系统从肌肉移行处抽脱离断，血管神经抽脱断裂也比较严重，内部潜在损害广泛，修复起来比较复杂，手术容易出现前臂筋膜室综合征，需要提前切开减压。

1. 完善术前准备，首先考虑断肢再植。

2. 断肢再植创面应用重组人酸性成纤维细胞生长因子喷洒创面，促进再植成活。

3. 断腕再植成活，腕部和前臂筋膜室切开减压处有皮肤缺损，每天换药并喷洒重组人酸性成纤维细胞生长因子促进肉芽组织新鲜，为植皮提供前期准备。前臂和腕部创面新鲜后，局部植皮，创面完全愈合（图 3.3.3、图 3.3.4）。

Case 3 Wrist detachment injury

◆ Cause of injury

The patient's left hand was crushed by the packaging machine and the machine belt twisted the arm, causing it to rotate and tear off.

◆ Signs and symptoms

Pale complexion, acute appearance, carried into the ward, blood pressure of 90/50 mmHg, fine pulse, heart rate of 110 beats per minute, left hand completely detached from the wrist joint, finger extension, wrist extension, finger flexion, and wrist flexion tendons extracted from the muscle belly, ulnar artery and radial artery and their accompanying veins long segment extracted and disconnected, ulnar nerve and median nerve free extracted by 11 cm, skin tear and defect of 4 cm × 3 cm on the back of the hand (Figure 3.3.1, Figure 3.3.2).

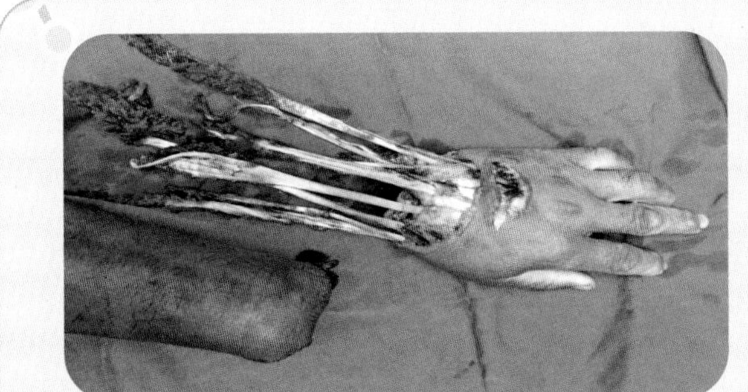

Figure 3.3.1 Tearing off of Hands Back

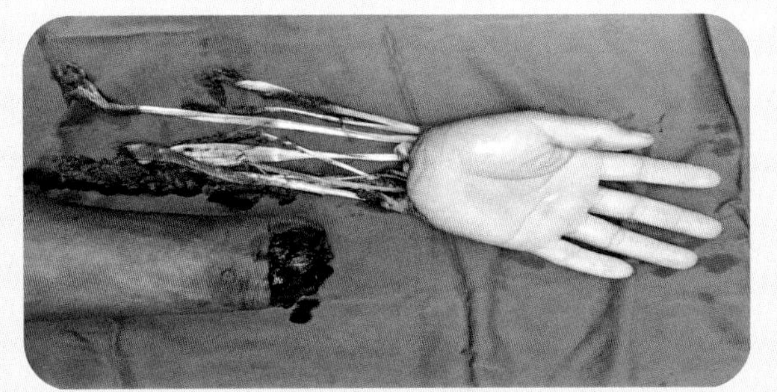

Figure 3.3.2 Palm Surface Condition

◆ Treatment plan

Such cases of surgery are often difficult to heal in one stage, and there will be different wounds that need to be repaired at a later date. Due to the detachment and rupture of the tendon system from the muscle migration site, the vascular and nerve detachment and rupture are also quite severe, with extensive potential internal damage and complex repair. Surgery is prone to the development of forearm compartment syndrome, requiring early incision and decompression.

1. Improve preoperative preparation, first consider limb replantation.

2. Recombinant human acidic fibroblast growth factor should be sprayed onto the wound surface for limb replantation to promote the survival of the replantation.

3. The severed wrist was successfully replanted, but there were skin defects at the decompression site of the wrist and forearm fascial compartments. Daily dressing changes and spraying of recombinant human acidic fibroblast growth factor were performed to promote fresh granulation tissue and provide preliminary preparation for skin grafting. After the forearm and wrist wounds were fresh, local skin grafting was performed, and the wounds fully healed (Figure 3.3.3, Figure 3.3.4).

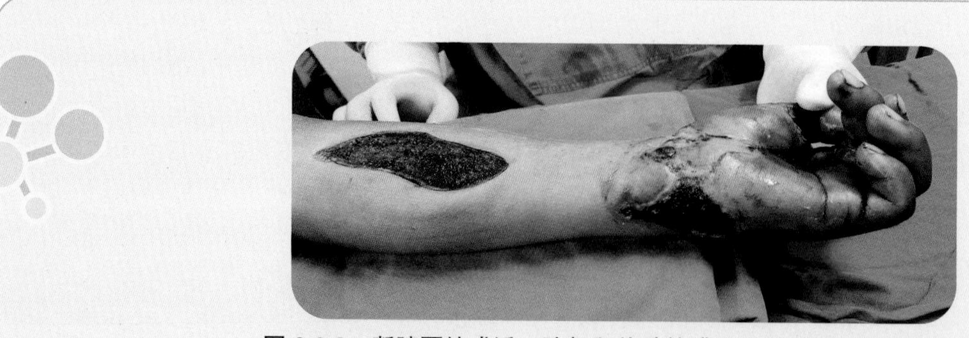

图 3.3.3　断腕再植成活，腕部和前臂筋膜室切开减压处有皮肤缺损

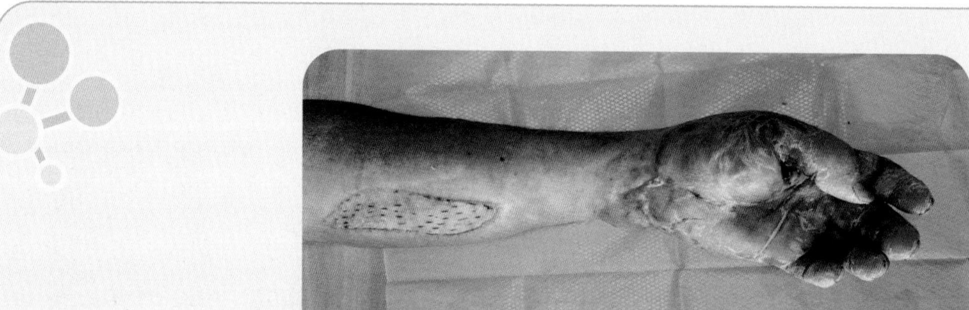

图 3.3.4　前臂和腕部创面新鲜后，局部植皮，创面完全愈合

（陈善亮　杨艳行）

案例四　小腿绞勒性离断

◆ 损伤原因

患者砍柴放木排时，右小腿被绳索勒断。

◆ 症状与体征

肢体离断 4 小时，入院时面色苍白，全身湿冷，表情淡漠，脉搏纤细，血压 70/40 mmHg，伴有失血性休克，右小腿从膝关节下 8 cm 处离断，断面整齐远端完整（图 3.4.1），腹部膨隆，移动性浊音，B 超显示脾大，既往有肝硬化腹水，白蛋白 21 g。

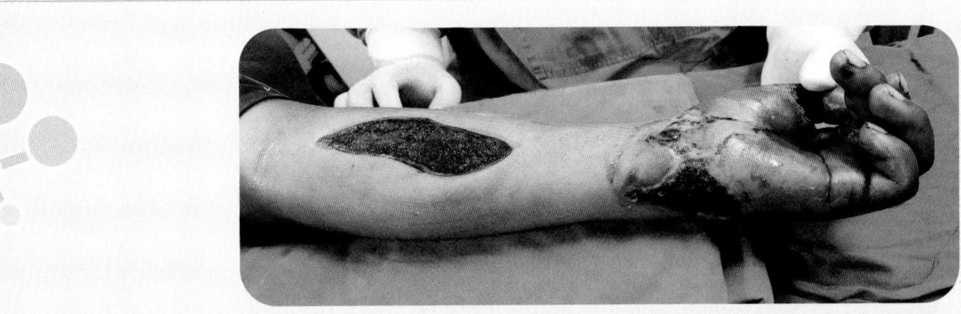

Figure 3.3.3 Successful replantation of severed wrist, with skin defects at the site of fascial compartment incision and decompression in the wrist and forearm

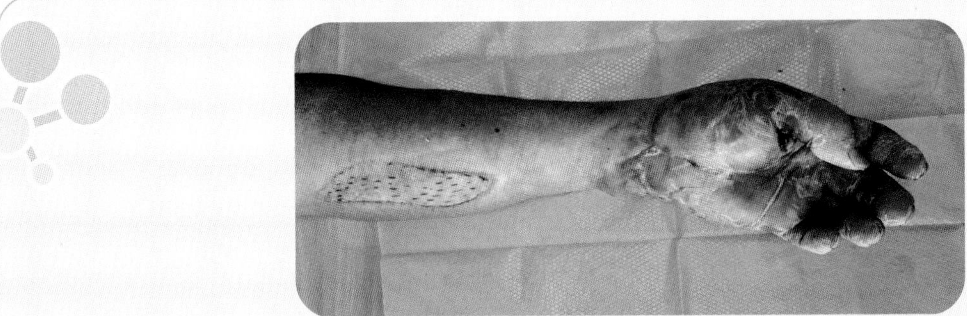

Figure 3.3.4 After fresh wounds on the forearm and wrist, local skin grafting was performed and the wounds fully healed

(Chen Shanliang, Yang Yanxing)

Case 4 Stranded separation of the lower leg

◆ Cause of injury

The patient's right calf was strangled by a rope while chopping wood and placing wooden planks.

◆ Signs and symptoms

Limb amputation occurred 4 hours ago. Upon admission, the patient had a pale complexion, a damp and cold body, a indifferent expression, a fine pulse, a blood pressure of 70/40 mmHg, and accompanied by hemorrhagic shock. The right calf was severed 8 cm below the knee joint, with a neat and intact distal section (Figure 3.4.1). The abdomen was distended, with a mobile voiced sound. B-ultrasound showed splenomegaly, and there was a history of ascites due to cirrhosis, with an albumin content of 21 g.

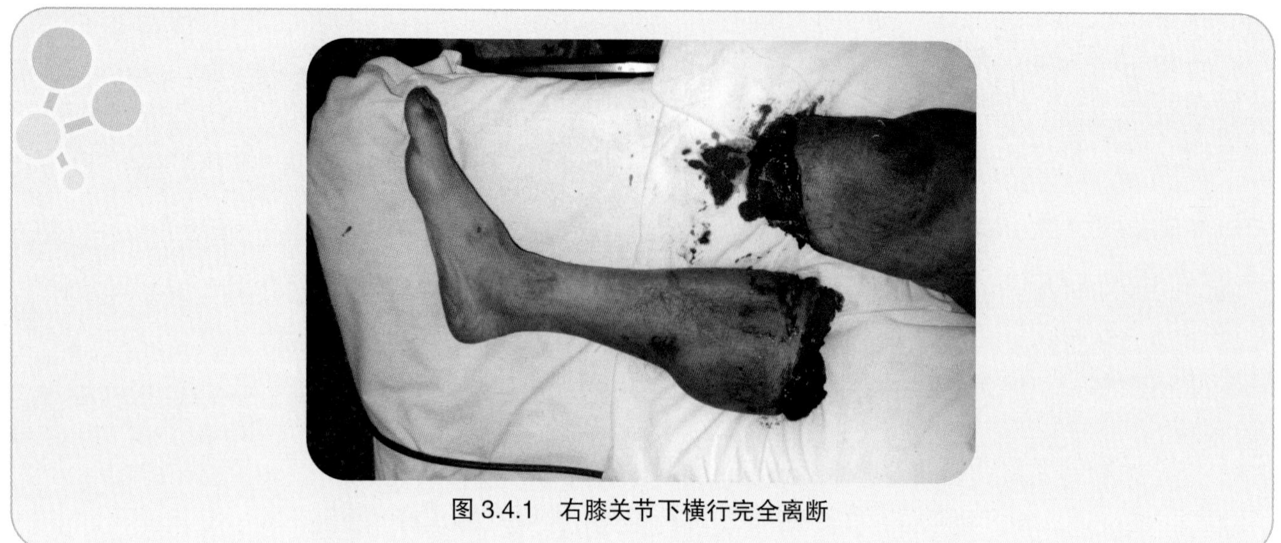
图 3.4.1　右膝关节下横行完全离断

◆ 治疗方案

1. 立即加压包扎止血，远端肢体放冰箱保存。

2. 开通静脉通道，配血型输血，输白蛋白，补液，积极治疗失血性休克。

3. 保肝护胃，纠正低蛋白血症，预防应激性溃疡。

4. 迅速纠正休克，生命体征平稳后，立即行清创断腿再植术。

5. 胫腓骨行钢板内固定术。

6. 配制重组人酸性成纤维细胞生长因子溶液喷洒肌肉断面，缝合肌肉修复血管着床。

7. 配制重组人酸性成纤维细胞生长因子血管冲洗液、灌洗血管至清水流出为止。

8. 吻合胫后动脉及其两条伴行静脉，大隐静脉，修复胫后神经，腓总神经。闭合伤口。

9. 由于这个案例有硬化腹水，加上本次严重的创伤，会加重肝脏损害而危及生命。发起多学科会诊，共同参与治疗。

10. 断肢再植术后，再植肢体血运良好（图 3.4.2）。术后 3 年，小腿肌肉中度萎缩，膝关活动良好，足趾肌力 4 级，足底感觉 S3，较健侧短缩（图 3.4.3）；可以抬起 50 kg 左右的重物，并且行走自如，穿增高矫形鞋，轻度拐行，仍可以上山砍柴（图 3.4.4）。

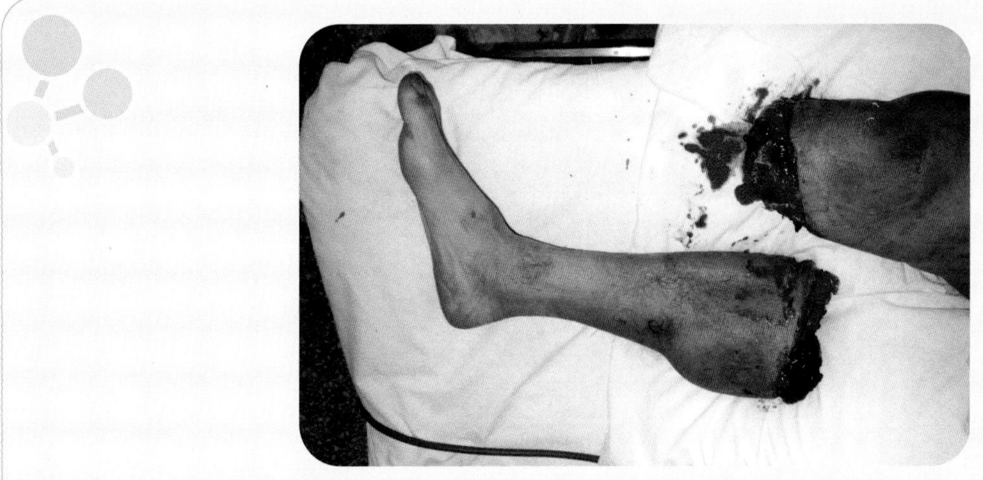

Figure 3.4.1 Complete transverse dissection of the right knee joint

◆ Treatment plan

1. Immediately apply pressure and bandage to stop bleeding, and store the distal limb in the refrigerator.

2. Open the venous channel, provide blood transfusion, albumin infusion, fluid replacement, and actively treat hemorrhagic shock.

3. Protect the liver and stomach, correct hypoalbuminemia, and prevent stress ulcers.

4. Quickly correct shock and perform debridement and leg replantation surgery immediately after vital signs stabilize.

5. Internal fixation of tibia and fibula with steel plate.

6. Configure recombinant human acidic fibroblast growth factor solution to spray on muscle sections, suture muscles to repair vascular implantation.

7. Prepare recombinant human acidic fibroblast growth factor vascular wash solution and wash the blood vessels until clear water flows out.

8. Anastomose the posterior tibial artery and its two accompanying veins, the great saphenous vein, to repair the posterior tibial nerve and common peroneal nerve. Close the wound.

9. Due to the presence of hardened ascites in this case, coupled with the severe trauma, it will exacerbate liver damage and endanger life. Initiate multidisciplinary consultations and participate in treatment together.

10. After the limb replantation surgery, the blood supply of the replanted limb was good (Figure 3.4.2). Three years after surgery, the calf muscles showed moderate atrophy, the knee joint was active, the toe muscle strength was at level 4, and the plantar sensation was S3, with shortening compared to the healthy side (Figure 3.4.3); It can lift a weight of about 50 kg and walk freely, wearing height correcting shoes, making slight turns, and still be able to go up the mountain to chop firewood (Figure 3.4.4).

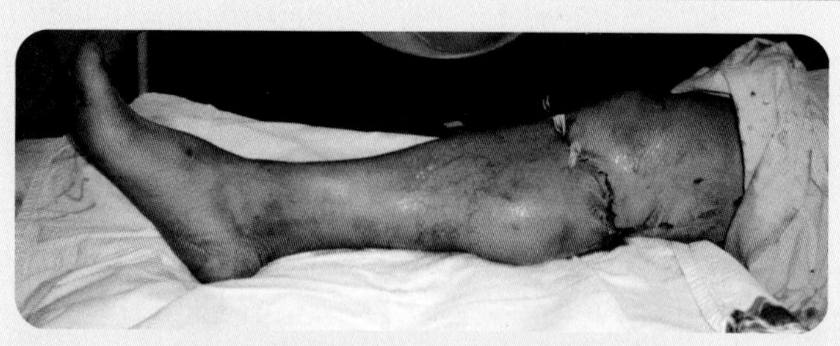

图 3.4.2　断肢再植术后，再植肢体血运良好

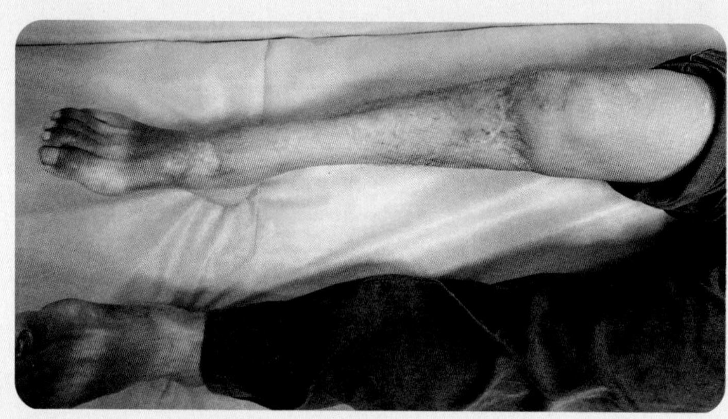

图 3.4.3　断肢再植术后 3 年，小腿肌肉中度萎缩，膝关活动良好，足趾肌力 4 级，足底感觉 S3，较健侧短缩 6 cm

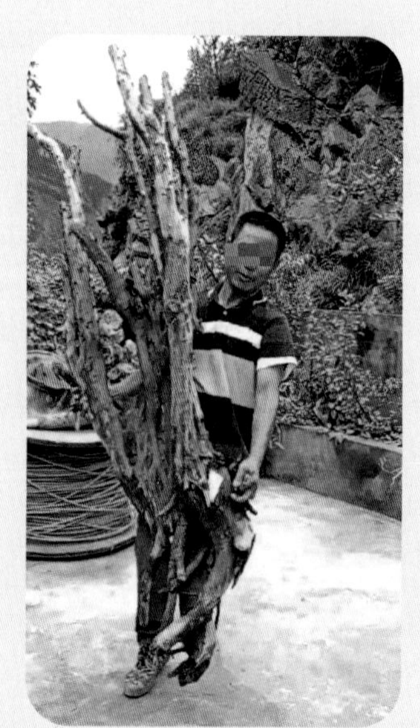

图 3.4.4　可以抬起 100 多斤重物，并且行走自如，穿增高矫形鞋，轻度拐行，仍可以上山砍柴

（陈善亮　高士强）

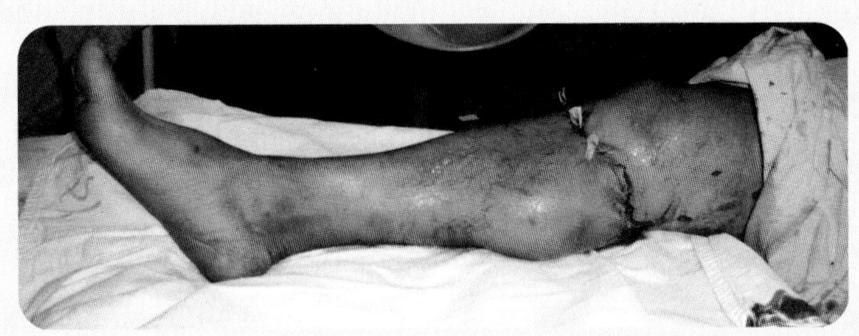

Figure 3.4.2 After limb replantation, the blood supply of the replanted limb is good

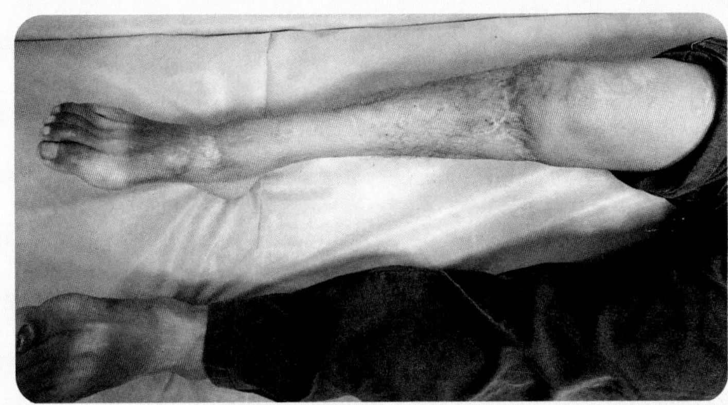

Figure 3.4.3 Three years after limb replantation, the calf muscles showed moderate atrophy, the knee joint was active, the toe muscle strength was at level 4, and the plantar sensation was S3, with a 6 cm shortening compared to the healthy side

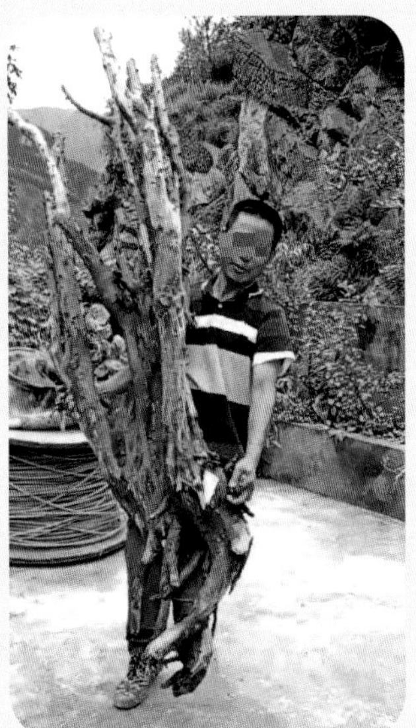

Figure 3.4.4 The person can lift over 100 pounds of weight and walk freely, wearing height correcting shoes and making slight turns. They can still go up the mountain to chop firewood

(Chen Shanliang, Gao Shiqiang)

案例五　手掌切割性离断

◆ 损伤原因

患者因操作铁板切割机不当，致左手掌切割性离断。

◆ 症状与体征

左手掌切断后剧痛难忍，伤口出血呈喷射状，工友用腰带捆扎前臂止血，伤后2小时急诊入院，面色苍白，血压80/40 mmHg，前臂中段有腰带捆扎，断端出血活跃，局部肿胀明显，断面有油污污染，远端完整无血运，断面从手掌中段离断（图3.5.1、图3.5.2）。

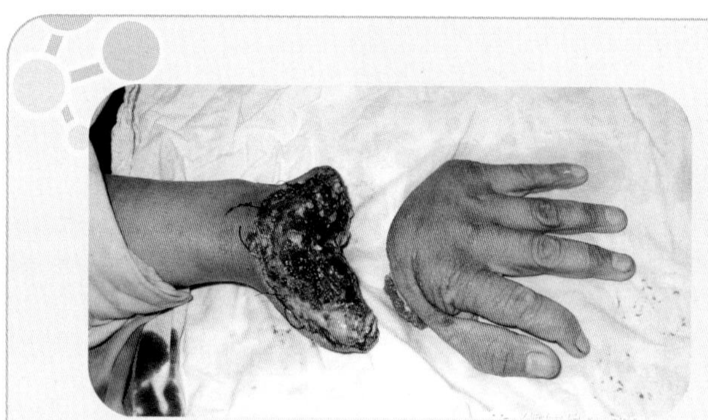

图3.5.1　左手掌横行完全离断，断端较齐，远端较完整，背侧情况

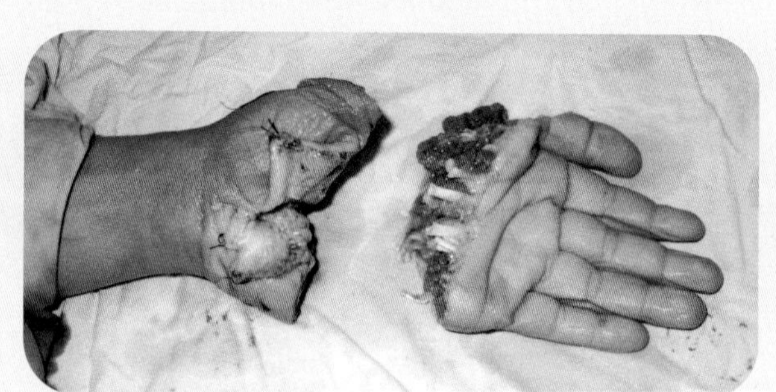

图3.5.2　手掌掌侧离断情况，远端苍白

◆ 治疗方案

1. 立即解开腰带止血措施，局部有较深皮肤压痕，给予厚棉垫加压包扎止血。

2. 积极建立静脉通道，抗休克。

3. 断掌远端放冰箱中低温保存。

4. 积极做好手术前准备。

5. 完善手术前准备后立即在臂丛麻醉下行清创再植术。

6. 清创术，克氏针骨支架建立，修复伸指肌腱，屈指深浅肌腱，修复腱鞘及手内在肌。

7. 配备重组人酸性成纤维细胞生长因子冲洗液喷洒断掌断面。

8. 显微镜下修剪手背静脉和掌浅弓，指总动脉吻合口，并用重组人酸性成纤维细胞生长因子冲洗液冲洗血管管腔，取10号显微针线吻合血管，缝合指神经，逐层缝合伤口，放置引流。

Case 5 Palm cutting detachment

◆ Cause of injury

The patient's left palm was cut off due to improper operation of the iron plate cutting machine.

◆ Signs and symptoms

After cutting off the left palm, the pain was unbearable, and the bleeding from the wound had sprayed out. A colleague tied the forearm with a belt to stop the bleeding. Two hours after the injury, the patient was admitted to the emergency department with a pale complexion and a blood pressure of 80/40 mmHg. The middle part of the forearm was tied with a belt, and the bleeding was active at the broken end with obvious local swelling. The section was contaminated with oil, and the distal end was intact without blood supply. The section was separated from the middle part of the palm (Figure 3.5.1, Figure 3.5.2).

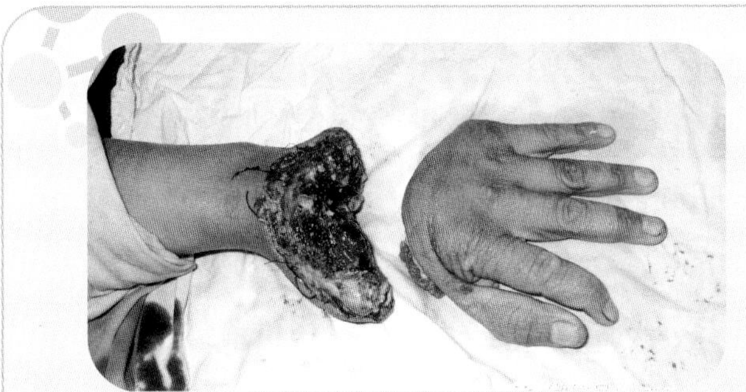

Figure 3.5.1 The left palm is completely severed horizontally, with the broken ends aligned and the distal end intact. The situation is on the dorsal side

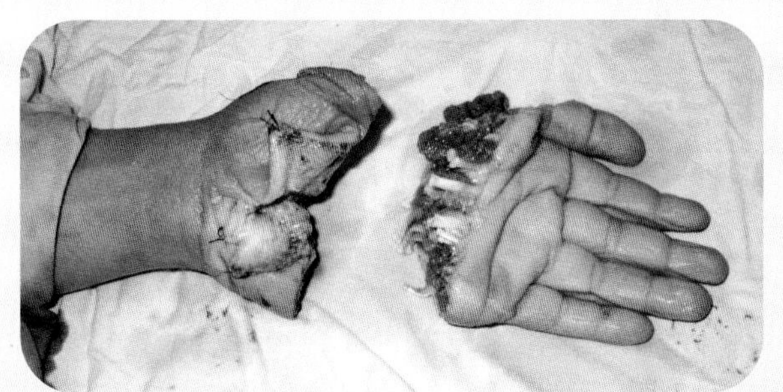

Figure 3.5.2 Palm side detachment, with pale distal end

◆ Treatment plan

1. Immediately undo the belt to stop bleeding. If there are deep skin indentations in the area, apply a thick cotton pad and apply pressure to bandage and stop bleeding.
2. Actively establish venous channels to prevent shock.
3. Store the severed palm at a low temperature in the refrigerator.
4. Actively prepare for surgery.
5. Immediately perform debridement and replantation surgery under brachial plexus anesthesia after completing preoperative preparations.
6. Debridement surgery, establishment of Kirschner wire bone scaffold, repair of extensor and flexor tendons, repair of tendon sheath and intrinsic hand muscles.
7. Equip with recombinant human acidic fibroblast growth factor rinse solution to spray the severed palm section.
8. Trim the dorsal vein and superficial arch of the hand under a microscope, and anastomose the common digital artery. Rinse the vascular lumen with recombinant human acidic fibroblast growth factor flushing solution. Take a 10 gauge microneedle to anastomose the blood vessels, suture the finger nerves, suture the wound layer by layer, and place drainage.

9. 术后扩容、解痉镇痛、抗感染治疗，每天换药时喷洒重组人酸性成纤维细胞生长因子。

10. 术后 7 天，被动活动指间关节，防止关节僵硬及肌腱粘连，术后 12 天拆线，1.5 个月拔出克氏针并进行功能训练。左手掌再植成活（图 3.5.3、图 3.5.4）。

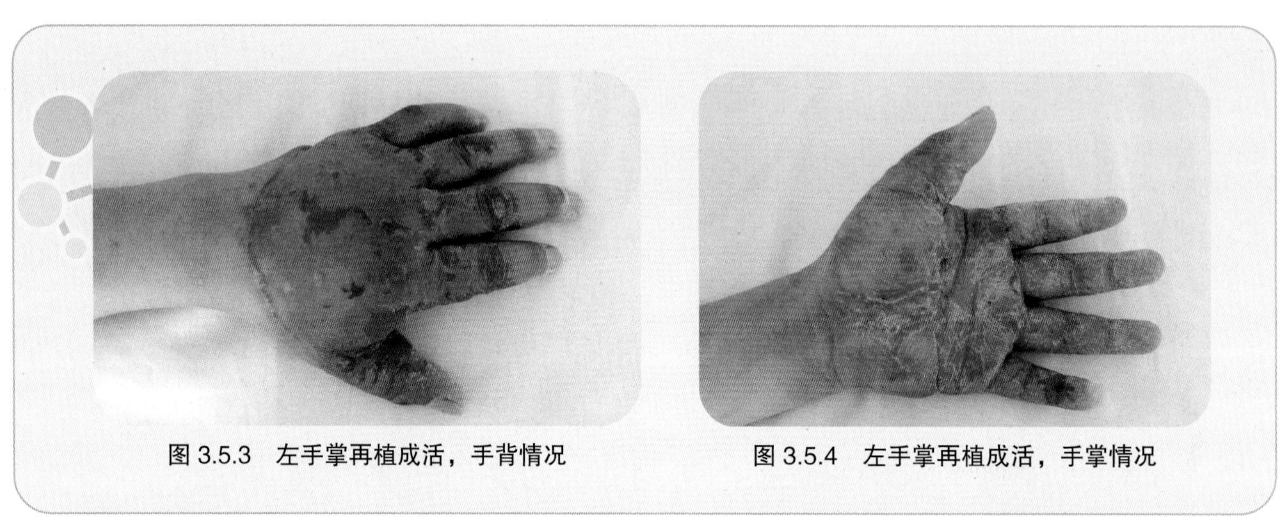

图 3.5.3　左手掌再植成活，手背情况

图 3.5.4　左手掌再植成活，手掌情况

（陈善亮　谭森录）

案例六　拇指示指切割性离断

◆ 损伤原因

患者左手因操作切纸机不当，致拇指、示指切割性离断。

◆ 症状与体征

左手拇指、示指切断后剧痛，局部出血不止，拇指、示指畸形不能活动，伤后工友用毛巾包扎止血而入院。左拇指完全离断，有少许皮带与示指相连，拇指无血运，远端苍白，示指离断，仅示指尺侧有部分皮蒂相连，血液反流迟缓，远端苍白，示指掌指关节面粉碎，拇指从第 1 掌骨远端离断，掌指关节完整，拇指、示指伸肌腱近端回缩，创面出血活跃，污染不重，断面整齐（图 3.6.1 ~ 图 3.6.3）。

9. Postoperative expansion, spasmolysis and analgesia, anti infection treatment, and daily spraying of recombinant human acidic fibroblast growth factor during dressing changes.

10. On the 7th day after surgery, passively move the interphalangeal joint to prevent joint stiffness and tendon adhesion. On the 12th day after surgery, remove the stitches, and at 1.5 months, remove the Kirschner wire and perform functional training. The left palm was successfully replanted (Figure 3.5.3, Figure 3.5.4).

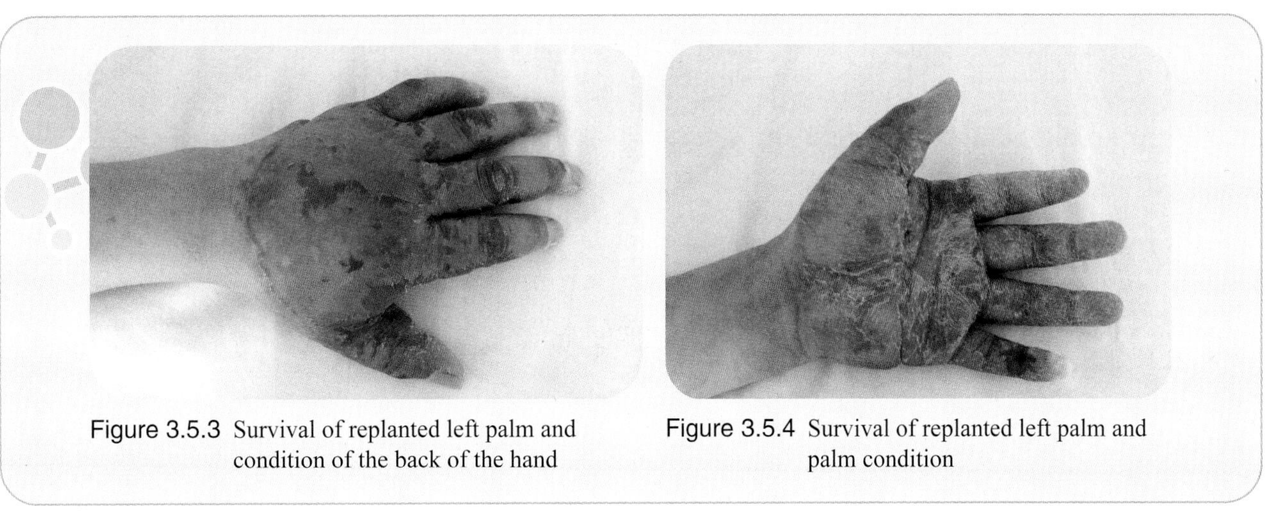

Figure 3.5.3 Survival of replanted left palm and condition of the back of the hand

Figure 3.5.4 Survival of replanted left palm and palm condition

(Chen Shanliang, Tan Senlu)

Case 6 Finger cutting detachment of thumb indicator

◆ Cause of injury

The patient's left hand suffered from cutting detachment of the thumb and index finger due to improper operation of the paper cutter.

◆ Signs and symptoms

After cutting off the left thumb and index finger, there was severe pain and continuous local bleeding. The thumb and index finger were deformed and unable to move. After the injury, the colleague used a towel to bandage and stop the bleeding, and was admitted to the hospital. The left thumb is completely severed, with a small amount of pedicle connected to the index finger. The thumb has no blood supply, and the distal end is pale. The index finger is severed, with only a portion of the pedicle connected to the ulnar side of the index finger. Blood reflux is slow, and the distal end is pale, indicating that the metacarpophalangeal joint is crushed. The thumb is severed from the distal end of the first metacarpal bone, and the metacarpophalangeal joint is intact. The proximal end of the extensor muscle of the thumb and index finger retracts, and the wound bleeding is active with minimal contamination and a neat cross-section (Figure 3.6.1-Figure 3.6.3).

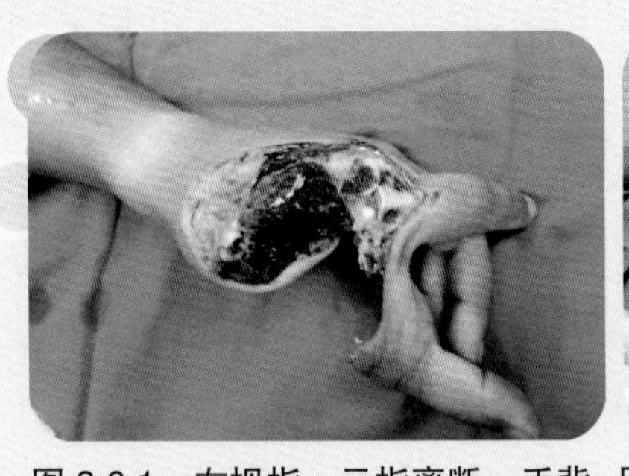

图 3.6.1 左拇指、示指离断，手背情况

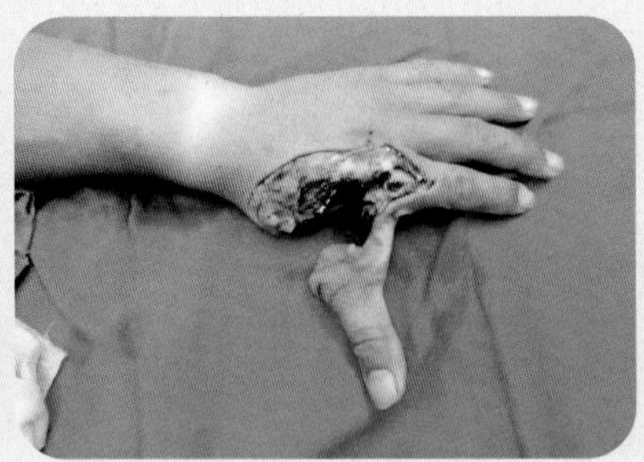

图 3.6.2 左拇指、示指离断，断面整齐，手背情况

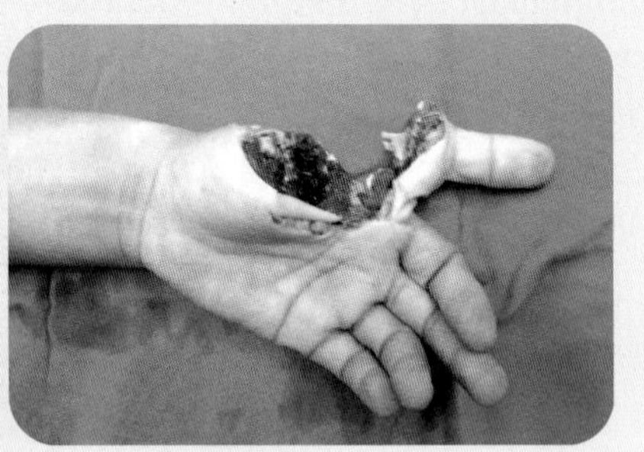

图 3.6.3 左拇指、示指离断，手掌情况

◆ 治疗方案

1. 患者入院后立即局部加压包扎止血。

2. 积极建立静脉通道，手部数字 X 射线摄影（DR）拍片。

3. 快速完善手术术前准备。

4. 在臂丛麻醉下行清创再植术，首先清创，建立骨支架，修复肌腱及肌肉，显露手背和拇指、示指动脉，取重组人酸性成纤维细胞生长因子配备冲洗液，冲洗血管喷洒创面，于显微镜下吻合 2 条动脉 3 条静脉。皮下放置橡皮条引流，闭合伤口，安返病房（图 3.6.4、图 3.6.5）。

5. 术后给予扩容、解痉镇痛、抗感染治疗，抬高患肢，2 天拔引流，12 天拆线康复出院，门诊随访对症治疗。

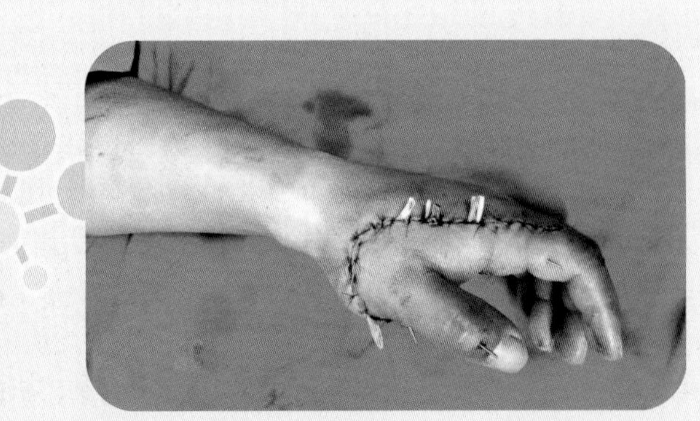

图 3.6.4 拇指、示指再植术后，血运良好，伤口深部放置引流条，手背情况

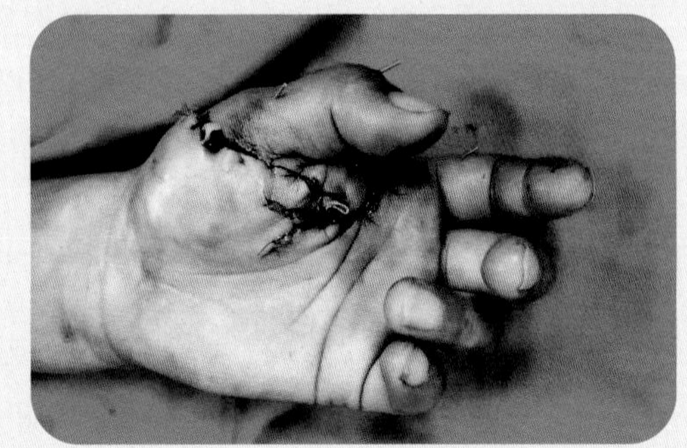

图 3.6.5 拇指、示指再植术后，掌侧、手掌情况

（陈善亮 彭发林）

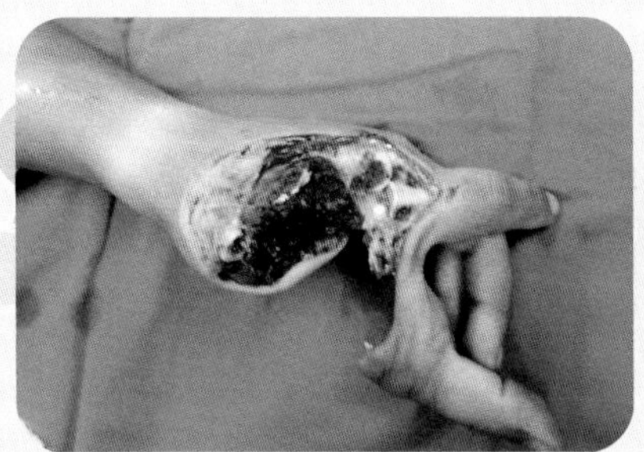

Figure 3.6.1 Left thumb and index finger disconnected, back of hand condition

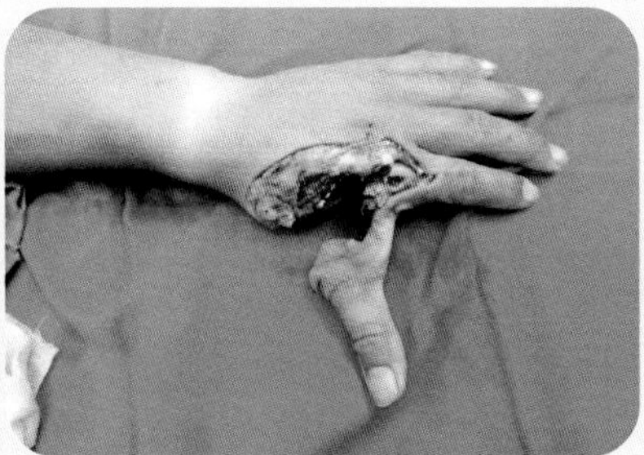

Figure 3.6.2 Left thumb and index finger disconnected, with neat cross-section and condition of the back of the hand

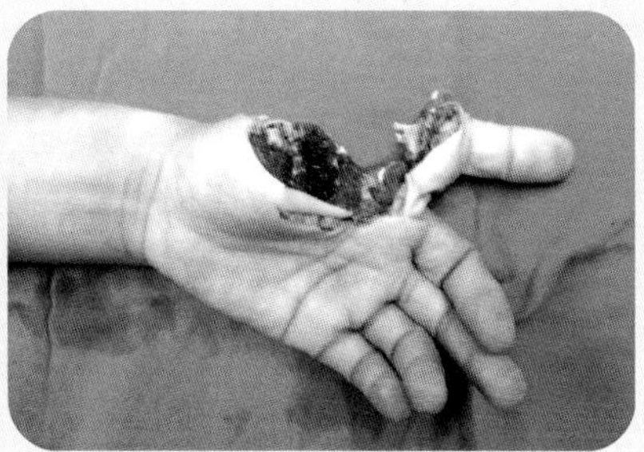

Figure 3.6.3 Left thumb and index finger disconnected, palm condition

◆ Treatment plan

1. Immediately apply local pressure and bandage to stop bleeding after the patient is admitted.
2. Actively establish venous access and perform digital X-ray (DR) imaging on the hands.
3. Quickly improve preoperative preparation for surgery.
4. Under brachial plexus anesthesia, debridement and replantation surgery are performed. Firstly, debridement is performed to establish a bone scaffold, repair tendons and muscles, expose the dorsal hand, thumb, and index finger arteries. Recombinant human acidic fibroblast growth factor is taken to prepare flushing solution, and the blood vessels are flushed and sprayed onto the wound. Two arteries and three veins are anastomosed under a microscope. Subcutaneous placement of rubber strips for drainage, closure of the wound, and safe return to the ward (Figure 3.6.4, Figure 3.6.5).
5. Postoperative treatment includes expansion, spasmolysis, analgesia, and anti infection therapy. The affected limb is elevated, and drainage is removed for 2 days. After 12 days of suture removal, the patient recovers and is discharged. Outpatient follow-up is provided for symptomatic treatment.

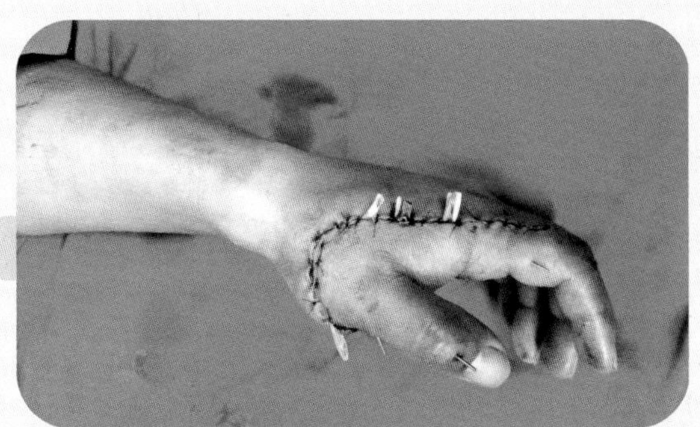

Figure 3.6.4 After thumb and index finger replantation surgery, the blood supply is good, a drainage strip is placed deep in the wound, and the condition of the back of the hand is good

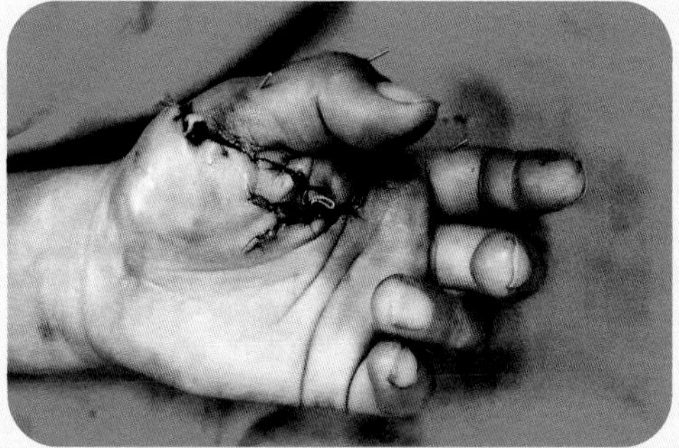

Figure 3.6.5 After thumb and index finger replantation, palmar and palmar conditions

(Chen Shanliang, Peng Falin)

案例七　双下肢毁损性离断

◆ 损伤原因

患者因车祸导致双下肢毁损性离断。

◆ 症状与体征

急性病容，面色苍白，指甲、口唇及眼睑结膜极度苍白，表情淡漠，全身湿冷，呼吸微弱、血压 60/40 mmHg，双下肢创面渗血活跃，右下肢从足踝区远端离断，远端毁损，距骨及跟骨缺损；左下肢从膝关节下端离断，腘窝和大腿后侧有大面积皮肤软组织缺损；小腿中段皮肤肌肉组织抽脱毁损严重，胫腓骨多段粉碎骨折，左侧足踝区完整，仅有少许挫灭腓肠肌相连，离断肢体苍白无血运（图 3.7.1 ~图 3.7.3）。

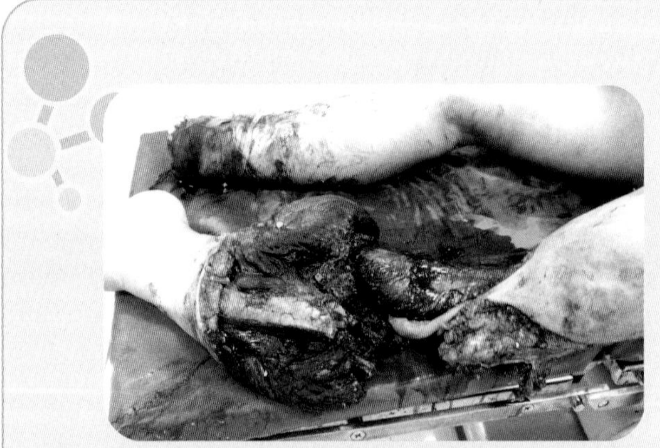

图 3.7.1　右下肢从足踝区远端毁损，近端完整；左下肢从大腿中下段和小腿中段节段毁损，足踝远端完整

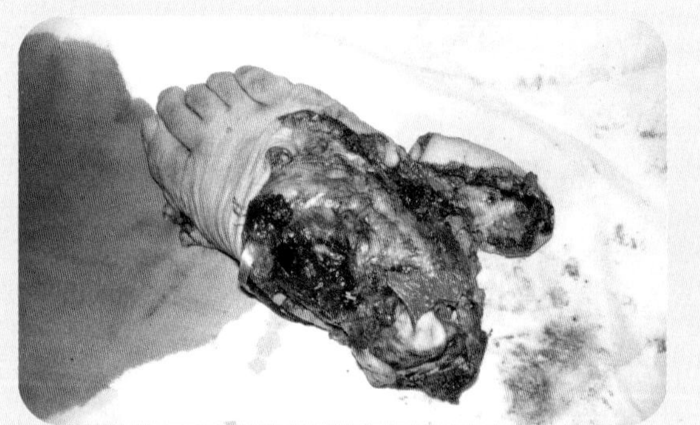

图 3.7.2　右足跟骨距骨毁损缺失、足背和足跟皮肤软组织缺损

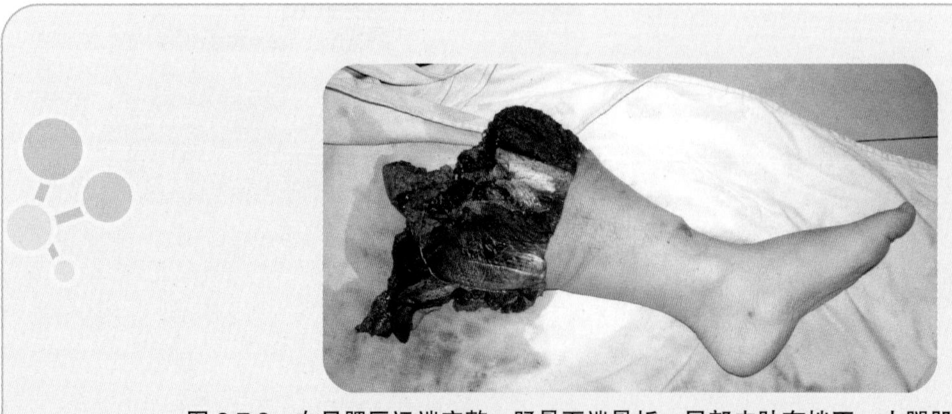

图 3.7.3　左足踝区远端完整，胫骨下端骨折，局部皮肤有挫灭，小腿肌肉抽脱挫灭

Case 7 Destructive separation of two lower limbs

◆ Cause of injury

The patient suffered a destructive separation of both lower limbs due to a car accident.

◆ Signs and symptoms

Acute appearance, pale complexion, extremely pale nails, lips, eyelids, and conjunctiva, indifferent expression, wet and cold all over the body, weak breathing, blood pressure of 60/40 mmHg, active bleeding from wounds in both lower limbs, distal detachment and destruction of the right lower limb from the ankle area, defects in the talus and calcaneus; The left lower limb is severed from the lower end of the knee joint, and there is a large area of skin and soft tissue defect in the popliteal fossa and posterior thigh; The skin and muscle tissue in the middle of the calf have been severely removed and damaged, with multiple comminuted fractures of the tibia and fibula. The left ankle area is intact, with only a slight contusion of the gastrocnemius muscle connection. The severed limb is pale and lacks blood circulation (Figure 3.7.1-Figure 3.7.3).

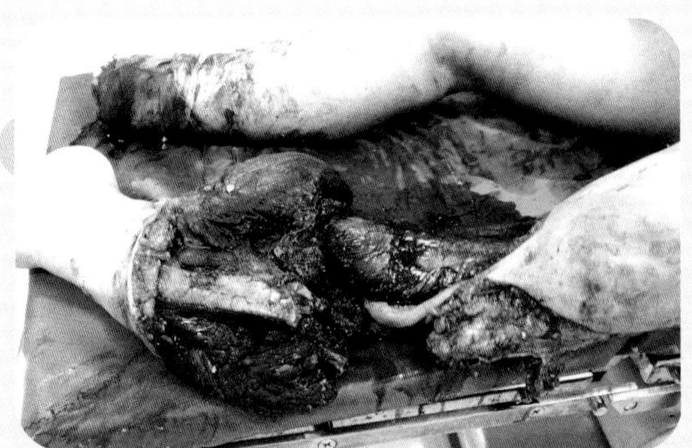

Figure 3.7.1 The right lower limb is damaged from the distal end of the ankle area, with the proximal end intact; The left lower limb is damaged in the middle and lower segments of the thigh and calf, while the distal end of the ankle is intact

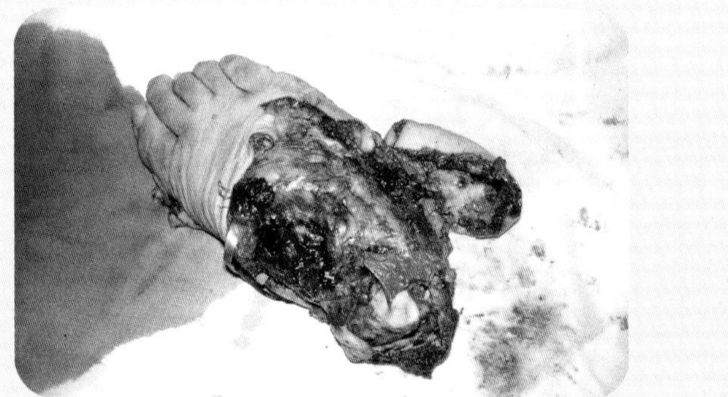

Figure 3.7.2 Right foot calcaneal bone destruction and loss, as well as skin and soft tissue defects in the dorsum and heel of the foot

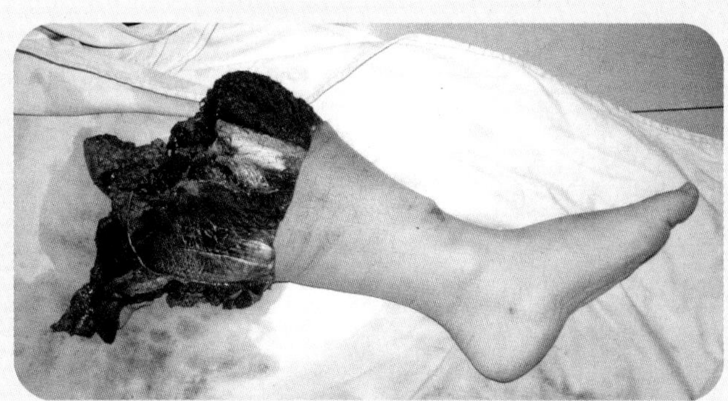

Figure 3.7.3 The distal end of the left ankle area is intact, the lower end of the tibia is fractured, and there is local skin contusion, as well as calf muscle detachment and contusion

第二部分 典型个案介绍

◆ 治疗方案

这类案例属于高能量损伤，在临床上十分少见，目前文献报道不多。

1. 入院积极止血，建立静脉通道，扩容补液，备血输血，以积极抗休克维持生命为主。

2. 全身检查是否有复合伤。

3. 下肢气压止血带止血。

4. 离断肢体远端冷储，肢体伤口临时消毒包扎，并抬高患肢。

5. 吸氧，备皮，导尿，完善手术前准备。

6. 生命体征平稳后，耐受麻醉和手术，行左大腿中下段截肢残端修复术。

7. 手术过程

7.1 清创、骨支架（左侧胫骨和右侧胫骨对接钢板固定），左侧胫前肌群远端和右侧胫前肌群近端缝合，左侧胫后肌群和右侧胫后肌群对接缝合。

7.2 血管神经修复：左侧胫前动脉及伴行静脉和右侧胫前动脉及伴行静脉吻合，左侧胫后动脉及伴行静脉和右侧胫后动脉及伴行静脉近端吻合，左侧胫后神经远端和右侧胫后神经近端吻左侧大隐静脉远端和右侧大隐静脉近端吻合，即胫前血管修复是在胫骨前交叉吻合，胫后血管修复是在胫骨后侧交叉吻合。组织间隙中重组人酸性成纤维细胞生长因子，放置引流条，缝合伤口，石膏固定。

8. 由于骨骼，肌肉血管神经都是交叉移位修复，在清创时对血管神经保留足够长度，避免交叉移位修复时不够长。左侧肢体移位右下肢再植后，血运良好，足背动脉搏动良好（图 3.7.4、图 3.7.5）。

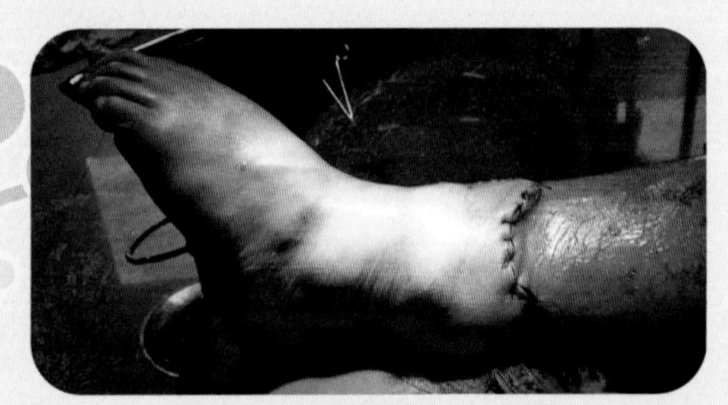

图 3.7.4　将左足远端和右足踝清创后，行肢体移位再植，左侧大腿中段截肢残端修复

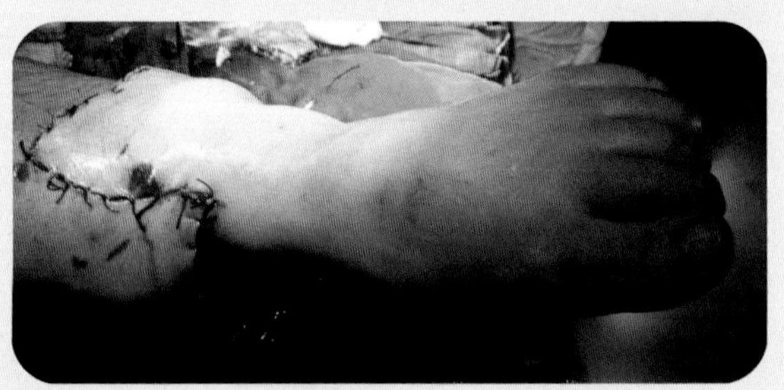

图 3.7.5　左侧肢体移位右下肢再植后，血运良好，足背动脉搏动良好

◆ Treatment plan

This type of case belongs to high-energy injury and is very rare in clinical practice. Currently, there are few literature reports on it.

1. Actively stop bleeding upon admission, establish venous channels, expand and replenish fluids, prepare blood for transfusion, and focus on actively resisting shock to maintain life.

2. Conduct a full body examination to check for any compound injuries.

3. Lower limb pneumatic tourniquet to stop bleeding.

4. Disconnect the distal limb for cold storage, temporarily disinfect and bandage the limb wound, and elevate the affected limb.

5. Oxygen inhalation, skin preparation, catheterization, and complete preoperative preparation.

6. After stabilizing vital signs, tolerate anesthesia and surgery, and perform left thigh middle and lower segment amputation and stump repair surgery.

7. Surgical process

7.1 Debridement and bone support (fixation of left and right tibia with steel plates), distal and proximal suturing of left anterior tibialis muscle group, and suturing of left posterior tibialis muscle group and right posterior tibialis muscle group.

7.2 Vascular and nerve repair: anastomosis of the left anterior tibial artery and associated vein with the right anterior tibial artery and associated vein, anastomosis of the left posterior tibial artery and associated vein with the proximal end of the right posterior tibial artery and associated vein, anastomosis of the distal end of the left posterior tibial nerve and the proximal end of the right posterior tibial nerve with the distal end of the left great saphenous vein and the proximal end of the right great saphenous vein, i.e., anterior tibial vascular repair is achieved by cross anastomosis in the anterior aspect of the tibia, and posterior tibial vascular repair is achieved by cross anastomosis in the posterior aspect of the tibia. Recombinant human acidic fibroblast growth factor in the interstitial space, placement of drainage strips, suturing of wounds, and plaster fixation.

8. Due to the fact that bones, muscles, blood vessels, and nerves are all repaired through cross displacement, sufficient length of blood vessels and nerves should be preserved during debridement to avoid insufficient repair time for cross displacement. After the left limb was displaced and the right lower limb was replanted, the blood supply was good and the dorsalis pedis artery pulsation was good (Figure 3.7.4, Figure 3.7.5).

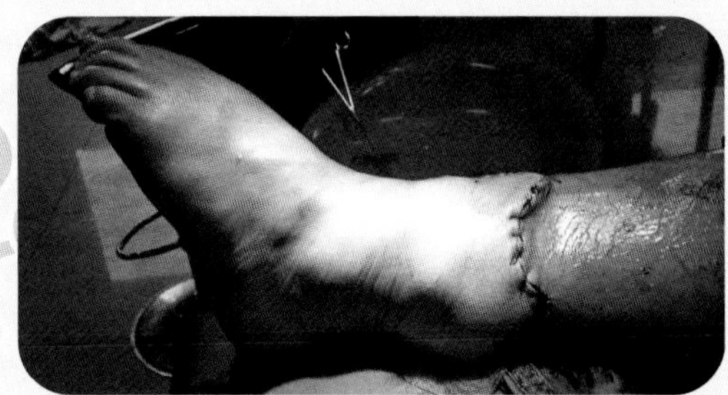

Figure 3.7.4 After debridement of the distal left foot and right ankle, limb displacement and replantation were performed, and the left thigh mid segment amputation stump was repaired

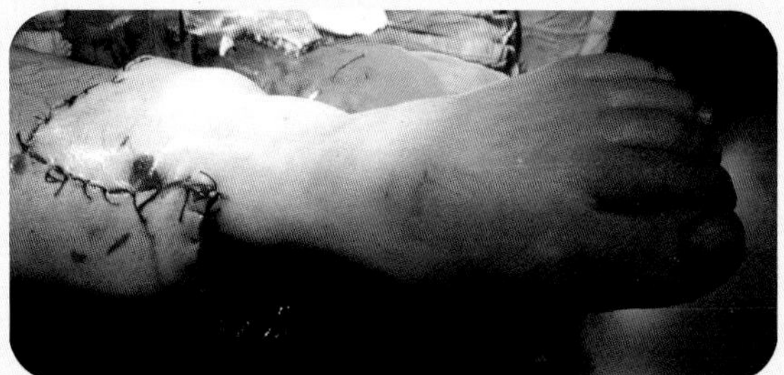

Figure 3.7.5 After left limb displacement and right lower limb replantation, the blood supply is good and the dorsalis pedis artery pulsation is good

9. 下肢移位再植手术，保留了一侧肢体，对侧肢体截肢后安装假肢。

10. 术后抗休克，预防血管痉挛、抗血栓和抗感染仍是关键。

11. 发起多学科会诊共同参与治疗。

（陈善亮　黄　鹏）

案例八　踝关节撕脱性离断

◆ 损伤原因

患者因铁板压砸，致左踝关节撕脱性离断。

◆ 症状与体征

铁板倒塌砸伤左足踝，左足踝区离断、外踝有 2 cm 皮带相连，皮缘有挫灭，参差不齐，胫前肌群和胫后肌群抽脱离断，胫前动脉和胫后动脉抽脱离断伴缺损，近端断端有血栓形成，内踝区有部分皮肤缺损，足远端无血运，足苍白，血液无反流，皮温凉，足远端无感觉，伤口污染严重，布满铁锈和泥沙（图 3.8.1）

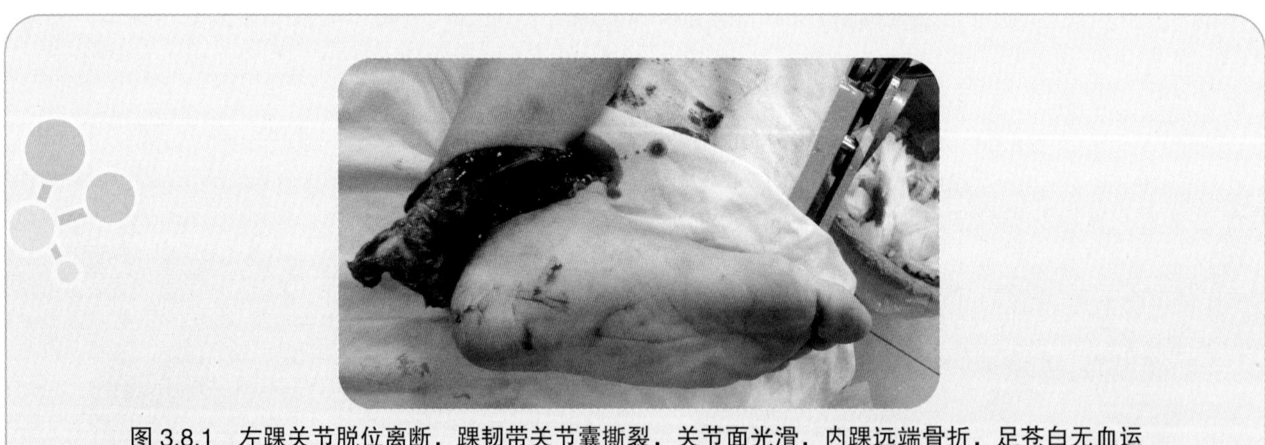

图 3.8.1　左踝关节脱位离断，踝韧带关节囊撕裂，关节面光滑，内踝远端骨折，足苍白无血运

◆ 治疗方案

1. 入院后消毒包扎止血，建立静脉通道，完善手术前准备。

2. 腰硬联合麻醉下行断踝再植术。

3. 手术过程

3.1 骨支架建立：由于踝关节开放性脱位性离断，骨关节面完整，关节复位后将撕裂关节周围韧带完全

9. Lower limb displacement and replantation surgery, with one limb preserved and the other limb amputated and repaired, followed by the installation of a prosthetic limb.

10. Postoperative anti shock measures, prevention of vascular spasm, anti thrombosis, and anti infection remain key.

11. Initiate multidisciplinary consultations to jointly participate in treatment.

(Chen Shanliang, Huang Peng)

Case 8 Ankle joint tear separation 

◆ Cause of injury

The patient suffered a torn and dislocated left ankle joint due to being hit by an iron plate.

◆ Signs and symptoms

The iron plate collapsed and injured the left ankle, with the left ankle area severed and a 2cm skin pedicle connected to the outer ankle. The skin was crushed and uneven, and the tibialis anterior and posterior muscle groups were detached and severed. The tibialis anterior and posterior arteries were detached and severed with defects, and there was thrombus formation at the proximal end. There was partial skin defect in the inner ankle area. There was no blood flow in the distal foot, pale foot, no blood reflux, warm skin, and no sensation in the distal foot. The wound was heavily contaminated and covered with rust and mud (Figure 3.8.1)

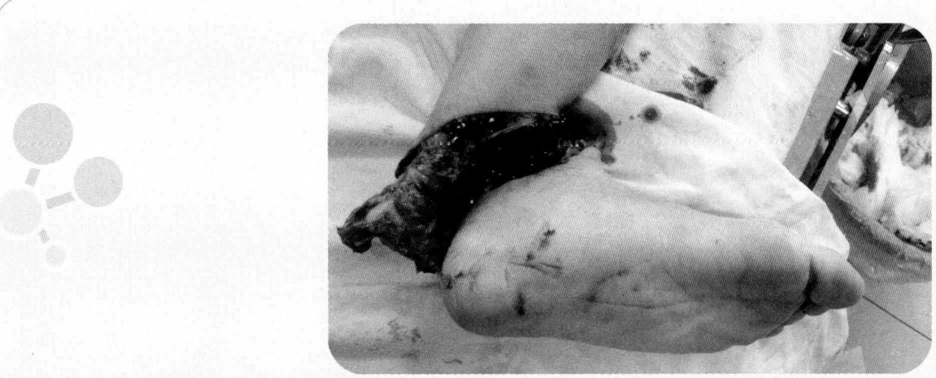

Figure 3.8.1 Left ankle dislocation and fracture, torn ankle ligament capsule, smooth joint surface, distal medial ankle fracture, pale foot with no blood supply

◆ Treatment plan

1. Disinfect, bandage and stop bleeding after admission, establish venous access, and improve preoperative preparation.

2. Limb replantation surgery under combined spinal and epidural anesthesia.

3. Surgical process

3.1 Establishment of bone scaffold: Due to open dislocation and detachment of the ankle joint, the bone joint surface is intact, and after joint reduction, the torn ligaments around the joint are completely repaired, maintaining

修复，保持肢体长度，有利于防止术后短缩拐行，修复离断肌腱肌肉组织，对因撕裂短缩的肌腱局部做肌腱延长或肌腱移位术。

3.2 神经修复：胫后神经两端松解后外膜 + 束膜缝合，修复浅表腓肠神经。

3.3 血管修复：这类损伤动脉和静脉大多数短缩，直接吻合血管不够长度，需要做血管移植术，切取对侧大隐静脉倒置后根据短缩程度分别移植于胫前和胫后动脉，大隐静脉顺行分别移植于胫前动脉和胫后动脉的两条伴行静脉，修复大隐静脉。应用重组人酸性成纤维细胞生长因子各组织间隙中，促进血管神经修复，肌腱和肌肉修复。

3.4 胫前皮肤撕脱缺损，面积 6 cm × 3 cm，局部应用负压封闭引流（VSD）治疗，并常规使用外用人重组酸性生长因子滴注冲洗创面，4 天后拆除 VSD 治疗，创面植皮（图 3.8.2）。

4. 手术后预防感染、预防血管痉挛和血栓形成，术后保温，抬高患肢，观察四大显微指标。

5. 手术后石膏固定 4 周，拆出石膏后行关节松动，训练康复治疗。

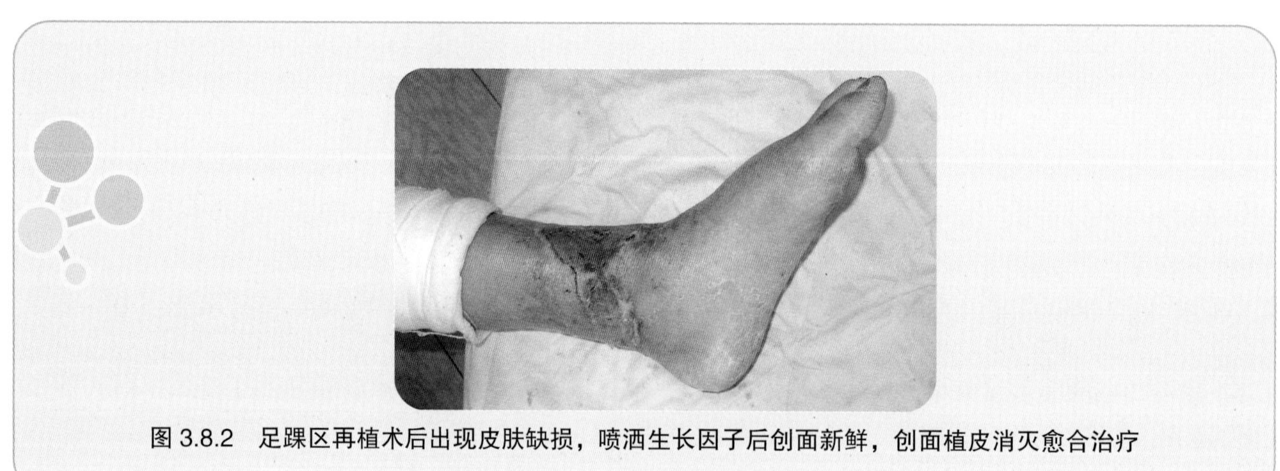

图 3.8.2　足踝区再植术后出现皮肤缺损，喷洒生长因子后创面新鲜，创面植皮消灭愈合治疗

（陈善亮　蒋良福）

案例九　手掌压轧性离断

◆ 损伤原因

患者右手腕部因打包带机绞勒，致手掌压轧性离断。

◆ 症状与体征

右手腕部离断后出血不止，伤后被工友用尼龙绳捆扎止血，右腕关节完全离断，桡侧伸腕肌、尺侧伸

limb length and preventing postoperative shortening and twisting. It is beneficial to repair the severed tendon and muscle tissue, and perform tendon lengthening or tendon displacement surgery on the tendon caused by tearing and shortening.

3.2 Neural repair: After loosening both ends of the posterior tibial nerve and suturing the outer membrane and bundle membrane, repair the superficial sural nerve.

3.3 Vascular repair: Most of the damaged arteries and veins are shortened, and direct anastomosis of the blood vessels is not long enough. Vascular transplantation is required. The contralateral great saphenous vein is inverted and transplanted into the anterior and posterior tibial arteries according to the degree of shortening. The great saphenous vein is transplanted into the two accompanying veins of the anterior and posterior tibial arteries in the anterograde direction to repair the great saphenous vein. The application of recombinant human acidic fibroblast growth factor promotes vascular and nerve repair, tendon and muscle repair in the interstitial spaces of various tissues.

3.4 The skin tear defect in front of the tibia, with an area of 6 cm × 3 cm, was treated locally with negative pressure closure drainage (VSD), and the wound was routinely rinsed with topical recombinant acidic growth factor infusion. After 4 days, the VSD was removed for treatment, and skin grafting was performed on the wound (Figure 3.8.2).

4. Prevent infection, vascular spasm, and thrombosis after surgery, keep warm after surgery, elevate the affected limb, and observe the four major microscopic indicators.

5. After the surgery, the plaster was fixed for 4 weeks. After removing the plaster, the joints became loose and underwent training and rehabilitation treatment.

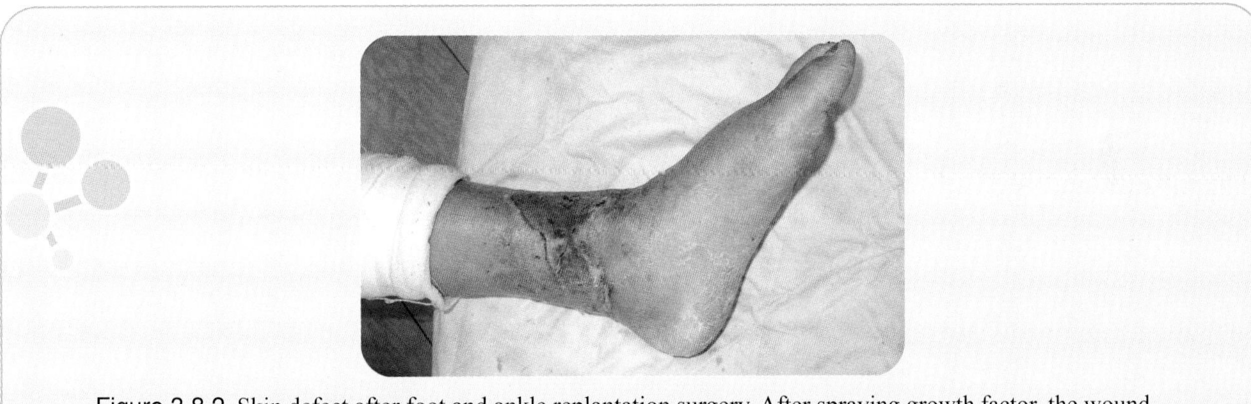

Figure 3.8.2 Skin defect after foot and ankle replantation surgery. After spraying growth factor, the wound is fresh and treated with skin grafting to eliminate and heal the wound

(Chen Shanliang, Jiang Liangfu)

Case 9 Palm compression induced fracture

◆ Cause of injury

The patient's right wrist was twisted by the strapping machine, causing the palm to be crushed and detached.

◆ Signs and symptoms

After the right wrist was severed, there was continuous bleeding. After the injury, the colleague tied it with

腕肌和示指伸肌腱从肌腱肌肉移行处抽脱离断，断端皮肤和离断肌腱，血管神经参差不齐，局部皮肤有挫灭，近排腕骨缺损（舟骨、月骨），腕背侧有 4 cm × 3 cm 皮肤缺损，尺骨桡骨远端关节面骨折伴缺损，离断手掌苍白无血运（图 3.9.1、图 3.9.2）。

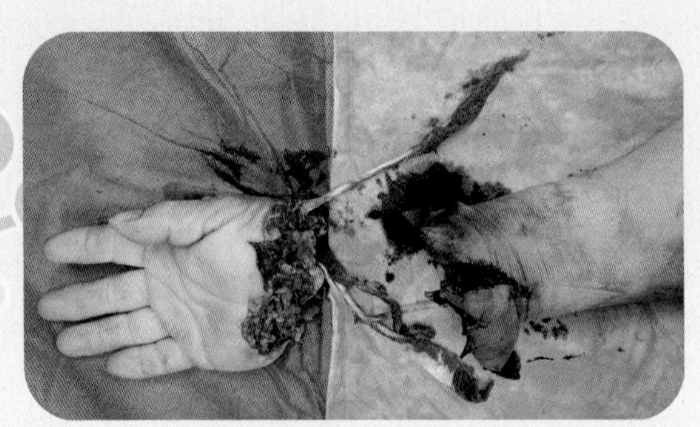

图 3.9.1　右手掌在腕关节处离断，肌腱从肌腹处抽脱，近端参差不齐，正中神经游离约 8 cm

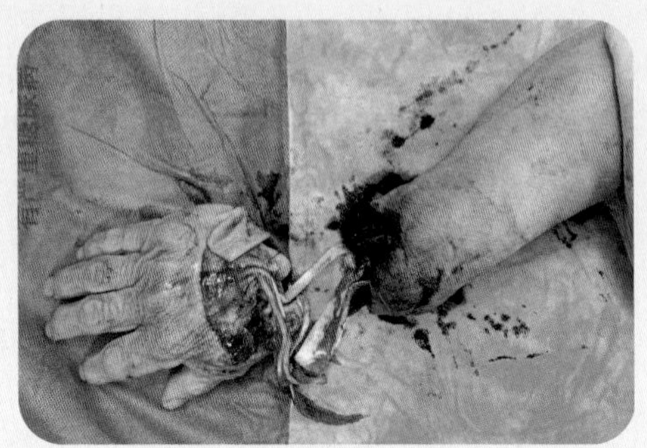

图 3.9.2　右手背有偏桡侧有皮肤软组织缺损，部分肌腱从肌腹处长段抽脱

◆ 治疗方案

该案例为绞勒撕脱性离断，肌腱、血管、神经撕脱性离断，损伤广泛。离断肢体出血活跃，现场止血减少出血量，防止出血性休克，十分关键。工友第一时间用尼龙绳捆扎离断肢体近端，有效减少出血量。

1. 入院立即行局部加压止血，松绑工友捆扎的尼龙绳，局部可见皮肤深深的压痕，（工友现场止血松紧度难以把握），并抬高患肢。

2. 迅速完善手术前准备，建立静脉通道，扩容补液，手术前准备结束后，立即进入手术室行断腕再植手术。

3. 采用臂丛神经阻滞麻醉。

4. 手术过程

4.1 骨支架建立：由于近排腕骨和桡骨远端骨折伴缺损，行腕关节融合，取 2.0 克氏针固定并融合，肌腱修复；修复桡侧伸腕肌腱，尺侧伸腕肌腱和伸指肌腱。修复桡侧屈腕肌腱尺侧屈腕和屈指深浅肌腱。修复正中神经、尺神经、桡神经手背支、尺神经手背支。

4.2 血管修复：依次吻合头静脉和贵要静脉手背支、尺动脉及两条伴行静脉，桡动脉两条伴行静脉及桡动脉，（血管吻合口和肌腱神经喷洒生长因子），创腔深部防止橡皮条引流，逐层缝合伤口，包扎伤口，石膏固定。

nylon rope to stop the bleeding. The right wrist joint was completely severed, and the radial extensor wrist muscle, ulnar extensor wrist muscle, and index finger extensor tendon were pulled and detached from the tendon muscle migration site. The skin and detached tendon at the severed end were uneven, and there were local skin contusions. There was a defect in the proximal wrist bone (navicular bone, lunate bone) and a 4 cm × 3 cm skin defect on the dorsal side of the wrist. The distal joint surface of the ulna and radius was fractured with defects. The severed palm was pale and had no blood supply (Figure 3.9.1, Figure 3.9.2).

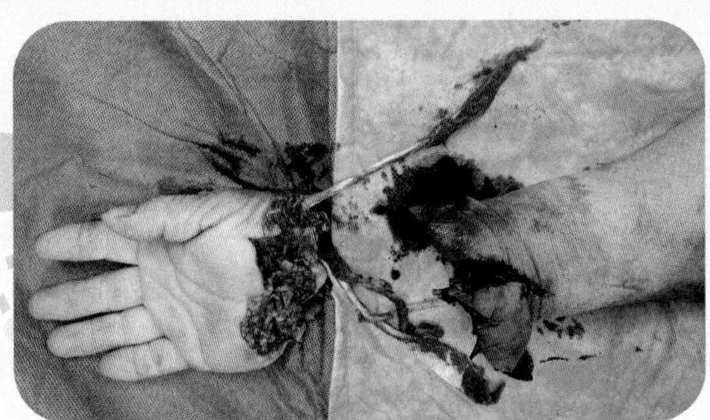

Figure 3.9.1 The right palm is severed at the wrist joint, and the tendon is pulled out from the muscle belly. The proximal end is uneven, and the median nerve is about 8 cm free

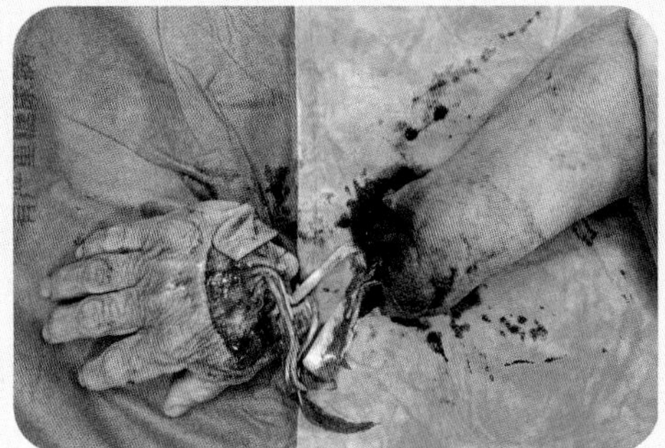

Figure 3.9.2 There is a skin and soft tissue defect on the radial side of the right back, and some tendons have been extracted from the long segment of the muscle belly

◆ Treatment plan

This case is a strangulation induced detachment, involving extensive damage to tendons, blood vessels, and nerves. It is crucial to have active bleeding in the severed limbs, stop bleeding on site to reduce the amount of bleeding, and prevent hemorrhagic shock. The colleague immediately tied the proximal end of the severed limb with nylon rope, effectively reducing the amount of bleeding.

1. Immediately apply local pressure to stop bleeding upon admission, loosen the nylon rope tied by the colleague, and deep skin marks can be seen locally (the tightness of the hemostasis on site is difficult to grasp), and raise the affected limb.

2. Quickly improve preoperative preparation, establish venous channels, expand and replenish fluids. After the preoperative preparation is completed, immediately enter the operating room for wrist replantation surgery.

3. Use brachial plexus block anesthesia.

4. Surgical process

4.1 Establishment of bone scaffold: Due to proximal wrist and distal radius fractures with defects, wrist joint fusion was performed, and 2.0 Kirschner wires were used for fixation and fusion, followed by tendon repair; Repair the radial extensor wrist tendon, ulnar extensor wrist tendon, and extensor finger tendon. Repair the radial flexor tendon, ulnar flexor tendon, and deep and shallow flexor tendon. Repair the median nerve, ulnar nerve, dorsal branch of radial nerve, and dorsal branch of ulnar nerve.

4.2 Vascular repair: sequentially anastomose the dorsal branch of the cephalic vein and the basilic vein, the ulnar artery, and two accompanying veins, as well as the two accompanying veins of the radial artery and the radial artery (vascular anastomosis site and tendon nerve spray growth factor), prevent rubber strip drainage in the deep part of the wound cavity, suture the wound layer by layer, wrap the wound, and fix it with plaster.

5. 手术后抗炎、扩容、解痉，预防血栓形成，镇痛，抗肿胀，神经营养。

6. 严密观察血液循环，抬高患肢，保温，加强换药，3 天拔引流条，换药时喷洒生长因子促进创面愈合。

7. 手背有皮肤缺损，行二次植皮（图 3.9.3、图 3.9.4）。

8. 术后 2 周行手部各关节松动训练。腕关节融合，3 个月后拔出克氏针。

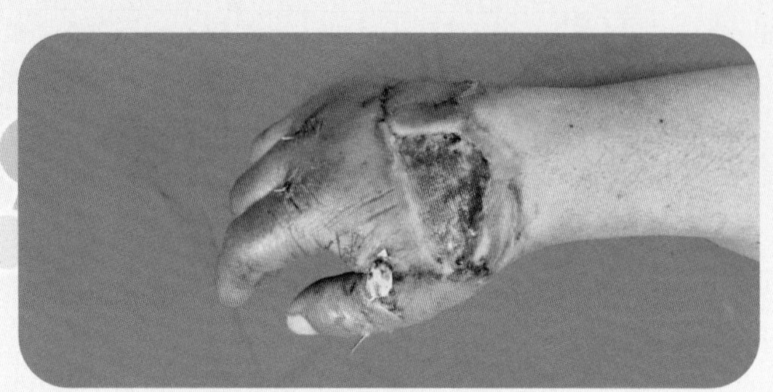

图 3.9.3　右手腕再植后成活，掌背侧有皮肤缺损，约 4 cm × 3 cm，经多次换药喷洒生长因子后创面新鲜，待植皮手术

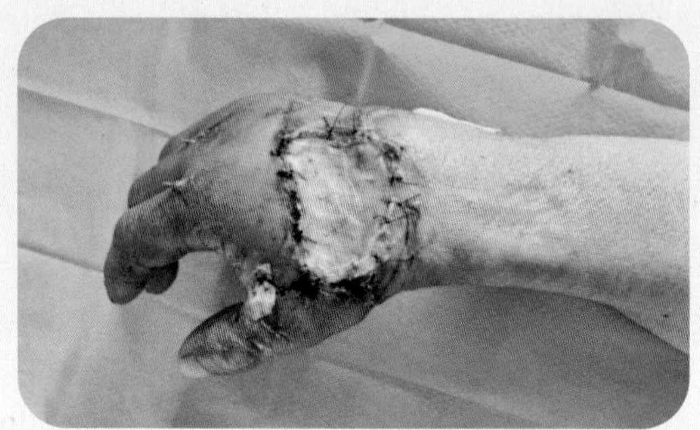

图 3.9.4　右侧腕背侧创面植皮成活。术后 20 天，再植手掌血运良好，克氏针固定可靠

（陈善亮　曹　辉）

案例十　右上臂撕脱性离断

◆ 损伤原因

患者右上臂卷入拉丝机中，致撕脱离断。

◆ 症状与体征

损伤后断臂近端喷射出血，伤后工友用毛巾加压包扎止血，急送来院就诊。入院时面色苍白，睑结膜，口唇及齿龈极度苍白，大汗淋漓，急性病容，表情淡漠，血压 80/45 mmHg。右上臂残端有毛巾捆扎，衣裤被鲜血浸透，断端皮肤有皮肤环绕勒伤，局部皮肤挫灭，上臂近端呈脱套状，局部空虚。肱骨干从中段离断，局部出血活跃，肩背部及右侧侧胸壁有大面积皮肤擦伤，局部压痛，肋骨无骨擦感骨擦音，呼吸音清。

右上臂从肱骨中段离断，肱骨斜行骨折，尺神经和正中神经长段逆行抽脱并缠绕在肱骨干上，肱动

5. After surgery, anti-inflammatory, dilating, spasmolytic, thrombotic prevention, analgesia, anti swelling, and nerve nutrition.

6. Carefully observe blood circulation, elevate the affected limb, keep warm, strengthen dressing changes, remove drainage strips within 3 days, and spray growth factors during dressing changes to promote wound healing.

7. There is a skin defect on the back of the hand, requiring secondary skin grafting (Figure 3.9.3, Figure 3.9.4).

8. Two weeks after surgery, perform hand joint mobilization training. Fusion of wrist joint, and removal of Kirschner wire after 3 months.

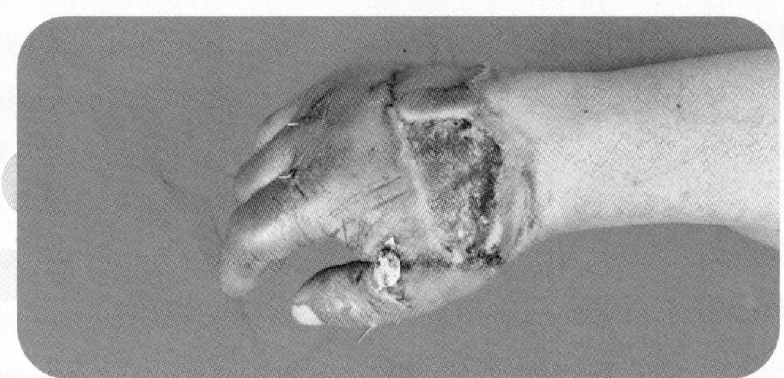

Figure 3.9.3 Survives after right wrist replantation, with a skin defect on the dorsal side of the palm, approximately 4 cm × 3 cm. After multiple dressing changes and growth factor sprays, the wound is fresh and awaiting skin grafting surgery

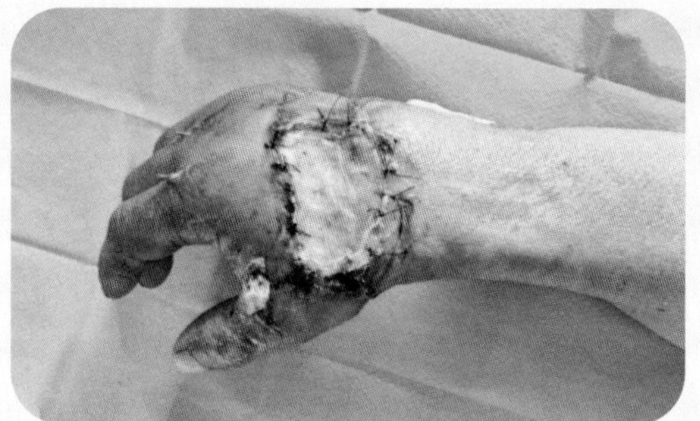

Figure 3.9.4 Survival of skin graft on the dorsal wound of the right wrist. 20 days after surgery, the blood supply of the replanted palm was good, and the Kirschner wire fixation was reliable

(Chen Shanliang, Cao Hui)

Case 10 Right upper arm tear separation

◆ Cause of injury

The patient's right upper arm was caught in the wire drawing machine, causing tearing and detachment.

◆ Signs and symptoms

After the injury, the proximal end of the severed arm was sprayed with bleeding. The injured worker used a towel to apply pressure and bandage to stop the bleeding, and was urgently sent to the hospital for treatment. At admission, the patient had a pale complexion, extremely pale eyelids, conjunctiva, lips, and gums, profuse sweating, acute appearance, indifferent expression, and blood pressure of 80/45 mmHg. The residual end of the right upper arm is tied with a towel, and the clothes and pants are soaked in blood. The skin at the broken end is surrounded and scratched, and the local skin is bruised. The proximal end of the upper arm is in a loose state, with a local void. The humeral shaft is severed from the middle, with active local bleeding. There are large areas of skin abrasions on the shoulder, back, and right chest wall, with local tenderness. There is no bone friction sensation in the ribs, and the breathing sounds are clear.

The right upper arm is severed from the middle of the humerus, with a diagonal fracture of the humerus. The long segments of the ulnar and median nerves are retrogradely extracted and wrapped around the humeral shaft. The brachial artery and accompanying veins are widely extracted and severed, with a proximal free distance of about

脉及伴行静脉广泛抽脱离断，近端游离约 15 cm，肱三头肌远端从止点处离断，肱二头肌从近端横行撕脱离断，前臂掌侧及桡背侧有大面积皮肤擦伤，局部有大面积瘀斑，远端苍白无血运，肘关节前侧有皮肤缺损。肘关节和前臂未触及骨擦感骨擦音，肘关节被动活动良好（图 3.10.1）。

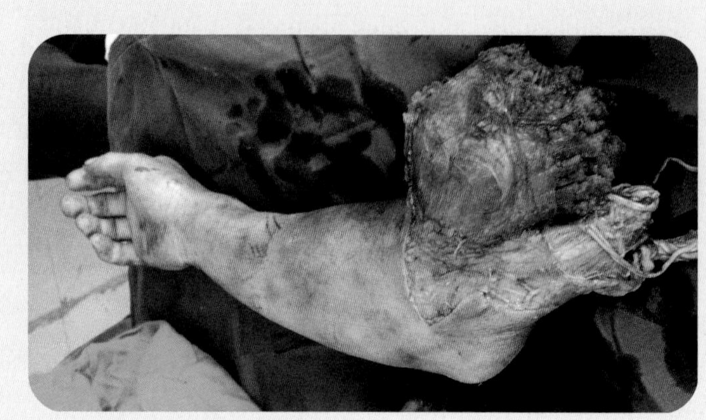

图 3.10.1　右前臂有大面积皮肤擦伤，皮肤散在瘀斑，尺神经和正中神经缠绕在肱骨干，肱二头肌断裂，局部污染重

◆ 治疗方案

右上臂完全离断，这类损伤出血凶猛，现场出血较多。入院时大多数伴有急性失血性休克。

1. 入院时局部加压止血或者上气囊止血带止血。

2. 积极建立静脉通道，快速补液，备血输血，抗休克等综合治疗。

3. 肢体远端厚棉垫包扎放冰箱低温保存。

4. 完善手术前准备。

5. 采用臂丛麻醉阻滞麻醉。

6. 手术过程

6.1 骨支架建立：肱骨干骨折采用七孔加压钢板固定。

6.2 肌肉修复：修复肱二头肌、肱肌和肱三头肌，修复血管神经着床。

6.3 神经修复：吻合桡神经、正中神经和尺神经。

6.4 血管修复：依次吻合头静脉、肱动脉两条伴行静脉及肱动脉，重组人酸性成纤维细胞生长因子冲洗血管吻合口，血管神经和肌间隙中喷洒生长因子。血管修复结束后，前臂出现广泛性肿胀，张力逐渐增高，尺动脉和桡动脉搏动减弱，反流迟缓，皮温低，皮肤苍白，考虑为缺血性痉挛急性期，故给予前臂切开筋膜室减压，前臂切开减压后，手部血运逐渐红润，桡动脉尺动脉搏动有力。闭合再植伤口，前臂减压切口 +

15 cm. The distal end of the triceps brachii is severed from the insertion point, and the biceps brachii is torn and severed laterally from the proximal end. There are large areas of skin abrasions on the palmar and dorsal sides of the forearm, with large areas of bruising locally. The distal end is pale and lacks blood supply, and there is a skin defect on the anterior side of the elbow joint. The elbow joint and forearm did not touch the bone friction sensation, and the passive movement of the elbow joint was good (Figure 3.10.1).

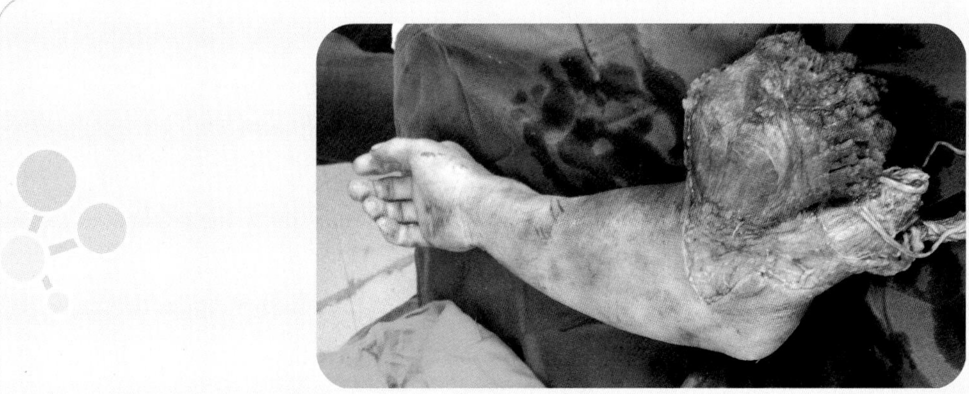

Figure 3.10.1 There is a large area of skin abrasion on the right forearm, with scattered bruising on the skin. The ulnar nerve and median nerve are wrapped around the humeral shaft, and the biceps brachii muscle is broken, with severe local contamination

◆ Treatment plan

The right upper arm is completely severed, and this type of injury causes severe bleeding, with more bleeding on site. Most patients are admitted with acute hemorrhagic shock.

1. Apply local pressure or use an airbag tourniquet to stop bleeding upon admission.

2. Actively establish venous channels, quickly replenish fluids, prepare blood for transfusion, and provide comprehensive treatment such as anti-shock.

3. Wrap the distal limbs with thick cotton pads and store them in a refrigerator at low temperature.

4. Improve preoperative preparation.

5. Use brachial plexus anesthesia and block anesthesia.

6. Surgical process

6.1 Establishment of bone scaffold: Brachial shaft fractures are fixed using a seven hole compression steel plate.

6.2 Muscle repair: Repair the biceps, brachii, and triceps muscles, and repair vascular and nerve implantation.

6.3 Neural repair: anastomosis of radial nerve, median nerve, and ulnar nerve.

6.4 Vascular repair: sequentially anastomose the two accompanying veins of the cephalic vein and brachial artery, as well as the brachial artery. Rinse the vascular anastomosis with recombinant human acidic fibroblast growth factor, and spray growth factor into the vascular nerve and muscle spaces. After the vascular repair was completed, there was widespread swelling in the forearm, gradually increasing tension, weakened pulsation of the ulnar and radial arteries, slow reflux, low skin temperature, and pale skin. It was considered to be an acute phase of ischemic spasm, so the forearm was incised into the fascial compartment for decompression. After the forearm was incised for decompression, the blood flow in the hand gradually turned red, and the radial and ulnar arteries had

VSD+ 生长因子滴注冲洗，石膏固定。

7. 手术后继续扩容、解痉，补充血容量，纠正休克，预防感染。由于大段肢体离断出血量多，手术后纠正休克十分关键。

8. 抬高患肢减轻肿胀，室内保温，加强换药，断肢伤口每天喷洒生长因子促进愈合，严密观察肢体血运。

9. 术后 3 天拔出再植伤口引流条，拆除前臂 VSD 装置。每天创面喷洒生长因子，加强换药，减张创面肉芽组织新鲜后，创面植皮（图 3.10.2 ~ 图 3.10.5）。2 周开始进行肩肘腕手功能训练。

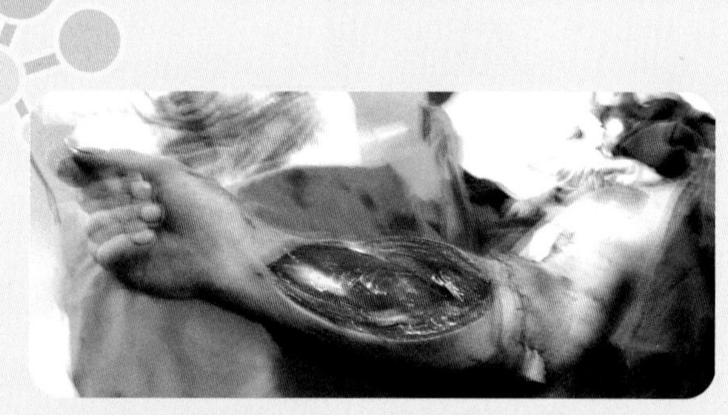

图 3.10.2 断肢再植后，前臂出现缺血性挛缩，影响肢体血运，术后及时切开减压，VSD 覆盖切口

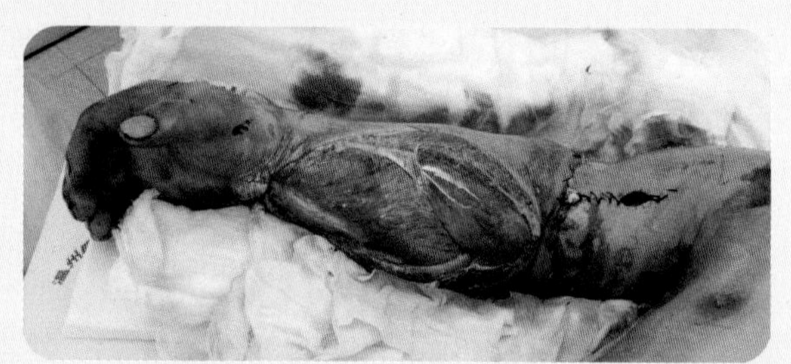

图 3.10.3 断肢再植后 10 天，前臂高度肿胀前臂肌肉水肿，肉芽组织不新鲜，每天更换敷料 2 次，并喷洒重组人酸性成纤维细胞生长因子

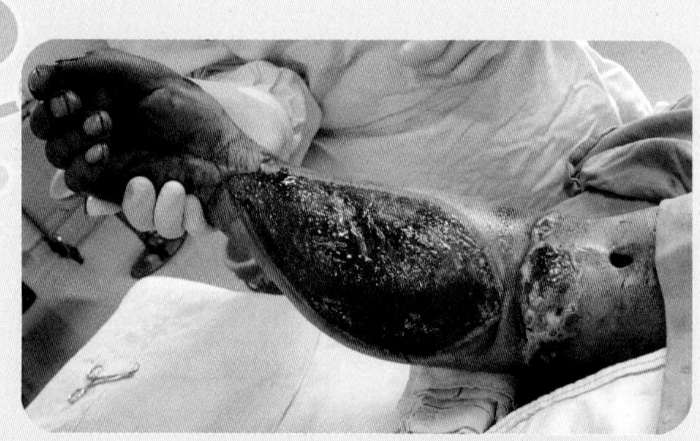

图 3.10.4 右前臂经过换药喷洒重组人酸性成纤维细胞生长因子后，前臂减张创面逐渐新鲜，肿胀减退，可以行植皮手术

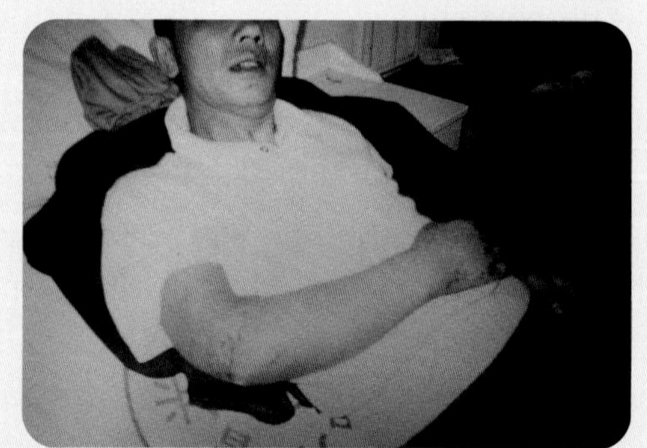

图 3.10.5 断肢再植 1.5 个月，再植成活，前臂减张创面植皮成活

（陈善亮　吴思苗）

strong pulsation. Close the replanted wound, perform forearm decompression incision + VSD + growth factor drip irrigation, and fix with plaster.

7. Continue to expand and relieve spasms after surgery, replenish blood volume, correct shock, and prevent infection. Correcting shock after surgery is crucial due to the high amount of bleeding caused by large limb amputation.

8. Raise the affected limb to reduce swelling, keep it warm indoors, strengthen dressing changes, spray growth factors daily on the severed limb wound to promote healing, and closely monitor limb blood circulation.

9. Three days after surgery, remove the replanted wound drainage strip and dismantle the forearm VSD device. Spray growth factors on the wound every day, strengthen dressing changes, reduce the tension of granulation tissue, and then graft skin onto the wound (Figure 3.10.2-Figure 3.10.5). Shoulder, elbow, wrist, and hand function training will begin in 2 weeks.

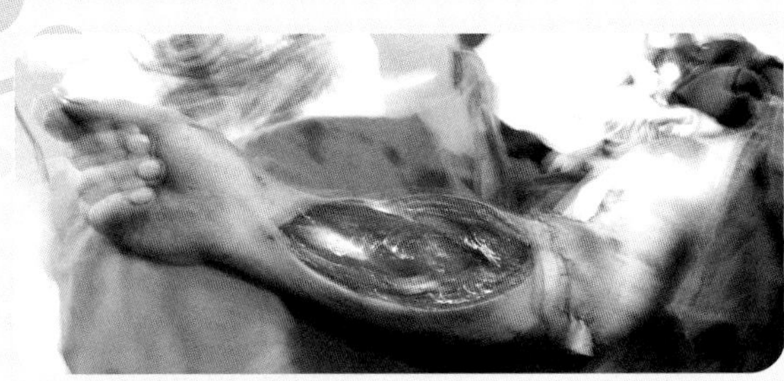

Figure 3.10.2 After limb replantation, ischemic contracture occurred in the forearm, affecting limb blood supply. After surgery, timely incision and decompression were performed, and VSD covered the incision

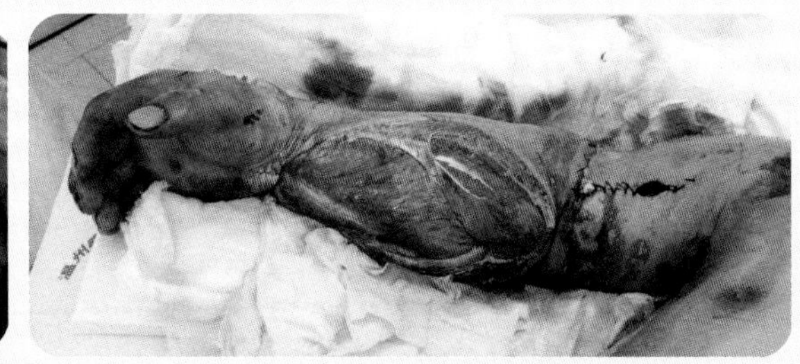

Figure 3.10.3 Ten days after limb replantation, the forearm is highly swollen, the forearm muscles are swollen, and the granulation tissue is not fresh. The dressing is changed twice a day and recombinant human acidic fibroblast growth factor is sprayed

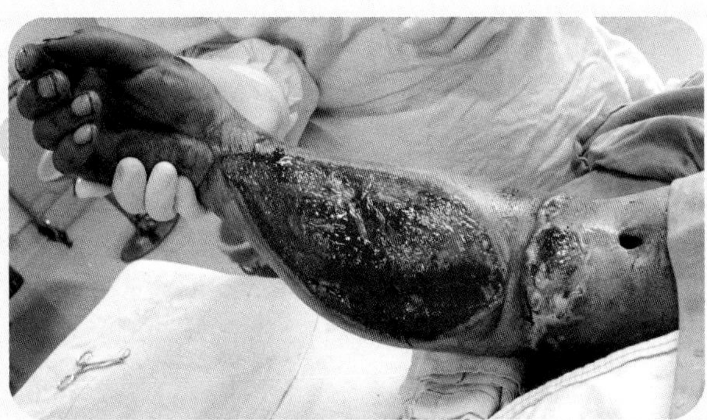

Figure 3.10.4 After changing the dressing and spraying recombinant human acidic fibroblast growth factor on the right forearm, the tension reducing wound on the forearm gradually becomes fresh, the swelling decreases, and skin grafting surgery can be performed

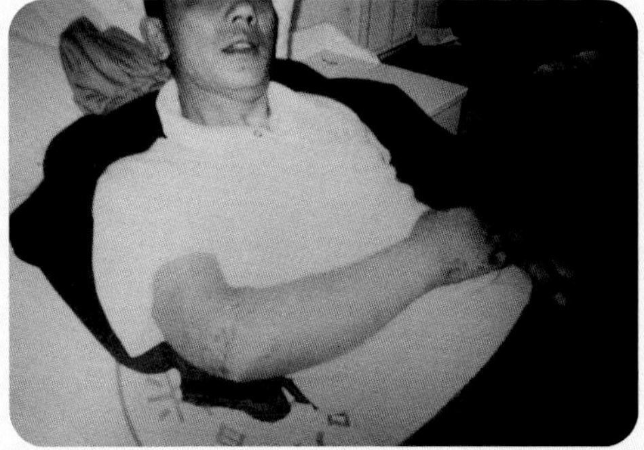

Figure 3.10.5 Limb replantation for 1.5 months, successful replantation, and successful skin grafting on the reduced tension wound of the forearm

(Chen Shanliang, Wu Simiao)

案例十一　孕妇上臂多段撕脱性离断

◆ 损伤原因

患者，女性，29 岁，怀孕 7 个月，高速发生车祸，左上肢和高速护栏碰撞，致上臂离断。

◆ 症状与体征

急性痛苦面容，面色苍白，血压 110/60 mmHg，无腹痛，阴道无出血，产科会诊胎心良好，无流产迹象。左上臂中段呈脱套状离断，肱骨干多段粉碎骨折伴缺损，上臂皮肤软组织呈套袖样脱套，肱二头肌和肱三头肌离断，肱动脉伴行静脉、头静脉和贵要静脉抽脱离断，局部出血活跃，正中神经、尺神经和桡神经抽脱离断，断端参差不齐。离断肢体远端苍白无血运，小鱼际肌处有 6 cm 斜行伤口，深达第 5 掌骨，尺神经深支离断，小鱼际肌离断，小指屈指深浅肌腱离断（图 3.11.1、图 3.11.2）。

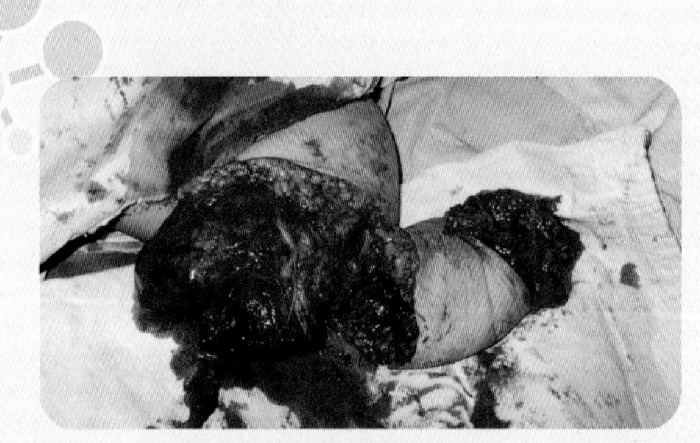

图 3.11.1　左上臂呈套袖样脱套离断、肱二头肌肱三头肌多段撕脱离断，血管神经长段抽脱

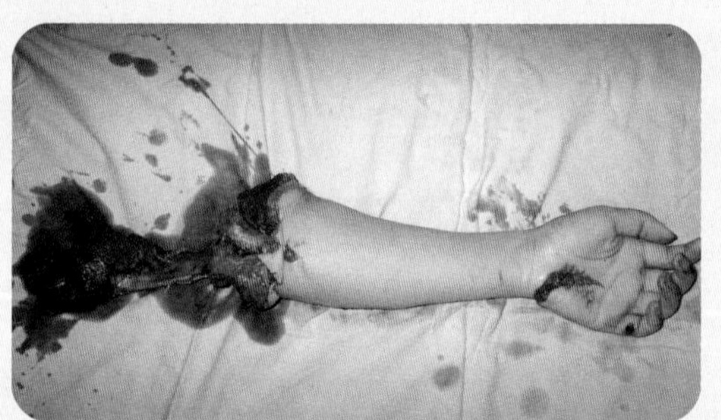

图 3.11.2　肱三头肌逆行撕脱，桡神经逆行抽脱离断 16 cm，肢体离断断面不整齐

◆ 治疗方案

该案例患者怀孕 7 个月，左上肢遭受高能量损伤，对治疗带来新的挑战，保护患者生命安全、保护胎儿安全、保护肢体成活。

1. 入院后积极建立静脉通道，上肢加压包扎止血，积极抗休克，离断肢体低温保存。同时发起产科会诊，会诊后无羊水破裂，阴道无流血。

2. 完善手术前准备，预在臂丛麻醉下行断肢再植手术。

3. 手术过程

3.1 骨支架建立：肱骨干短缩 10 cm、6 孔加压钢板固定。

Case 11 Multiple segment tearing and detachment of the upper arm in pregnant women

◆ Cause of injury

Patient, female, 29 years old, 7 months pregnant, had a car accident on the highway. Her left upper limb collided with the highway guardrail, causing her upper arm to be severed.

◆ Signs and symptoms

Acute painful facial appearance, pale complexion, blood pressure 110/60 mmHg, no abdominal pain, no vaginal bleeding, obstetric consultation shows good fetal heart rate, no signs of miscarriage. The middle section of the left upper arm is dislocated, with multiple comminuted fractures of the humeral shaft accompanied by defects. The skin and soft tissue of the upper arm are dislocated in a sleeve like manner. The biceps and triceps muscles are dislocated, and the brachial artery is accompanied by veins such as the cephalic vein and the basilic vein. Local bleeding is active, and the median nerve, ulnar nerve, and radial nerve are dislocated with uneven ends. The distal end of the severed limb is pale and lacks blood supply. There is a 6 cm oblique wound at the small fish border muscle, reaching as deep as the 5th metacarpal bone. The deep branch of the ulnar nerve is severed, the small fish border muscle is severed, and the deep and shallow flexor tendons of the little finger are severed (Figure 3.11.1, Figure 3.11.2).

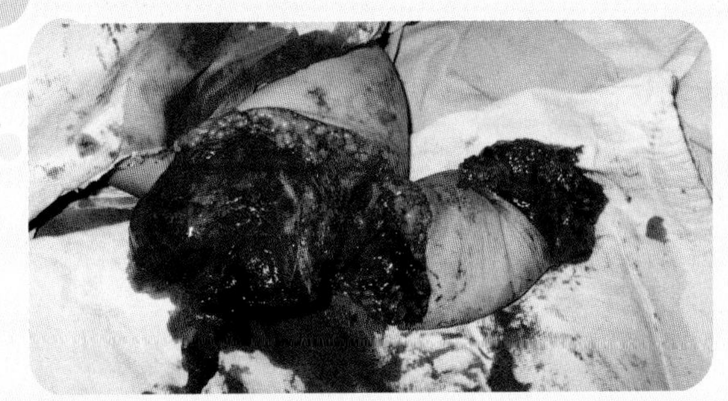

Figure 3.11.1 The left upper arm shows a sleeve like detachment, with multiple segments of the biceps and triceps muscles torn apart and severed, and long segments of blood vessels and nerves extracted

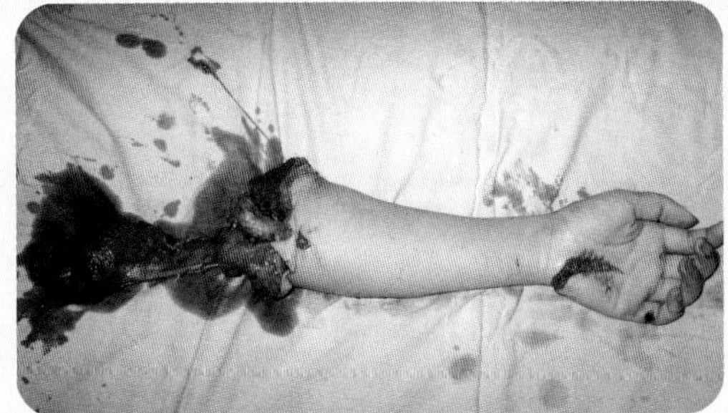

Figure 3.11.2 Retrograde tear of the triceps brachii, retrograde extraction of the radial nerve, and a 16 cm transection, resulting in an irregular cross-section of the severed limb

◆ Treatment plan

The patient in this case was 7 months pregnant and suffered high-energy damage to the left upper limb, which posed new challenges to treatment and protected the patient's life safety, fetal safety, and limb survival.

1. After admission, actively establish a venous channel, apply pressure and bandage to stop bleeding in the upper limbs, actively resist shock, and store the severed limbs at low temperature. At the same time, an obstetric consultation was initiated, and after the consultation, there was no amniotic fluid rupture or vaginal bleeding.

2. Improve preoperative preparation and perform limb replantation surgery under brachial plexus anesthesia.

3. Surgical process

3.1 Establishment of bone scaffold: Brachial shaft shortened by 10 cm and fixed with 6-hole compression steel plate.

3.2 肌肉修复：肱三头肌、肱二头肌、肱肌和部分三角肌缝合，修复血管神经着床。

3.3 神经修复：修剪神经断端，依次缝合桡神经、尺神经、正中神经、臂内侧皮神经，修复小鱼际肌及手掌部尺神经深支。

3.4 血管修复：修建血管吻合口，配备重组人酸性成纤维细胞生长因子冲洗液，冲洗血管管腔，依次吻合两条肱静脉、肱动脉、头静脉、肘正中静脉，重组人酸性成纤维细胞生长因子喷洒肌间隙，伤口深部放置引流条，逐层缝合伤口，包扎伤口，石膏固定。

4. 手术后严密监测胎心变化，观察是否有迟发子宫破裂，迟发流产可能。

5. 手术后继续扩容解痉，补充血容量，纠正休克，预防感染。

6. 严密观察生命体征，抬高患肢，减轻肿胀，肢体血运变化。

7. 加强换药，术后 3 天拔出引流条，半个月后拆线。

8. 石膏固定 4 周，去除石膏后功能训练（图 3.11.3）。

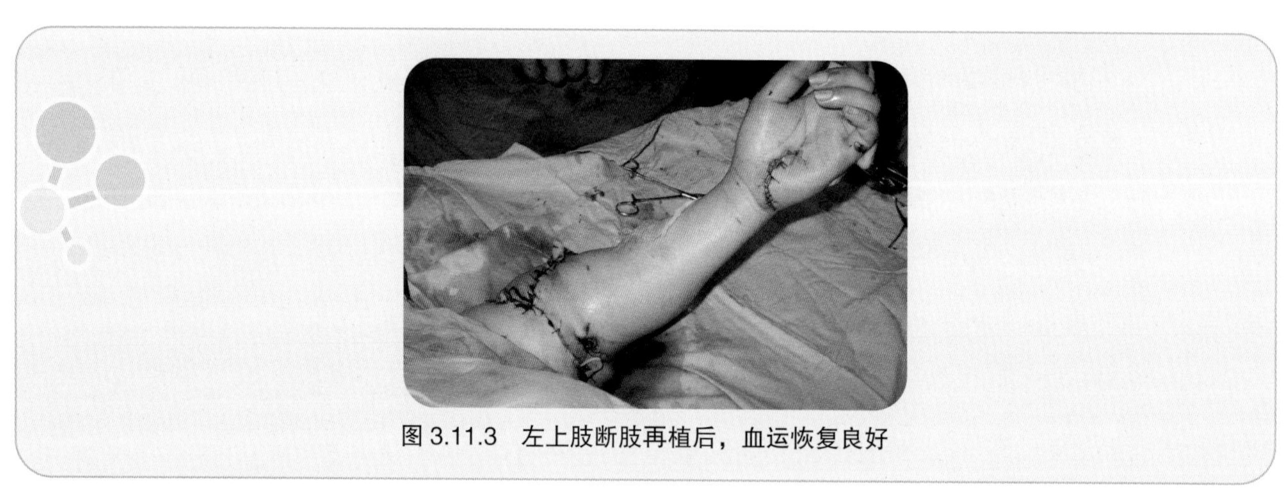

图 3.11.3　左上肢断肢再植后，血运恢复良好

（陈善亮　皮艳青）

案例十二　上臂部撕脱性离断

◆ 损伤原因

患者戴手套工作时，被卷入机器中，致右上臂撕脱性离断。

◆ 症状与体征

急性病容，剧痛难忍，衣裤被鲜血湿透，严重贫血貌，面色、齿龈、眼睑、口唇苍白，全身湿冷，心率增快，

3.2 Muscle repair: Suture of triceps, biceps, brachii, and partial deltoid muscles to repair vascular and nerve implantation.

3.3 Neural repair: Trim the nerve stump, suture the radial nerve, ulnar nerve, median nerve, and medial cutaneous nerve of the arm in sequence, repair the small fish border muscle and deep branch of the ulnar nerve in the palm.

3.4 Vascular repair: Construct vascular anastomosis, equip with recombinant human acidic fibroblast growth factor flushing solution, flush the vascular lumen, sequentially anastomose two brachial veins, brachial artery, cephalic vein, and median cubital vein, spray recombinant human acidic fibroblast growth factor into the muscle space, place drainage strips deep in the wound, suture the wound layer by layer, bandage the wound, and fix it with plaster.

4. After surgery, closely monitor changes in fetal heart rate and observe whether there is a possibility of delayed uterine rupture or delayed miscarriage.

5. Continue to expand and relieve spasms after surgery, replenish blood volume, correct shock, and prevent infection.

6. Monitor vital signs closely, elevate the affected limb, reduce swelling, and monitor changes in limb blood circulation.

7. Strengthen dressing changes, remove the drainage strip 3 days after surgery, and remove the stitches half a month later.

8. Gypsum fixation for 4 weeks, functional training after removal of gypsum (Figure 3.11.3).

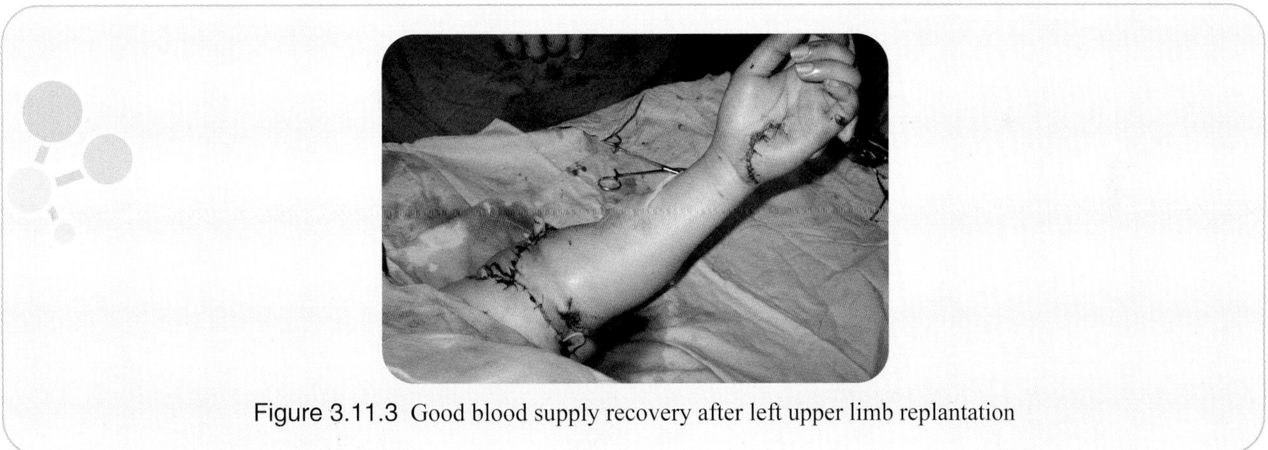

Figure 3.11.3 Good blood supply recovery after left upper limb replantation

(Chen Shanliang, Pi Yanqing)

Case 12 Tearing and detachment of upper arm

◆ Cause of injury

The patient was caught in the machine while wearing gloves at work, causing tearing and detachment of the right upper arm.

◆ Signs and symptoms

Acute appearance, unbearable pain, clothes soaked in blood, severely anemic appearance, pale complexion,

血压 70/40 mmHg，表情淡漠。右上臂上段完全离断，肱二头肌和肱三头肌从肌腱移行处撕脱离断，三角肌从肌腹中段撕脱离断。肱动脉及伴行静脉从腋窝处撕脱离断，正中神经尺神经桡神经从肱骨中段撕脱离断，肌皮神经从肩部撕脱离断，肱骨干从中段骨折离断，远端环形脱套状离断，断端整齐，远端皮肤有大面积皮肤瘀斑及擦皮伤，前臂尺桡骨骨擦音、骨擦感阳性，被动反常活动，手背有大面积擦伤，远端肢体完整，苍白无血运（图 3.12.1 ～图 3.12.4）。右侧上腹部有大面积擦皮伤。

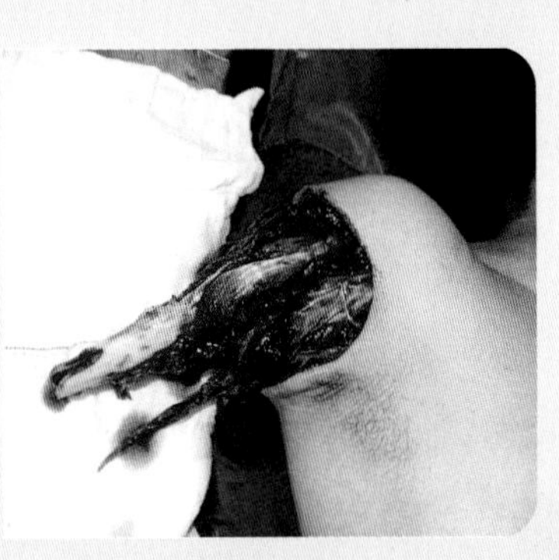

图 3.12.1　右上臂上段有撕脱创面，肱动脉及伴行静脉长段撕脱断裂，搏动性出血，肱二头肌和肱三头肌呈条索状撕脱离断，肱骨干横行骨折，断端皮肤整齐

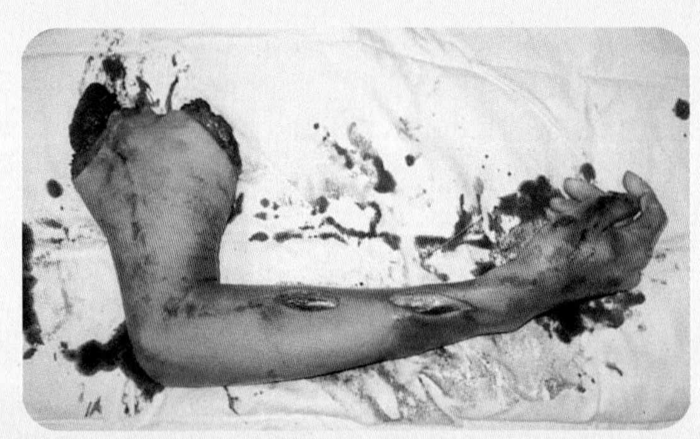

图 3.12.2　右上肢远端较为完整，皮肤有大面积瘀斑及擦伤，上臂呈脱套状离断，尺桡骨骨擦感、骨擦音阳性，远端苍白无血运

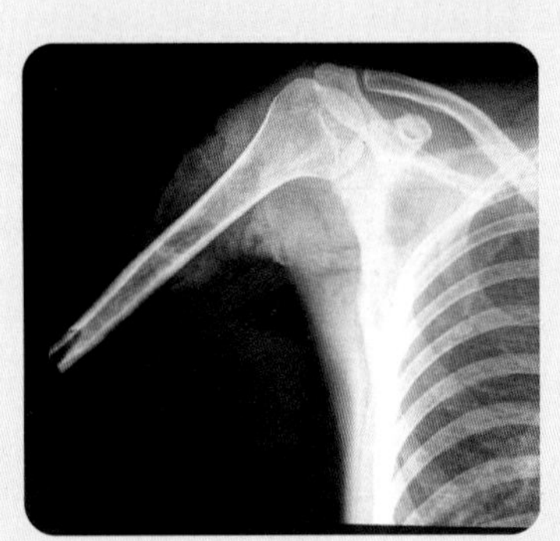

图 3.12.3　右上臂中段骨折、断端粉碎性骨折

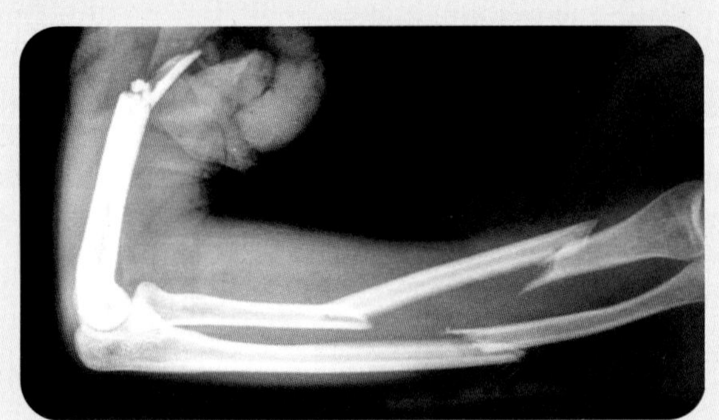

图 3.12.4　桡骨两段骨折，尺骨中段骨折

◆ 治疗方案

这类患肢高位离断伤，血管粗大，离断后出血凶猛，入院时大多伴有失血性休克，积极包扎止血，抗

gums, eyelids, lips, wet and cold whole body, increased heart rate, blood pressure of 70/40 mmHg, indifferent expression. The upper part of the right upper arm is completely severed, and the biceps and triceps muscles are torn off and severed from the tendon transition. The deltoid muscle is torn off and severed from the mid segment of the muscle belly. The brachial artery and accompanying veins are torn and severed from the axilla, the median nerve, ulnar nerve, and radial nerve are torn and severed from the middle section of the humerus, the cutaneous nerve is torn and severed from the shoulder, the humeral shaft is fractured and severed from the middle section, and the distal end is detached in a circular shape with neat ends. There are large areas of skin bruising and abrasions on the distal skin. The ulnar and radial bones of the forearm have positive abrasions and bone abrasions, passive abnormal movement, and large areas of abrasions on the back of the hand. The distal limb is intact and pale without blood circulation (Figure 3.12.1- Figure 3.12.4). There is a large area of abrasions on the upper right abdomen.

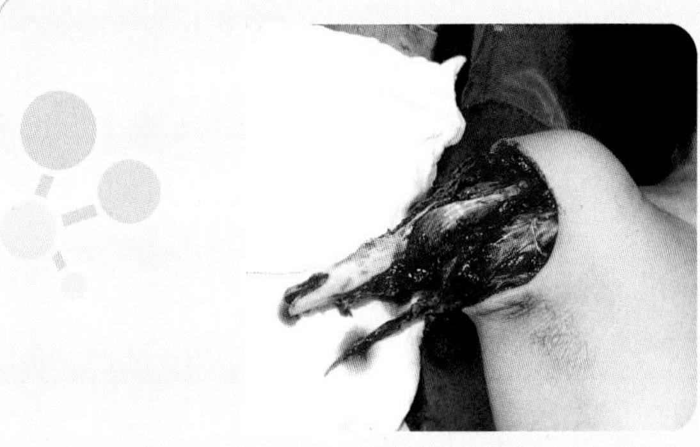

Figure 3.12.1 There is a torn wound in the upper right upper arm, with a long segment of the brachial artery and accompanying vein torn off and broken, pulsating bleeding. The biceps and triceps muscles are torn off and broken in a cord like manner, and the humeral shaft is horizontally fractured with neat skin at the broken end

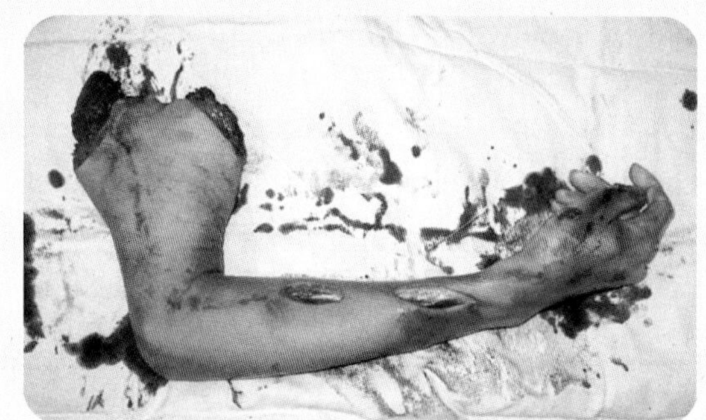

Figure 3.12.2 The distal end of the right upper limb is relatively intact, with large areas of bruising and abrasions on the skin. The upper arm is detached and broken, and there is a positive bone friction sensation and sound in the radius and ulna. The distal end is pale and lacks blood circulation

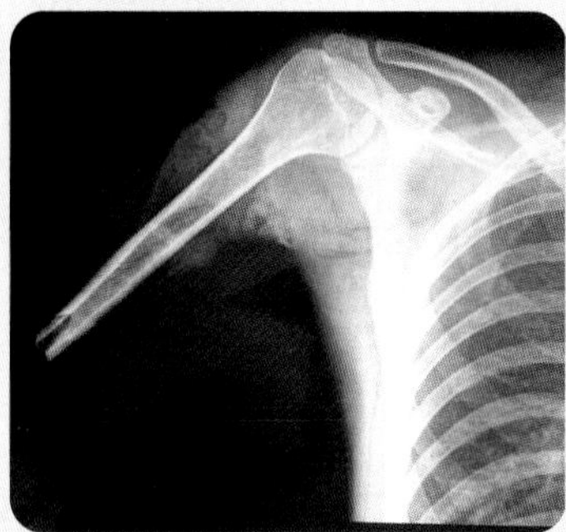

Figure 3.12.3 Middle right upper arm fracture and comminuted fracture at the fracture end

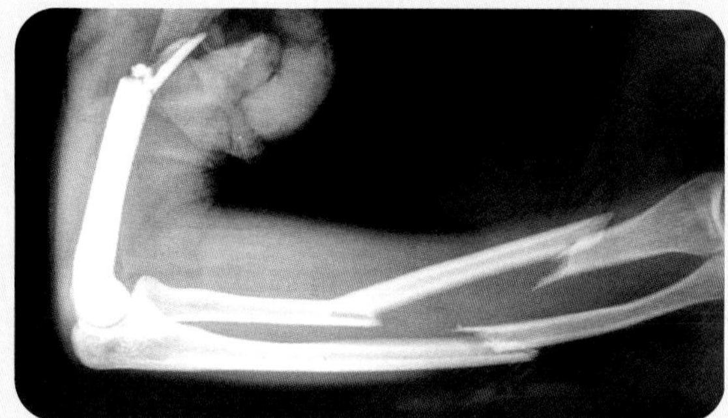

Figure 3.12.4 Two segment radius fracture and mid segment ulna fracture

◆ Treatment plan

This type of high position amputation injury of the affected limb has large blood vessels and fierce bleeding after amputation. When admitted, it is often accompanied by hemorrhagic shock. Active bandaging to stop bleeding

休克仍是治疗的关键，近端血管广泛抽脱离断，用血管钳钳夹止血有效而彻底，然后加压包扎。

1. 积极建立静脉通道，快速补液，备血输血，完善相关检查，排查胸腹部复合伤。

2. 肢体远端临时包扎放冰箱中保存。

3. 纠正休克后，完善手术前检查，进入手术室行断臂再植术。

4. 选用全身麻醉。

5. 此案例属于高位断臂，而且前臂有多段粉碎性骨折，手术可分为两组人员同时进行，一组人员行近端清创，显露血管神经肌肉组织，短缩肱骨备再植时用；另一组人员行尺桡骨骨折切开复位钢板内固定，桡骨两段骨折，采用加长锁定钢板植入固定，前臂尺桡骨骨折复位固定后。前臂骨折手术结束后，两组合一组进行断肢再植手术。

6. 手术过程

6.1 骨支架建立：肱骨短缩 5 cm。骨折复位后采用 6 孔锁定加压钢板植入固定。

6.2 肌肉修复：修复肱二头肌、肱三头肌、三角肌及胸大肌肱骨头，修复血管着床。

6.3 神经修复：依次缝合桡神经、正中神经、尺神经、肌皮神经、臂内侧皮神经。

6.4 血管修复：配备生长因子冲洗液，并用重组人酸性成纤维细胞生长因子冲洗液冲洗血管管腔，依次吻合肱动脉及两条伴行静脉、头静脉。创面深部放置四条橡皮条引流，逐层缝合伤口，包扎，术终，应用过肩长臂石膏固定。

7. 手术后积极抗休克、扩容、解痉抗炎镇痛，仍是术后重要工作之一，尽管手术前已经纠正休克，由于手术时间久，骨折断端、手术切口，仍会有大量液体渗出，所以术后 3 天仍是抗休克治疗的关键（图 3.12.5）。

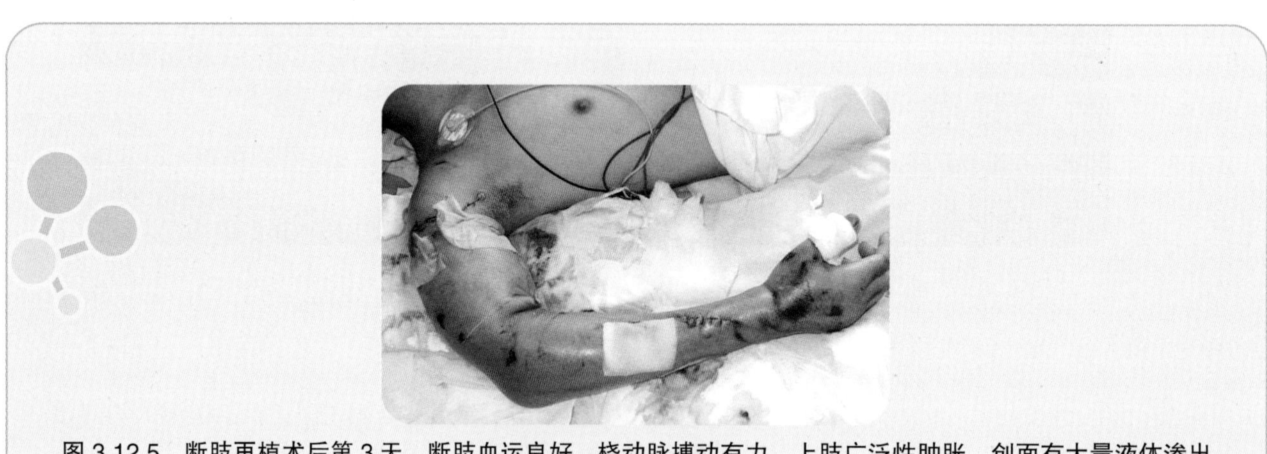

图 3.12.5　断肢再植术后第 3 天，断肢血运良好，桡动脉搏动有力，上肢广泛性肿胀，创面有大量液体渗出

is still the key to treatment. The proximal blood vessels are widely extracted and detached, and effective and thorough hemostasis is achieved by clamping with vascular clamps, followed by pressure bandaging.

1. Actively establish venous channels, quickly replenish fluids, prepare blood transfusions, complete relevant examinations, and investigate chest and abdominal composite injuries.

2. Temporarily wrap the distal end of the limb and store it in the refrigerator.

3. After correcting shock, complete preoperative examination and enter the operating room for arm replantation surgery.

4. Use general anesthesia.

5. This case belongs to a high-level severed arm, and there are multiple comminuted fractures in the forearm. The surgery can be performed simultaneously by two groups of personnel. One group of personnel performs proximal debridement to expose vascular, nerve, and muscle tissue, which is used for shortening the humerus for replanting; Another group of personnel underwent open reduction and internal fixation with steel plates for fractures of the radius and ulna. Two segments of the radius were fractured and fixed with extended locking steel plates implanted. After reduction and fixation of the forearm radius and ulna fractures. After the forearm fracture surgery, a combination of two groups will undergo limb replantation surgery.

6. Surgical process

6.1 Establishment of bone scaffold: humeral shortening of 5 cm. After fracture reduction, a 6-hole locking compression steel plate was implanted for fixation.

6.2 Muscle repair: Repair the biceps, triceps, deltoid, and pectoralis major muscles of the humeral head, and repair vascular implantation.

6.3 Neural repair: Suture the radial nerve, median nerve, ulnar nerve, cutaneous nerve, and medial brachial nerve in sequence.

6.4 Vascular repair: Equipped with growth factor flushing solution, and using recombinant human acidic fibroblast growth factor flushing solution to flush the vascular lumen, sequentially anastomose the brachial artery and two accompanying veins, as well as the cephalic vein. Four rubber strips were placed deep in the wound for drainage, and the wound was sutured layer by layer, bandaged, and fixed with shoulder and long arm plaster at the end of the surgery.

7. Actively anti shock, volume expansion, antispasmodic, anti-inflammatory and analgesic treatment after surgery is still one of the important postoperative tasks. Although shock has been corrected before surgery, due to the long operation time, there will still be a large amount of fluid leakage from the fracture site and surgical incision. Therefore, 3 days after surgery is still the key to anti shock treatment (Figure 3.12.5).

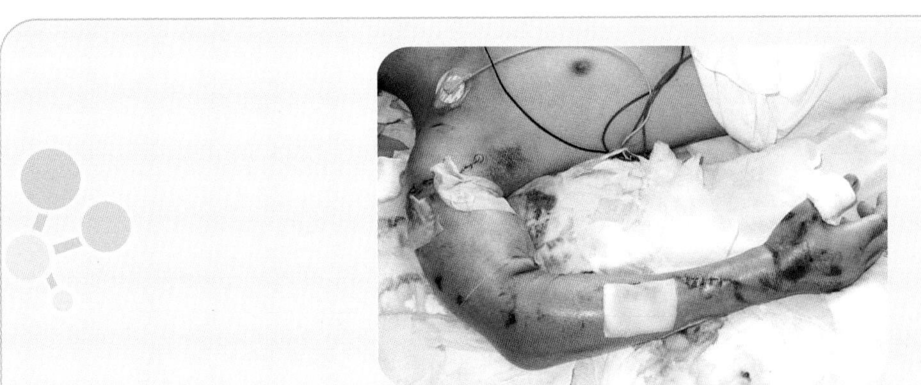

Figure 3.12.5 On the third day after limb replantation, the blood supply of the severed limb was good, the radial artery pulsation was strong, the upper limb was extensively swollen, and there was a large amount of fluid leakage from the wound

8. 病室保温，抬高患肢，加强换药，严格观察肢体血运及肿胀，加强护理及心理疏导，积极预防断肢再植术后并发症。

9. 术后 3 天被动手部关节训练，断肢再植成活后 15 天，循序渐进地进行大关节松动以预防关节僵硬、肌肉萎缩，早起神经营养及周围神经康复治疗。

10. 术后换药时伤口常规喷洒重组人酸性成纤维细胞生长因子促进伤口愈合。

（陈善亮）

案例十三　腕部切割性离断

◆ 损伤原因

患者左手被钢板切割机切伤，致腕部切割性离断。

◆ 症状与体征

左手腕关节离断后剧痛，出血不止，伤后工友用腰带扎住前臂止血，现场出血不多，急诊送来院，左腕部从近排腕骨处离断，断端整齐，断面污染较轻，关节面切割性骨折伴缺损，手腕远端完整，苍白无血运，肘关节远端有皮带捆扎止血（图 3.13.1、图 3.13.2）。

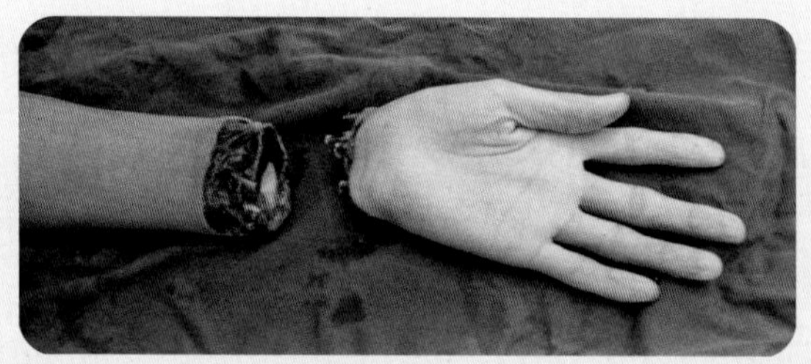

图 3.13.1　左腕关节处完全离断，断端整齐完整，远端苍白无血运

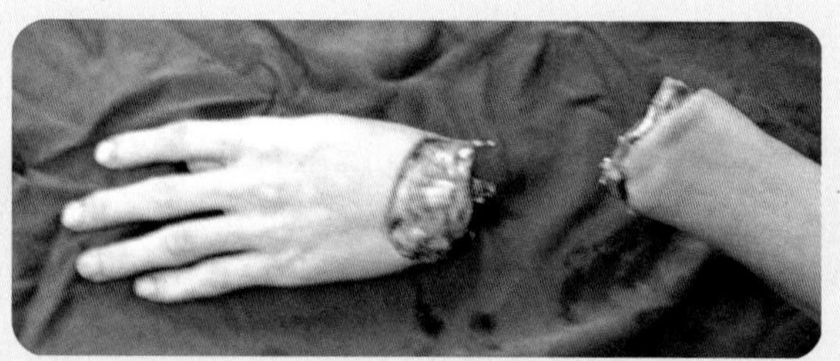

图 3.13.2　断端关节面缺损，皮肤回缩

◆ 治疗方案

该案例为低位断肢再植，通过精细显微外科修复手术大多数会获得良好功能康复。

1. 入院采取止血加压包扎，松开自行捆绑的止血带（由于工友捆扎的止血带压力容易损伤局部皮肤甚至深部组织），远端送冰箱低温保存。

8. Keep the ward warm, elevate the affected limb, strengthen dressing changes, strictly observe limb blood flow and swelling, strengthen nursing and psychological counseling, and actively prevent complications after limb replantation surgery.

9. Three days after surgery, passive hand joint training was performed. Fifteen days after the limb was successfully replanted, large joint loosening was gradually performed to prevent joint stiffness and muscle atrophy. Early neurotrophic and peripheral nerve rehabilitation treatment were also administered.

10. During postoperative dressing changes, the wound is routinely sprayed with recombinant human acidic fibroblast growth factor to promote wound healing.

(Chen Shanliang)

Case 13 Severely severed wrist

◆ Cause of injury

The patient's left hand was cut by a steel plate cutting machine, resulting in wrist amputation.

◆ Signs and symptoms

After the left wrist joint was severed, there was severe pain and continuous bleeding. After the injury, the colleague tied the forearm with a belt to stop the bleeding. There was not much bleeding on site, and the patient was sent to the hospital for emergency treatment. The left wrist was severed from the proximal wrist bone, with a neat fracture end and light contamination of the section. The joint surface was cut and fractured with defects, and the distal end of the wrist was intact, pale and without blood circulation. The distal end of the elbow joint was tied with a belt to stop bleeding (Figure 3.13.1, Figure 3.13.2).

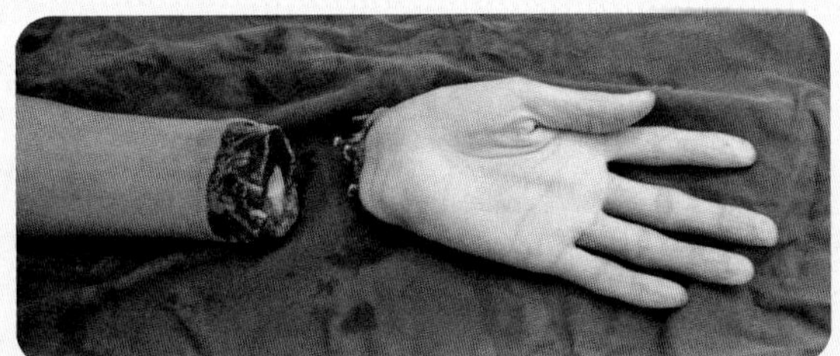

Figure 3.13.1 The left wrist joint is completely severed, with the severed end neat and intact, and the distal end pale and bloodless

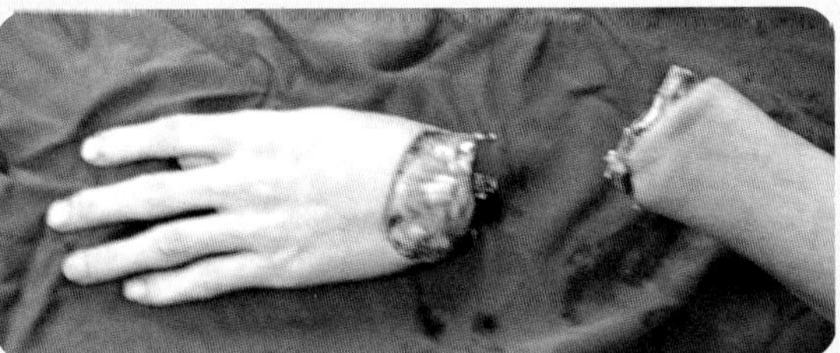

Figure 3.13.2 Fracture joint surface defect, skin retraction

◆ Treatment plan

This case is a low limb replantation, and most cases will achieve good functional recovery through fine microsurgical repair surgery.

1. Upon admission, hemostasis and pressure bandaging were performed, and the self bound tourniquet was loosened (due to the pressure of the tourniquet tied by a colleague, it can easily damage local skin or even deep tissues). The distal part was sent to a refrigerator for low-temperature storage.

2. 建立静脉通道，快速静脉补液，完善手术前检查。

3. 选用臂丛神经阻滞麻醉，三角肌下上气囊止血带。

4. 手术过程

4.1 骨支架建立：去除近排腕骨及桡骨尺骨关节面，取两枚 2.0 粗克氏针纵行固定并融合腕关节，修复骨膜覆盖融合腕关节。

4.2 肌腱修复：依次修复伸腕肌腱、拇长伸肌腱及示指、中指、环指、小指肌腱。修复屈腕肌腱、拇长屈肌腱及示指、中指、环指、小指屈指深浅肌腱，修补腱鞘和血管神经着床。

4.3 神经修复：依次修复正中神经、尺神经、尺神经手背支和桡神经鼻咽窝支。

4.4 血管修复：配制生长因子冲洗液，并用重组人碱性成纤维细胞生长因子冲洗液冲洗血管管腔，依次吻合桡动脉尺动脉及其伴行静脉，吻合头静脉及贵要静脉。动脉静脉比例为 2 ∶ 6。血管神经肌肉间隙中喷洒重组人酸性成纤维细胞生长因子，伤口深部放置引流条，逐层缝合伤口，包扎，石膏外固定。

5. 手术后以预防休克为主，补充血容量，积极抗炎预防血管痉挛和血栓形成，抗肿胀。

6. 病室保温，抬高患肢，加强换药，严格观察肢体血运及肿胀，加强护理及心理疏导，积极预防断肢再植术后并发症。

7. 该部位断腕是肌腱肌肉移行处，所有肌腱都从此处通过，术后极容易出现肌腱神经粘连，手术后早起进行主动加被动功能训练可有效预防肌腱神经粘连。

8. 手术后 12 天拆线；4 周去掉石膏，并进行康复训练；3 个月拔出克氏针（图 3.13.3）。

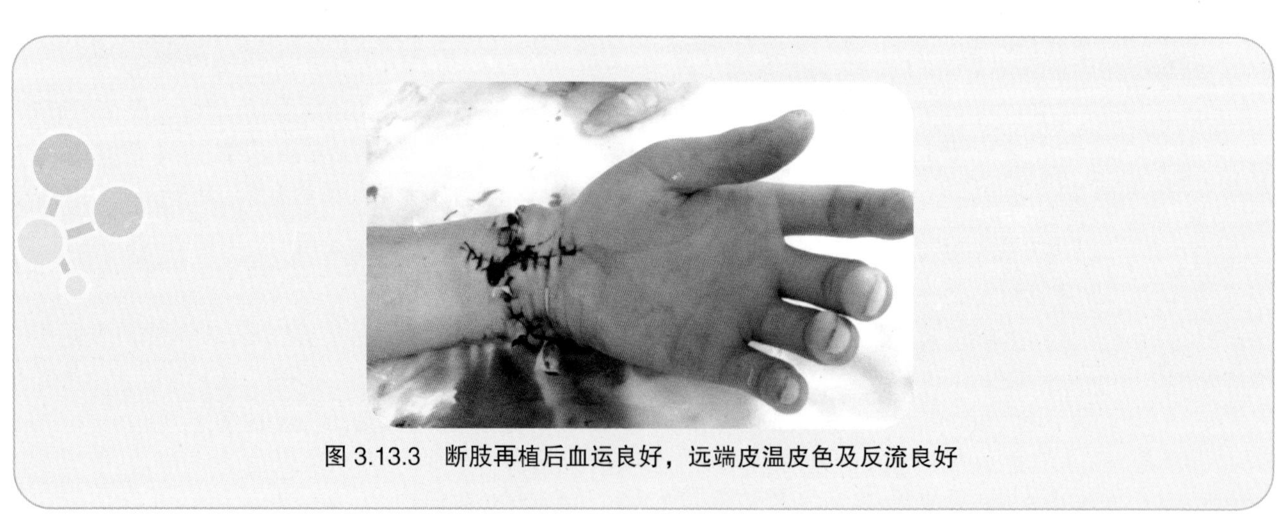

图 3.13.3　断肢再植后血运良好，远端皮温皮色及反流良好

（陈善亮）

2. Establish a venous channel for rapid intravenous fluid replacement and improve preoperative examinations.

3. Use brachial plexus block anesthesia and upper deltoid balloon tourniquet.

4. Surgical process

4.1 Establishment of bone scaffold: Remove the proximal wrist bone and the joint surface of the radius and ulna, take two 2.0 thick Kirschner wires for longitudinal fixation and fusion of the wrist joint, and repair the periosteum covering the fused wrist joint.

4.2 Tendon repair: sequentially repair the extensor carpi tendon, extensor hallucis longus tendon, as well as the tendons of the index finger, middle finger, ring finger, and little finger. Repair the flexor tendons of the wrist, flexor hallucis longus, as well as the deep and shallow flexor tendons of the index finger, middle finger, ring finger, and little finger. Repair the tendon sheath and vascular nerve implantation.

4.3 Neural repair: Repair the median nerve, ulnar nerve, ulnar nerve dorsal branch, and radial nerve nasopharyngeal fossa branch in sequence.

4.4 Vascular repair: Prepare growth factor flushing solution and flush the vascular lumen with recombinant human alkaline fibroblast growth factor flushing solution. Then, anastomose the radial artery ulnar artery and its accompanying veins, and anastomose the cephalic vein and basilic vein in sequence. The ratio of arteries to veins is 2 ∶ 6. Spray recombinant human acidic fibroblast growth factor into the gaps between blood vessels, nerves, and muscles, place drainage strips deep in the wound, suture the wound layer by layer, bandage it, and fix it externally with plaster.

5. After surgery, the main focus is on preventing shock, supplementing blood volume, actively anti-inflammatory measures to prevent vascular spasm and thrombosis, and anti-swelling.

6. Keep the ward warm, elevate the affected limb, strengthen dressing changes, strictly observe limb blood flow and swelling, strengthen nursing and psychological counseling, actively prevent complications after limb replantation surgery.

7. The wrist fracture in this area is the site of tendon and muscle migration, through which all tendons pass. Postoperative tendon and nerve adhesions are highly likely to occur. Early active and passive functional training after surgery can effectively prevent tendon and nerve adhesions.

8. Remove the stitches 12 days after surgery; Remove the plaster for 4 weeks and undergo rehabilitation training; Remove the Kirschner wire within 3 months (Figure 3.13.3).

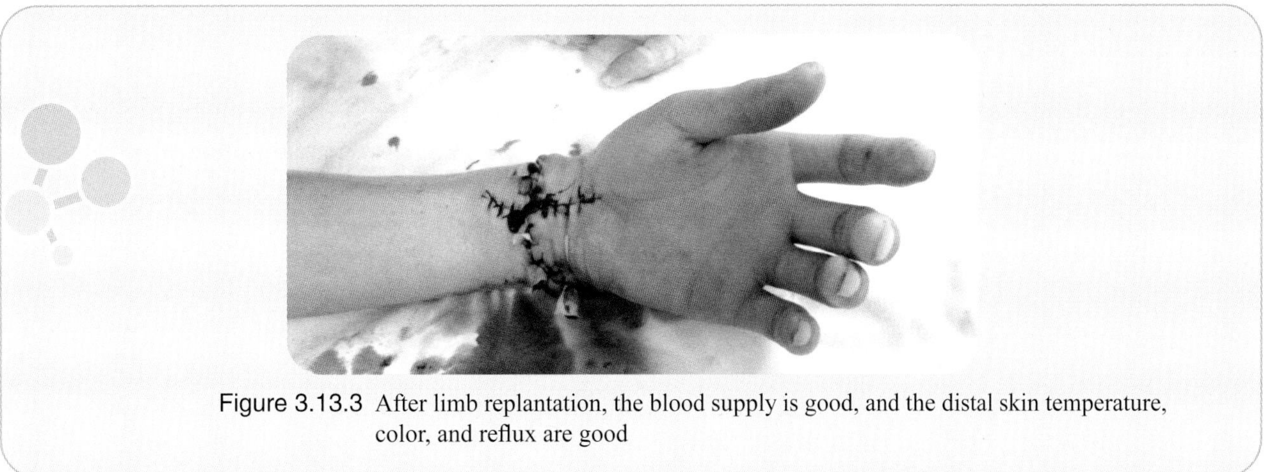

Figure 3.13.3 After limb replantation, the blood supply is good, and the distal skin temperature, color, and reflux are good

(Chen Shanliang)

案例十四　前臂刀砍伤性离断

◆ 损伤原因

患者因斗殴刀砍伤，致上肢不全离断。

◆ 症状与体征

刀砍伤后出血不止，剧痛难忍，伤后用毛巾包扎急诊入院。面色苍白、口唇、眼睑及指甲极度苍白，全身湿冷，在血压 75/35 mmHg，右侧三角肌有 12 cm 横行伤口，深达肌层，三角肌横行断裂，伤口出血活跃，前臂中段横行离断，仅前臂掌侧有 4 cm 皮蒂相连，尺骨桡骨横行骨折，桡骨粉碎性骨折；前臂伸肌群和屈肌群完全离断，桡神经尺神经和正中神经完全断裂，桡动脉尺动脉及其伴行静脉完全断裂；远端血液反流迟缓，活动完全障碍，感觉丧失（图 3.14.1、图 3.14.2）。

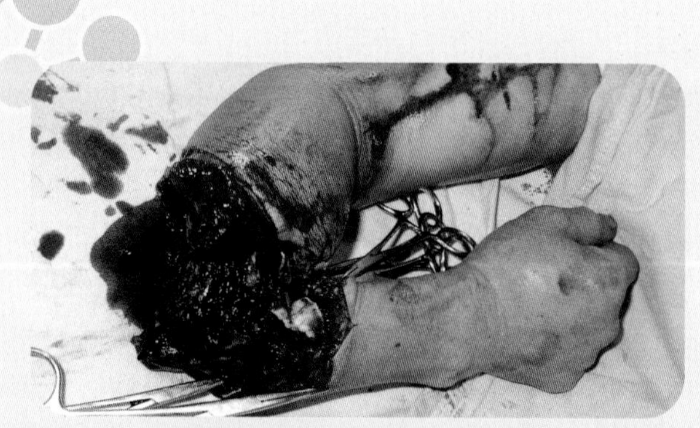

图 3.14.1　右前臂中段横行离断，断端整齐，畸形，可见横断肌肉和骨折

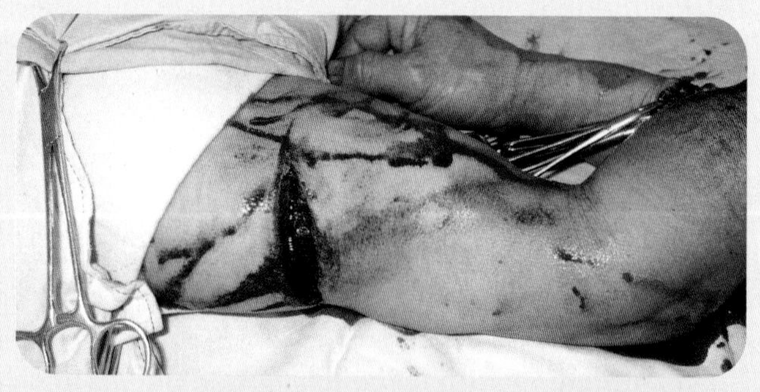

图 3.14.2　右上臂有 12 cm 横行伤口，深达肱骨打结节，三角肌大部分断裂，局部出血活跃，前臂畸形

◆ 治疗方案

1. 入院后立即钳夹止血局部加压包扎，抬高患肢。

2. 快速建立静脉通道，快速补液，备血输血，纠正休克，完善手术前准备，纠正休克后急诊行断肢再植手术。

3. 选用臂丛神经阻滞麻醉。

4. 先清创，修复三角肌及闭合肩部伤口。

5. 手术过程

5.1 骨支架建立：桡骨尺骨短缩 2 cm，骨折复位后，应用 7 孔锁定加压钢板植入固定。

Case 14 Forearm knife induced amputation

◆ Cause of injury

The patient suffered a knife wound during a fight, resulting in incomplete upper limb amputation.

◆ Signs and symptoms

After the knife cut, the bleeding continued and the pain was unbearable. The patient was admitted to the emergency department with a towel wrapped around the wound. Pale complexion, extremely pale lips, eyelids, and nails, damp and cold throughout the body, with a blood pressure of 75/35 mmHg. There is a 12 cm transverse wound on the right deltoid muscle, deep into the muscle layer, with transverse rupture of the deltoid muscle and active bleeding from the wound. The middle part of the forearm is transverse and disconnected, with only a 4 cm pedicle connected to the palmar side of the forearm. There is a transverse fracture of the ulna and radius, and a comminuted fracture of the radius; The extensor and flexor muscle groups of the forearm are completely severed, the radial nerve ulnar nerve and median nerve are completely severed, and the radial artery ulnar artery and its accompanying veins are completely severed; Remote blood reflux is delayed, activity is completely impaired, and sensation is lost (Figure 3.14.1, Figure 3.14.2).

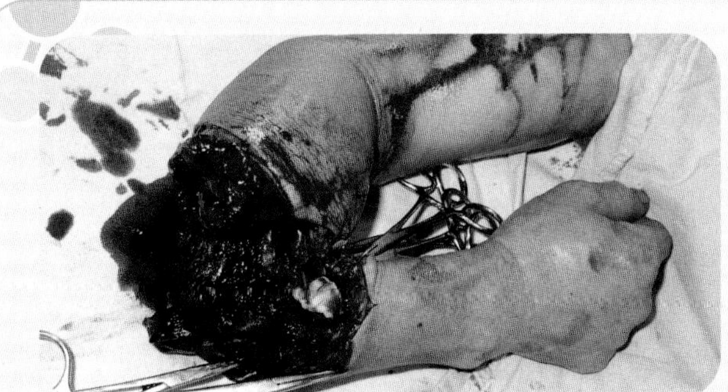

Figure 3.14.1 Transverse fracture of the middle section of the right forearm, with neat and deformed ends, showing transverse muscles and fractures

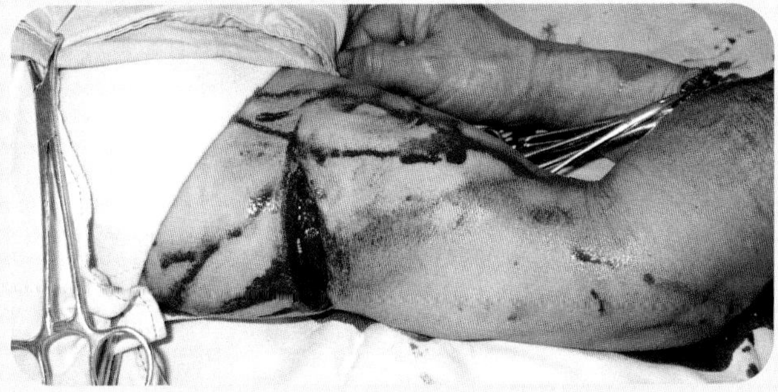

Figure 3.14.2 There is a 12 cm transverse wound on the right upper arm, reaching deep into the humeral tuberosity. Most of the deltoid muscle is broken, with active local bleeding and forearm deformity

◆ Treatment plan

1. Immediately clamp and stop bleeding, apply local pressure and bandage, and elevate the affected limb upon admission.

2. Quickly establish a venous channel, replenish fluids quickly, prepare blood for transfusion, correct shock, improve preoperative preparation, and perform emergency limb replantation surgery after correcting shock.

3. Use brachial plexus block anesthesia.

4. First, clean the wound, repair the deltoid muscle, and close the shoulder wound.

5. Surgical process

5.1 Establishment of bone scaffold: The radius and ulna are shortened by 2 cm. After fracture reduction, a 7-hole locking compression steel plate is implanted for fixation.

5.2 肌肉修复：依次修复掌侧屈腕屈指肌群、伸腕伸指肌群，修补血管神经着床。

5.3 神经修复：依次缝合正中神经，尺神经桡神经及皮神经。

5.4 血管修复：配制重组人酸性成纤维细胞生长因子冲洗液，并用重组人酸性成纤维细胞生长因子冲洗血管管腔。依次吻合桡动脉及其两条伴行静脉、尺动脉及其两条伴行静脉，吻合头静脉及贵要静脉，血管神经肌肉间隙中喷洒生长因子，创腔深部放置引流条，逐层缝合伤口，包扎伤口，石膏固定。

6. 病室保温，抬高患肢，加强换药，严格观察肢体血运及肿胀，加强护理及心理疏导，积极预防断肢再植术后并发症。

7. 该案例是在肌肉部位断裂，断肢再植后血运丰富，愈合较快，术后要早期行功能训练，大多数可获得很好的功能和外形（图 3.14.3）。

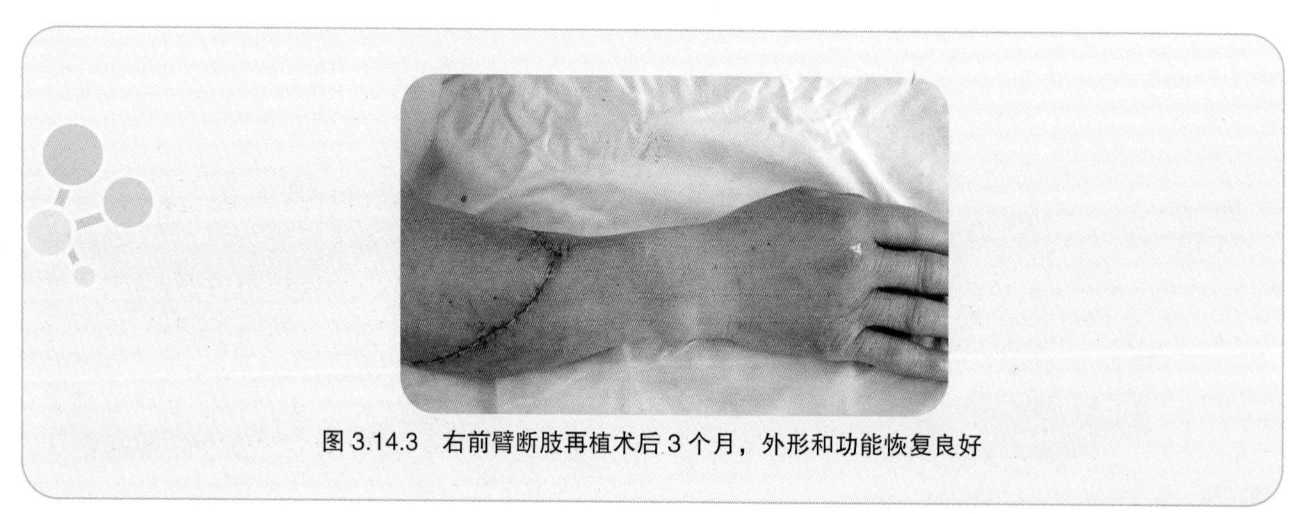

图 3.14.3　右前臂断肢再植术后 3 个月，外形和功能恢复良好

（陈善亮　陈皮紫涵）

案例十五　拇指指端缺损

◆ 损伤原因

患者左手因机器挤压，致拇指指端缺损。

◆ 症状与体征

左手拇指剧痛，局部出血不止，拇指指端缺损，指骨外露末节活动受限，甲板缺失，甲床裂伤，指骨无骨折，断端有油污，创缘不齐。

◆ 治疗方案

指端缺损修复方法很多，可以根据主刀医生本人经验采取不同的方法修复。本案例在臂丛麻醉下，采用了指背侧方筋膜蒂移植修复指端缺损，也取得了良好效果。

5.2 Muscle repair: sequentially repair the palmar wrist flexor muscle group, wrist extensor muscle group, and repair vascular and nerve implantation.

5.3 Neural repair: Suture the median nerve, ulnar nerve, radial nerve, and cutaneous nerve in sequence.

5.4 Vascular repair: Prepare recombinant human acidic fibroblast growth factor flushing solution and flush the vascular lumen with recombinant human acidic fibroblast growth factor. Sequentially anastomose the radial artery and its two accompanying veins, the ulnar artery and its two accompanying veins, anastomose the cephalic vein and the basilic vein, spray growth factors in the vascular nerve muscle gap, place drainage strips deep in the wound cavity, suture the wound layer by layer, bandage the wound, and fix it with plaster.

6. Keep the ward warm, elevate the affected limb, strengthen dressing changes, strictly observe limb blood flow and swelling, strengthen nursing and psychological counseling, and actively prevent complications after limb replantation surgery.

7. This case involves a muscle fracture, and after limb replantation, the blood supply is abundant and healing is fast. Early functional training is required after surgery, and most patients can achieve good function and appearance (Figure 3.14.3).

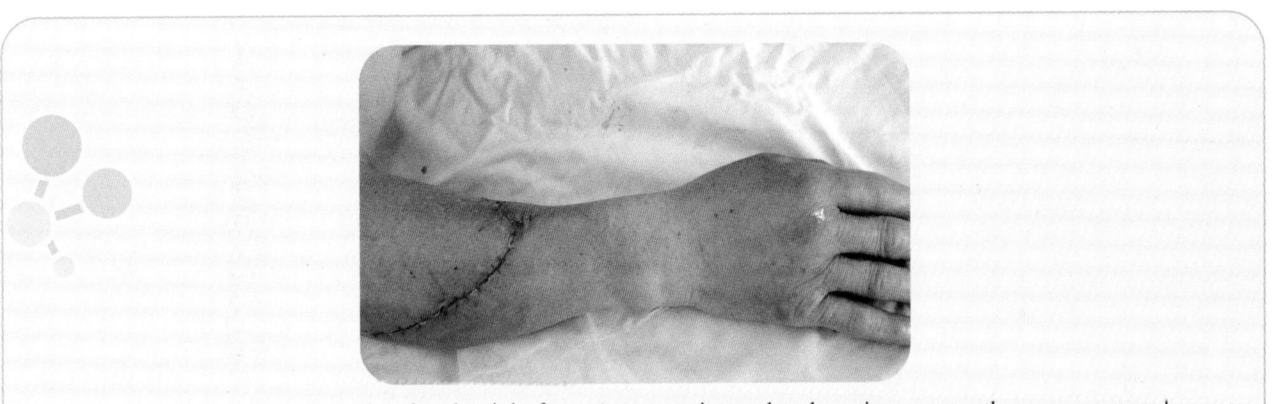

Figure 3.14.3 Three months after the right forearm amputation and replantation surgery, the appearance and function have recovered well

(Chen Shanliang, Chen Pi Zihan)

Case 15 Thumb tip defect

◆ Cause of injury

The patient's left hand was crushed by the machine, resulting in a missing thumb tip.

◆ Signs and symptoms

Severe pain in the left thumb, continuous local bleeding, missing tip of the thumb, limited movement of the distal phalanx exposed, missing deck, nail bed laceration, no fracture of the phalanx, oil stains on the broken end, and uneven wound margin.

◆ Treatment plan

There are many methods for repairing fingertip defects, and different methods can be adopted based on the experience of the surgeon in charge. In this case, under brachial plexus anesthesia, the dorsal fascial pedicle transplantation was used to repair the fingertip defect, and good results were also achieved.

1. 皮瓣设计，示指侧方为轴线，蒂长 2 cm，筋膜蒂宽 0.3 cm，解剖面筋膜浅层，旋转 180° 移植于受区（图 3.15.1）。

2. 供区全厚皮肤移植，局部不留瘢痕，外观美观，保证了手指长度。

3. 术后给予扩容、解痉、抗感染治疗，伤口加强换药。

4. 甲床通过喷洒重组人酸性成纤维细胞生长因子后，很快逐渐上皮化，局部干燥，2 个月后指甲生成。

5. 术后 7 天开始关节活动训练。皮瓣移植术后第 12 天，皮瓣成活（图 3.15.2）。

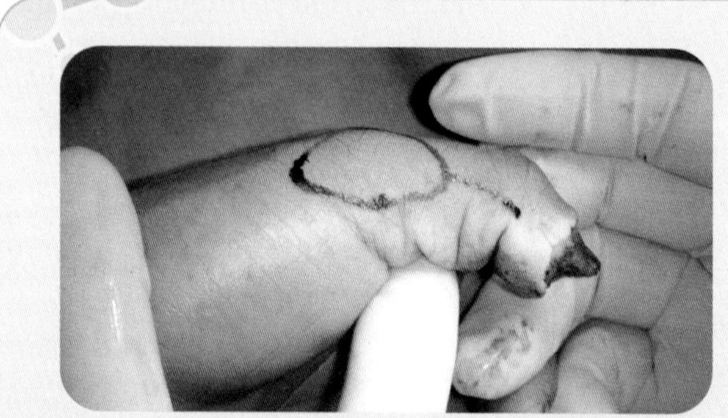

图 3.15.1　指端缺损情况，指背侧方筋膜皮瓣设计示意

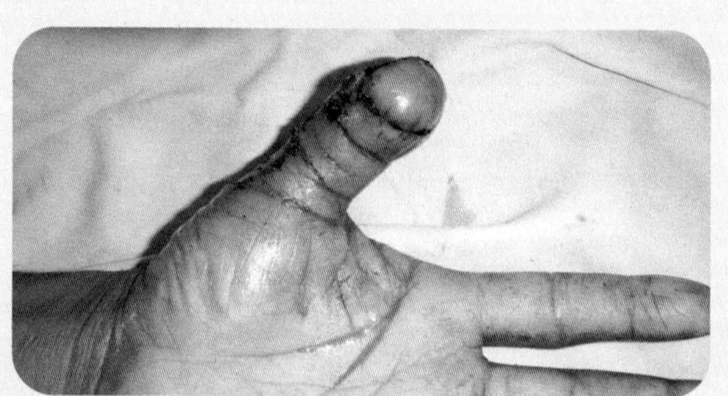

图 3.15.2　皮瓣移植术后第 12 天，皮瓣成活

（陈善亮　刘　江）

案例十六　拇指远端指间关节皮肤缺损

◆ 损伤原因

患者右手因模具压伤，致拇指远端指间关节皮肤缺损。

◆ 症状与体征

右手拇指剧痛，肿胀并渐加重，局部出血。右拇指末节指间关节背侧 1 cm × 1.5 cm 皮肤缺损，边界不清楚，伸肌腱止点不全断裂，关节面外露，垂指畸形，伸指活动受限，屈指活动良好；指甲部分缺损，甲床破裂（图 3.16.1）。

1. Skin flap design, with the index finger side as the axis, a pedicle length of 2 cm, and a fascial pedicle width of 0.3 cm. Dissect the superficial gluten membrane and rotate 180 ° to transplant it into the recipient area (Figure 3.15.1).

2. Full thickness skin transplantation in the donor area, without leaving scars locally, with a beautiful appearance and ensuring finger length.

3. After surgery, provide expansion, spasmolysis, and anti-infection treatment, and strengthen wound dressing changes.

4. After spraying recombinant human acidic fibroblast growth factor on the nail bed, it quickly gradually epithelialized, locally dried, and nails formed after 2 months.

5. Joint activity training will begin 7 days after surgery. On the 12th day after the skin flap transplantation, the skin flap survived (Figure 3.15.2).

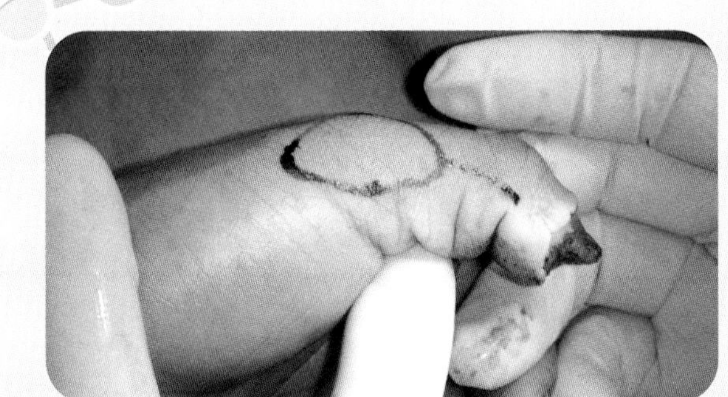

Figure 3.15.1 Fingertip defect situation, schematic diagram of the design of the dorsal lateral fascia skin flap of the finger

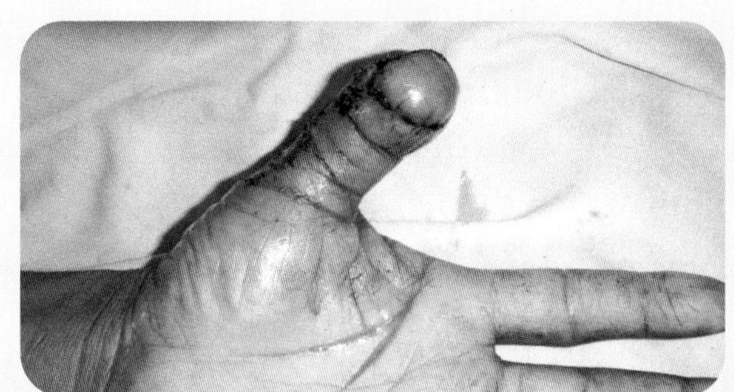

Figure 3.15.2 On the 12th day after skin flap transplantation, the skin flap survived

(Chen Shanliang, Liu Jiang)

Case 16 Skin defect of distal interphalangeal joint of thumb

◆ Cause of injury

The patient's right hand was injured due to mold compression, resulting in skin defects at the distal interphalangeal joint of the thumb.

◆ Signs and symptoms

The right thumb is severely painful, swollen and gradually worsening, with local bleeding. A 1 cm × 1.5 cm skin defect on the dorsal side of the distal interphalangeal joint of the right thumb, with unclear boundaries, incomplete rupture of the extensor tendon insertion point, exposed joint surface, drooping finger deformity, limited finger extension activity, and good finger flexion activity; Partial nail defect and nail bed rupture (Figure 3.16.1).

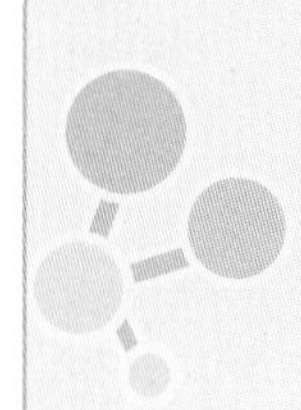

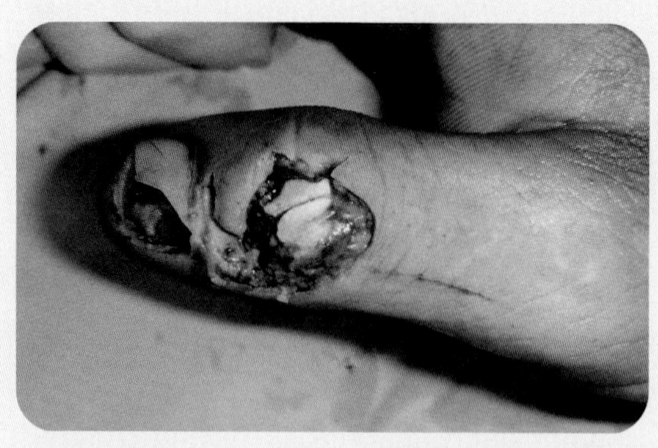

图 3.16.1　右手拇指背侧皮肤缺损，肌腱断裂外露，关节面外露

◆ 治疗方案

该手指皮肤缺损，选用了最近的手指背筋膜皮瓣移植，其优点是，临近取材，解剖表浅，皮肤松弛，可直接缝合，易于成活。

1. 皮瓣设计，拇指背侧方为轴线，蒂长 2 cm、蒂宽 0.3 cm，解剖面为筋膜浅层，旋转 180° 行受供区缝合（图 3.16.2）。供区全厚皮肤移植并打包缝合。末节关节 1.0 克氏针穿入固定。

2. 术后给予扩容、解痉、抗感染治疗，伤口加强换药，每天换药常规喷洒重组人酸性成纤维细胞生长因子促进创口愈合。

3. 术后 7 天开始训练掌指关节，3 周后拔出克氏针并进行末节关节康复训练（图 3.16.3）。

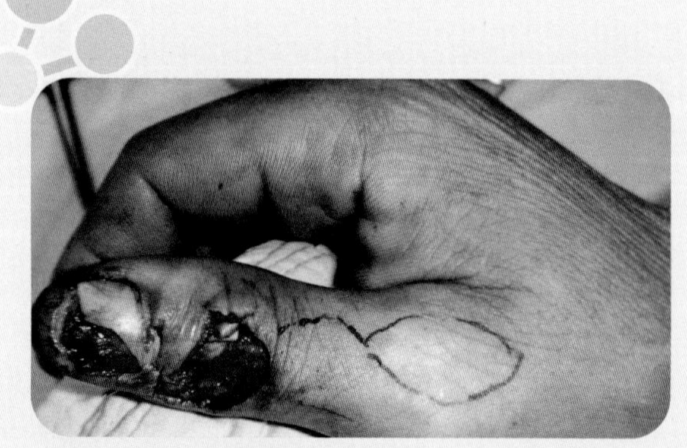

图 3.16.2　肌腱和甲床修复后，皮瓣设计示意

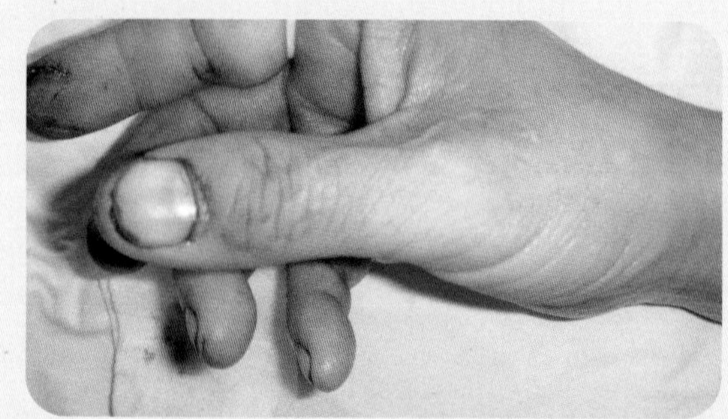

图 3.16.3　皮瓣移植术后 3 个月，指甲美观，皮瓣移植修复后受供区美观，关节活动灵活

（陈善亮）

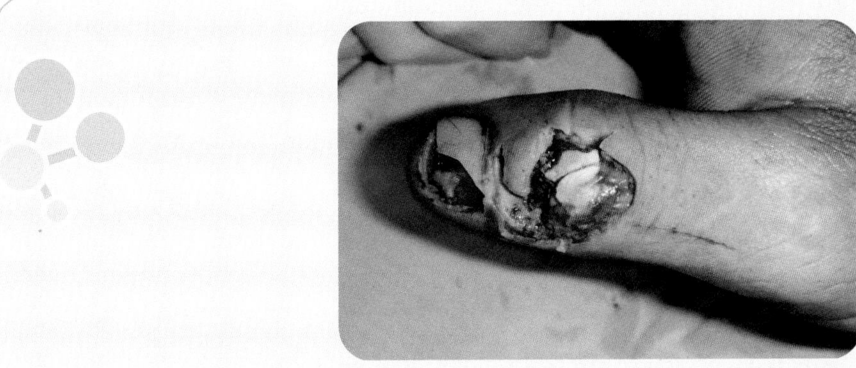

Figure 3.16.1 Right thumb dorsal skin defect, tendon rupture exposed, joint surface exposed

◆ Treatment plan

The skin defect of the finger was treated with the recent dorsal fascia skin flap transplantation, which has the advantages of being close to the sample, shallow dissection, loose skin, and can be directly sutured, making it easy to survive.

1. Skin flap design, with the dorsal side of the thumb as the axis, a pedicle length of 2 cm and a pedicle width of 0.3 cm, the anatomical surface is the superficial fascia, and the donor site is sutured by rotating 180 ° (Figure 3.16.2). Full thickness skin transplantation and packaging suturing in the donor area. 1.0 Kirschner wire is inserted into the distal joint for fixation.

2. Postoperative treatment includes expansion, spasmolysis, and anti-infection therapy. The wound dressing should be changed regularly, and recombinant human acidic fibroblast growth factor should be sprayed daily to promote wound healing.

3. Training of the metacarpophalangeal joint began 7 days after surgery, and 3 weeks later, the Kirschner wire was removed and rehabilitation training was performed on the distal joint (Figure 3.16.3).

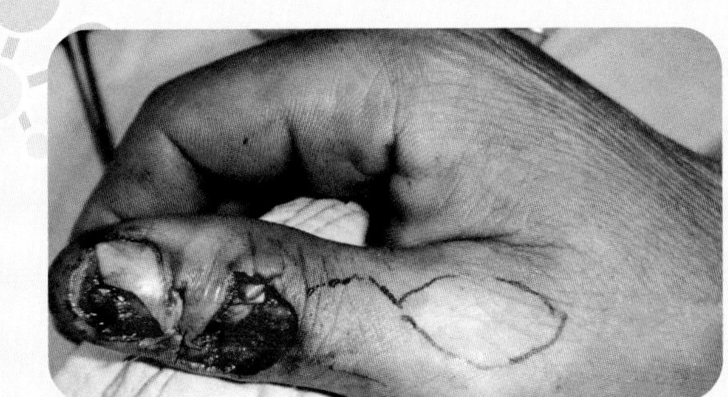

Figure 3.16.2 Schematic diagram of flap design after tendon and nail bed repair

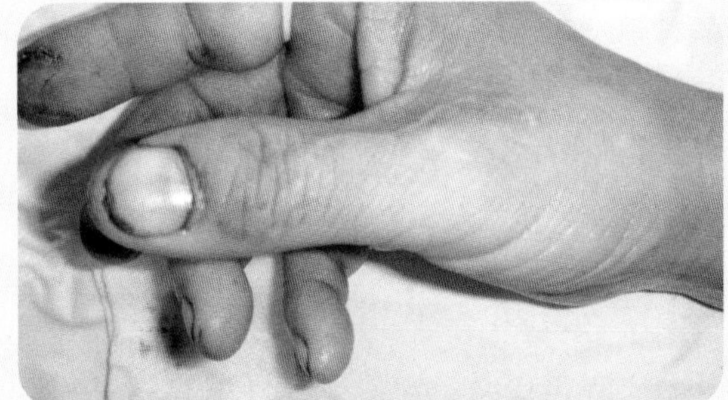

Figure 3.16.3 Three months after skin flap transplantation, the nails are aesthetically pleasing, the donor site is aesthetically pleasing after skin flap transplantation repair, and the joints are flexible in movement

(Chen Shanliang)

案例十七　示指中指环指热压伤皮肤缺损

◆ 损伤原因

患者右手因 150℃高温热压伤，致示指、中指、环指皮肤缺损。

◆ 症状与体征

右手示指、中指和环指肿胀，疼痛伴活动受限。示指、中指和环指的指间关节背侧各有 2 cm × 1.5 cm 皮肤坏死。局部皮肤皮革样变，质地较硬，坏死皮肤边界清楚，示指、中指和环指深屈活动受限。

◆ 治疗方案

热压伤患者，由于压伤后皮肤坏死界限不清楚，大多数需要择期手术，有充分的时间选择不同的皮瓣修复缺损。

1. 手术过程

1.1 清创及关节固定：根据坏死边界将坏死皮肤及肌腱切除，并结扎活动出血点，骨关节外露（图 3.17.1），取 1.0 克氏针顺行固定示指、中指和环指指间关节。

1.2 皮瓣设计：示指和中指采用指背筋膜皮瓣移植，中指采用掌背筋膜皮瓣移植，示指、环指为开放隧道，中指为闭合隧道。示指、中指轴线为指背正中线，蒂长 1.5 cm、蒂宽 0.3 cm，解剖面为肌腱浅层。中指皮瓣轴线为第 2 掌骨和第 3 掌骨间隙，蒂长 3.5 cm，解剖面肌腱浅层，旋转点距指蹼 1.5 cm。

1.3 皮瓣移植：依次解剖每个皮瓣，并结扎活动出血点，解剖结束后皮瓣旋转并行受供区缝合，皮瓣下放置橡皮条引流，闭合隧道。于下腹部切取全厚皮肤移植皮瓣供区并打包缝合，闭合腹部切口包扎伤口，术终（图 3.17.2）。

2. 术后抬高患肢，加强换药并喷洒生长因子促进伤口愈合，包扎松紧度适中，24 小时拔出引流条。常规扩容、解痉镇痛、抗感染治疗（图 3.17.3）。

3. 术后 12 天拆线，4 周后拔出克氏针，进行关节松动康复，择期肌腱修复（图 3.17.4、图 3.17.5）。

Case 17 Skin defect caused by heat pressure injury on the middle finger of the finger

◆ Cause of injury

The patient's right hand was injured by 150°C high temperature thermal compression, resulting in skin defects on the index finger, middle finger, and ring finger.

◆ Signs and symptoms

Swelling of the index finger, middle finger, and ring finger of the right hand, accompanied by pain and restricted movement. There is 2 cm × 1.5 cm of skin necrosis on the dorsal side of the interphalangeal joints of the index finger, middle finger, and ring finger. Localized leather like changes in the skin, with a harder texture, clear boundaries of necrotic skin, and limited deep flexion activity of the index finger, middle finger, and ring finger.

◆ Treatment plan

Patients with thermal compression injuries often require elective surgery due to unclear boundaries of skin necrosis after compression, allowing ample time to choose different skin flaps for defect repair.

1. Surgical process

1.1 Debridement and joint fixation: Remove the necrotic skin and tendons according to the necrotic boundary, ligate the active bleeding point, expose the bone and joint (Figure 3.17.1), and use a 1.0 gram needle to fix the interphalangeal joints of the index finger, middle finger, and ring finger in a forward direction.

1.2 Skin flap design: The index finger and middle finger are transplanted with dorsal fascia skin flaps, while the middle finger is transplanted with dorsal fascia skin flaps. The index finger and ring finger are open tunnels, while the middle finger is a closed tunnel. The axis of the index finger and middle finger is the midline of the dorsal finger, with a pedicle length of 1.5 cm and a pedicle width of 0.3 cm. The anatomical surface is the superficial layer of the tendon. The axis of the middle finger flap is the gap between the second and third metacarpal bones, with a pedicle length of 3.5 cm and a superficial tendon layer on the anatomical surface. The rotation point is 1.5 cm away from the finger web.

1.3 Skin flap transplantation: Dissect each skin flap in sequence and ligate the active bleeding point. After dissection, rotate the skin flap and suture the donor area. Place a rubber strip under the skin flap for drainage and close the tunnel. Cut a full-thickness skin graft flap from the lower abdomen and package it for suturing. Close the abdominal incision and wrap the wound, and the surgery ends (Figure 3.17.2).

2. After surgery, raise the affected limb, strengthen dressing changes, and spray growth factors to promote wound healing. The tightness of the bandage should be moderate, and the drainage strip should be removed within 24 hours. Conventional expansion, spasmolysis and analgesia, and anti infective treatment (Figure 3.17.3).

3. The stitches were removed 12 days after surgery, and the Kirschner wire was removed 4 weeks later for joint loosening rehabilitation and elective tendon repair (Figure 3.17.4, Figure 3.17.5).

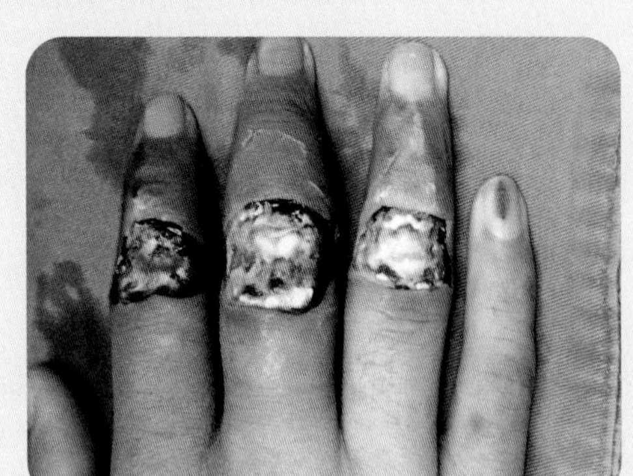

图 3.17.1　右手示指、中指、环指指背皮肤坏死清创后，肌腱部分缺损，骨关节外露

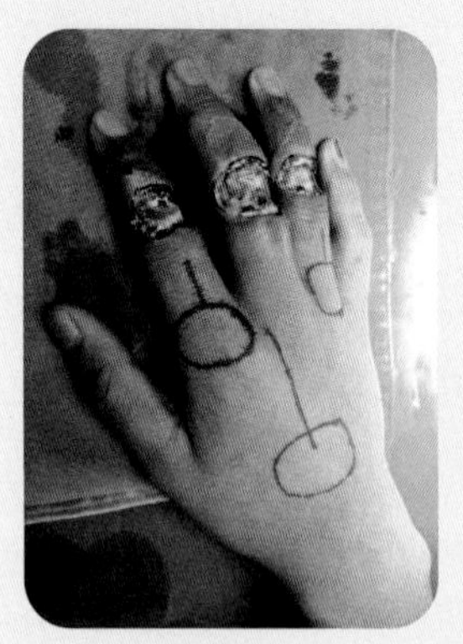

图 3.17.2　右手示指和环指设计指背筋膜蒂皮瓣，中指设计掌背筋膜蒂皮瓣

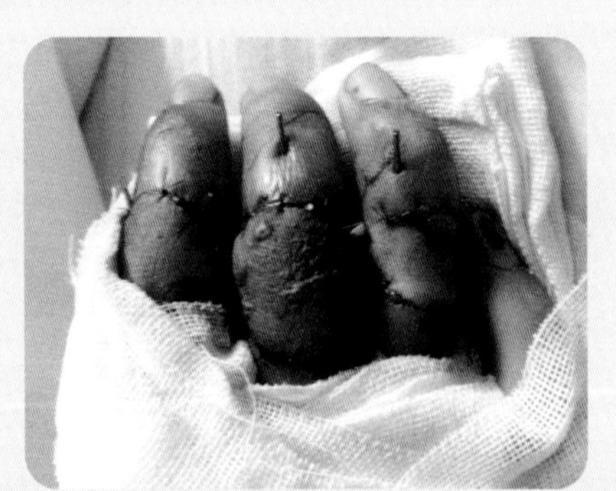

图 3.17.3　皮瓣移植术后 5 天，中指皮瓣出现水疱，并逐渐干结

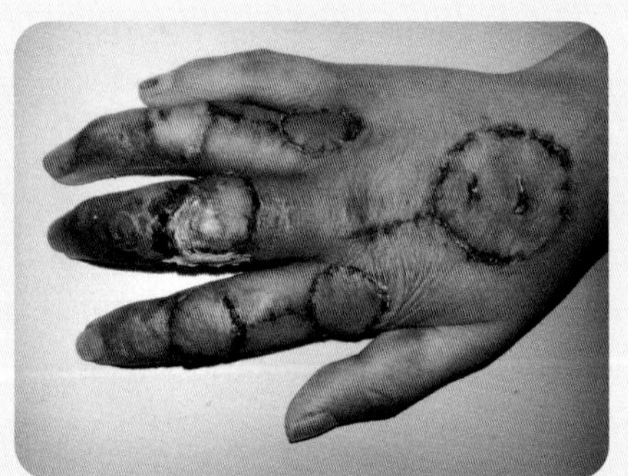

图 3.17.4　皮瓣移植术后 15 天、切口结痂逐渐脱落

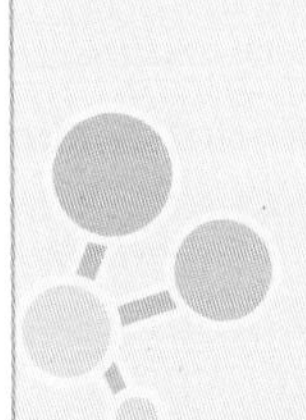

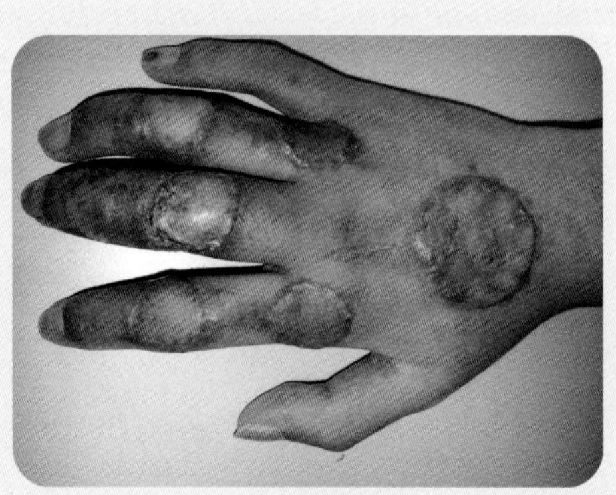

图 3.17.5　皮瓣移植术后 30 天、皮瓣成活，局部肿胀消退，关节康复训练，择期肌腱修复

（陈善亮）

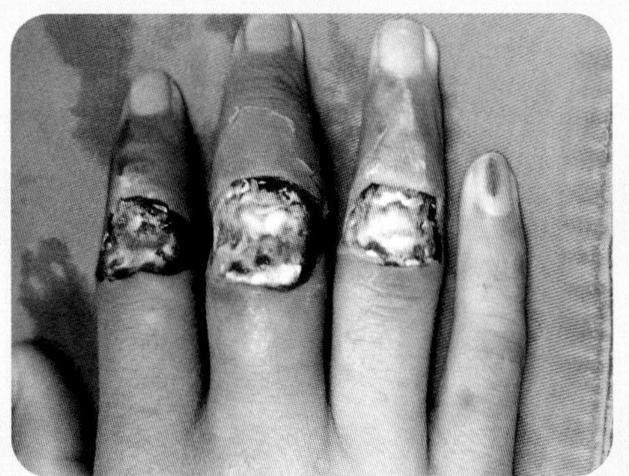

Figure 3.17.1 After debridement and necrosis of the skin on the back of the index finger, middle finger, and ring finger of the right hand, there is a partial defect in the tendons and exposed bone joints

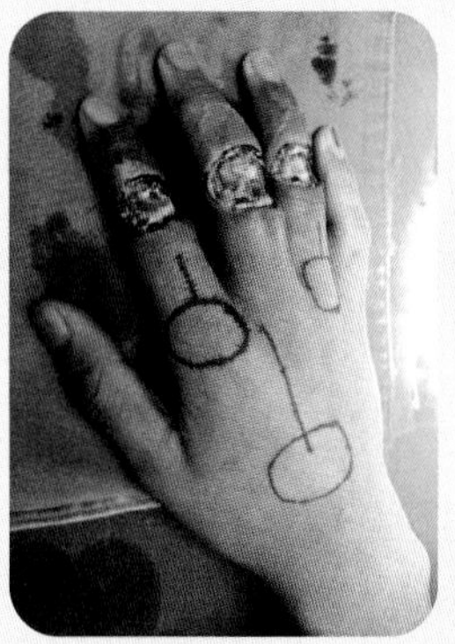

Figure 3.17.2 Right hand index finger and ring finger design with dorsal fascia pedicle flap, middle finger design with dorsal fascia pedicle flap

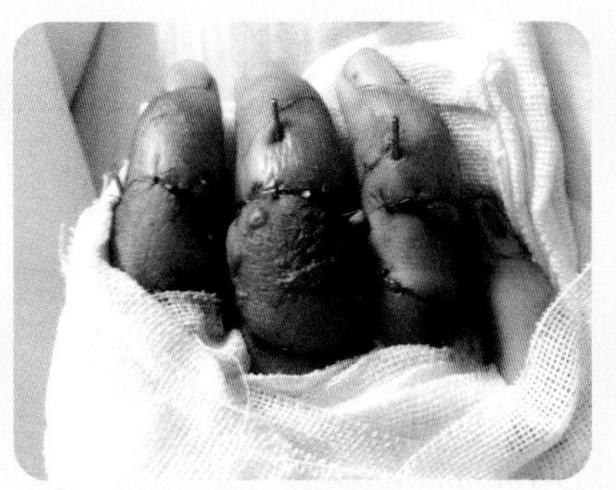

Figure 3.17.3 Five days after flap transplantation, blisters appeared on the middle finger flap and gradually dried up

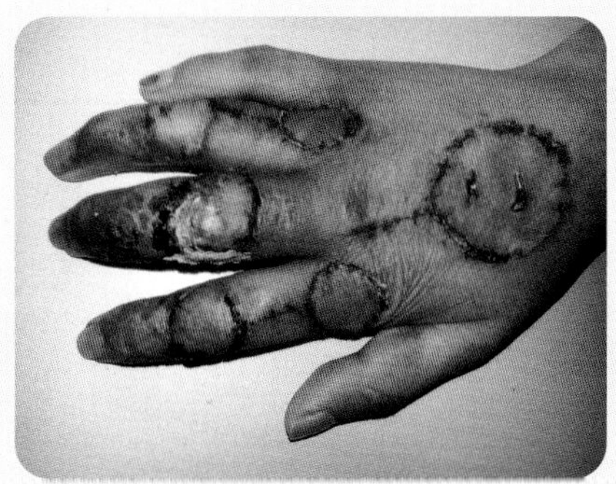

Figure 3.17.4 15 days after skin flap transplantation, the scab on the incision gradually falls off

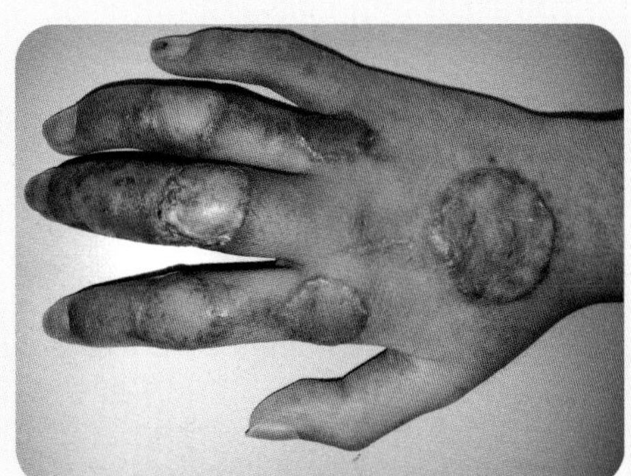

Figure 3.17.5 30 days after flap transplantation, flap survival, local swelling resolution, joint rehabilitation training, and elective tendon repair

(Chen Shanliang)

案例十八 拇指背侧皮肤缺损

◆ 损伤原因

患者左手因机器压伤，致拇指背侧皮肤缺损。

◆ 症状与体征

左手掌肿胀明显，手掌背侧伤口出血不止，拇指深屈活动受限。左手背广泛性肿胀，以拇指为主，拇指背侧有 6 cm 不规则伤口，深达近节指骨，近节指骨骨擦感、骨擦音阳性，拇指掌背皮肤有挫灭，血运差，拇长伸肌腱断裂，拇指背伸活动受限。

◆ 治疗方案

1. 急诊在臂丛麻醉下行清创骨折复位内固定术，肌腱修复术。术后拇指掌背皮肤出现坏死，并行坏死皮肤切除，局部喷洒生长因子促进创面新鲜，为皮瓣移植做准备。

2. 手术过程

2.1 皮瓣设计：顺行皮瓣，以第 2 掌骨桡侧缘为轴线，解剖面深筋膜浅层，蒂宽 0.3 cm，皮蒂内含第 2 掌骨背动脉（图 3.18.1）。

2.2 皮瓣移植：依次切开皮肤及皮下组织，解剖游离第 2 掌骨背动脉（图 3.18.2），结扎活动出血点，游离闭合隧道，将皮瓣从隧道拉出，受供区缝合，缝合前喷洒重组人酸性成纤维细胞生长因子，皮瓣下放橡皮条引流。于前臂内侧切取全厚皮肤移植皮瓣供区并缝合，植皮区加压包扎，术终。

3. 术后抬高患肢，严密观察皮瓣血运，换药时喷洒生长因子，24 小时拔出引流条。

4. 由于皮蒂内含第 2 掌骨背动脉，有效地供应皮瓣血运，术后无须扩容、解痉镇痛、抗感染治疗（图 3.18.3、图 3.18.4）。

5. 术后 12 天拆线，1 个月后拔出克氏针并进行康复训练。

Case 18 Skin defect on the dorsal side of the thumb

◆ Cause of injury

The patient's left hand was injured by a machine, resulting in a skin defect on the back of the thumb.

◆ Signs and symptoms

The swelling of the left palm is obvious, the wound on the back of the palm is bleeding continuously, and the deep flexion movement of the thumb is restricted. Widespread swelling on the back of the left hand, mainly on the thumb. There is an irregular wound of 6 cm on the back side of the thumb, reaching deep into the proximal phalanx. The proximal phalanx bone has a positive rubbing sensation and bone rubbing sound. The skin on the back of the thumb palm has been bruised, with poor blood supply. The extensor pollicis longus tendon is broken, and the thumb's dorsiflexion is restricted.

◆ Treatment plan

1. Emergency treatment includes debridement, fracture reduction, internal fixation, and tendon repair under brachial plexus anesthesia. After surgery, the skin on the dorsal side of the thumb showed necrosis, and the necrotic skin was removed in parallel. Local spraying of growth factors was used to promote wound freshness and prepare for skin flap transplantation.

2. Surgical process

2.1 Skin flap design: A anterograde skin flap is used, with the radial edge of the second metacarpal bone as the axis, the anatomical plane is deep and superficial, the pedicle is 0.3 cm wide, and the pedicle contains the dorsal artery of the second metacarpal bone (Figure 3.18.1).

2.2 Skin flap transplantation: Cut open the skin and subcutaneous tissue in sequence, dissect and free the second dorsal metacarpal artery (Figure 3.18.2), ligate the active bleeding point, free and close the tunnel, pull out the skin flap from the tunnel, suture the donor area, spray recombinant human acidic fibroblast growth factor before suturing, and place a rubber strip under the skin flap for drainage. Cut and suture a full-thickness skin graft on the inner side of the forearm, apply pressure to the graft area, and wrap it up at the end of the surgery.

3. After surgery, elevate the affected limb, closely observe the blood flow of the skin flap, spray growth factors during dressing changes, and remove the drainage strip 24 hours later.

4. Due to the inclusion of the second dorsal metacarpal artery in the pedicle, it effectively supplies blood flow to the skin flap, and there is no need for postoperative dilation, spasmolysis, analgesia, or anti infection treatment (Figure 3.18.3, Figure 3.18.4).

5. The stitches were removed 12 days after surgery, and one month later, the Kirschner wire was removed and rehabilitation training was conducted.

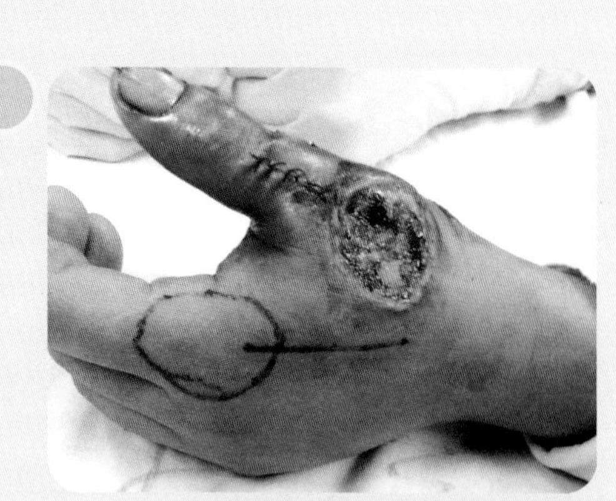

图 3.18.1　掌骨开放性骨折术后出现皮肤坏死，缺损面积 2.5 cm × 3 cm，第 2 掌骨背皮瓣移植示意

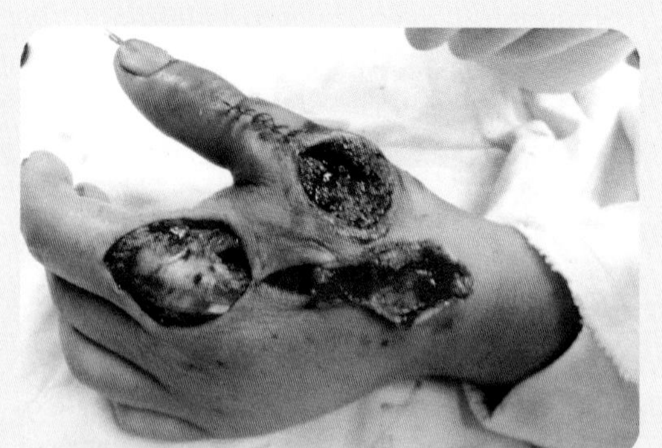

图 3.18.2　皮瓣解剖游离后

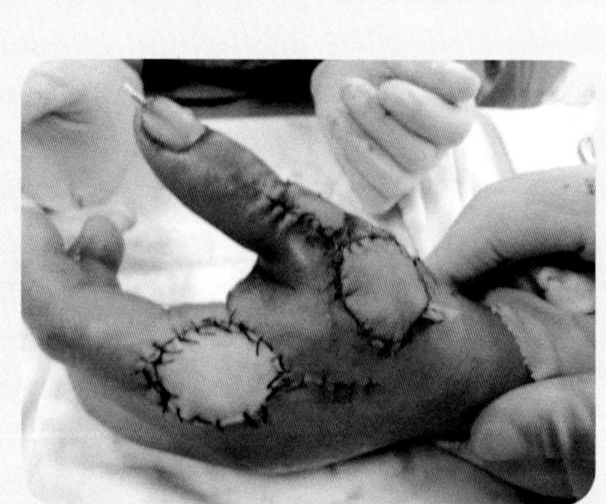

图 3.18.3　皮瓣移植后血运良好，供区全厚皮肤移植

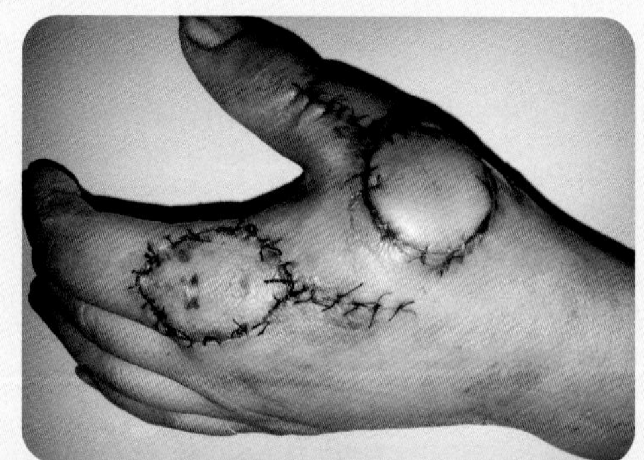

图 3.18.4　术后 1 周，移植皮瓣和全厚植皮成活

（陈善亮）

案例十九　中指环指热压伤皮肤坏死

◆ 损伤原因

患者右手因模具热压伤，致中指、环指皮肤坏死。

◆ 症状与体征

右手中指、环指和小指压伤后疼痛伴深屈活动受限 3 天。中指、环指和小指指背侧有圆形皮肤坏死，中指、示指坏死皮肤各约 1.5 cm × 2 cm，小指坏死皮肤 1 cm × 0.5 cm，局部皮革样变，边界清楚，无红肿及渗出。中指、环指和小指深屈活动受限。

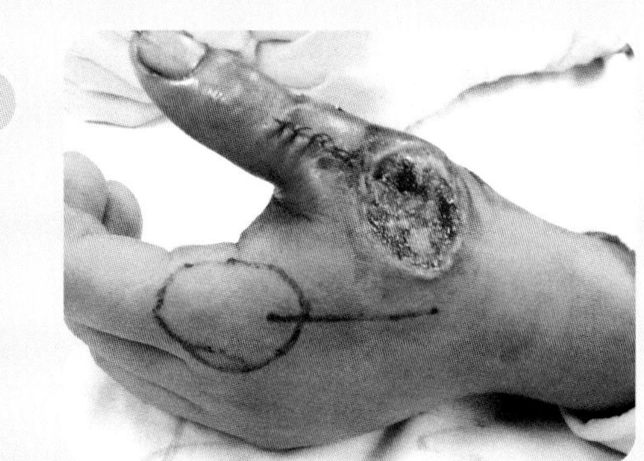

Figure 3.18.1 Skin necrosis occurred after surgery for open fracture of the metacarpal bone, with a defect area of 2.5 cm × 3 cm. Schematic diagram of the second metacarpal dorsal skin flap transplantation

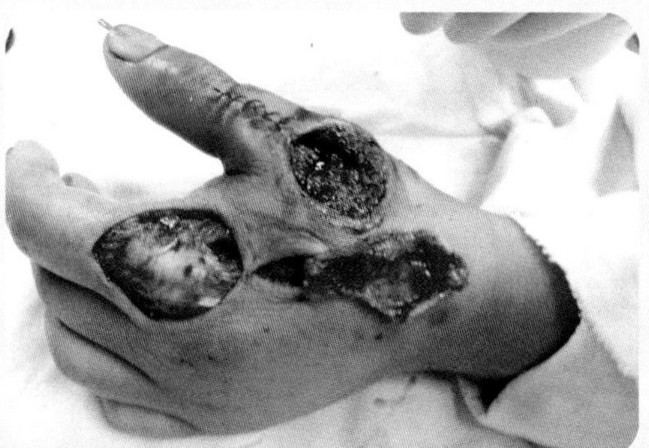

Figure 3.18.2 Dissection and Release of Skin Flap

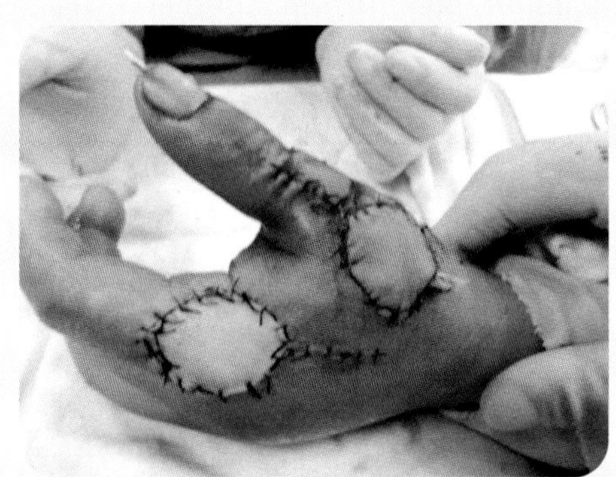

Figure 3.18.3 Good blood supply after skin flap transplantation, full-thickness skin transplantation in the donor area

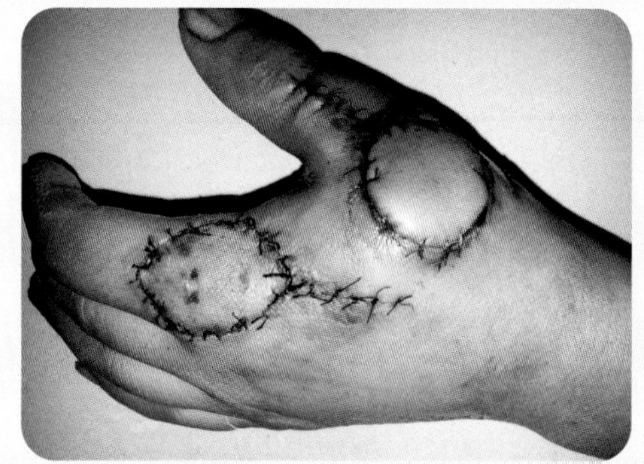

Figure 3.18.4 One week after surgery, survival of transplanted skin flap and full-thickness skin graft

(Chen Shanliang)

Case 19 Skin necrosis caused by finger thermal compression injury

◆ Cause of injury

The patient's right hand suffered from mold hot pressing injury, resulting in skin necrosis of the middle finger and ring finger.

◆ Signs and symptoms

Pain accompanied by restricted deep flexion movement for 3 days after compression injury to the middle finger, ring finger, and little finger of the right hand. There is circular skin necrosis on the back of the middle finger, ring finger, and little finger. The necrotic skin on the middle finger and index finger is about 1.5 cm × 2 cm each, and the necrotic skin on the little finger is 1 cm × 0.5 cm. The local leather like changes have clear boundaries, no redness, swelling, or exudation. The deep flexion movement of the middle finger, ring finger, and little finger is restricted.

◆ 治疗方案

该案例热压伤后3天入院，坏死皮肤界限基本清楚，入院后完善术前检查，在臂丛麻醉下行坏死皮肤切除，行掌背筋膜蒂皮瓣移植。

1. 手术过程

1.1 清创：切除中指、环指坏死皮肤，保留肌腱及腱周膜，小指三度坏死区域不大，约0.3 cm×0.3 cm，局部敷用生长因子干粉剂油纱包扎可以愈合。

1.2 皮瓣设计：中指皮瓣采用第2掌骨与第3掌骨间为轴线，旋转点距指蹼1.5 cm，解剖面为筋膜浅层。环指皮瓣采用第4掌骨与第5掌骨间为轴线，旋转点距指蹼1.5 cm，解剖面为筋膜浅层。

1.3 皮瓣移植：依次切开皮肤及皮下组织，保留0.3 cm筋膜蒂，采用开放隧道，皮瓣解剖游离后，解剖面喷洒外用重组人碱性成纤维细胞生长因子，皮瓣受区供区缝合，皮瓣下放置橡皮条引流，掌背皮瓣全厚皮肤游离移植并缝合（图3.19.1、图3.19.2）。

2. 术后抬高患肢，观察皮瓣血运，预防感染，由于皮瓣内有掌背动脉，术后无须解痉治疗，换药时喷洒重组人酸性成纤维细胞生长含因子促进伤口愈合，术后24小时拔出引流条。

3. 术后12天拆线，并进行康复训练。

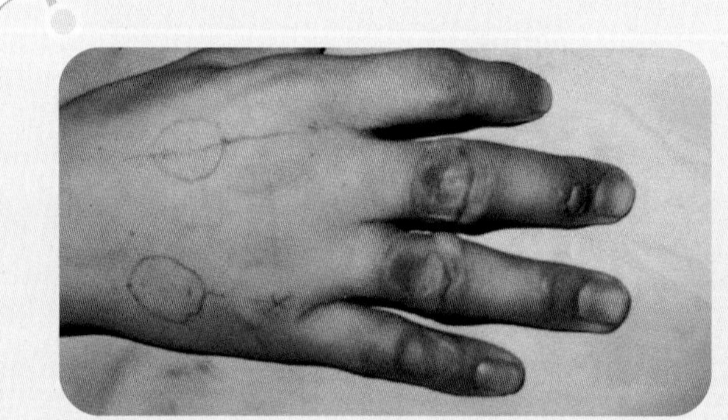

图3.19.1 坏死皮肤及皮瓣设计示意

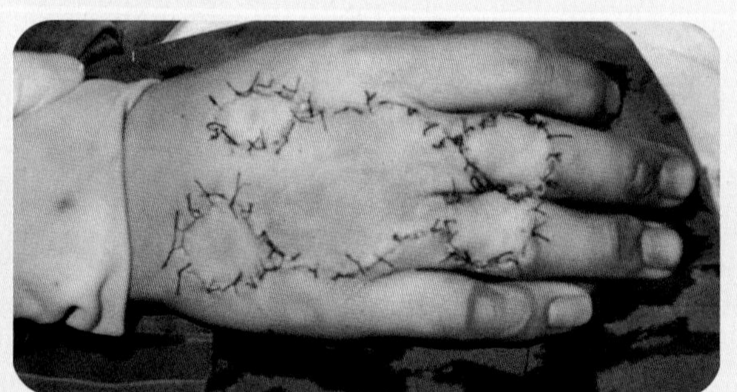

图3.19.2 设计的掌背筋膜蒂皮瓣移植示意

（陈善亮）

案例二十 示指中指掌侧皮肤缺损

◆ 损伤原因

患者右手因机器挤压伤，致示指、中指掌侧皮肤缺损。

◆ Treatment plan

The case was admitted to the hospital 3 days after thermal compression injury, and the boundaries of necrotic skin were basically clear. After admission, preoperative examinations were completed, and necrotic skin was removed under brachial plexus anesthesia, followed by palmar dorsal fascia flap transplantation.

1. Surgical process

1.1 Debridement: Remove the necrotic skin of the middle finger and ring finger, preserve the tendon and periaponeurosis. The third degree necrosis area of the little finger is not large, about 0.3 cm × 0.3 cm. Local application of growth factor dry powder oil gauze can heal.

1.2 Skin flap design: The middle finger skin flap adopts the axis between the second and third metacarpal bones, with a rotation point 1.5 cm away from the finger web, and the anatomical surface is the superficial fascia. The ring finger flap adopts the axis between the 4th and 5th metacarpal bones, with a rotation point 1.5 cm away from the finger web, and the anatomical surface is the superficial fascia.

1.3 Skin flap transplantation: Cut open the skin and subcutaneous tissue in sequence, preserve the 0.3 cm fascial pedicle, use an open tunnel, dissect and free the skin flap, spray recombinant human basic fibroblast growth factor on the anatomical surface, suture the donor area of the skin flap, place a rubber strip under the skin flap for drainage, and transplant and suture the full-thickness skin of the palmar dorsal skin flap (Figure 3.19.1, Figure 3.19.2).

2. After surgery, raise the affected limb and observe the blood flow of the skin flap to prevent infection. Due to the presence of the dorsal palmar artery in the skin flap, there is no need for spasmolytic treatment after surgery. When changing dressing, spray recombinant human acidic fibroblast growth factor to promote wound healing, and remove the drainage strip 24 hours after surgery.

3. Remove the stitches 12 days after surgery and undergo rehabilitation training.

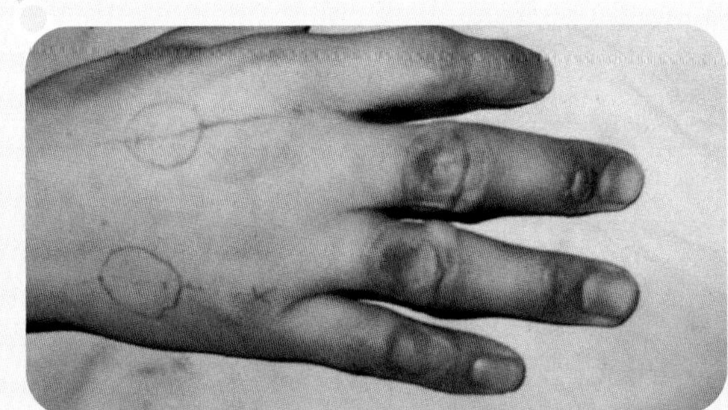

Figure 3.19.1 Schematic diagram of necrotic skin and flap design

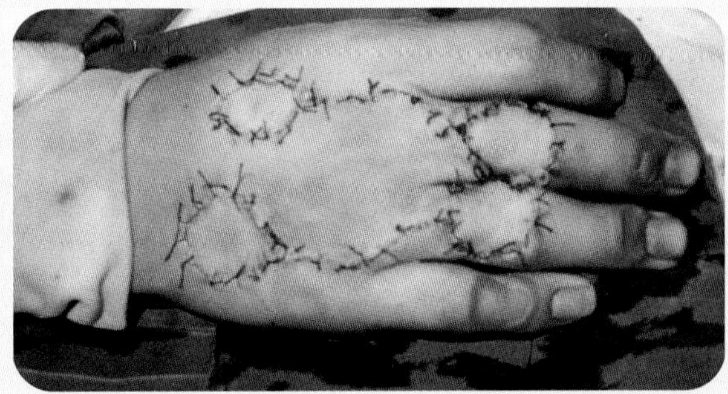

Figure 3.19.2 Schematic diagram of palmar dorsal fascia pedicle flap transplantation designed

(Chen Shanliang)

Case 20 Skin defect on the palmar side of the middle finger of the index finger

◆ Cause of injury

The patient's right hand was injured by machine compression, resulting in skin defects on the palmar side of the index finger and middle finger.

◆ 症状与体征

右手示指、中指疼痛，出血伴肿胀，活动受限。示指和中指掌侧皮肤缺损，示指皮肤缺损 1.5 cm × 1.5 cm，中指皮肤缺损 2 cm × 1.8 cm。局部肌腱和腱鞘外露，示指、中指屈伸活动略受限，指端感觉和血运良好（图 3.20.1）。

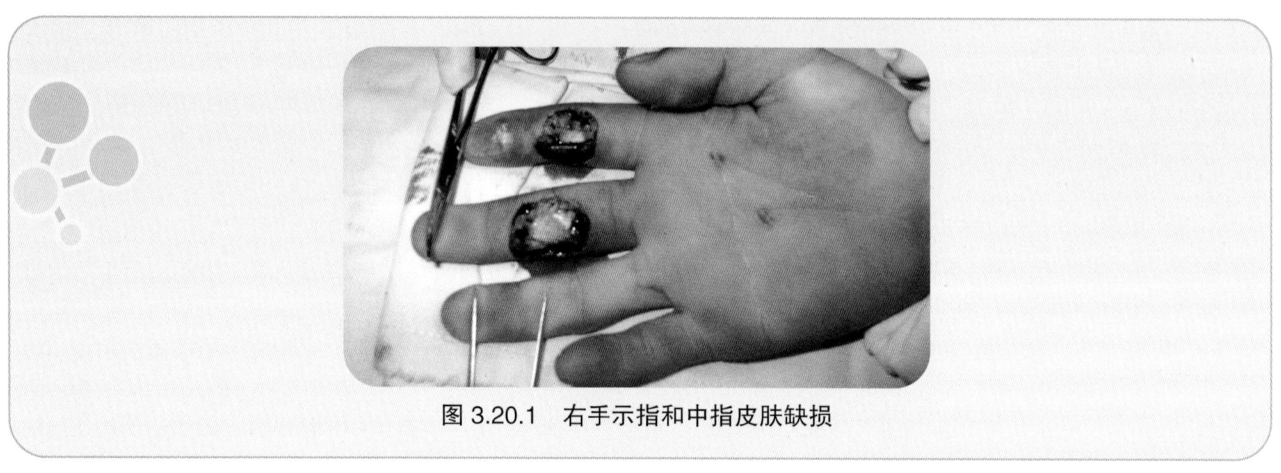
图 3.20.1　右手示指和中指皮肤缺损

◆ 治疗方案

1. 臂丛麻醉下急诊入院一期清创，一期皮瓣移植消灭创面。

2. 手术过程

2.1 皮瓣设计：以示指和中指侧中线为轴线，解剖面为筋膜浅层，旋转点为指间关节处，采用开放隧道，蒂长 2 cm、蒂宽 0.3 cm。

2.2 皮瓣移植：依次解剖皮瓣并结扎活动出血点，解剖结束后，创面喷洒生长因子，并行受供区缝合，皮瓣下放置橡皮条引流（图 3.20.2）。于下腹壁切取全厚皮肤移植到示指和中指供区并缝合。局部打包包扎。

3. 术后抬高患肢，观察皮瓣血运，每天换药喷洒外用重组人碱性成纤维细胞生长因子，术后 24 小时拔出引流条。

4. 术后 7 天骨关节主被动活动，12 天拆线，并进行全面康复训练（图 3.20.3）。

◆ Signs and symptoms

Pain in the index finger and middle finger of the right hand, accompanied by bleeding and swelling, and limited mobility. Skin defects on the palm side of the index finger and middle finger, with a skin defect of 1.5 cm × 1.5 cm on the index finger and 2 cm × 1.8 cm on the middle finger. Local tendons and tendon sheaths are exposed, and the flexion and extension activities of the index finger and middle finger are slightly restricted. The fingertip sensation and blood supply are good (Figure 3.20.1).

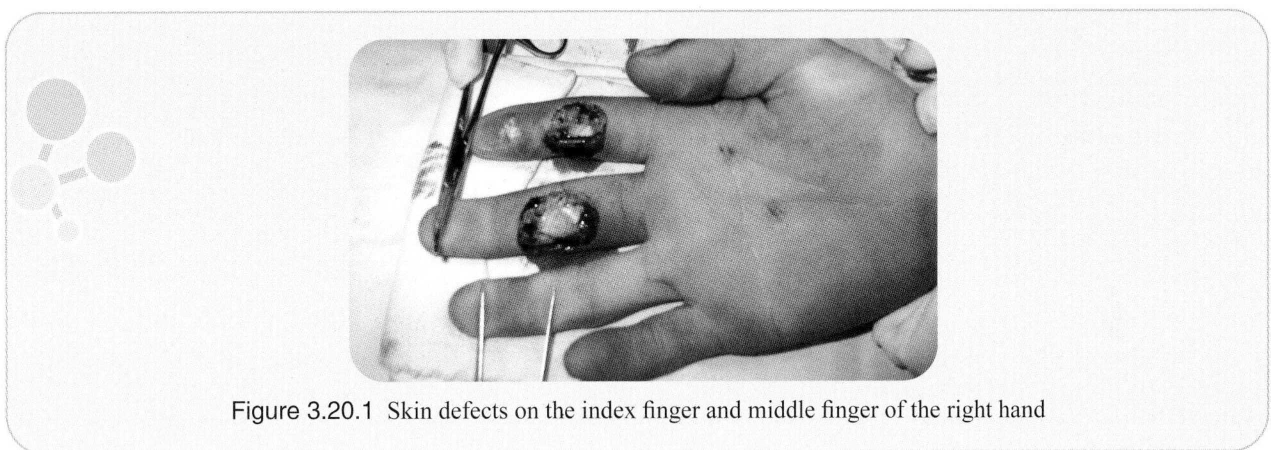

Figure 3.20.1 Skin defects on the index finger and middle finger of the right hand

◆ Treatment plan

1. Emergency admission under brachial plexus anesthesia with first stage debridement and first stage skin flap transplantation to eliminate the wound.

2. Surgical process

2.1 Skin flap design: Taking the midline of the index finger and middle finger as the axis, the anatomical surface is the superficial fascia, the rotation point is at the interphalangeal joint, and an open tunnel is used with a pedicle length of 2 cm and a pedicle width of 0.3 cm.

2.2 Skin flap transplantation: Dissect the skin flap in sequence and ligate the active bleeding point. After dissection, spray growth factor on the wound and suture the donor area. Place a rubber strip under the skin flap for drainage (Figure 3.20.2). Cut the full thickness skin from the lower abdominal wall and transplant it to the donor area of the index finger and middle finger, and suture it. Partial packaging and bandaging.

3. After surgery, raise the affected limb, observe the blood flow of the skin flap, change the dressing daily, spray external recombinant human basic fibroblast growth factor, and remove the drainage strip 24 hours after surgery.

4. After 7 days of surgery, active and passive bone and joint movements were performed, and stitches were removed 12 days later, followed by comprehensive rehabilitation training (Figure 3.20.3).

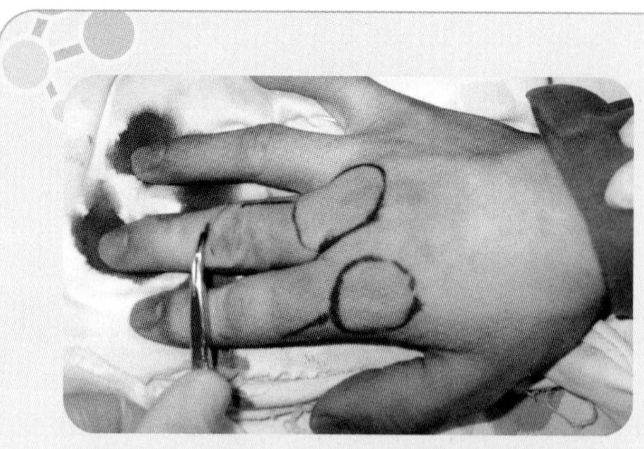
图 3.20.2　设计示指和中指指背筋膜皮瓣示意

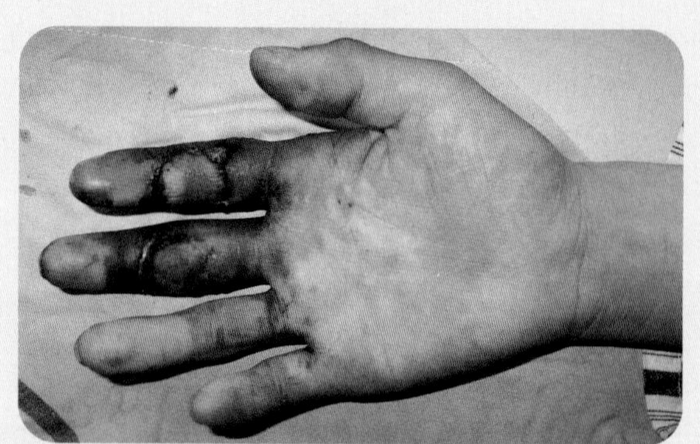
图 3.20.3　皮瓣移植成活后

（陈善亮）

案例二十一　示指指背皮肤缺损

◆ 损伤原因

患者右手因拉丝机刮伤，致示指指背皮肤缺损。

◆ 症状与体征

右手示指剧痛，出血不止，肿胀并逐渐加重。示指中远节背侧皮肤软组织缺损，边界整齐，污染较轻，伸指肌腱外露无断裂，示指伸屈活动良好（图 3.21.1）。皮肤缺损面积 3.5 cm × 1.5 cm。

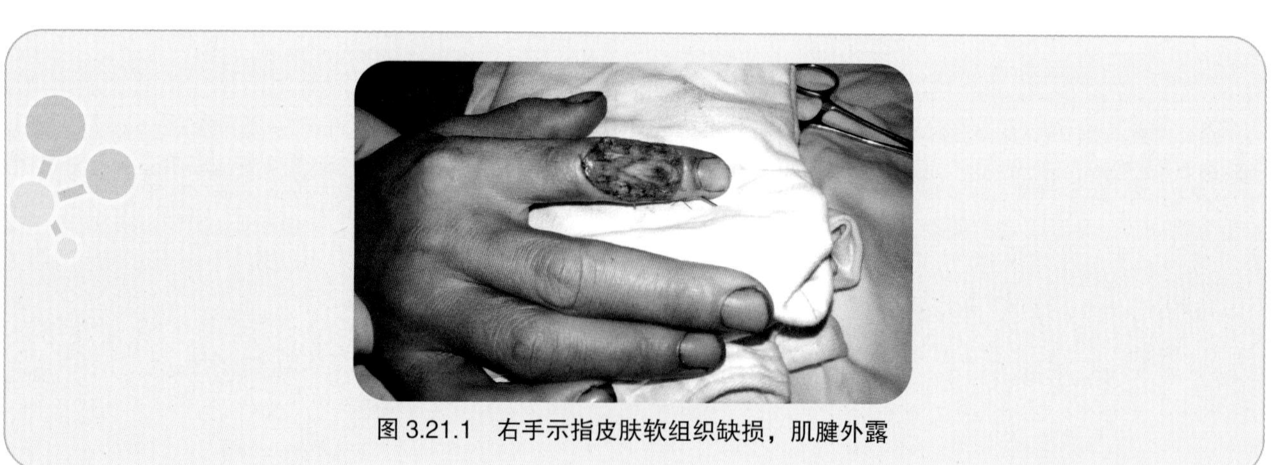
图 3.21.1　右手示指皮肤软组织缺损，肌腱外露

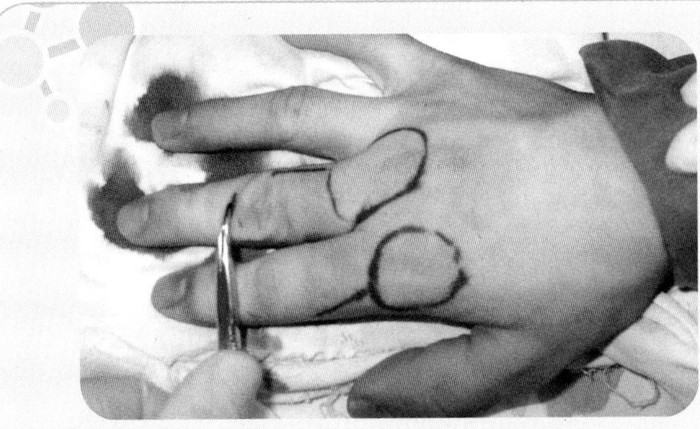

Figure 3.20.2 Schematic diagram of the design of the index finger and middle finger dorsal fascia flap

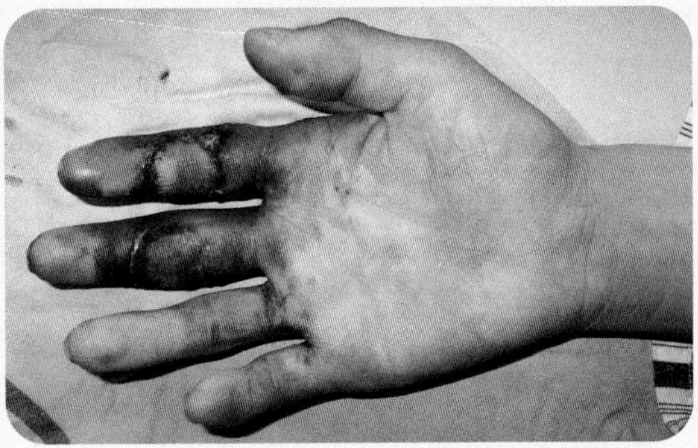

Figure 3.20.3 After successful flap transplantation

(Chen Shanliang)

Case 21 Skin defect on the back of the index finger

◆ Cause of injury

The patient's right hand was scratched by a wire drawing machine, resulting in a skin defect on the back of the index finger.

◆ Signs and symptoms

The right index finger is experiencing severe pain, continuous bleeding, swelling, and gradually worsening. The skin and soft tissue on the dorsal side of the middle and distal segments of the index finger are missing, with neat boundaries and mild contamination. The extensor tendon is exposed without rupture, and the index finger has good flexion and extension activity (Figure 3.21.1). The area of skin defect is 3.5 cm × 1.5 cm.

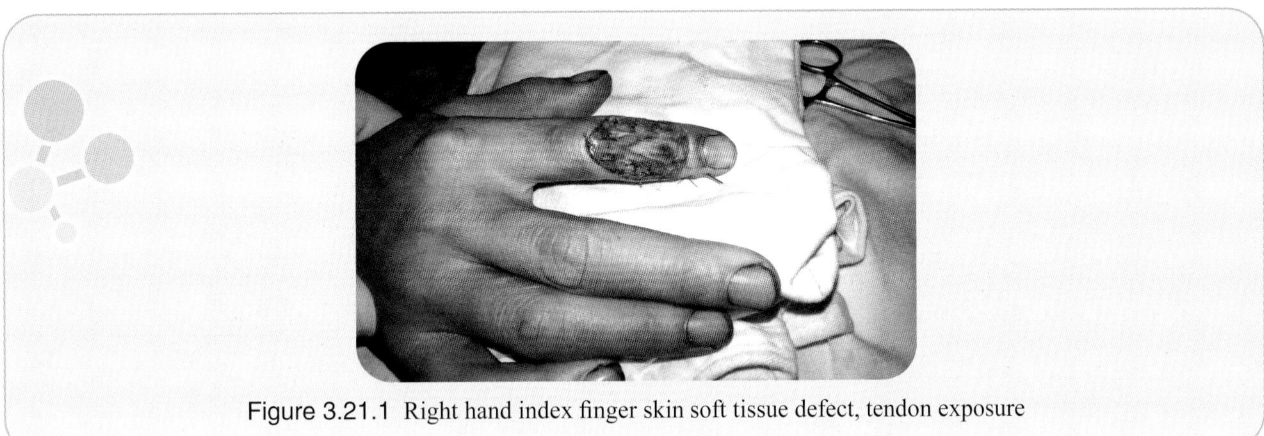

Figure 3.21.1 Right hand index finger skin soft tissue defect, tendon exposure

◆ 治疗方案

1. 臂丛麻醉下急诊入院一期清创，一期皮瓣移植消灭创面。

2. 手术过程

2.1 皮瓣设计：以示指指背侧中线为轴线，解剖面为筋膜浅层，旋转点距创缘 1 cm 处。蒂长 1.5 cm、蒂宽 0.35 cm（图 3.21.2）。

2.2 皮瓣移植：开放隧道，依次解剖皮瓣并结扎切口内分支血管，皮瓣解剖后，创面喷洒生长因子，并行受区供区缝合，皮瓣下放置橡皮条引流。供区切口直接缝合。

3. 术后抬高患肢，观察皮瓣血运，每天换药喷洒外用重组人酸性成纤维细胞生长因子，术后 24 小时拔出引流条。

4. 术后 7 天骨关节主被动活动，12 天拆线，并进行全面康复训练（图 3.21.3）。

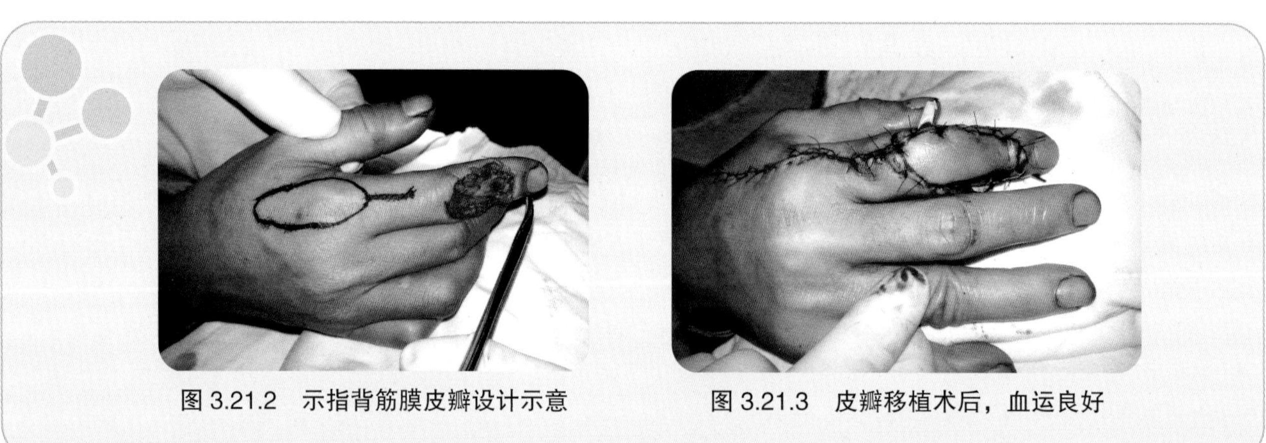

图 3.21.2 示指背筋膜皮瓣设计示意

图 3.21.3 皮瓣移植术后，血运良好

（陈善亮）

案例二十二 示指甲床缺损指骨外露

◆ 损伤原因

患者左手因钢管压伤，致示指甲床缺损指骨外露。

◆ 症状与体征

左手示指剧痛，出血不止，肿胀伴活动受限。示指末节甲床缺损，缺损面积 1.5 cm × 1.5 cm，指骨外露，末节指骨骨擦感、骨擦音阳性，末节关节活动受限，指背皮肤有擦伤，示指广泛性肿胀，局部污染不重（图 3.22.1）。

◆ Treatment plan

1. Emergency admission under brachial plexus anesthesia with first stage debridement and first stage skin flap transplantation to eliminate the wound.

2. Surgical process

2.1 Skin flap design: Using the midline of the dorsal side of the finger as the axis, the anatomical surface is the superficial layer of the fascia, and the rotation point is 1 cm away from the wound edge. The pedicle is 1.5 cm long and 0.35 cm wide (Figure 3.21.2).

2.2 Skin flap transplantation: Open the tunnel, dissect the skin flap in sequence and ligate the branch blood vessels inside the incision. After dissecting the skin flap, spray growth factor on the wound, suture the donor area in parallel, and place a rubber strip under the skin flap for drainage. The incision in the supply area is directly sutured.

3. After surgery, raise the affected limb, observe the blood flow of the skin flap, change the dressing daily, spray external recombinant human acidic fibroblast growth factor, and remove the drainage strip 24 hours after surgery.

4. After 7 days of surgery, active and passive bone and joint movements were performed, and stitches were removed 12 days later, followed by comprehensive rehabilitation training (Figure 3.21.3).

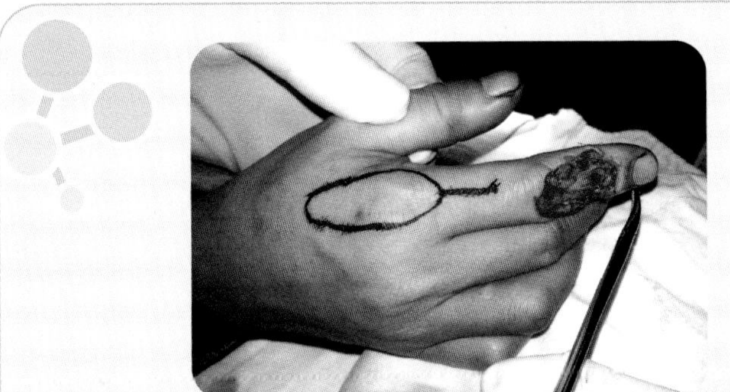

Figure 3.21.2 Schematic diagram of the design of the index finger dorsal fascia skin flap

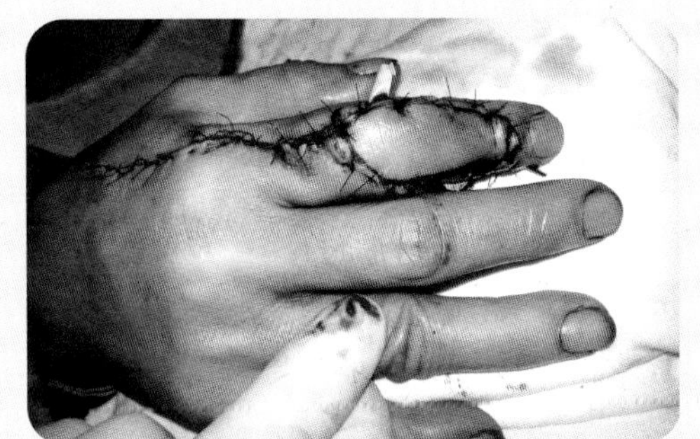

Figure 3.21.3 Good blood flow after flap transplantation

(Chen Shanliang)

Case 22 Nail bed defect with exposed finger bones

◆ Cause of injury

The patient's left hand was injured by a steel tube, resulting in a nail bed defect and exposed finger bones.

◆ Signs and symptoms

Severe pain in the left index finger, continuous bleeding, swelling with restricted movement. There is a defect in the nail bed of the distal phalanx of the index finger, with a defect area of 1.5 cm × 1.5 cm. The phalanx is exposed, and the bone friction sensation and bone friction sound of the distal phalanx are positive. The joint movement of the distal phalanx is limited, and there is abrasion on the skin of the back of the finger. The index finger is widely swollen, and the local contamination is not significant (Figure 3.22.1).

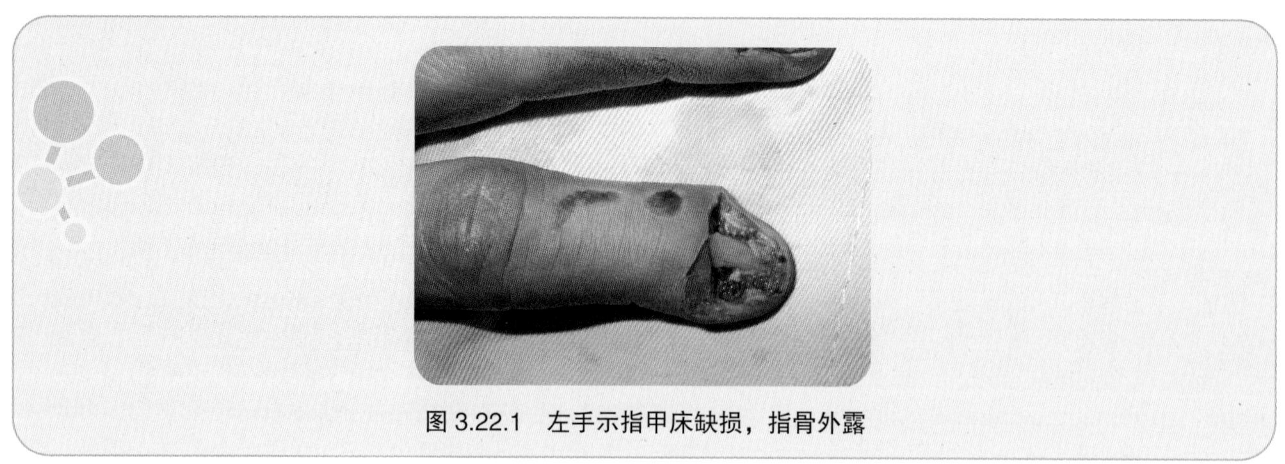

图 3.22.1　左手示指甲床缺损，指骨外露

◆ 治疗方案

1. 臂丛麻醉下急诊入院一期清创，一期皮瓣移植消灭创面，首先骨折复位，取 1.0 克氏针固定。

2. 手术过程

2.1 皮瓣设计：示指指背中线为轴线，避开皮肤擦伤处，解剖面为筋膜浅层，旋转点距创缘 1.5 cm 处，蒂长 1.5 cm、蒂宽 0.3 cm。

2.2 皮瓣移植：依次解剖皮瓣，开放隧道，皮瓣解剖完毕后，创面喷洒生长因子，行受区供区缝合。供区全厚皮肤移植（图 3.22.2）。

3. 术后抬高患肢，观察皮瓣血运，每天换药喷洒外用重组人酸性成纤维细胞生长因子促进伤口愈合。

4. 术后 12 天拆线，1 个月后拔克氏针，并进行全面康复训练。

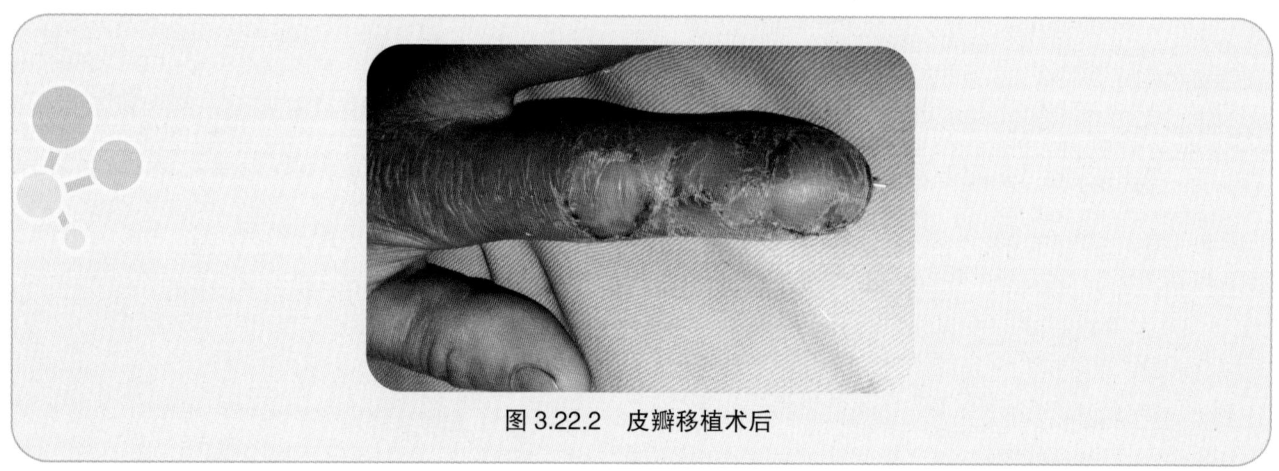

图 3.22.2　皮瓣移植术后

（陈善亮）

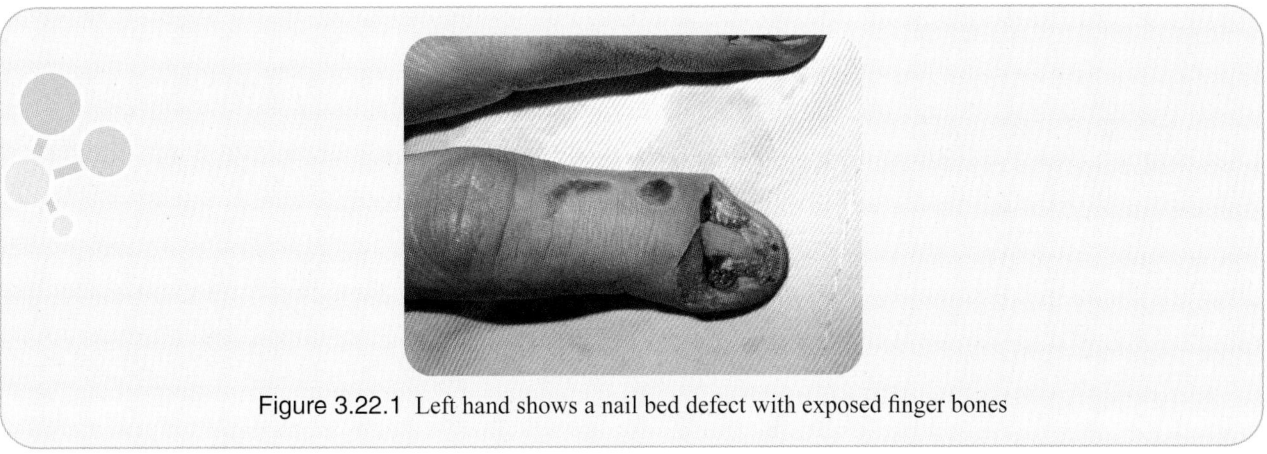

Figure 3.22.1 Left hand shows a nail bed defect with exposed finger bones

◆ Treatment plan

1. Emergency admission under brachial plexus anesthesia for first stage debridement, first stage skin flap transplantation to eliminate the wound, first fracture reduction, and fixation with 1.0 gram Kirschner wire.

2. Surgical process

2.1 Skin flap design: The midline of the index finger is used as the axis, avoiding skin abrasions. The anatomical surface is the superficial layer of the fascia, and the rotation point is 1.5 cm away from the wound edge. The pedicle is 1.5 cm long and 0.3 cm wide.

2.2 Skin flap transplantation: Dissect the skin flap in sequence, open the tunnel, and after the dissection of the skin flap is completed, spray growth factors on the wound surface and suture the donor site in the receiving area. Full thickness skin transplantation in the donor area (Figure 3.22.2).

3. After surgery, elevate the affected limb, observe the blood flow of the skin flap, and change the dressing daily to spray external recombinant human acidic fibroblast growth factor to promote wound healing.

4. Remove the stitches 12 days after surgery, remove the Kirschner wire one month later, and undergo comprehensive rehabilitation training.

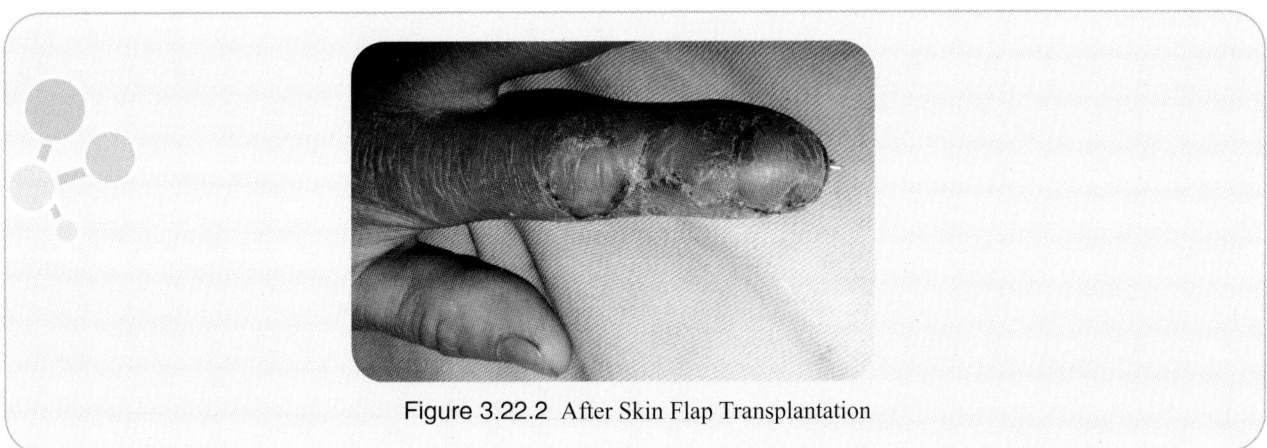

Figure 3.22.2 After Skin Flap Transplantation

(Chen Shanliang)

案例二十三　示指指间关节皮肤软组织缺损

◆ 损伤原因

患者右手因模具挤压伤，致示指指间关节皮肤软组织缺损。

◆ 症状与体征

右手示指疼痛，出血不止。右示指末节指间关节桡侧有 1.5 cm × 0.8 cm 创面，桡侧指动脉和指神经断裂，屈指深肌腱部分断裂，指端桡侧感觉消失，末节指间关节活动受限（图 3.23.1）。

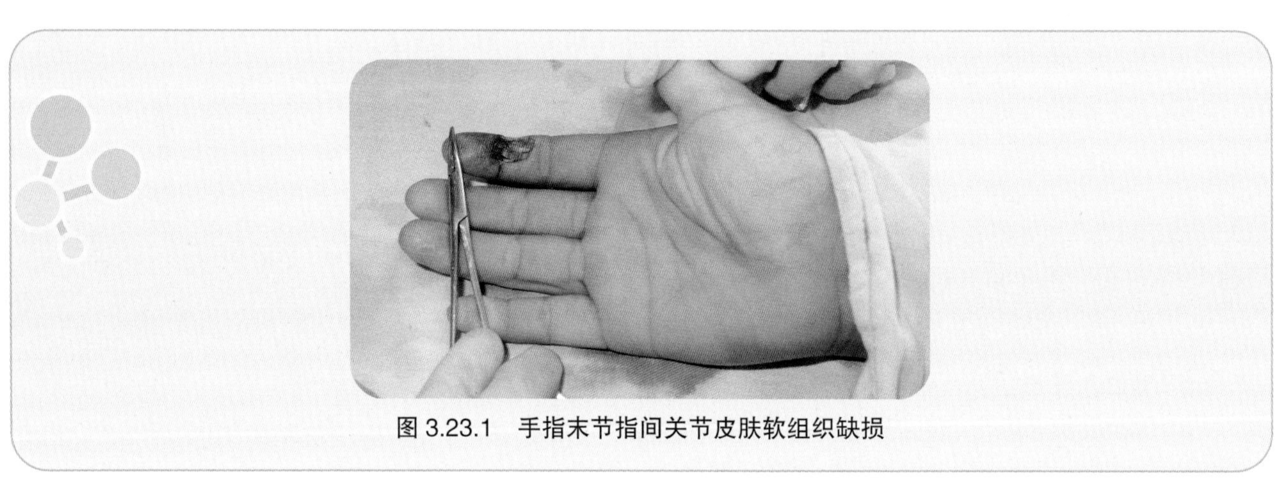

图 3.23.1　手指末节指间关节皮肤软组织缺损

◆ 治疗方案

1. 臂丛麻醉急诊一期清创，血管神经肌腱修复。

2. 手术过程

2.1 皮瓣设计：以示指桡侧中线为轴线，解剖面为筋膜浅层，旋转点在中指间关节处，蒂长 1.8 cm、蒂宽 0.3 cm 并保留部分皮蒂。

2.2 皮瓣移植：依次解剖并游离皮瓣，皮瓣解剖完毕后，创面喷洒生长因子，并行受供区缝合，皮瓣供区全厚皮肤移植。石膏固定于功能位（图 3.23.2、图 3.23.3）。

3. 术后抬高患肢，观察皮瓣血运，每天换药喷洒外用重组人酸性成纤维细胞生长因子促进伤口愈合。

4. 术后 12 天拆线，石膏固定 4 周，去石膏后并进行全面康复训练。

Case 23 Skin and soft tissue defects in the interphalangeal joint of the index finger

◆ Cause of injury

The patient's right hand suffered from compression injury caused by a mold, resulting in skin and soft tissue defects in the interphalangeal joint.

◆ Signs and symptoms

The right index finger is painful and bleeding continuously. There is a 1.5 cm × 0.8 cm wound on the radial side of the distal interphalangeal joint of the right index finger. The radial finger artery and nerve are broken, and the deep flexor tendon is partially broken. The sensation on the radial side of the fingertip disappears, and the movement of the distal interphalangeal joint is restricted (Figure 3.23.1).

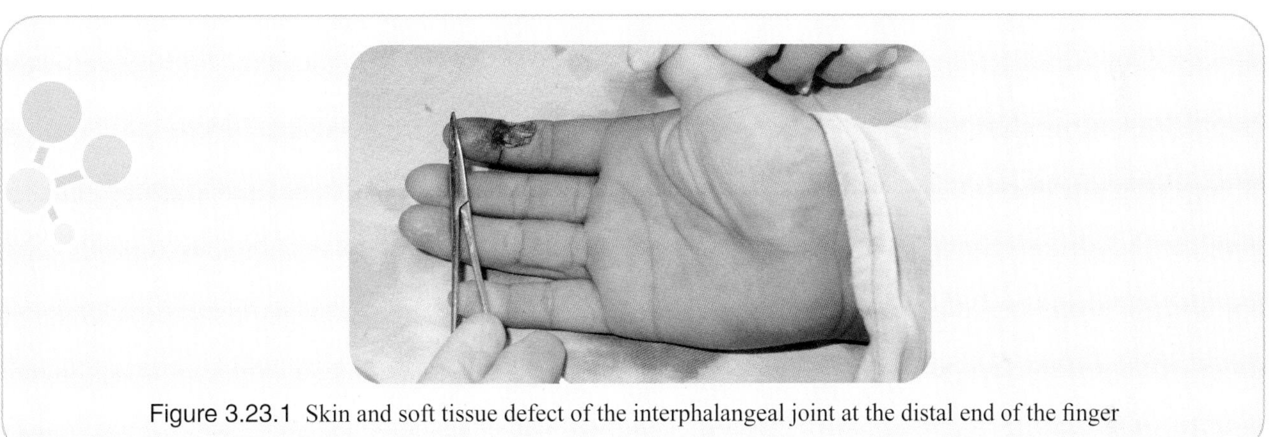

Figure 3.23.1 Skin and soft tissue defect of the interphalangeal joint at the distal end of the finger

◆ Treatment plan

1. Emergency first stage debridement of brachial plexus anesthesia, vascular, nerve, and tendon repair.

2. Surgical process

2.1 Skin flap design: Taking the radial midline of the finger as the axis, the anatomical surface is the superficial fascia, the rotation point is at the interphalangeal joint, the pedicle length is 1.8 cm, the pedicle width is 0.3 cm, and part of the skin pedicle is retained.

2.2 Skin flap transplantation: Dissect and free the skin flap in sequence. After the dissection of the skin flap is completed, spray growth factors on the wound surface, suture the donor area in parallel, and transplant the full-thickness skin of the skin flap donor area. Gypsum is fixed in the functional position (Figure 3.23.2, Figure 3.23.3).

3. After surgery, elevate the affected limb, observe the blood flow of the skin flap, and change the dressing daily to spray external recombinant human acidic fibroblast growth factor to promote wound healing.

4. The stitches were removed 12 days after surgery, and the plaster was fixed for 4 weeks. After removing the plaster, comprehensive rehabilitation training was conducted.

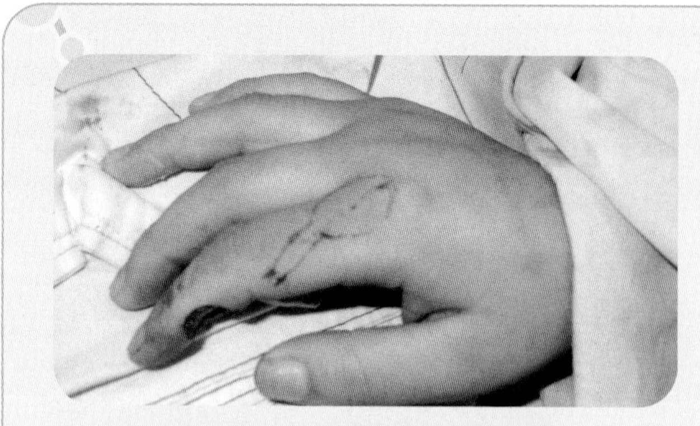

图 3.23.2　示指背筋膜皮瓣示意

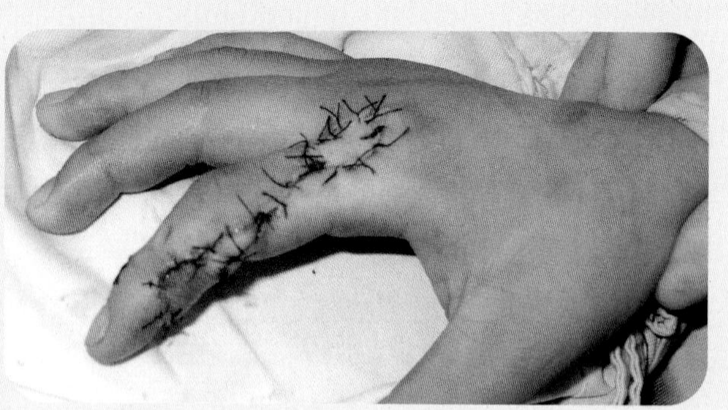

图 3.23.3　皮瓣移植后

（陈善亮）

案例二十四　拇指指腹缺损骨外露

◆ 损伤原因

患者左手因高温热压伤，致拇指指腹缺损、骨外露。

◆ 症状与体征

左手拇指压伤后剧痛，肿胀并渐加重，曾在当地医院换药治疗，伤口不能愈合。拇指指腹干瘪萎缩，指腹残留未愈合创面，末节指骨外露，末节关节僵硬，深屈活动受限，皮肤软缺损面积 1.5 cm × 2.5 cm，指端感觉消失（图 3.24.1、图 3.24.2）。

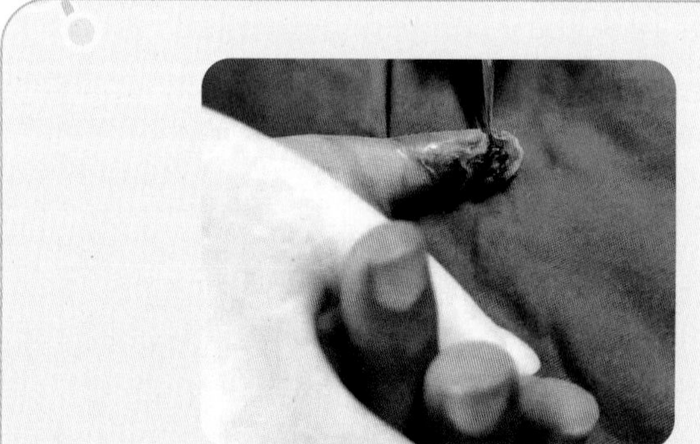

图 3.24.1　左手拇指指腹瘪陷，指骨外露

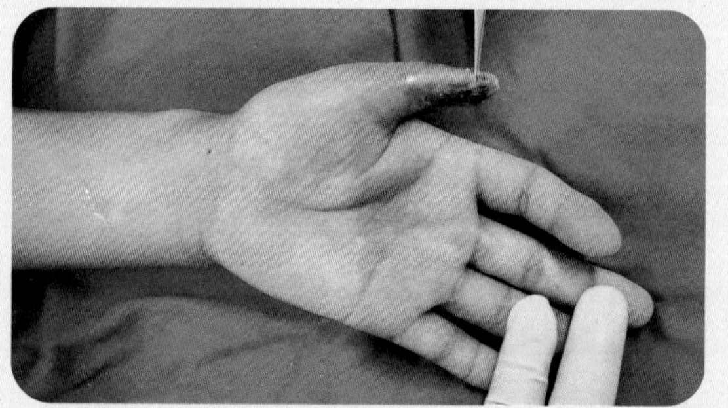

图 3.24.2　左手拇指侧位，扁平纤细，关节强直

◆ 治疗方案

该患者为陈旧外伤，伤后在当地医院换药治疗，伤口都是瘢痕替代，指骨外露，瘢痕无生长能力覆盖指骨，

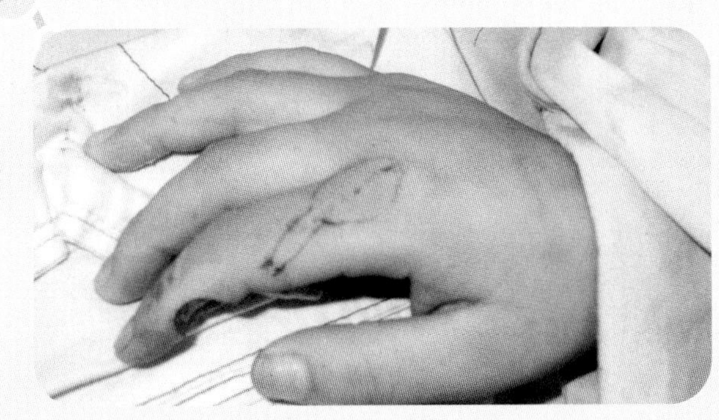

Figure 3.23.2 Schematic diagram of the dorsal fascia flap of the index finger

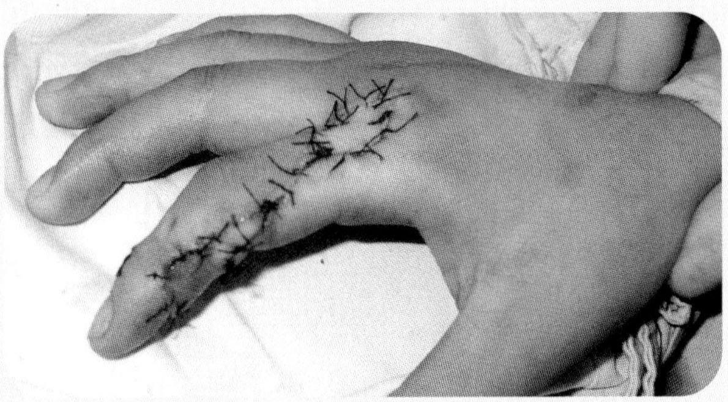

Figure 3.23.3 After Skin Flap Transplantation

(Chen Shanliang)

Case 24 Thumb pulp defect with bone exposure

◆ Cause of injury

The patient's left hand was injured by high temperature and heat pressure, resulting in a defect in the fingertip and exposed bone.

◆ Signs and symptoms

After the left thumb was crushed, there was severe pain, swelling, and gradually worsening. I had to change the dressing at a local hospital for treatment, but the wound could not heal. The thumb's fingertip is withered and atrophied, with residual unhealed wounds on the fingertip. The distal phalanx is exposed, the distal phalanx joint is stiff, and deep flexion activity is limited. The soft skin defect area is 1.5 cm × 2.5 cm, and the fingertip sensation disappears (Figure 3.24.1, Figure 3.24.2).

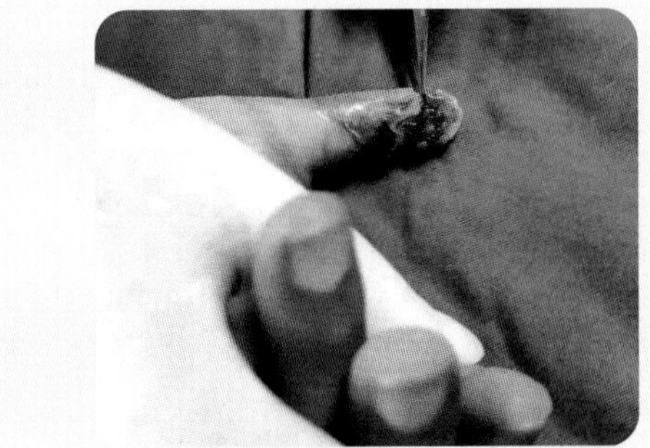

Figure 3.24.1 Left thumb with depressed fingertip and exposed phalanx

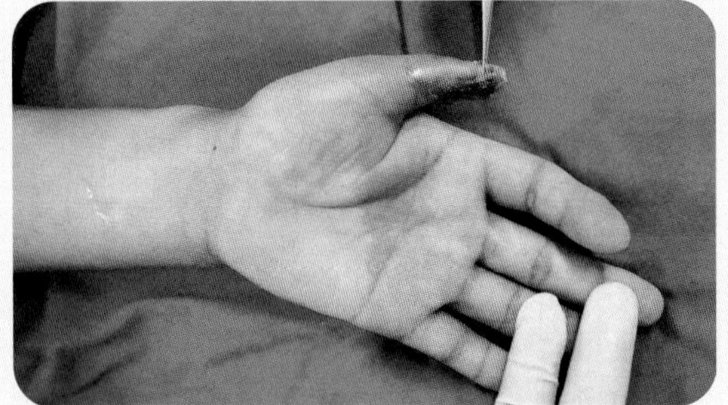

Figure 3.24.2 Left thumb side view, flat and slender, joint stiffness

◆ Treatment plan

The patient had an old trauma and was treated with dressing changes at a local hospital after the injury. The wounds were all scar replacements, with exposed phalanges and no ability for scar growth to cover the phalanges.

瘢痕硬化关节僵硬，末节功能丧失。治疗主要切除部分瘢痕，皮瓣移植覆盖指骨。

1. 采用臂丛神经阻滞麻醉。

2. 手术过程

2.1 清创：切除菲薄硬化瘢痕，修剪裸露干瘪坏死指骨，修剪伤口边缘。

2.2 皮瓣设计：采用示指背皮瓣，以第 2 掌骨桡侧缘为轴线，蒂长 4 cm、蒂宽 0.3 cm。

2.3 皮瓣移植：解剖面为筋膜浅层，皮瓣采用闭合隧道，依次解剖皮瓣，解剖结束后，创面外用重组人酸性成纤维细胞生长因子，并行受供区缝合，于前臂内侧切取全厚皮肤移植于皮瓣受区，闭合切口，包扎伤口，术终（图 3.24.3、图 3.24.4）。

3. 术后抬高患肢，观察皮瓣血运，每天换药重组人酸性成纤维细胞生长因子促进伤口愈合（图 3.24.5）。

4. 术后 12 天拆线，石膏固定 4 周，去石膏后并进行全面康复训练。

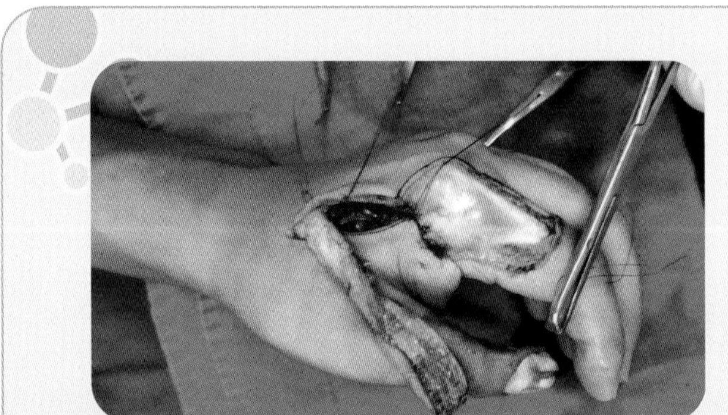

图 3.24.3　皮瓣完全解剖游离

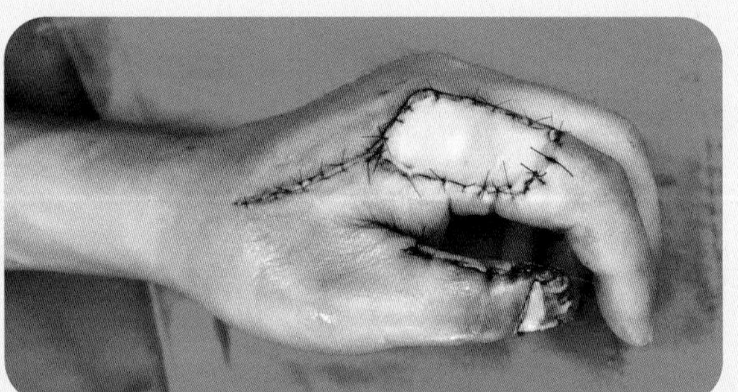

图 3.24.4　皮瓣和游离植皮术后

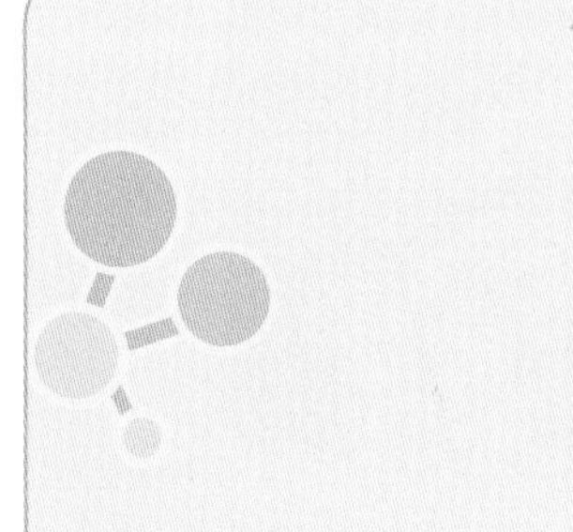

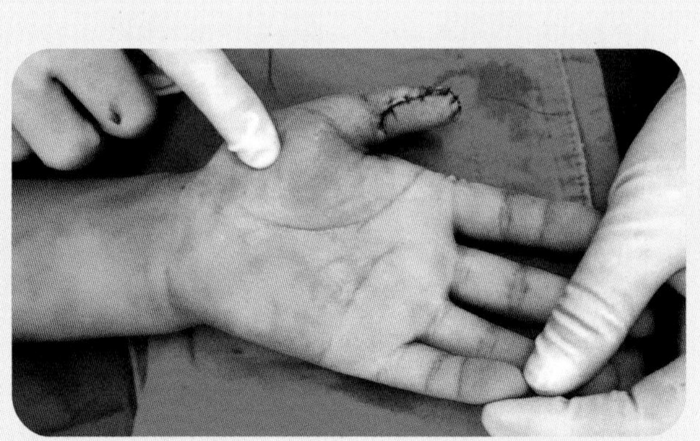

图 3.24.5　皮瓣移植术后第 3 天，皮瓣血运外形良好

（陈善亮）

The scars hardened and the joints became stiff, resulting in loss of distal end function. The treatment mainly involves removing partial scars and transplanting skin flaps to cover the finger bones.

1. Use brachial plexus block anesthesia.

2. Surgical process

2.1 Debridement: Remove thin and hardened scars, trim exposed withered and necrotic finger bones, and trim the edges of the wound.

2.2 Skin flap design: The index finger dorsal skin flap is used, with the radial edge of the second metacarpal bone as the axis, a pedicle length of 4 cm, and a pedicle width of 0.3 cm.

2.3 Skin flap transplantation: The anatomical surface is the superficial layer of the fascia, and the skin flap is dissected sequentially using a closed tunnel. After dissection, recombinant human acidic fibroblast growth factor is applied externally to the wound, and the donor site is sutured. Full thickness skin is cut from the inner side of the forearm and transplanted into the skin flap recipient site. The incision is closed, the wound is wrapped, and the surgery is completed (Figure 3.24.3, Figure 3.24.4).

3. After surgery, raise the affected limb, observe the blood flow of the skin flap, and change the dressing of recombinant human acidic fibroblast growth factor every day to promote wound healing (Figure 3.24.5).

4. The stitches were removed 12 days after surgery, and the plaster was fixed for 4 weeks. After removing the plaster, comprehensive rehabilitation training was conducted.

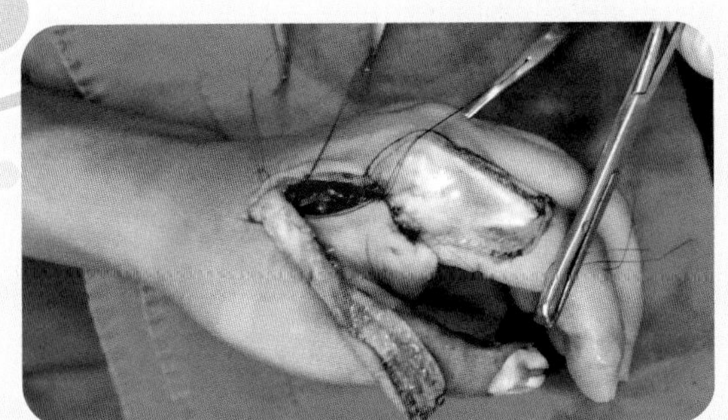

Figure 3.24.3 Fully dissected and free flap

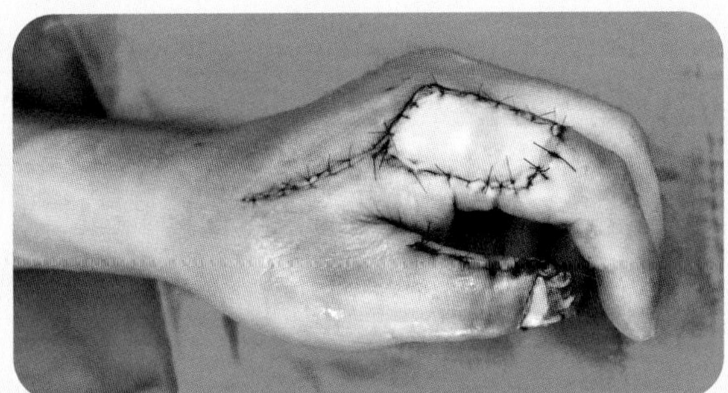

Figure 3.24.4 After Skin Flap and Free Skin Transplantation

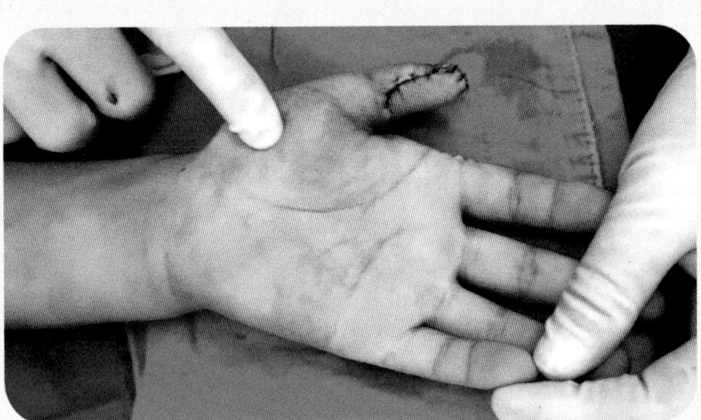

Figure 3.24.5 On the third day after the skin flap transplantation, the blood flow and appearance of the skin flap are good

(Chen Shanliang)

案例二十五　足内侧擦伤皮肤缺损

◆ 损伤原因

患者因车祸拖行摩擦伤，致左足内侧皮肤大面积缺损。

◆ 症状与体征

左足剧痛难忍，出血、肿胀并逐渐加重。左足蹞趾和足内侧，有两处不规则伤口，皮缘有挫灭伤，伤口内有泥沙，深达骨膜，内踝有挫伤，足内侧创面 7 cm × 4 cm，足蹞趾指内侧创面 3.5 cm × 3.0 cm，足趾活动良好（图 3.25.1）。足部无骨折。

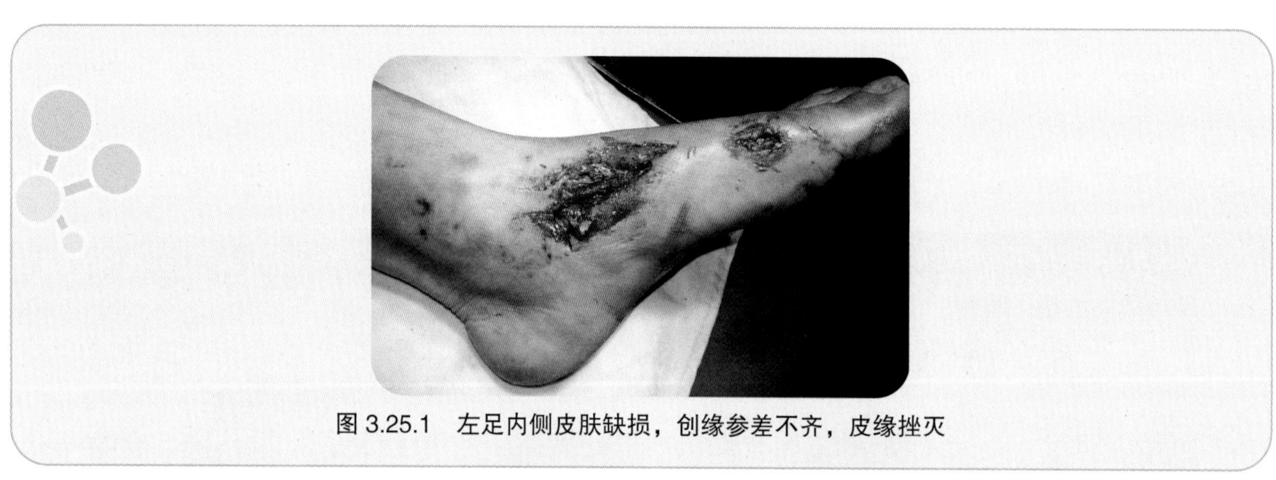

图 3.25.1　左足内侧皮肤缺损，创缘参差不齐，皮缘挫灭

◆ 治疗方案

由于足部创面在地下摩擦伤，皮肤创缘坏死界限不清。局部污染重，直接皮瓣移植有感染概率，此类损伤分为两期手术覆盖创面。

1. 一期清创预防感染 + 外用重组人酸性成纤维细胞生长因子冲洗 +VSD 治疗，负压治疗 5 天，拆除 VSD 并行胫后动脉内踝上穿支皮瓣移植（图 3.25.2、图 3.25.3）。

2. 手术过程

2.1 皮瓣设计：胫骨内侧缘于内踝跟腱连线为皮瓣轴线，内踝尖偏后侧为旋转点，解剖面为筋膜浅层，蒂宽 3 cm。采用开放隧道，由于受区为 2 个创面，皮瓣设计了串联皮瓣，即一蒂两瓣（图 3.25.4）。皮瓣大小面积，近端蒂面积 7 cm × 3.5 cm，远端蒂面积 2 cm × 3 cm。

2.2 皮瓣移植：依次切开皮肤皮下脂肪达肌筋膜浅层，将大隐静脉包含在皮瓣内，结扎皮瓣血管分支，皮瓣游离解剖完毕后观察皮瓣远端血运，远端蒂皮瓣血运良好。皮瓣近端蒂为开放隧道，远端蒂为闭合隧道，

Case 25 Scratches and skin defects on the inner side of the foot

◆ Cause of injury

The patient suffered from dragging and friction injuries in a car accident, resulting in a large area of skin defect on the inner side of the left foot.

◆ Signs and symptoms

The left foot is severely painful, with bleeding, swelling, and gradually worsening. There are two irregular wounds on the left toe and inner side of the foot, with a bruise on the skin edge and mud inside the wound, reaching deep into the periosteum. There is also a bruise on the inner ankle, with a 7 cm × 4 cm wound on the inner side of the foot and a 3.5 cm × 3.0 cm wound on the inner side of the toe. The toe is well moved (Figure 3.25.1). No fractures in the foot.

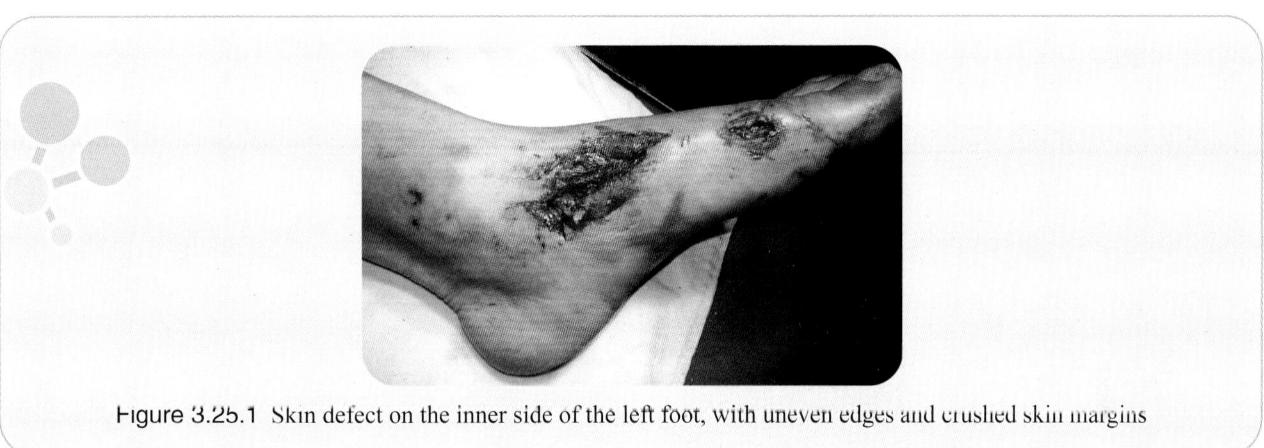

Figure 3.25.1 Skin defect on the inner side of the left foot, with uneven edges and crushed skin margins

◆ Treatment plan

Due to the friction wound on the foot underground, the boundary of skin wound necrosis is unclear. Local pollution is severe, and direct skin flap transplantation has a probability of infection. This type of injury is divided into two stages of surgical coverage of the wound.

1. First stage debridement for infection prevention + external application of recombinant human acidic fibroblast growth factor flushing + VSD treatment, negative pressure treatment for 5 days, removal of VSD and transplantation of the medial malleolus perforator flap of the posterior tibial artery (Figure 3.25.2, Figure 3.25.3).

2. Surgical process

2.1 Skin flap design: The inner side of the tibia is connected to the Achilles tendon of the medial malleolus as the axis of the skin flap, and the posterior side of the medial malleolus tip is the rotation point. The anatomical plane is the superficial layer of the fascia, and the pedicle width is 3 cm. Using an open tunnel, as the receiving area consists of two wounds, a series of skin flaps were designed, namely one pedicle and two flaps (Figure 3.25.4). The size and area of the skin flap are 7 cm × 3.5 cm for the proximal pedicle and 2 cm × 3 cm for the distal pedicle.

2.2 Skin flap transplantation: Cut open the subcutaneous fat of the skin to the superficial layer of the fascia, include the great saphenous vein in the skin flap, ligate the vascular branches of the skin flap, and observe the blood flow of the distal end of the skin flap after dissection. The blood flow of the distal pedicle flap is good. The proximal pedicle of the skin flap is an open tunnel, and the distal pedicle is a closed tunnel. The wound is sprayed

创面喷洒外用重组人酸性成纤维细胞生长因子促进愈合，将皮瓣从闭合隧道中穿过，行受供区缝合，皮瓣下放置三条橡皮条引流，防止皮下血肿形成（图 3.25.5）。由于皮瓣供区直接闭合伤口困难，于小腿外侧切取中厚皮片移植于皮瓣供区并缝合，皮瓣移植后局部血运良好，包扎伤口，石膏托固定足踝部，术终。

3. 术后抬高患肢减轻肿胀，保温，日光灯照射，严密观察皮瓣血运，每天更换敷料一次，换药时常规喷洒外用重组人酸性成纤维细胞生长因子，皮瓣蒂部宽松包扎，包扎过紧容易压迫皮蒂影响皮瓣血供，48 小时拔出引流条（图 3.25.6）。

4. 扩容、解痉，补充血容量，增加皮瓣灌注量，常规镇痛，预防因疼痛引起血管痉挛。

5. 术后 12 天拆线，并下地逐渐负重行走，恢复踝关节功能，局部弹力治疗。

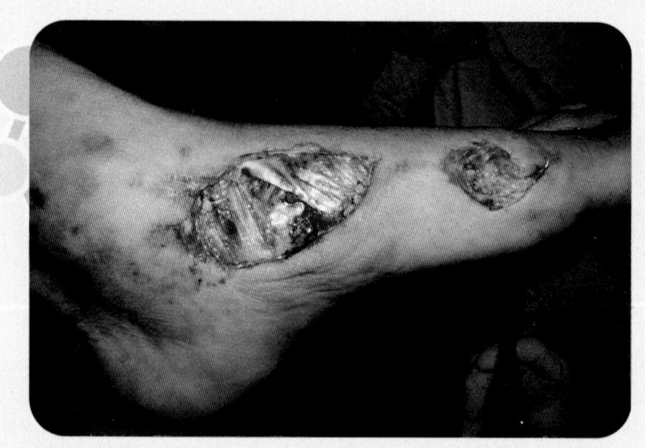

图 3.25.2　清创后韧带撕裂，足舟骨部分缺损

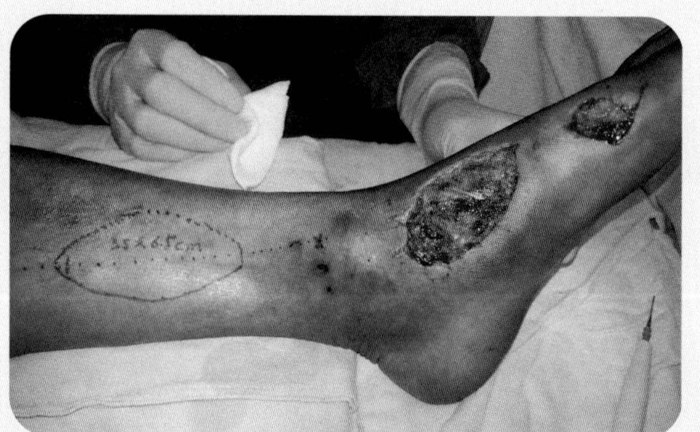

图 3.25.3　创面生长因子+VSD 负压治疗 5 天，有部分肉芽组织生长

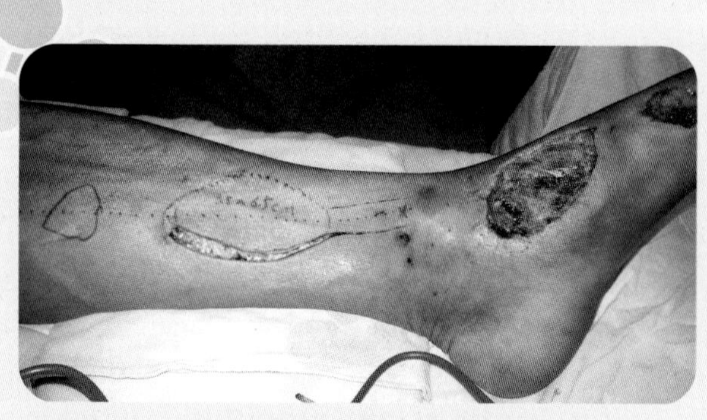

图 3.25.4　胫后动脉内踝上穿支皮瓣设计示意

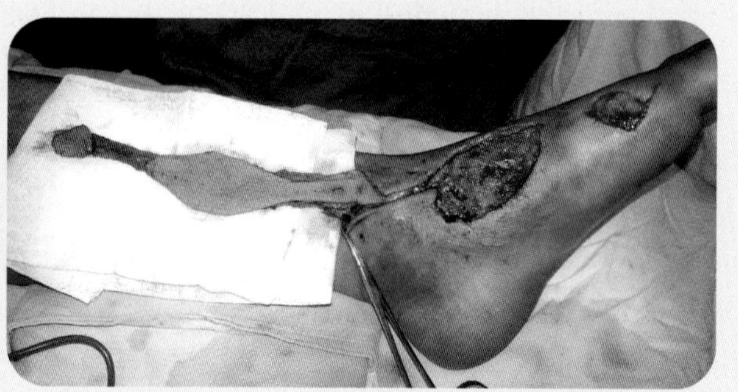

图 3.25.5　皮瓣完全游离解剖，采用开放隧道

with recombinant human acidic fibroblast growth factor to promote healing. The skin flap is passed through the closed tunnel and sutured at the donor site. Three rubber strips are placed under the skin flap for drainage to prevent subcutaneous hematoma formation (Figure 3.25.5). Due to the difficulty of directly closing the wound in the skin flap donor area, a medium thick skin graft was cut from the outer side of the calf and transplanted into the skin flap donor area and sutured. After the skin flap transplantation, the local blood supply was good, the wound was bandaged, and the ankle was fixed with a plaster cast. The surgery was completed.

3. After surgery, elevate the affected limb to reduce swelling, keep it warm, expose it to fluorescent light, closely observe the blood flow of the skin flap, change the dressing once a day, and spray recombinant human acidic fibroblast growth factor externally during dressing change. Loose wrapping of the skin flap pedicle can easily compress the pedicle and affect the blood supply of the skin flap. Remove the drainage strip within 48 hours (Figure 3.25.6).

4. Expand capacity, relieve spasms, replenish blood volume, increase flap perfusion, provide routine analgesia, and prevent vascular spasm caused by pain.

5. After 12 days of surgery, remove the stitches and gradually walk with weight-bearing to restore ankle joint function, followed by local elasticity treatment.

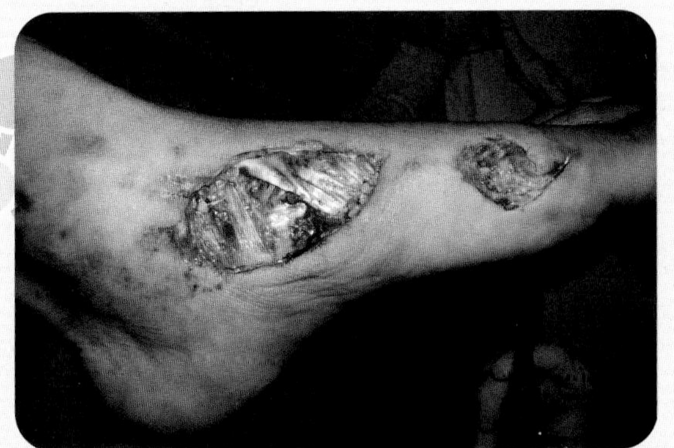

Figure 3.25.2 Posterior ligament tear after debridement, partial defect of talus bone

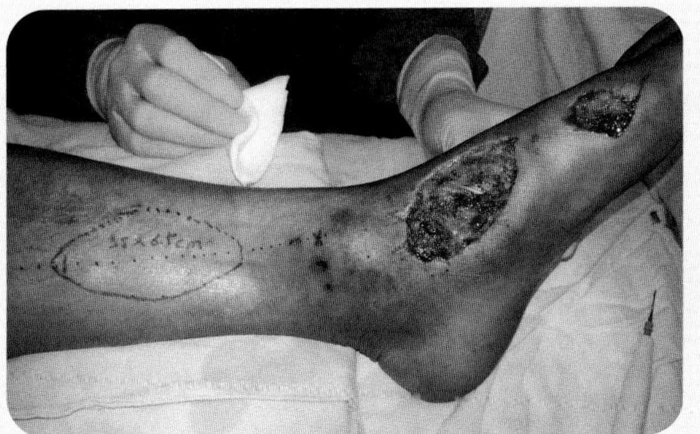

Figure 3.25.3 After 5 days of negative pressure treatment with wound growth factor and VSD, some granulation tissue grew

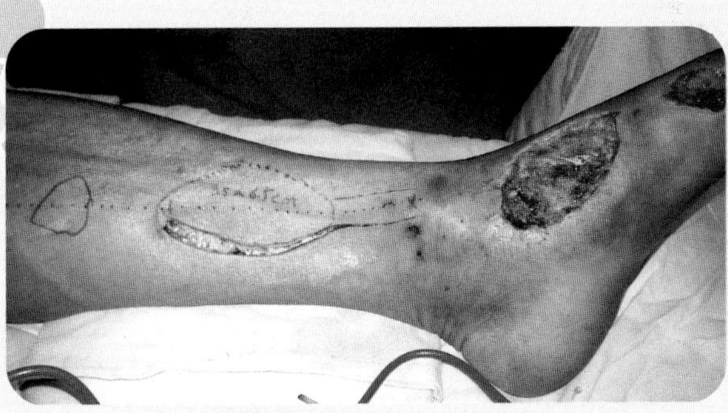

Figure 3.25.4 Schematic design of the medial malleolus perforator flap of the posterior tibial artery

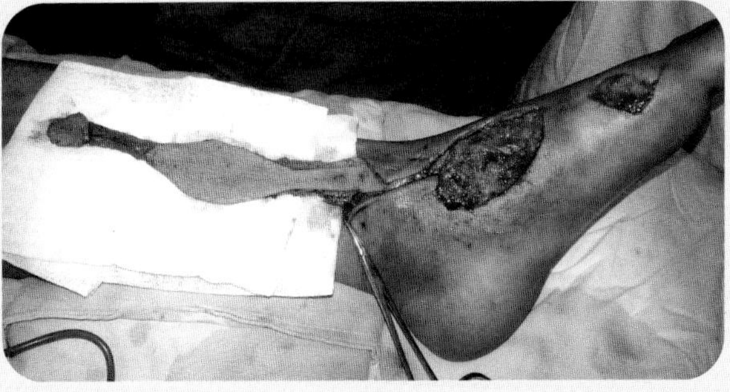

Figure 3.25.5 Fully free dissection of the skin flap using an open tunnel

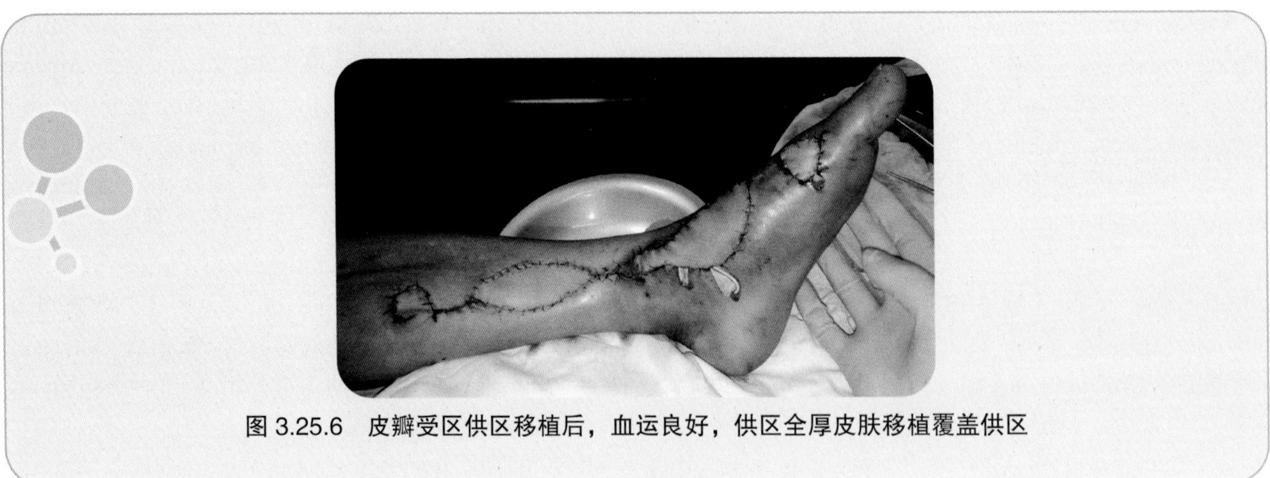

图 3.25.6　皮瓣受区供区移植后，血运良好，供区全厚皮肤移植覆盖供区

（陈善亮）

案例二十六　手背文身

◆ 发病原因

手背文身 8 年，曾经去文身漂洗 3 次，仍不能去除。

◆ 症状与体征

手背文身处紫外线照射不适感，时有瘙痒，局部皮肤硬化，凹凸不平，轻度触痛，拇指背侧感觉减退，拇指、示指深屈活动良好（图 3.26.1）。

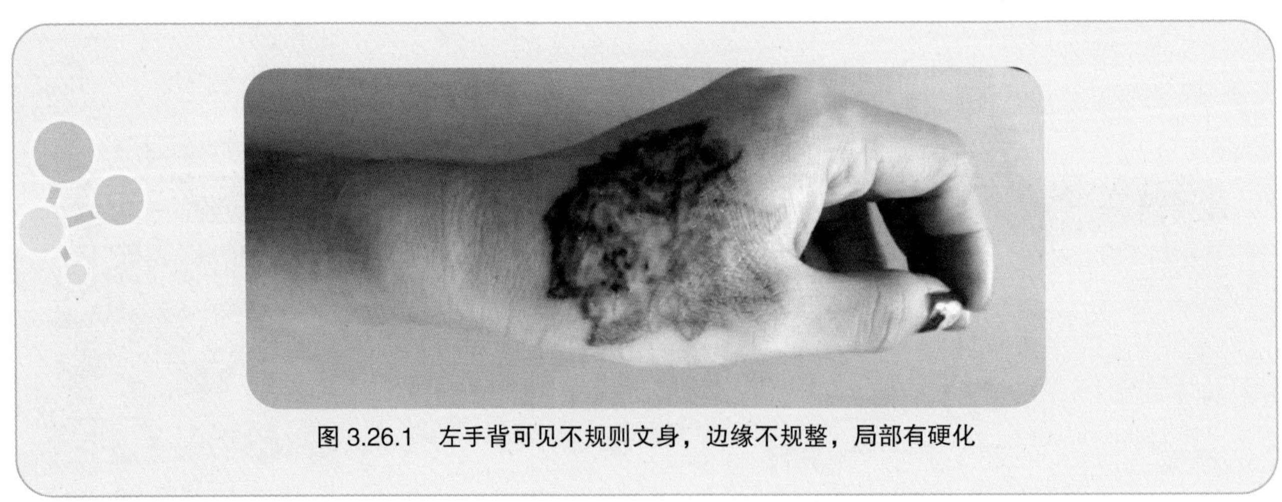

图 3.26.1　左手背可见不规则文身，边缘不规整，局部有硬化

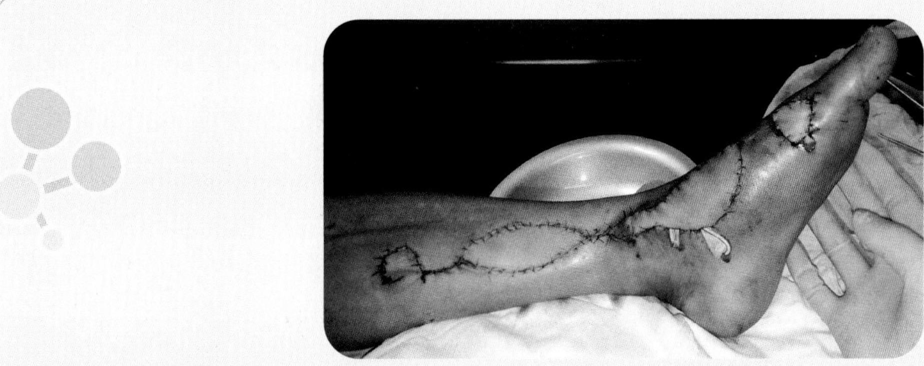

Figure 3.25.6 After transplantation of the skin flap to the donor site, the blood supply is good, and the full-thickness skin graft covers the donor site

(Chen Shanliang)

Case 26 Tattoo on the back of the hand

◆ Cause of onset

I have had a tattoo on my back of my hand for 8 years and have had it washed three times, but it still cannot be removed.

◆ Signs and symptoms

The tattoo on the back of the hand feels uncomfortable when exposed to ultraviolet radiation, with occasional itching, local skin hardening, unevenness, mild tenderness, decreased sensation on the back of the thumb, and good deep flexion and movement of the thumb and index finger (Figure 3.26.1).

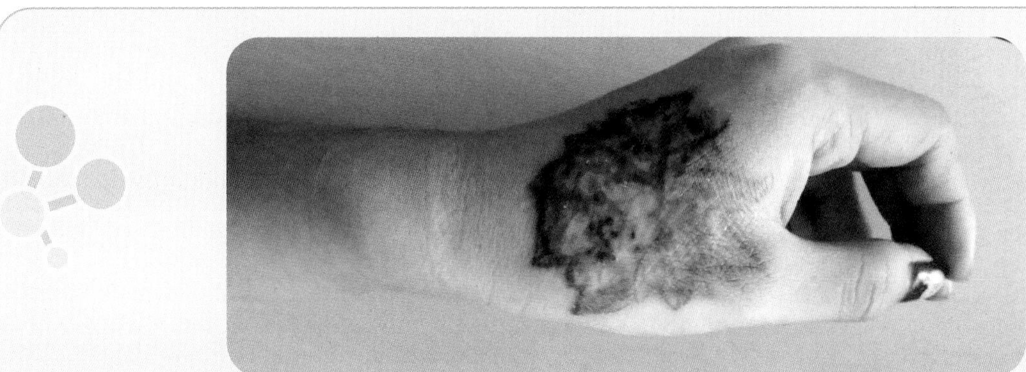

Figure 3.26.1 Irregular tattoo visible on the back of the left hand, with irregular edges and localized hardening

◆ 治疗方案

该案例曾经做过 3 次文身漂洗，由于文的较深，漂洗失败。

1. 患者文身处有瘙痒不适感，漂洗后局部皮肤有硬化。

2. 手术切除是唯一解决办法。手术要点：①硬化皮肤全层切除；②局部止血彻底；③移植皮肤精密缝合，减少瘢痕形成；④创面喷洒外用重组人酸性成纤维细胞生长因子；⑤全厚皮肤移植，局部加压包扎（图 3.26.2 ~ 图 3.26.4）。

3. 术后 7 天换药，12 天拆线。瘢痕压力治疗。

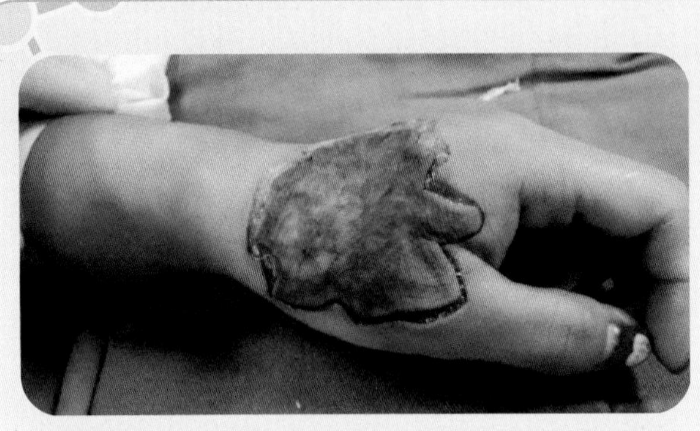

图 3.26.2 根据文身边缘，全层切除文身皮肤

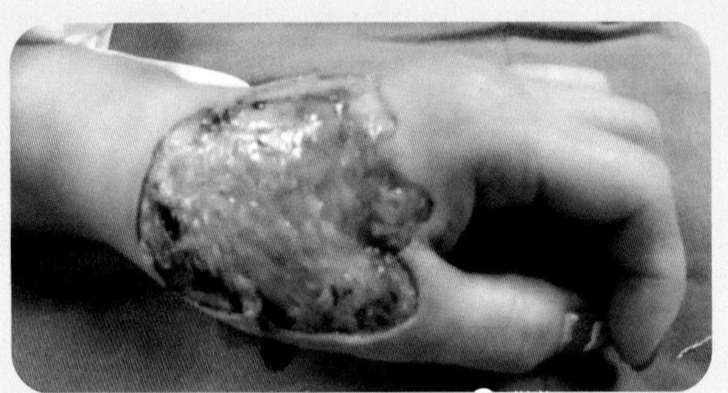

图 3.26.3 文身皮肤全层切除后，由于较深，皮下脂肪颜色蓝

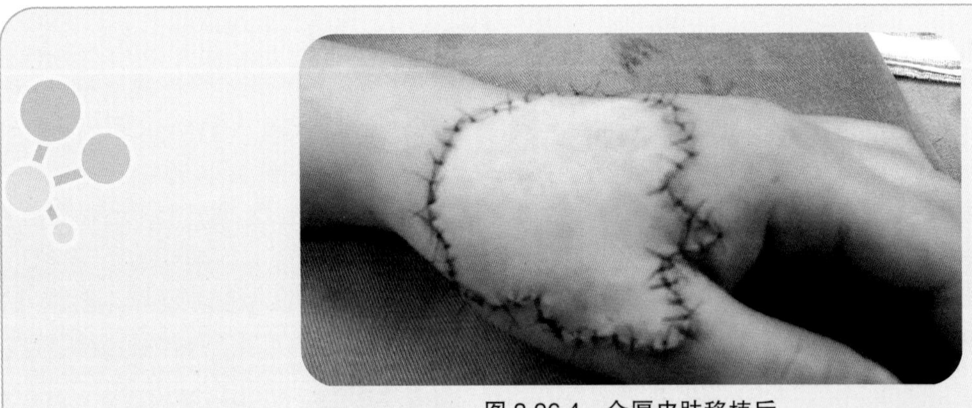

图 3.26.4 全厚皮肤移植后

（陈善亮）

案例二十七 拇指缺损

◆ 损伤原因

患儿，男性，2 岁，左手因打谷机打伤，致拇指离断。

◆ 症状与体征

左手拇指被打谷机打伤，在当地医院行清创再植，再植指术后 3 天，再植指完全坏死并切除。左手拇

◆ Treatment plan

This case has undergone 3 tattoo rinses, but due to the depth of the text, the rinses failed.

1. The patient has itching and discomfort at the tattoo site, and the local skin has hardened after rinsing.

2. Surgical resection is the only solution. Surgical points: ① Complete excision of hardened skin; ② Complete local hemostasis; ③ Precision suturing of transplanted skin to reduce scar formation; ④ External application of recombinant human acidic fibroblast growth factor for wound spraying; ⑤ Full thickness skin transplantation with local pressure bandaging (Figure 3.26.2-Figure3.26.4).

3. Change dressing 7 days after surgery and remove stitches 12 days later. Scar pressure treatment.

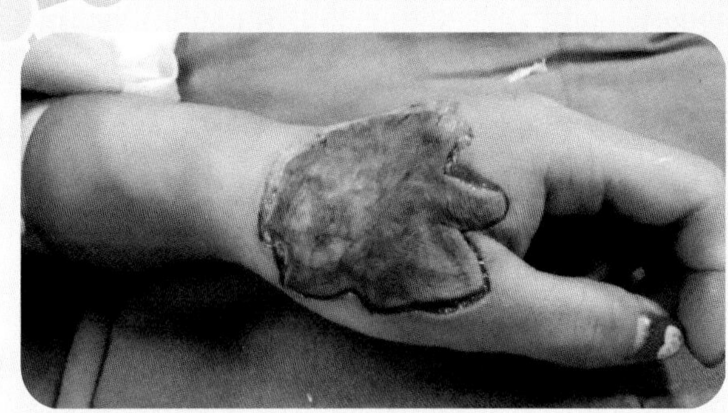

Figure 3.26.2 Total excision of tattoo skin based on the edge of the tattoo

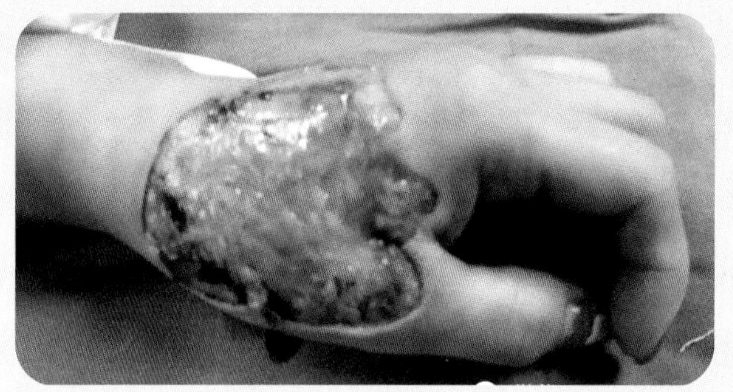

Figure 3.26.3 After complete excision of the tattoo skin, due to its depth, the subcutaneous fat color is blue

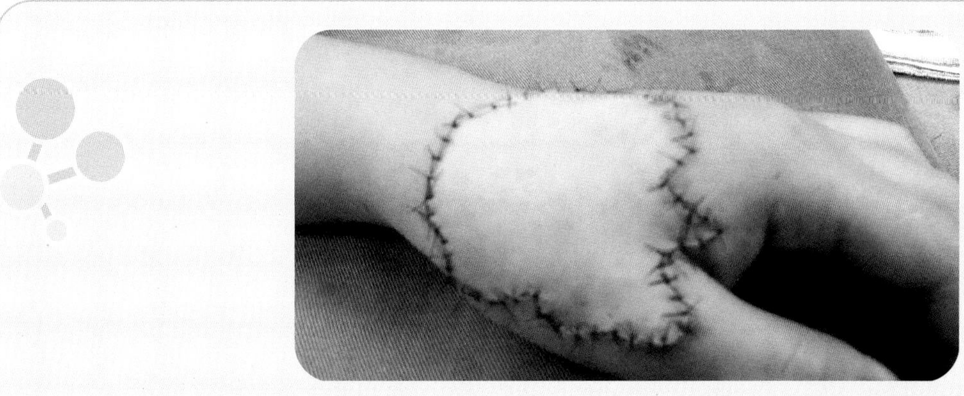

Figure 3.26.4 After full thickness skin transplantation

(Chen Shanliang)

Case 27 Thumb defect

◆ Cause of injury

Child, male, 2 years old, left hand injured by a threshing machine, resulting in thumb detachment.

◆ Signs and symptoms

The left thumb was injured by a threshing machine and underwent debridement and replantation at a local

指从掌指间关节以远端完全缺失，掌骨头缺失，局部创面有白色脓汁，创口周围皮肤红肿明显，腕关节和示指、中指、环指、小指活动良好（图 3.27.1）。

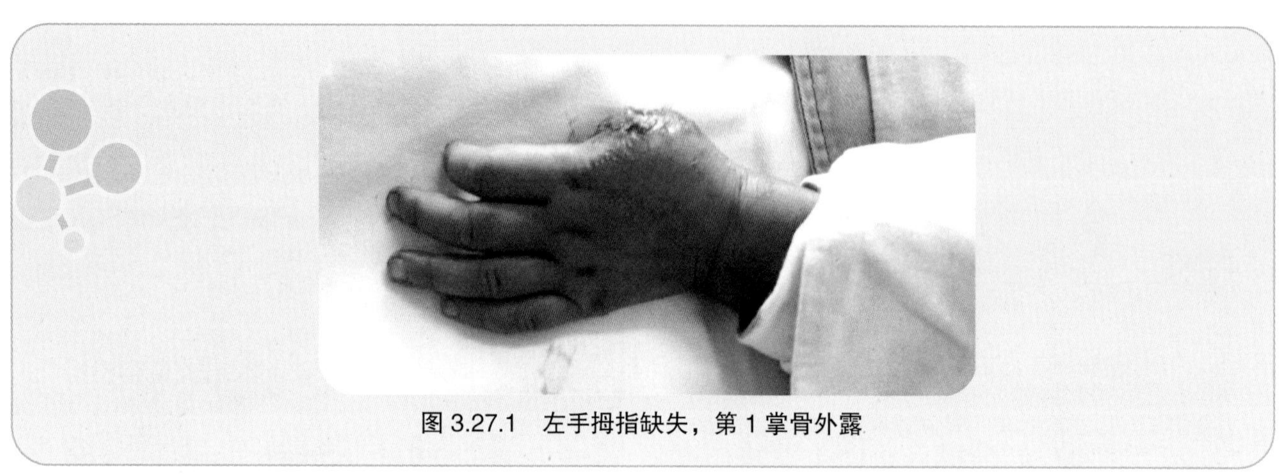

图 3.27.1　左手拇指缺失，第 1 掌骨外露

◆ 治疗方案

儿童拇指完全缺损少见，儿童由于处于发育阶段，选择拇指再造要统筹考虑，既要考虑拇指外观，还要考虑功能及随着孩子生长发育问题。该案例患儿第 2 足趾短小，不适合第 2 足趾移植，采用䠀趾甲皮瓣 + 髂骨移植，因为髂骨没有骨骺不会生长，故采用足䠀趾移植术。该手术最大优点是恢复手拇指缺失后复原，有利于患儿的心理和身体健康发育；缺点是牺牲了一个足䠀趾。

1. 手术过程

1.1 拇指受区切口设计：清创，切除无生机组织，修剪创缘并结扎活动出血点。显露拇指双侧指神经，于鼻咽窝处 3 cm 切口，显露头静脉、桡动脉鼻咽窝支，桡神经浅支，拇长伸肌腱，拇外展肌腱，于拇对掌纹处 2 cm 切口，显露拇长屈肌腱断端，从腱鞘中向远端拉出备用。手部受区准备结束。

1.2 足䠀趾供区切口设计：于左足䠀趾跖趾关节处设计 V 型切口，在䠀趾趾蹼处设计舌型皮瓣作为拇指虎口用，足䠀趾跖趾关节代替拇指的掌指关节，按切口设计依次切开皮肤及皮下，显露足䠀趾足背静脉、皮神经、足䠀长伸肌腱、足背动脉及伴行静脉。显露足底趾神经及足䠀长屈肌腱。根据肌腱，血管神经长度并依次断开，跖趾关节下 1.5 cm 平面切断跖骨头，足䠀趾完全游离。

1.3 足趾移植受供区对接：取 1.5 克氏针纵行跖骨掌骨固定并行跖趾关节侧副韧带缝合；肌腱缝合，拇长屈肌腱和足䠀长屈肌腱缝合，拇长伸肌腱和足䠀长伸肌腱缝合，腱鞘缝合。趾指神经缝合，趾神经和指

hospital. Three days after the replantation, the replanted finger completely died and was removed. The left thumb is completely missing from the distal end of the metacarpophalangeal joint, with a missing metacarpal head. There is white pus on the local wound, and the skin around the wound is visibly red and swollen. The wrist joint, index finger, middle finger, ring finger, and little finger are moving well (Figure 3.27.1).

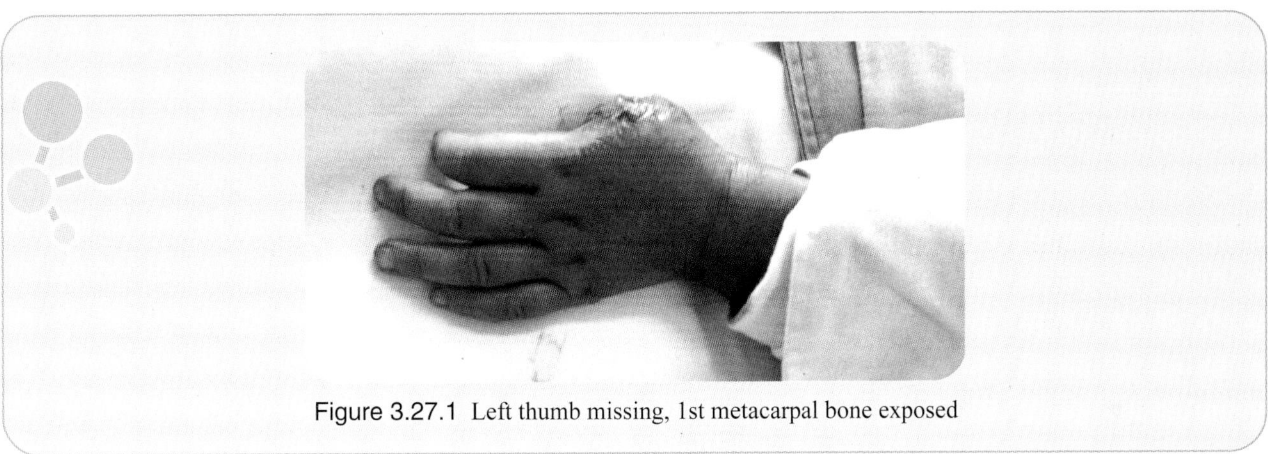

Figure 3.27.1 Left thumb missing, 1st metacarpal bone exposed

◆ Treatment plan

Complete thumb loss in children is rare. As children are in the developmental stage, the choice of thumb reconstruction should be considered comprehensively, taking into account not only the appearance of the thumb but also its function and development as the child grows. The second toe of the patient in this case is short and not suitable for transplantation. A toenail skin flap and iliac bone transplantation were used, as the iliac bone does not have epiphyseal plates and cannot grow. Therefore, toe transplantation was performed. The biggest advantage of this surgery is to restore the missing hand and thumb, which is beneficial for the psychological and physical health development of the child; The disadvantage is sacrificing one toe.

1. Surgical process

1.1 Design of incision for thumb receiving area: Debridement, removal of non living tissue, trimming of wound margin, and ligation of active bleeding points. Expose the bilateral finger nerves of the thumb, make a 3 cm incision at the nasopharyngeal fossa, expose the cephalic vein, radial artery nasopharyngeal fossa branch, superficial branch of radial nerve, extensor hallucis longus tendon, abductor hallucis tendon, make a 2 cm incision at the palm print of the thumb, expose the broken end of the flexor hallucis longus tendon, and pull it out of the tendon sheath towards the distal end for later use. Hand reception area preparation is completed.

1.2 Design of toe donor site incision: A V-shaped incision is designed at the metatarsophalangeal joint of the left toe, and a tongue shaped skin flap is designed at the toe web as the thumb's tiger mouth. The metatarsophalangeal joint of the toe replaces the metacarpophalangeal joint of the thumb, and the skin and subcutaneous tissue are sequentially cut according to the incision design to expose the dorsal vein, cutaneous nerve, extensor tendon, dorsal artery, and accompanying vein of the toe. Expose the plantar nerve and flexor tendon of the foot. According to the length of the tendons, blood vessels, and nerves, they are sequentially severed. The metatarsal head is cut at a plane 1.5 cm below the metatarsophalangeal joint, and the toes are completely free.

1.3 Docking of toe transplantation donor site: Use a 1.5 gram needle to fix the metatarsal and metacarpal bones longitudinally, and suture the collateral ligaments on the metatarsophalangeal joint side; Tendon suture, suture of flexor hallucis longus tendon and flexor hallucis longus tendon, suture of extensor hallucis longus tendon and

神经缝合，足䠞趾背神经和拇指桡神经皮支缝合。血管修复，足背动脉及伴行静脉和手部鼻咽窝桡动脉及伴行静脉吻合，足䠞趾背静脉和头静脉吻合。创面喷洒外用重组人酸性成纤维细胞生长因子，逐层缝合切口并包扎，石膏托固定，术终。

2. 儿童手术后容易恐惧医护人员，常规给予人工冬眠 3 天，待渡过血管痉挛期，停用冬眠疗法，以保证足趾移植顺利成活。

3. 术后常规抬高患肢，保温，日光灯照射，给予扩容、解痉镇痛、抗感染治疗，严密观察移植足趾“四大显微指标”。伤口 3 天内无须换药。换药时会增加患儿哭闹，诱发血管痉挛，所以术后尽量减少伤口换药。

4. 术后 7 天可以下地负重活动，12 天拆线，1 个月拔出克氏针，并进行主被动康复训练（图 3.27.2、图 3.27.3）。

5. 术后 1 年随访，移植拇指伸曲活动良好，患儿可以持笔、可自由翻阅纸张，移植拇指与示指灵活拿捏电线，虎口开大良好，可拿捏水杯（图 3.27.4 ~ 图 3.27.8）。术后随访 5 年，移植足趾外形几乎接近对侧手指，感觉正常，屈伸活动自如，翻阅纸张和穿针引线自如，DR 复查，骨骺随着患儿生长速度健康生长（图 3.27.9）。足䠞趾缺损不影响患儿走路跑步，步态和健康人无区别。

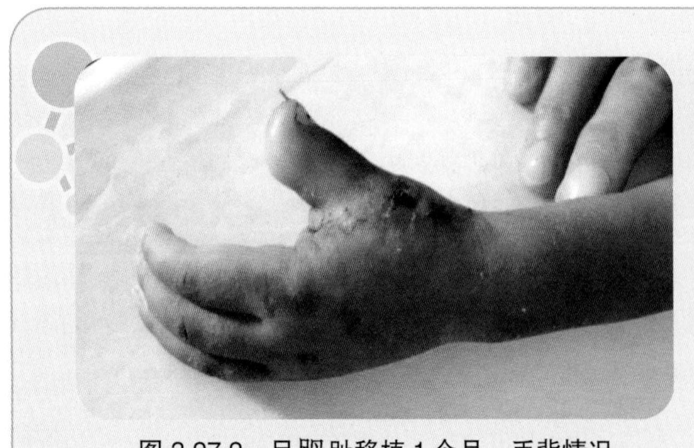

图 3.27.2　足䠞趾移植 1 个月，手背情况

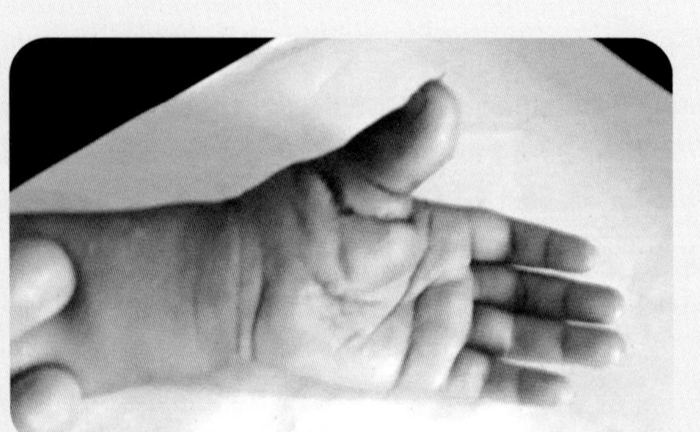

图 3.27.3　足䠞趾移植 1 个月，手掌情况

extensor hallucis longus tendon, suture of tendon sheath. Suture of toe and finger nerves, suture of toe and finger nerves, suture of dorsal toe nerve and radial thumb nerve cutaneous branches. Vascular repair, anastomosis of the dorsal artery and accompanying veins of the foot and the radial artery and accompanying veins of the nasopharynx fossa in the hand, and anastomosis of the dorsal vein and cephalic vein of the toe. Spray recombinant human acidic fibroblast growth factor on the wound surface, suture the incision layer by layer and wrap it, fix it with a plaster tray, and end the operation.

2. Children are prone to fear of medical staff after surgery, and are routinely given artificial hibernation for 3 days. After passing the vasospasm period, hibernation therapy is stopped to ensure the smooth survival of toe transplantation.

3. After surgery, the affected limb is routinely elevated, kept warm, and exposed to fluorescent light. Treatment includes expansion, spasmolysis, analgesia, and anti infection therapy. The "four major microscopic indicators" of the transplanted toe are closely observed. The wound does not require dressing change within 3 days. Changing dressings can increase crying and trigger vascular spasms in the patient, so postoperative dressing changes should be minimized as much as possible.

4. After 7 days of surgery, weight-bearing activities can be carried out on the ground. The stitches will be removed on 12 days, and the Kirschner wire will be removed after 1 month, followed by active and passive rehabilitation training (Figure 3.27.2, Figure 3.27.3).

5. One year follow-up after surgery showed that the transplanted thumb had good extension and flexion activity, and the child could hold a pen and freely flip through paper. The transplanted thumb and index finger were able to flexibly grasp the wires, and the tiger's mouth was well opened. The child could also hold a water cup (Figure 3.27.4-Figure3.27.8). After a 5-year follow-up after surgery, the transplanted toe almost resembled the contralateral finger in appearance and felt normal. It could move freely in flexion and extension, flip through paper and thread with ease. DR re examination showed that the epiphyseal plate grew healthily with the child's growth rate (Figure 3.27.9). Foot defects do not affect the walking and running of children, and their gait is no different from that of healthy individuals.

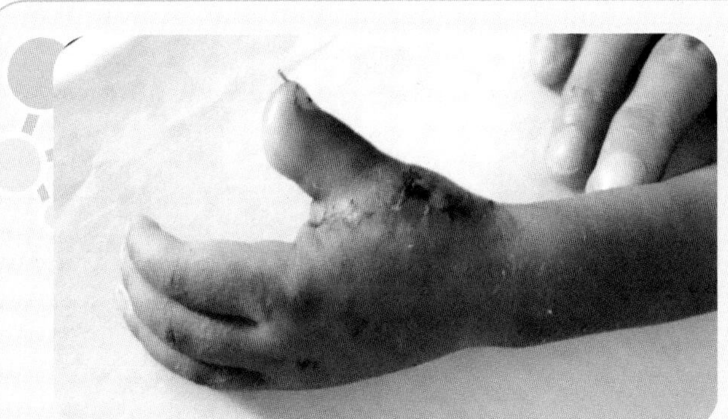

Figure 3.27.2 One month after finger transplantation, condition of the back of the hand

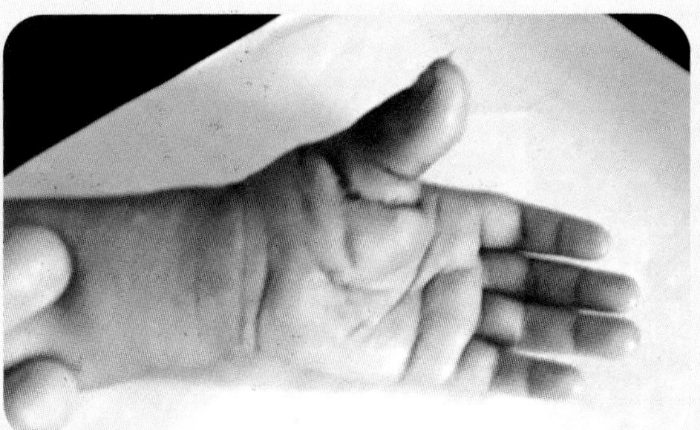

Figure 3.27.3 Palm condition after one month of finger transplantation

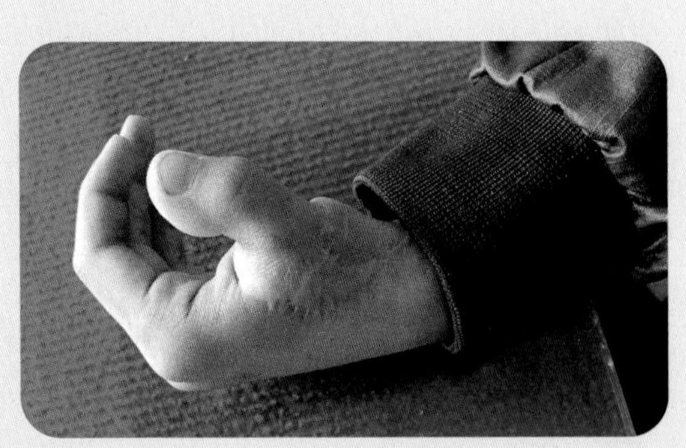

图 3.27.4　手术后 1 年随访，移植拇指伸曲活动良好

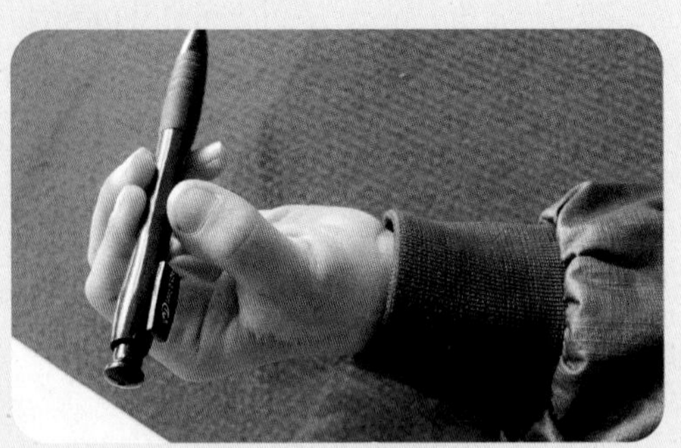

图 3.27.5　可以持笔

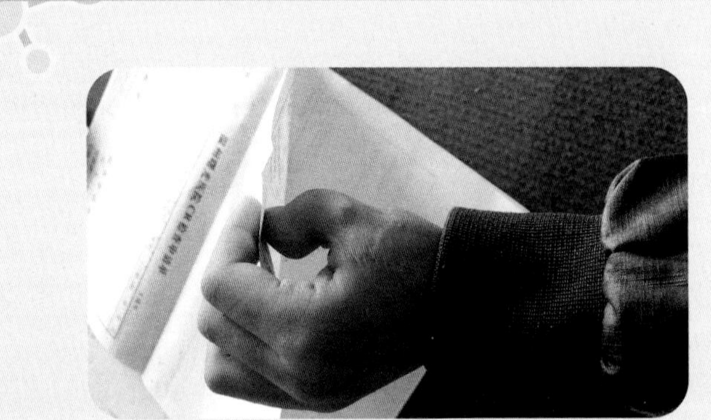

图 3.27.6　可自由翻阅纸张

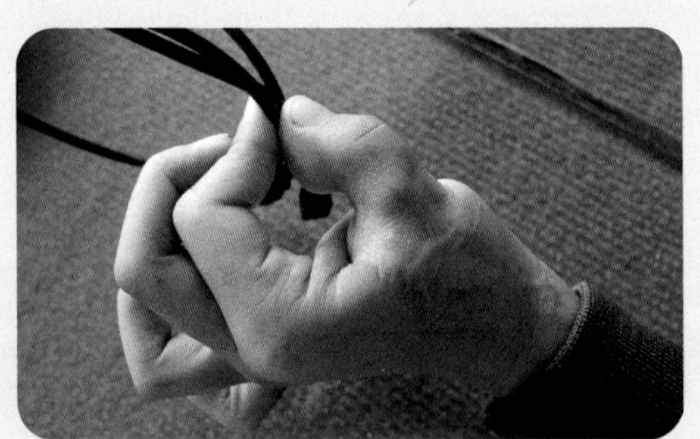

图 3.27.7　移植拇指与示指灵活拿捏电线

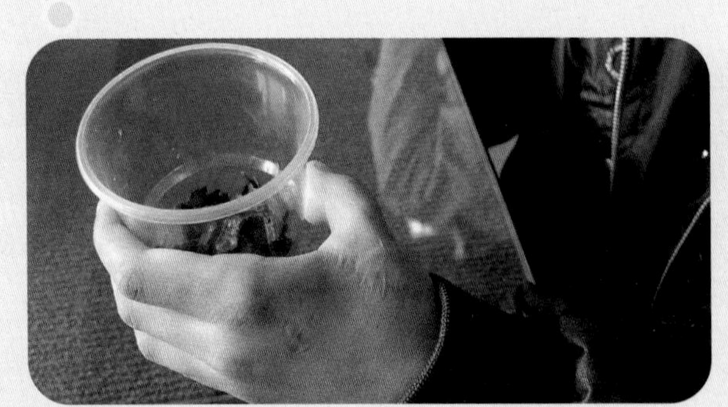

图 3.27.8　虎口开大良好，可拿捏水杯

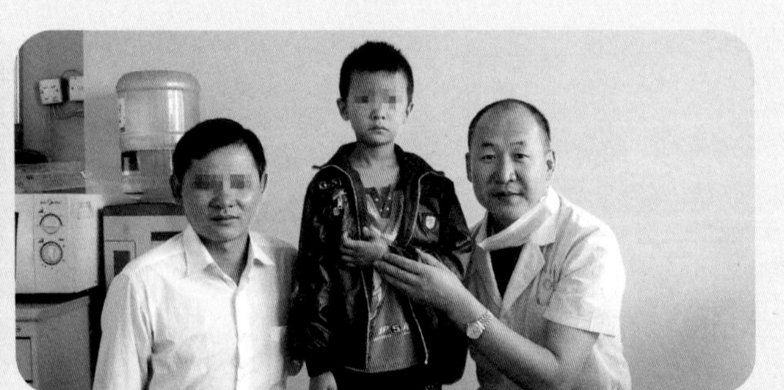

图 3.27.9　患儿 5 岁时随访

（陈善亮　黄　鹏）

案例二十八　足背皮肤缺损

◆ 损伤原因

患者右足因被石头砸伤，致第 3 足趾缺失、足背皮肤缺损。

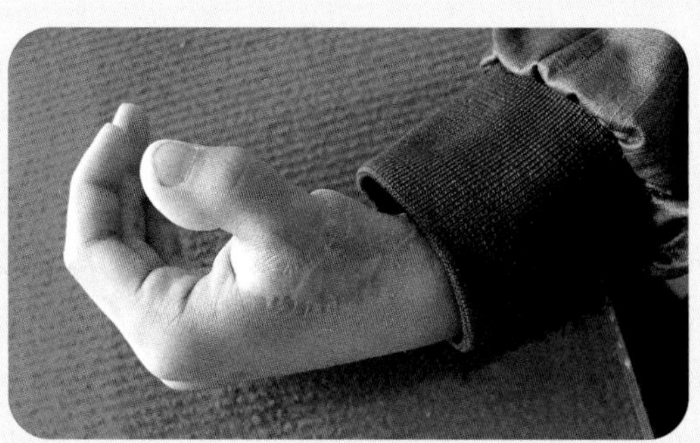

Figure 3.27.4 One year follow-up after surgery shows good extension and flexion activity of the transplanted thumb

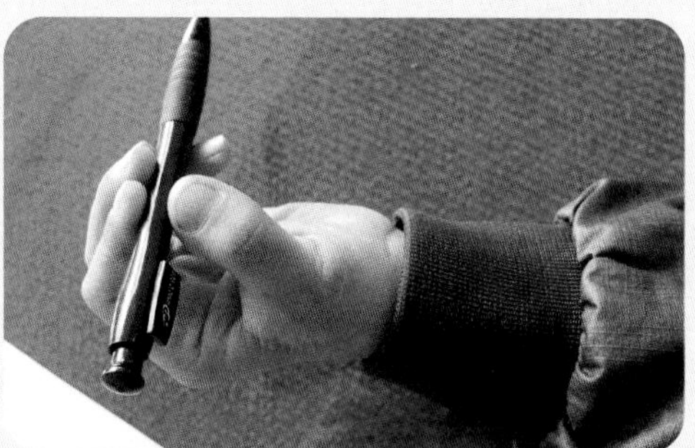

Figure 3.27.5 Can hold a pen

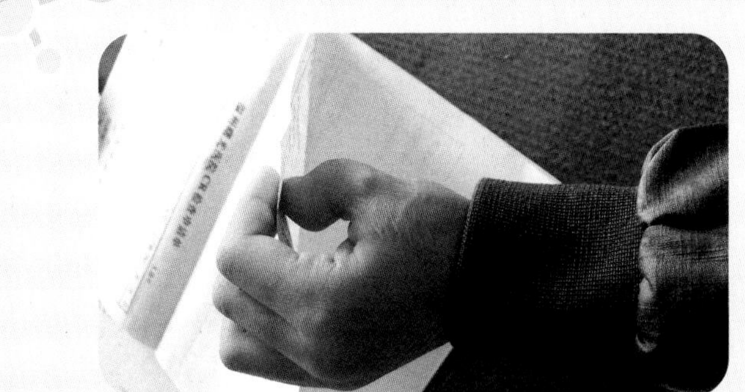

Figure 3.27.6 Free flipping of paper

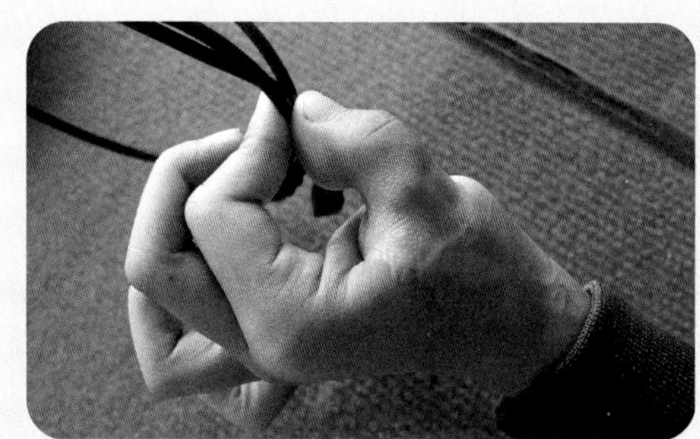

Figure 3.27.7 Transplanted thumb and indicator finger flexibly gripping wires

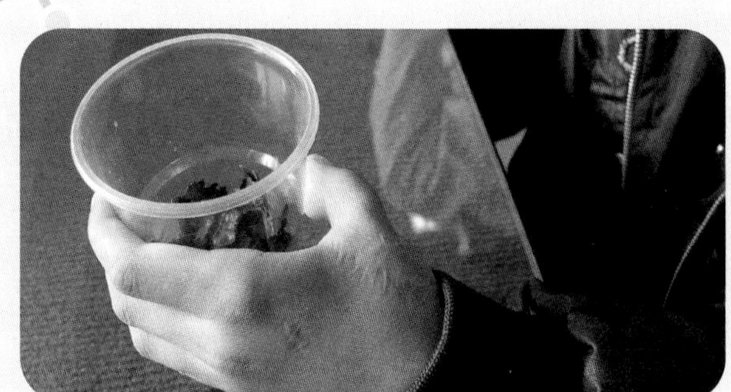

Figure 3.27.8 The tiger's mouth is wide open and good, it can hold a water cup

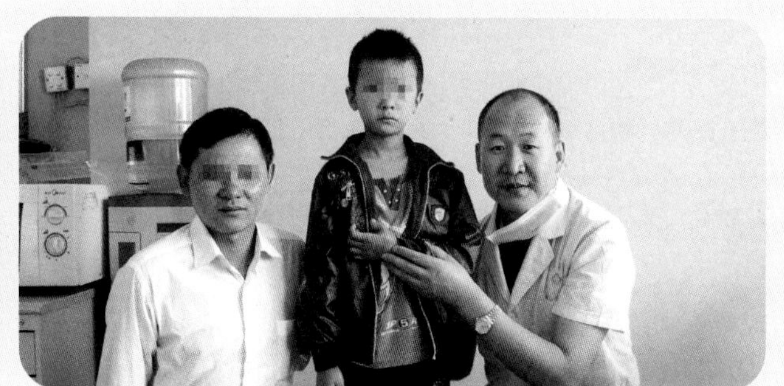

Figure 3.27.9 Follow up of the patient at the age of 5

(Chen Shanliang,Huang Peng)

Case 28 Skin defect on the back of the foot

◆ Cause of injury

The patient's right foot was injured by a stone, resulting in the loss of the third toe and skin defects on the back of the foot.

◆ 症状与体征

右足第 3 足趾毁损性缺损，第 2、第 4 足趾不全离断，仅足趾底部皮肤相连，足趾有血运，近节趾骨粉碎骨折，足背皮肤挫灭伴缺失，缺失面积约 4 cm × 4 cm，足踇趾和第 5 足趾无损伤。

◆ 治疗方案

1. 急诊入院行清创足趾再植手术。足背部 VSD+ 外用重组人酸性成纤维细胞生长因子冲洗治疗，促进创面肉芽组织新鲜，扩容解痉治疗促进再植足趾成活。

2. VSD+ 外用重组人酸性成纤维细胞生长因子冲洗治疗 5 天，去掉 VSD，足背创面新鲜（图 3.28.1）。

3. 右足背经过负压治疗后，创面新鲜，于局部麻醉下行中厚皮片移植，术后 12 天拆线（图 3.28.2）。1.5 个月后取出克氏针，并进行功能训练。

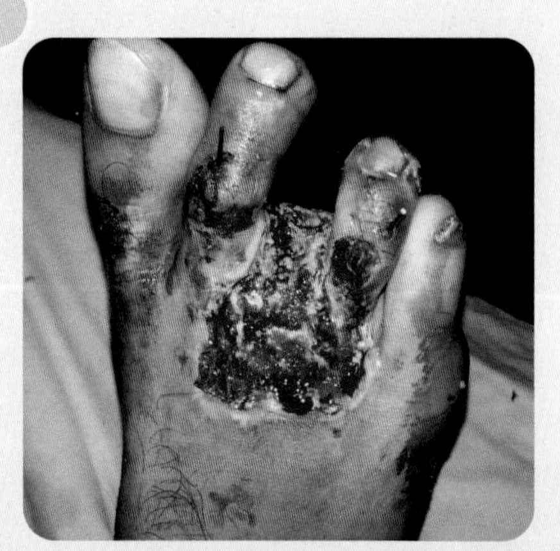

图 3.28.1 足背创面重组人酸性成纤维细胞生长因子 +VSD 治疗后，创面新鲜，待植皮

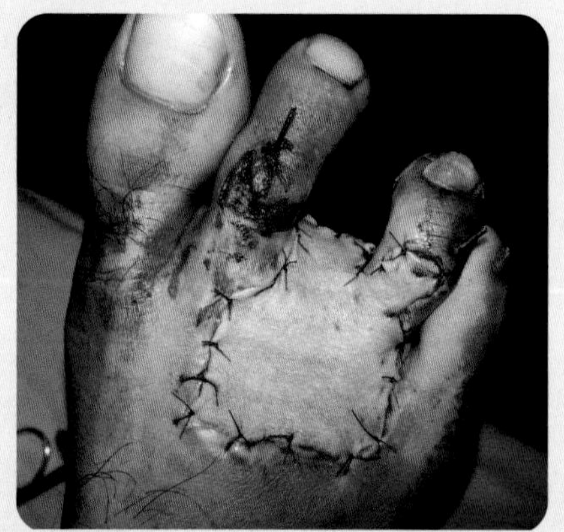

图 3.28.2 足背采用中厚皮片移植

（陈善亮）

案例二十九 上臂大面积撕脱伤

◆ 损伤原因

患者因车祸致左前臂大面积撕脱损伤。

◆ Signs and symptoms

Damaged defect of the third toe of the right foot, incomplete detachment of the second and fourth toes, only the skin at the bottom of the toe is connected, the toe has blood supply, the proximal phalanx bone is crushed and fractured, the skin on the back of the foot is crushed and missing, with a missing area of about 4 cm × 4 cm, and there is no damage to the toes and the fifth toe.

◆ Treatment plan

1. Emergency admission for debridement and toe replantation surgery. The treatment of VSD on the dorsum of the foot and external application of recombinant human acidic fibroblast growth factor flushing promotes the freshness of granulation tissue in the wound, and the expansion and spasmolysis treatment promotes the survival of replanted toes.

2. VSD + topical recombinant human acidic fibroblast growth factor flushing treatment for 5 days, removing VSD and keeping the foot dorsal wound fresh (Figure 3.28.1).

3. After negative pressure treatment on the back of the right foot, the wound was fresh and a medium thick skin graft was transplanted under local anesthesia. The suture was removed 12 days after surgery (Figure 3.28.2). After 1.5 months, remove the Kirschner wire and conduct functional training.

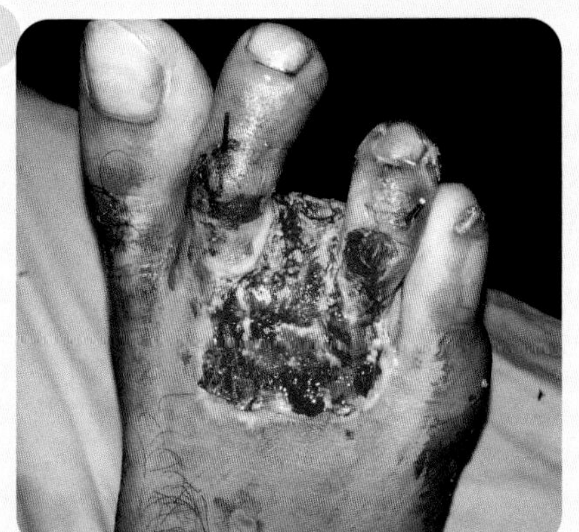

Figure 3.28.1 After treatment with recombinant human acidic fibroblast growth factor + VSD on the foot dorsal wound, the wound is fresh and ready for skin grafting

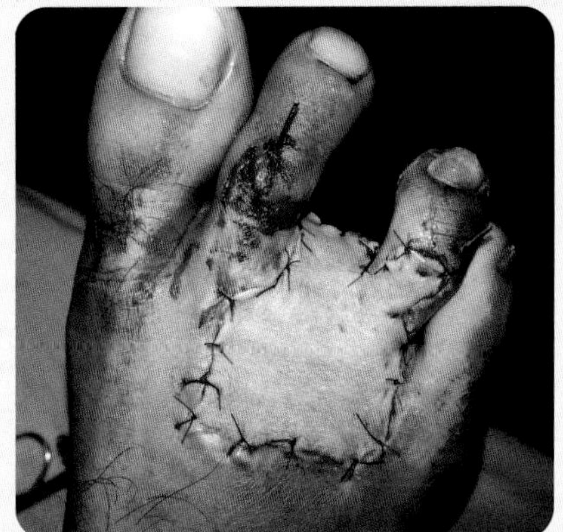

Figure 3.28.2 Transplantation of medium thick skin graft on the dorsum of the foot

(Chen Shanliang)

Case 29 Large area upper arm tear injury

◆ Cause of injury

The patient suffered extensive tearing and injury to the left forearm due to a car accident.

◆ 症状与体征

车祸伤后左前臂出血不止，剧痛难忍，肿胀并逐渐加重。左前臂背侧有大面积皮肤逆行撕脱性损伤，撕脱皮肤表皮有大面积擦伤，皮肤有挫灭，伸肌群有撕脱伤，部分肌群有挫灭伤（图 3.29.1）。伤口布满泥沙。

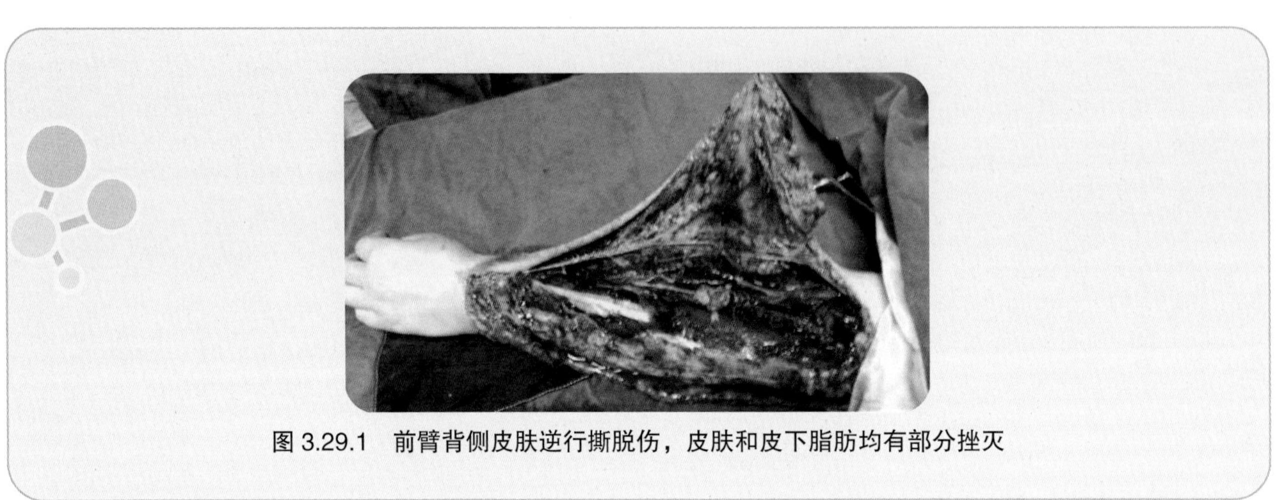

图 3.29.1　前臂背侧皮肤逆行撕脱伤，皮肤和皮下脂肪均有部分挫灭

◆ 治疗方案

1. 急诊入院加压包扎止血，并完善手术前准备，建立静脉通道，补充血容量。

2. 手术过程

2.1 一期：臂丛麻醉行清创，修剪清除无生机组织，结扎活动出血点，修复撕脱肌肉组织。修剪逆行撕脱皮下脂肪，将皮肤修剪成中厚皮肤，并将皮肤切开数个小孔洞，有利于皮下渗出引流，并预防原位回植皮肤浮起。重组人酸性成纤维细胞生长因子喷洒创面，将撕脱皮肤原位回植并缝合，应用 VSD+ 外用重组人酸性成纤维细胞生长因子冲洗。

2.2 二期：由于逆行撕脱皮肤有严重擦伤，回植皮肤大面积坏死，行坏死皮肤一次性清创切除，并再次行 VSD 负压 + 重组人酸性成纤维细胞生长因子冲洗，待肉芽组织新鲜后植皮。

2.3 三期：创面肉芽组织新鲜，创面皮肤缺损面积 28 cm × 9 cm，于大腿切取中厚皮片游离移植前臂创面，创面喷洒外用重组人酸性成纤维细胞生长因子，受区和供区应用油纱覆盖创面，并加压包扎。术后 7 天打开前臂植皮区，植皮全部成活（图 3.29.2 ~ 图 3.29.6）。

3. 术后抬高患肢减轻肿胀，康复理疗，并逐渐加强前臂功能训练。

◆ Signs and symptoms

After the car accident injury, the left forearm was bleeding continuously, causing unbearable pain and swelling that gradually worsened. There is a large area of skin reverse tearing injury on the dorsal side of the left forearm, with extensive abrasions on the peeled skin epidermis, skin contusion, tearing injury on the extensor muscle group, and contusion injury on some muscle groups (Figure 3.29.1). The wound is covered in mud and sand.

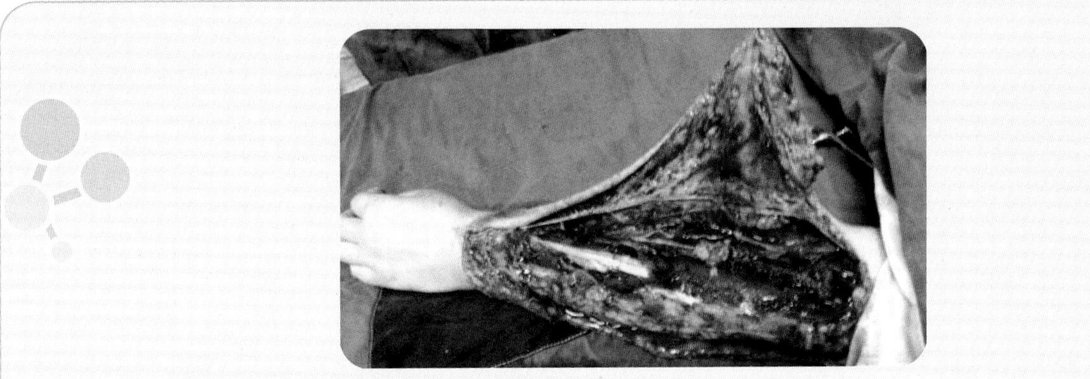

Figure 3.29.1 Retrograde skin tear injury on the back of the forearm, with partial destruction of both the skin and subcutaneous fat

◆ Treatment plan

1. Emergency admission with pressure bandaging to stop bleeding, and complete preoperative preparation, establish venous access, and supplement blood volume.

2. Surgical process

2.1 Phase 1: Brachial plexus anesthesia for debridement, trimming and removal of lifeless tissue, ligation of active bleeding points, and repair of torn muscle tissue. Pruning the reverse peeling off of subcutaneous fat, trimming the skin into medium thick skin, and cutting several small holes in the skin to facilitate subcutaneous exudation and drainage, and prevent the skin from floating up after in situ transplantation. Recombinant human acidic fibroblast growth factor is sprayed onto the wound, and the torn skin is replanted in situ and sutured. VSD and topical recombinant human acidic fibroblast growth factor are applied for rinsing.

2.2 Phase II: Due to severe abrasions caused by retrograde tearing of the skin, a large area of necrotic skin was replanted. A one-time debridement and excision of the necrotic skin was performed, followed by VSD negative pressure and recombinant human acidic fibroblast growth factor flushing. After the granulation tissue was fresh, skin grafting was performed.

2.3 Phase III: Fresh granulation tissue from the wound, with a skin defect area of 28 cm × 9 cm. A medium thick skin graft was cut from the thigh and freely transplanted onto the forearm wound. Recombinant human acidic fibroblast growth factor was sprayed topically on the wound, and oil gauze was used to cover the wound in both the recipient and donor areas, followed by pressure bandaging. Seven days after surgery, the forearm skin graft area was opened and all grafts survived (Figure 3.29.2- Figure 3.29.6).

3. After surgery, elevate the affected limb to reduce swelling, receive rehabilitation therapy, and gradually strengthen forearm function training.

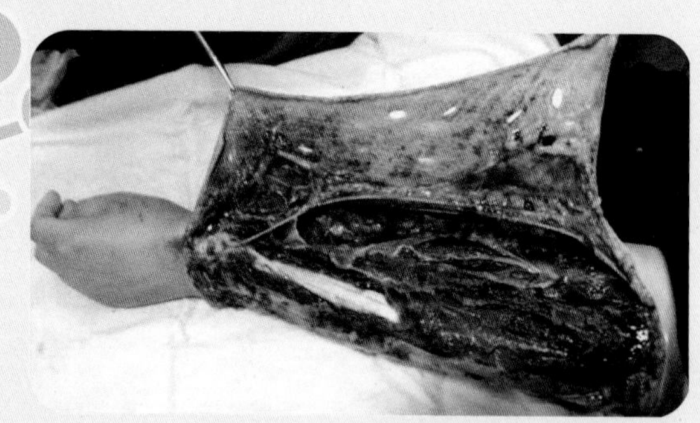

图 3.29.2 撕脱皮肤皮下脂肪剪除，修剪成中厚皮片

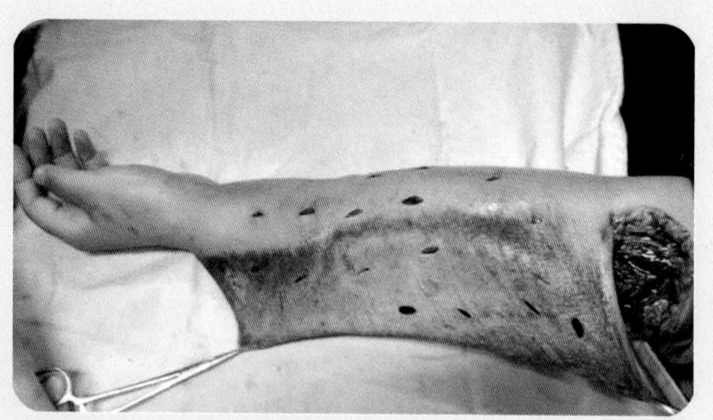

图 3.29.3 清创修剪皮下脂肪，并切开数个孔洞，防止皮下出血浮起

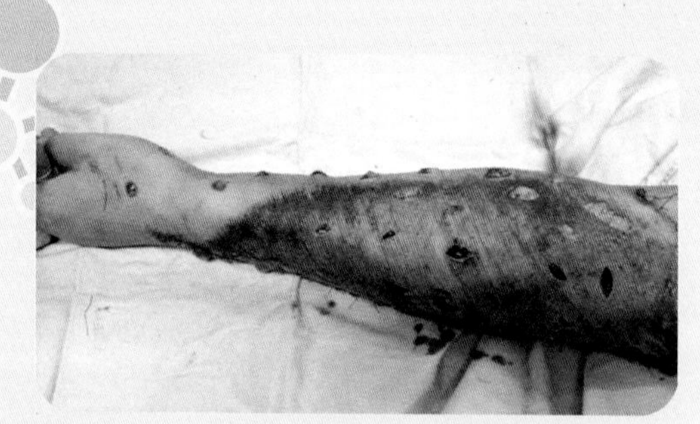

图 3.29.4 将逆行撕脱皮肤原位缝合，临时覆盖创面，VSD+ 重组人酸性成纤维细胞生长因子冲洗治疗

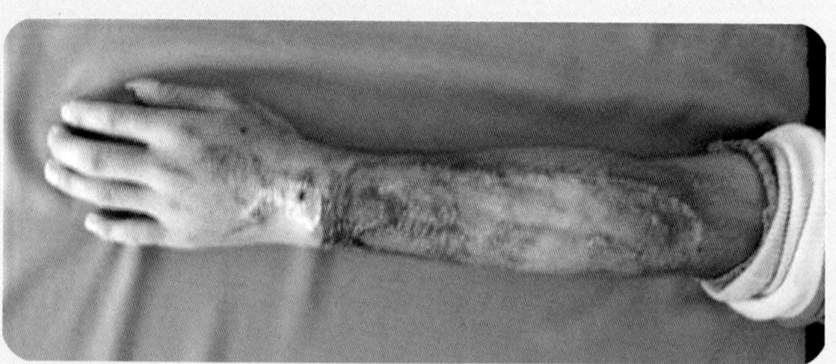

图 3.29.5 原位回植皮肤大部分坏死，坏死皮肤切除后，行中厚皮肤移植并成活，术后 1 个月

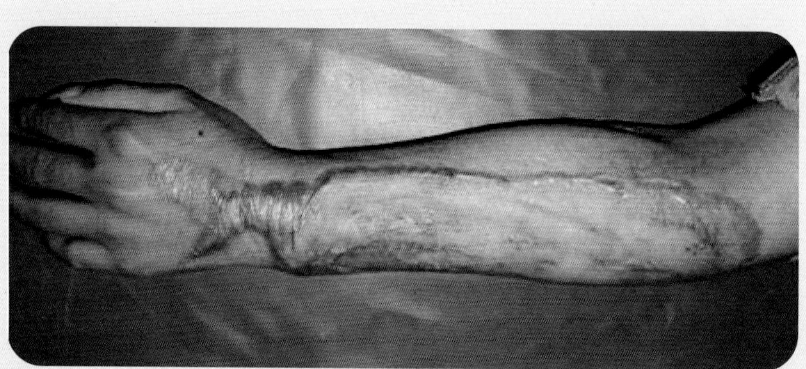

图 3.29.6 植皮成活后，外形和功能良好，手术后 3 个月，瘢痕逐渐软化

（陈善亮）

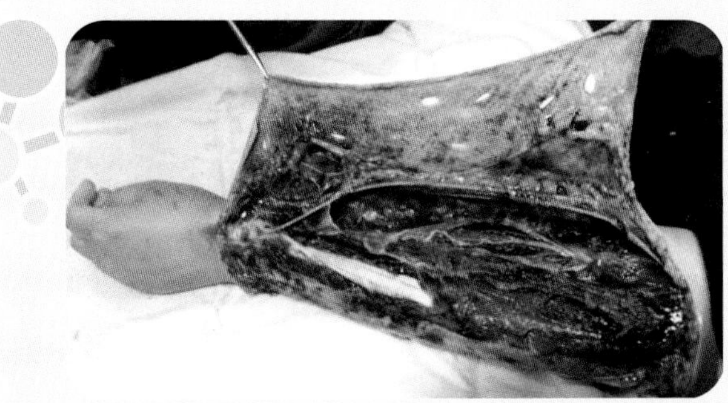

Figure 3.29.2 Peel off subcutaneous fat from the skin and trim it into medium thickness skin patches

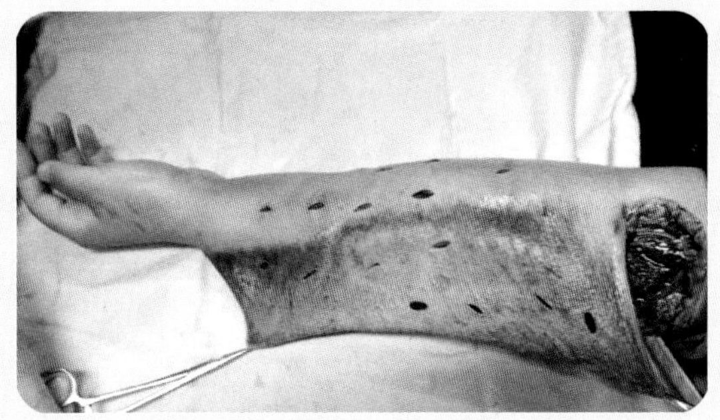

Figure 3.29.3 Debridement and trimming of subcutaneous fat, with several incisions to prevent subcutaneous bleeding and floating

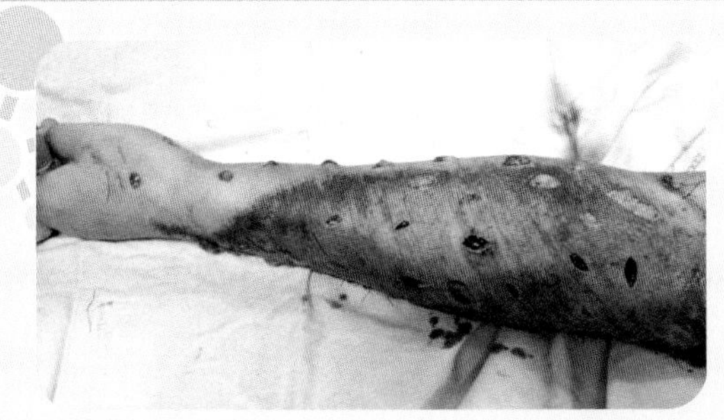

Figure 3.29.4 In situ suturing of retrograde tear off skin, temporary covering of wound, VSD + recombinant human acidic fibroblast growth factor flushing treatment

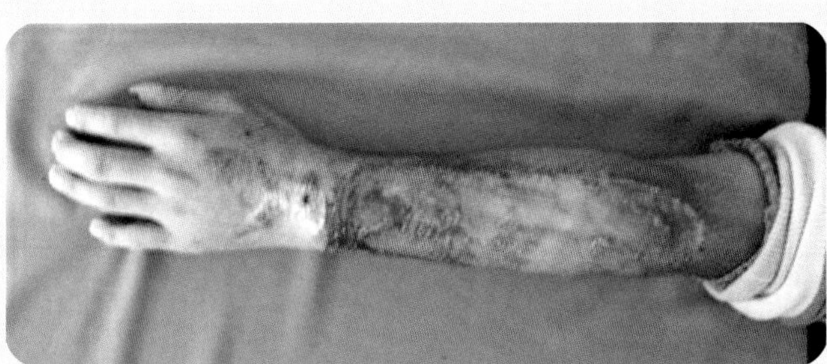

Figure 3.29.5 Most of the skin transplanted in situ was necrotic. After the necrotic skin was removed, a medium thick skin transplant was performed and survived. One month after surgery

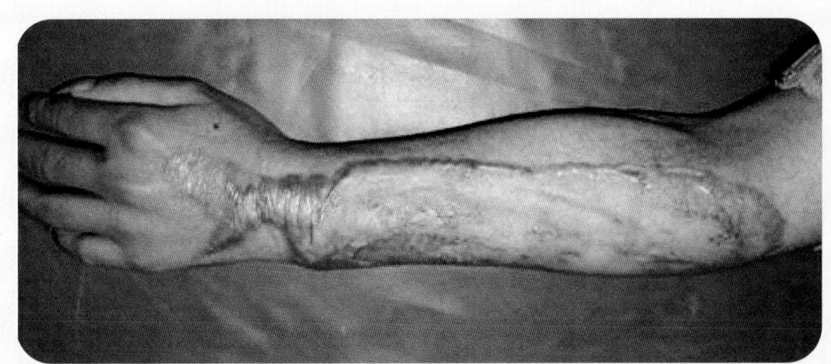

Figure 3.29.6 After skin grafting, the appearance and function are good. Three months after surgery, the scar gradually softens

(Chen Shanliang)

案例三十　足背逆行撕脱伤

◆ 损伤原因

患者因被滚木砸伤，致右足背逆行撕脱伤。

◆ 症状与体征

右足剧痛，肿胀并逐渐加重，出血不止，不敢负重行走。右足背肿胀明显，足背有不规则逆行皮肤撕脱，撕脱皮肤有挫灭，无血运，第 2 至第 4 足趾青紫，足趾活动受限，第 2、第 3 近节趾骨骨擦感及骨擦音阳性，足趾趾端血液反流迟缓（图 3.30.1）。足背创面 6 cm × 5 cm 局部污染严重，趾端感觉减退，创缘不齐。

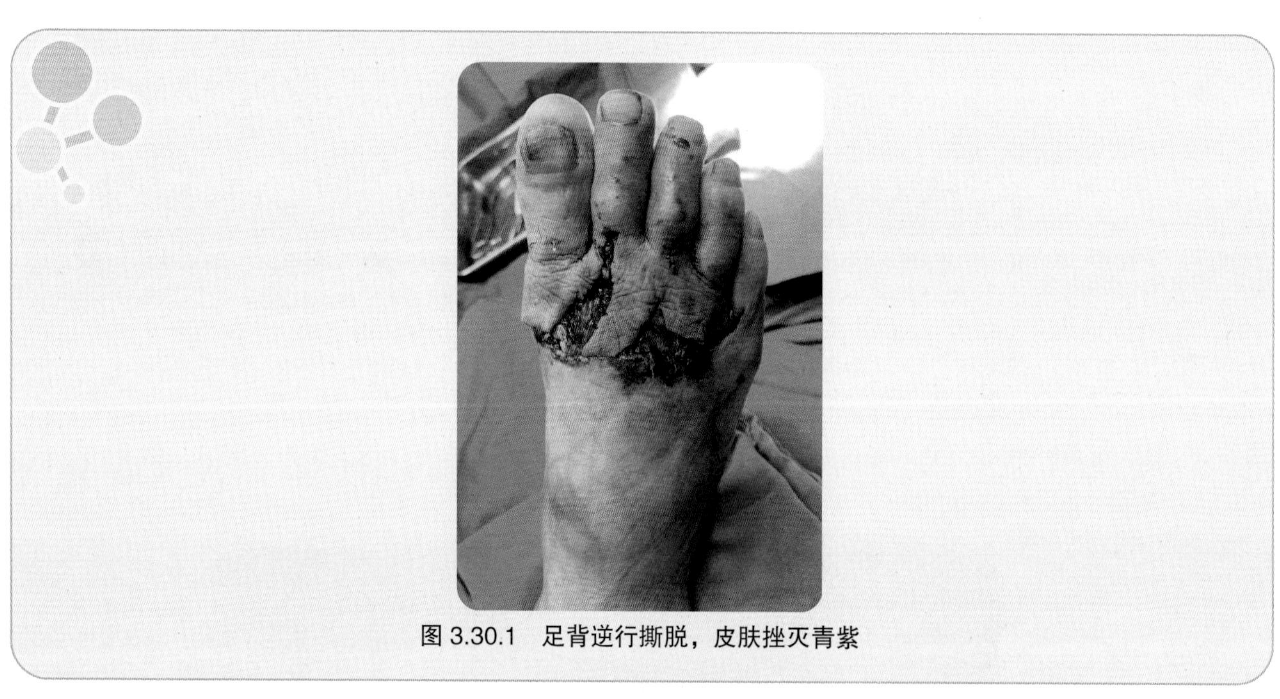

图 3.30.1　足背逆行撕脱，皮肤挫灭青紫

◆ 治疗方案

1. 急诊入院并完善手术前准备，建立静脉通道。

2. 腰硬联合麻醉下，行清创，骨折复位克氏针内固定术，逆行撕脱皮肤削薄翻转回植术，局部喷洒重组人酸性成纤维细胞生长因子油纱覆盖创面，局部加压包扎（图 3.30.2、图 3.30.3）。

3. 术后 5 天，原位回植皮肤坏死，予以清创切除坏死皮肤。采用 VSD+ 外用重组人酸性成纤维细胞生长因子冲洗治疗，VSD 治疗 4 天，创面新鲜，达到植皮条件，并在局部麻醉下行中厚皮片游离移植，术后 7 天，植皮成活（图 3.30.4、图 3.30.5）。

4. 手术后 1 个月，拔出克氏针并进行功能训练。

Case 30 Retrograde avulsion injury on the back of the foot

◆ Cause of injury

The patient suffered a retrograde avulsion injury to the back of the right foot due to being hit by a rolling wood.

◆ Signs and symptoms

Severe pain in the right foot, swelling and gradually worsening, continuous bleeding, and reluctance to walk with heavy loads. There is obvious swelling on the back of the right foot, and there is irregular retrograde skin tearing off on the back of the foot. The torn skin is bruised and there is no blood flow. The second to fourth toes are blue and purple, and the movement of the toes is limited. The bone friction sensation and bone friction sound of the second and third proximal phalanges are positive, and the blood reflux at the toe end of the toes is delayed (Figure 3.30.1). The 6 cm × 5 cm wound on the back of the foot is severely contaminated locally, with decreased sensation at the toe and uneven edges of the wound.

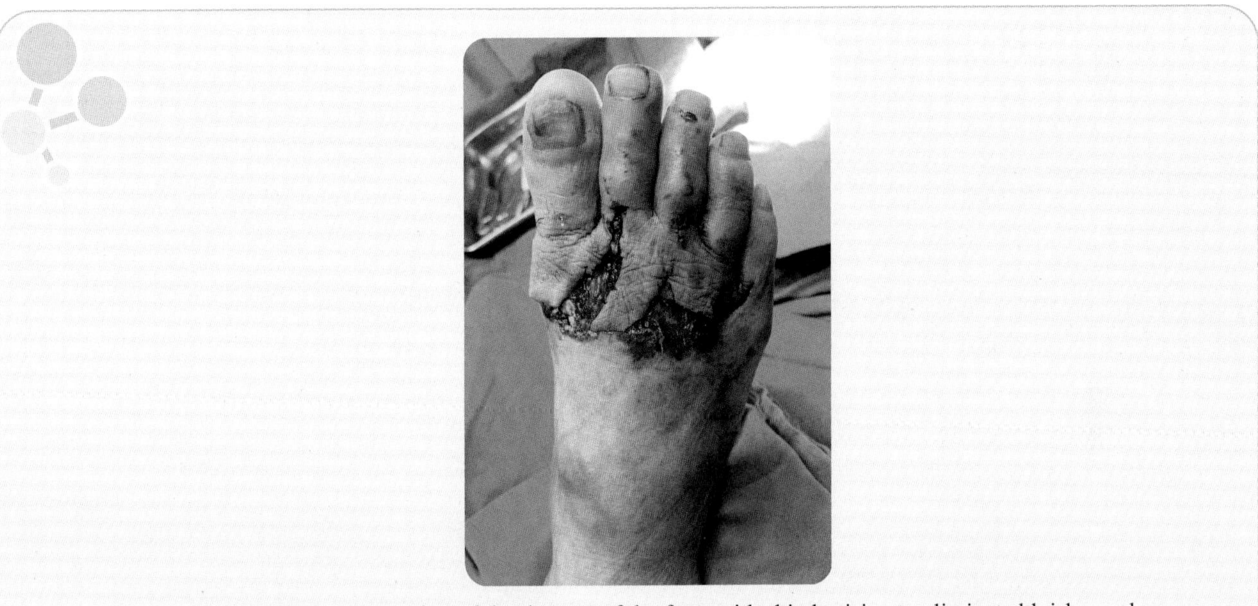

Figure 3.30.1 Retrograde tearing of the dorsum of the foot, with skin bruising to eliminate bluish purple

◆ Treatment plan

1. Emergency admission and complete preoperative preparation, establish venous access.

2. Under combined spinal and epidural anesthesia, debridement, fracture reduction with Kirschner wire internal fixation, retrograde skin peeling, thinning, flipping, and replanting were performed. The wound was locally sprayed with recombinant human acidic fibroblast growth factor oil gauze and pressure bandaged (Figure 3.30.2, Figure 3.30.3).

3. Five days after surgery, the necrotic skin was replanted in situ and debridement was performed to remove the necrotic skin. VSD + topical recombinant human acidic fibroblast growth factor flushing treatment was used. After 4 days of VSD treatment, the wound was fresh and met the conditions for skin grafting. Under local anesthesia, medium thick skin grafts were freely transplanted. Seven days after surgery, the skin grafts survived (Figure 3.30.4, Figure 3.30.5).

4. One month after surgery, remove the Kirschner wire and perform functional training.

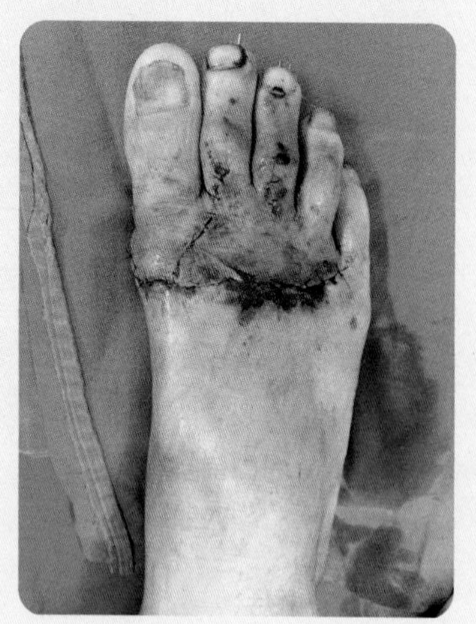
图 3.30.2 清创后原位回植，骨折复位闭合克氏针固定

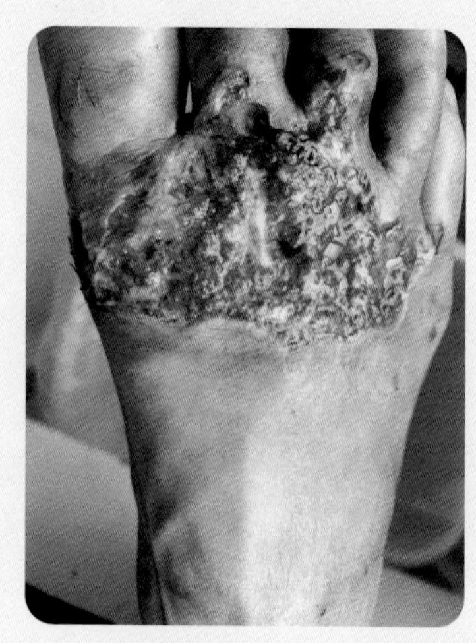
图 3.30.3 足背皮肤坏死，坏死皮肤切除，局部肉芽组织不新鲜

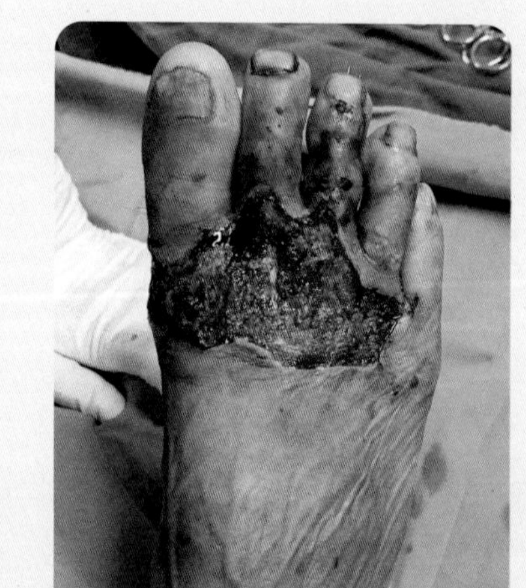
图 3.30.4 VSD+ 外用重组人酸性成纤维细胞生长因子冲洗，创面肉芽组织新鲜，待植皮

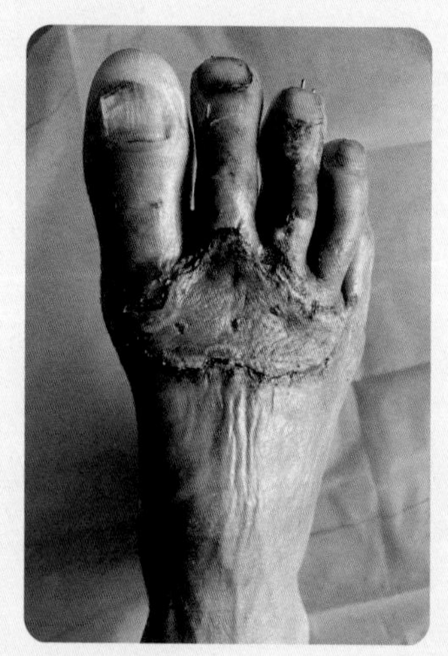
图 3.30.5 足背行中厚皮肤移植，术后 7 天移植皮肤成活

（陈善亮）

案例三十一　前臂大面积皮肤缺损

◆ 损伤原因

患者因车祸在地面上摩擦，致右前臂大面积皮肤缺损。

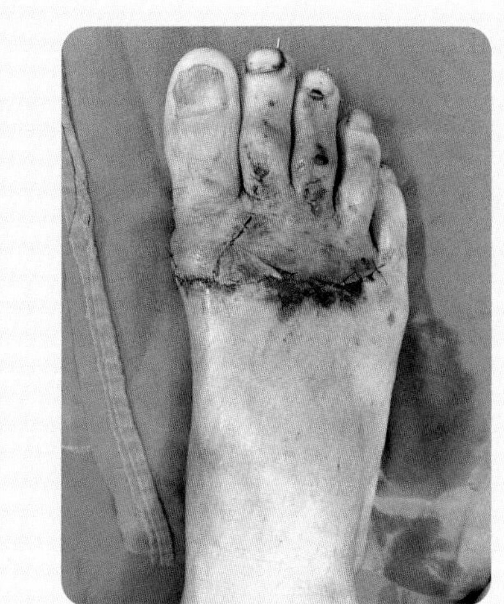
Figure 3.30.2 In situ replantation after debridement, fracture reduction and closure with Kirschner wire fixation

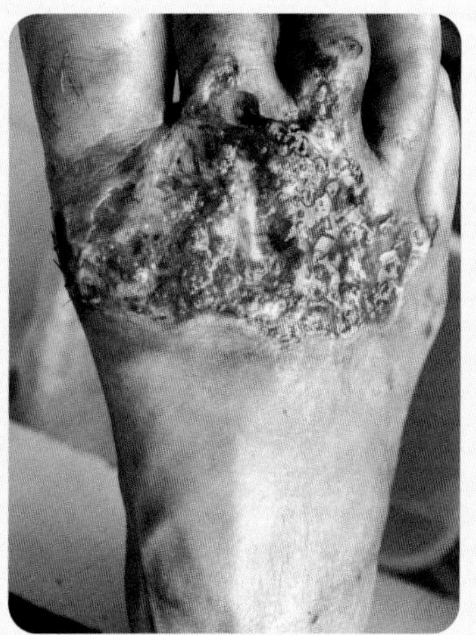
Figure 3.30.3 Necrosis of dorsum pedis skin, excision of necrotic skin, local granulation tissue not fresh

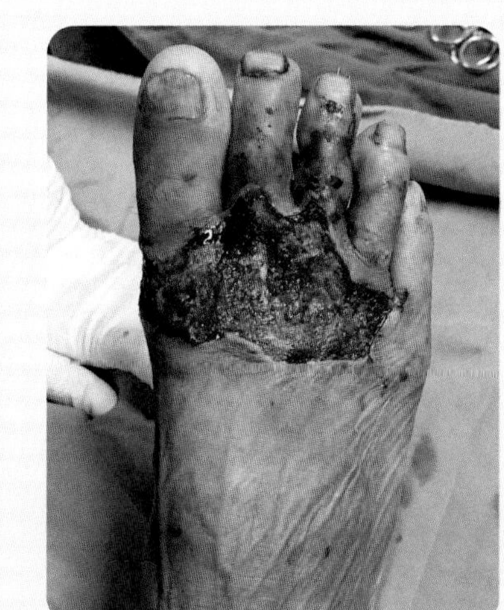
Figure 3.30.4 VSD+topical recombinant human acidic fibroblast growth factor rinsing, fresh granulation tissue of the wound, ready for skin grafting

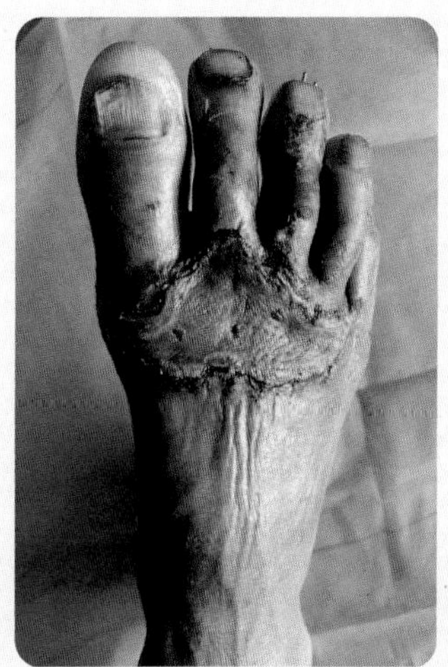
Figure 3.30.5 Mid thick skin transplantation performed on the dorsum of the foot, and the transplanted skin survived 7 days after surgery

(Chen Shanliang)

Case 31 Large area skin defect on the forearm

◆ Cause of injury

The patient suffered a large skin defect on the right forearm due to friction on the ground caused by a car accident.

◆ 症状与体征

右前臂出血不止，剧痛难忍，肿胀并逐渐加重。右前臂掌侧面有大面积擦伤创面，创面缺损面积34 cm × 8 cm，深达屈指前肌群，尺侧屈腕肌、屈指浅肌、掌长肌肌腹部分缺损，创缘边缘参差不齐，创面渗血活跃，中环、小指屈伸活动受限，手指血运良好，尺侧一个半指感觉减退。拇指近节背侧有 3 cm 裂伤，深达拇长伸肌腱，创缘不齐，伤口污染严重。创面布满泥沙。

◆ 治疗方案

1. 急诊入院完善术前准备后，立即在臂丛麻醉下行清创，结扎活动出血点，修复撕裂肌肉，并应用VSD+ 外用重组人酸性成纤维细胞生长因子滴注冲洗治疗。

2. 第一次 VSD 负压治疗 4 天，创面新鲜程度不够，创面凹凸不平，每天喷洒重组人酸性成纤维细胞生长因子，覆盖油纱。7 天后肉芽组织新鲜（图 3.31.1）。在大腿前侧切取中厚皮片游离移植，5 天后植皮完全成活（图 3.31.2）。

3. 术后 3 天开始手部功能训练，预防关节僵硬和肌腱粘连，该部位皮肤缺损，应常规选用中厚或者全厚皮肤游离移植，超薄皮片移植弹性差，不耐磨，易挛缩。

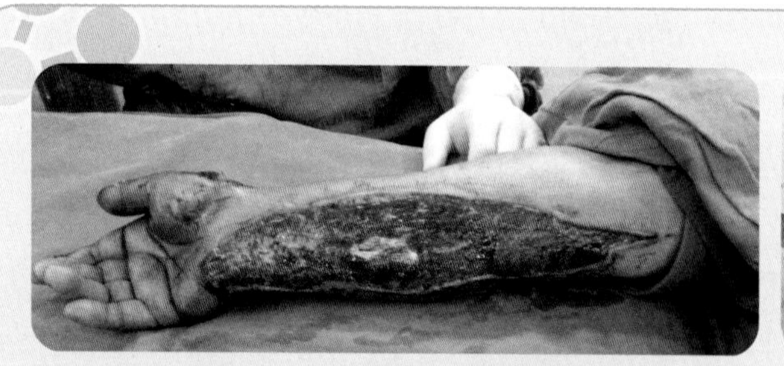

图 3.31.1　经过 VSD 治疗后，创面新鲜，肉芽组织饱满

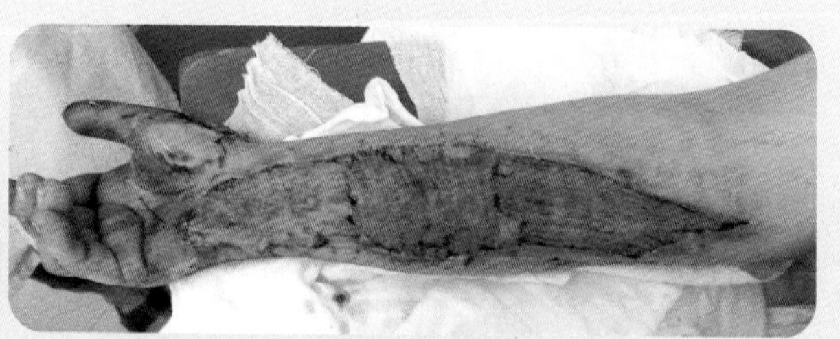

图 3.31.2　中厚皮片游离移植术后 5 天，植皮成活

（陈善亮）

案例三十二　下肢大面积撕脱伤伴皮肤缺损

◆ 损伤原因

患者因车祸导致右小腿复合外伤。

◆ Signs and symptoms

The right forearm is bleeding profusely, with unbearable pain and swelling that gradually worsens. There is a large area of abrasion wound on the palmar side of the right forearm, with a defect area of 34 cm × 8 cm, reaching deep into the anterior flexor muscle group. The ulnar flexor wrist muscle, superficial flexor finger muscle, and palmar longus muscle are partially deficient. The edge of the wound is uneven, and there is active bleeding from the wound. The flexion and extension of the middle ring and little finger are restricted, and the blood flow of the fingers is good. The sensation of one and a half fingers on the ulnar side is reduced. There is a 3cm laceration on the dorsal side of the proximal segment of the thumb, reaching deep into the extensor hallucis longus tendon, with uneven edges and severe wound contamination. The wound is covered with mud and sand.

◆ Treatment plan

1. After completing preoperative preparation for emergency admission, immediate debridement was performed under brachial plexus anesthesia, the bleeding point was ligated, the torn muscle was repaired, and VSD + topical recombinant human acidic fibroblast growth factor infusion and flushing treatment were applied.

2. The first VSD negative pressure treatment lasted for 4 days, but the wound was not fresh enough and uneven. Recombinant human acidic fibroblast growth factor was sprayed daily and covered with oil gauze. After 7 days, the granulation tissue was fresh (Figure 3.31.1). A medium thick skin graft was cut from the front of the thigh for free transplantation, and after 5 days, the skin graft completely survived (Figure 3.31.2).

3. Hand function training should be started 3 days after surgery to prevent joint stiffness and tendon adhesion. For skin defects in this area, medium or full thickness free skin transplantation should be routinely selected. Ultra thin skin grafts have poor elasticity, are not wear-resistant, and are prone to contraction.

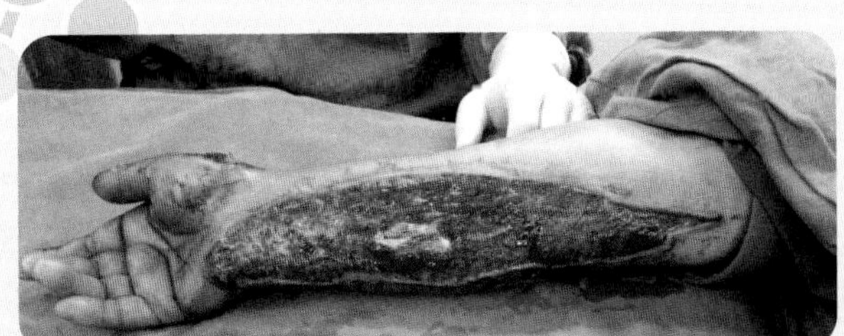

Figure 3.31.1 After VSD treatment, the wound is fresh and the granulation tissue is plump

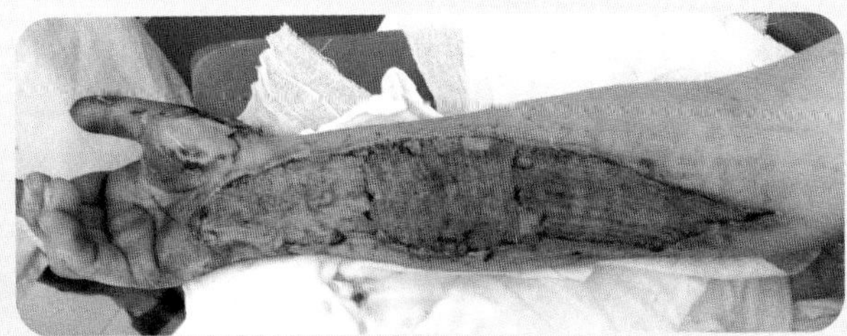

Figure 3.31.2 Five days after the free transplantation of medium thick skin graft, the skin graft survived

(Chen Shanliang)

Case 32 Large scale tearing injury of lower limbs with skin defects

◆ Cause of injury

The patient suffered a compound injury to the right calf due to a car accident.

◆ 症状与体征

右下肢剧痛难忍，出血不止，肿胀并逐渐加重，不能站立行走。右下肢广泛性肿胀，下肢见多处不规则伤口，髌前有 8 cm 伤口，深达髌骨，髌骨无骨折，髌韧带部分撕裂，胫前有两处伤口，各约 4 cm、2 cm，深达胫骨，胫腓骨无骨折。右小腿内测有 22 cm 纵行伤口，腓肠肌部分撕裂，小腿皮肤广泛性脱套并游离（图 3.32.1 ~ 图 3.32.3）。深浅筋膜潜行游离右足踝部，皮肤有多处不规则擦皮伤，足背动脉波动良好，足趾感觉减退，右小腿皮肤血液反流迟缓。伤口渗血活跃，右膝关节和足踝关节活动略受限，被动活动良好，右足趾皮肤血液反流略迟缓。

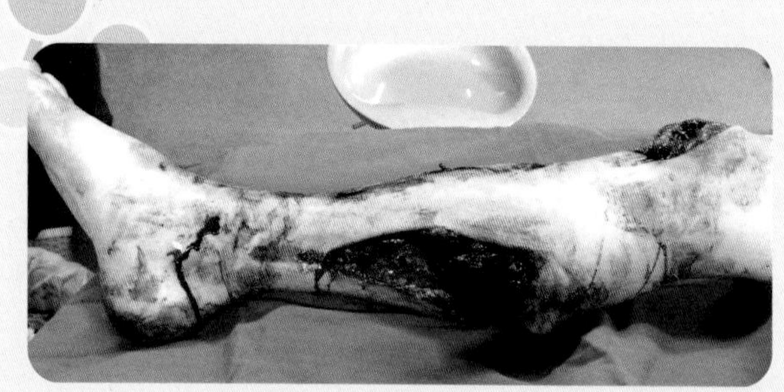

图 3.32.1　右小腿有大面积撕脱伤口，腓肠肌有部分断裂

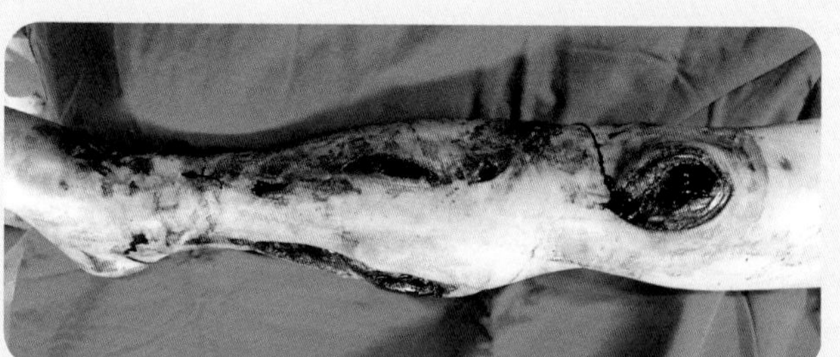

图 3.32.2　右髌骨前和胫前有多处伤口，有多处皮肤擦伤

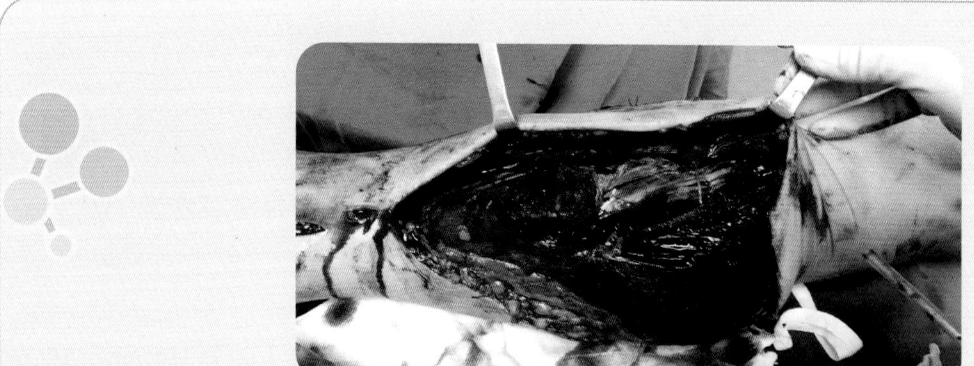

图 3.32.3　右小腿皮肤广泛性脱套，脂肪大面积挫灭，肌肉组织部分撕脱，肌肉组织水肿

◆ 治疗方案

大面积皮肤撕脱伴皮肤缺损，促进创面新鲜为植皮提供时间窗，VSD+ 外用重组人酸性成纤维细胞生长因子创面滴注，仍是最为有效方法之一。

◆ Signs and symptoms

The pain in the right lower limb is unbearable, with continuous bleeding, swelling that gradually worsens, and inability to stand and walk. There is extensive swelling in the right lower limb, with multiple irregular wounds visible. There is an 8 cm wound in front of the patella, reaching deep into the patella without fracture. The patellar ligament is partially torn, and there are two wounds in front of the tibia, each about 4 cm and 2 cm deep into the tibia without fracture. There is a 22 cm longitudinal wound on the right lower leg, with partial tearing of the gastrocnemius muscle and widespread detachment and detachment of the calf skin (Figure 3.32.1- Figure 3.32.3). The deep and shallow fascia is subducting and free in the right ankle, with multiple irregular abrasions on the skin, good fluctuations in the dorsalis pedis artery, decreased sensation in the toes, and delayed skin blood reflux in the right calf. The wound has active bleeding, with slightly restricted movement in the right knee and ankle joints, good passive movement, and slightly delayed skin blood reflux in the right toe.

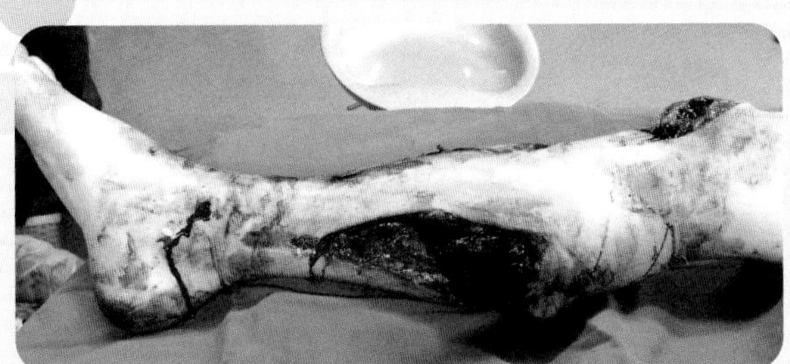

Figure 3.32.1 Large area tear off wound on the right calf, with partial rupture of the gastrocnemius muscle

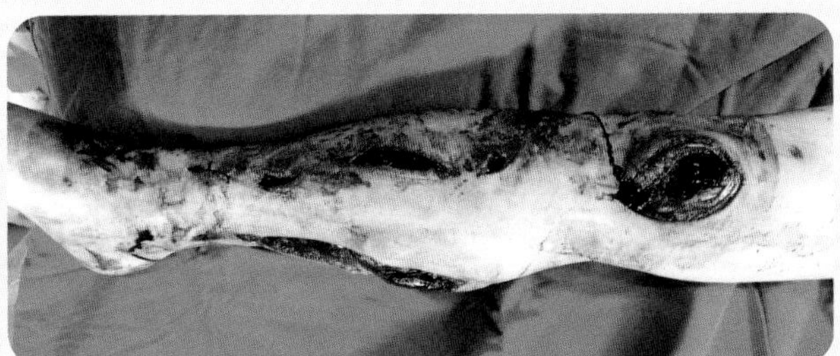

Figure 3.32.2 Multiple wounds and skin abrasions on the anterior right patella and anterior tibia

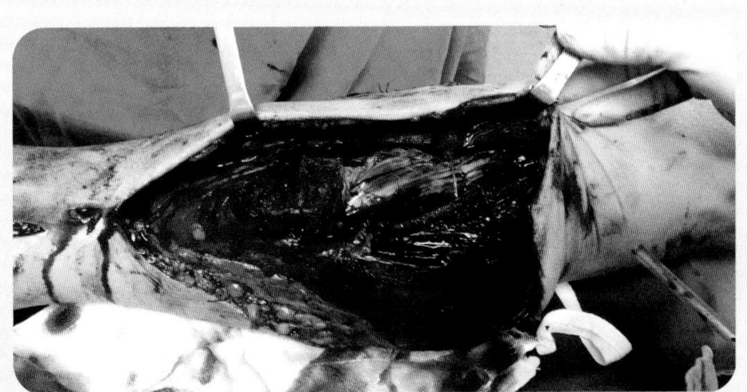

Figure 3.32.3 Widespread skin detachment of the right calf, extensive fat depletion, partial tearing of muscle tissue, and muscle tissue edema

◆ Treatment plan

One of the most effective methods is to promote the freshness of the wound and provide a time window for skin grafting through extensive skin peeling and skin defects. VSD + topical application of recombinant human acidic fibroblast growth factor wound infusion remains one of the most effective methods.

1. 手术过程，此案例复杂，需要几期手术方能消灭创面。

1.1 一期：急诊行清创，肌肉肌腱修复，髌韧带修复，撕脱皮肤回植，VSD+ 重组人酸性成纤维细胞生长因子冲洗治疗，预防感染，预防并发症发生（图 3.32.4、图 3.32.5）。

1.2 二期：小腿内侧有皮肤缺损，直接缝合困难，创面肉芽组织新鲜程度不够，植皮条件不够，需要再次应用 VSD+ 外用重组人酸性成纤维细胞生长因子创面滴注冲洗（图 3.32.6、图 3.32.7）。

1.3 三期：经过 2 次负压治疗，创面肉芽组织新鲜，故给予中厚皮片植皮手术，植皮成活（图 3.32.8）。

2. 下肢大面积撕脱性损伤，皮肤肌肉组织损害严重，术后往往会出现严重的粘连，关节松动，早期康复可有效恢复下肢功能。

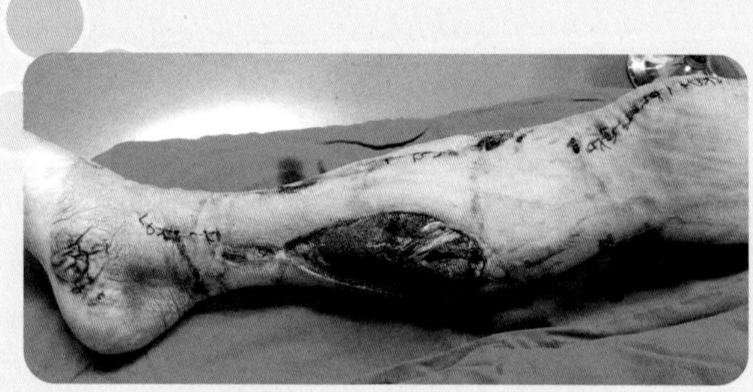

图 3.32.4 一期清创、肌肉修复、脱套皮肤原位回植，VSD 治疗

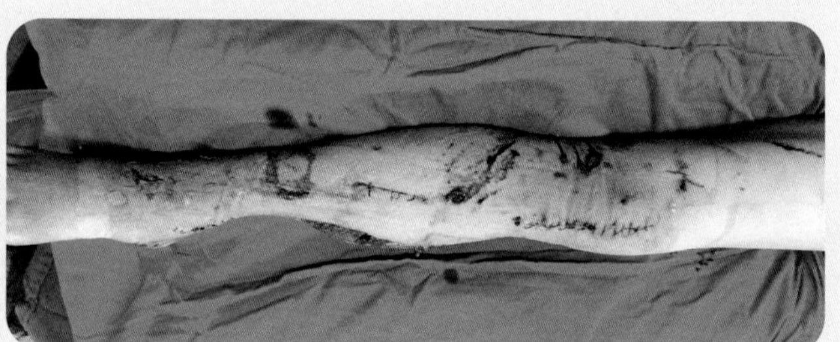

图 3.32.5 一期清创治疗后，皮肤血运良好、下肢中度肿胀

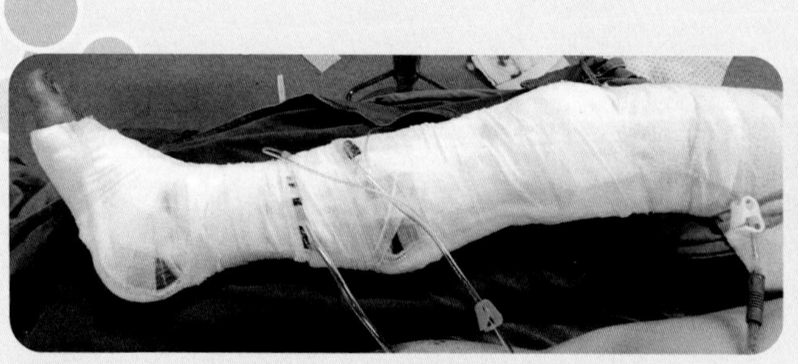

图 3.32.6 二期 VSD+ 外用重组人酸性成纤维细胞生长因子冲洗治疗，石膏固定

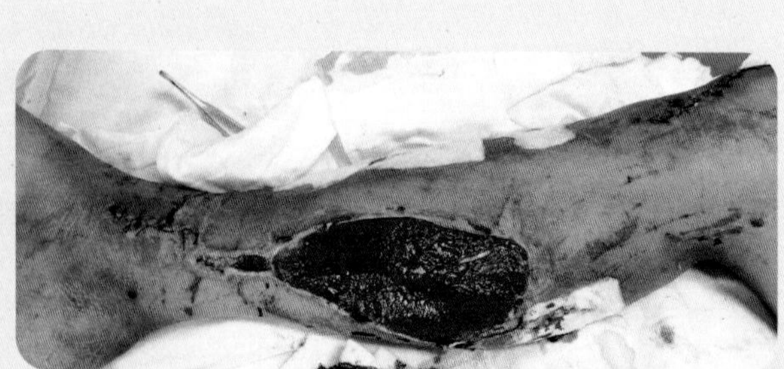

图 3.32.7 二期 VSD+ 外用重组人酸性成纤维细胞生长因子冲洗，创面肉芽组织新鲜，待植皮

1. The surgical process is complex in this case and requires several surgeries to eliminate the wound.

1.1 Phase 1: Emergency debridement, muscle tendon repair, patellar ligament repair, skin flap replantation, VSD + recombinant human acidic fibroblast growth factor flushing treatment to prevent infection and complications (Figure 3.32.4, Figure 3.32.5).

1.2 Phase II: There is a skin defect on the inner side of the calf, which is difficult to suture directly. The freshness of the granulation tissue on the wound is insufficient, and the conditions for skin grafting are not sufficient. It is necessary to apply VSD + topical recombinant human acidic fibroblast growth factor wound drip irrigation again (Figure 3.32.6, Figure 3.32.7).

1.3 Phase III: After 2 negative pressure treatments, the granulation tissue on the wound was fresh, so a medium thick skin graft surgery was performed, and the skin graft survived (Figure 3.32.8).

2. Large scale tearing injury of the lower limbs, severe damage to skin and muscle tissue, often leading to severe adhesion and joint loosening after surgery. Early rehabilitation can effectively restore lower limb function.

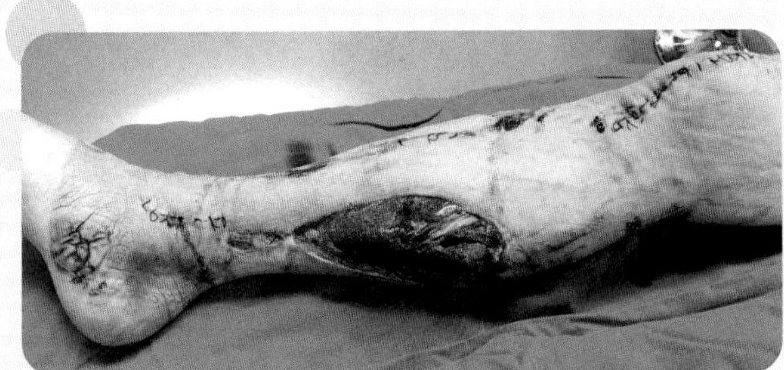

Figure 3.32.4 Phase I debridement, muscle repair, in situ skin grafting, VSD treatment

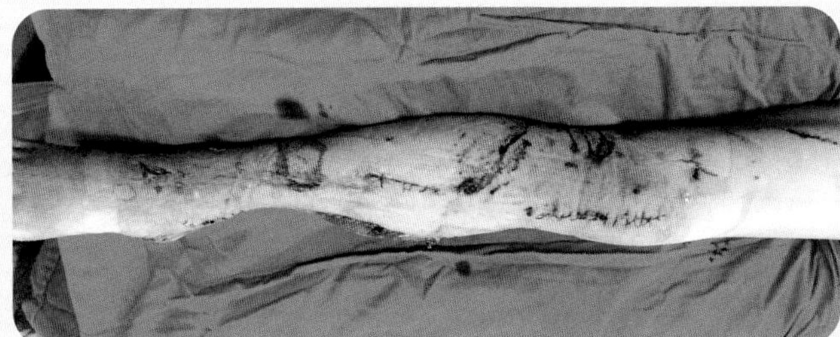

Figure 3.32.5 After the first stage of debridement treatment, the skin blood supply is good and there is moderate swelling in the lower limbs

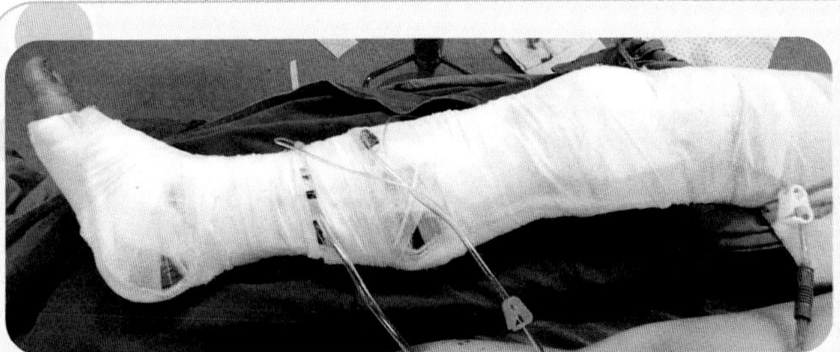

Figure 3.32.6 Phase II VSD + topical recombinant human acidic fibroblast growth factor flushing treatment, gypsum fixation

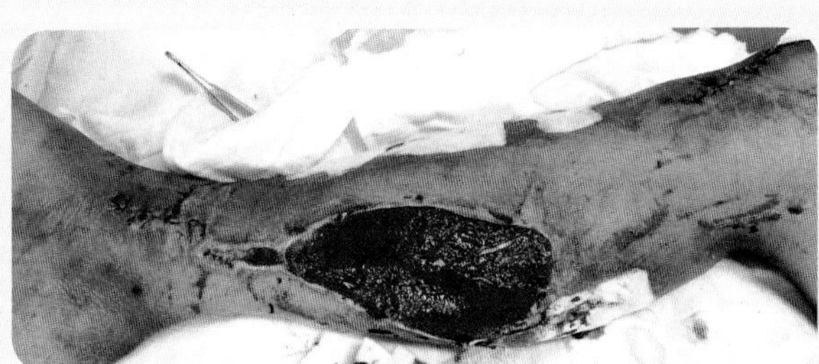

Figure 3.32.7 Phase II VSD+external application of recombinant human acidic fibroblast growth factor flushing, fresh granulation tissue of the wound, ready for skin grafting

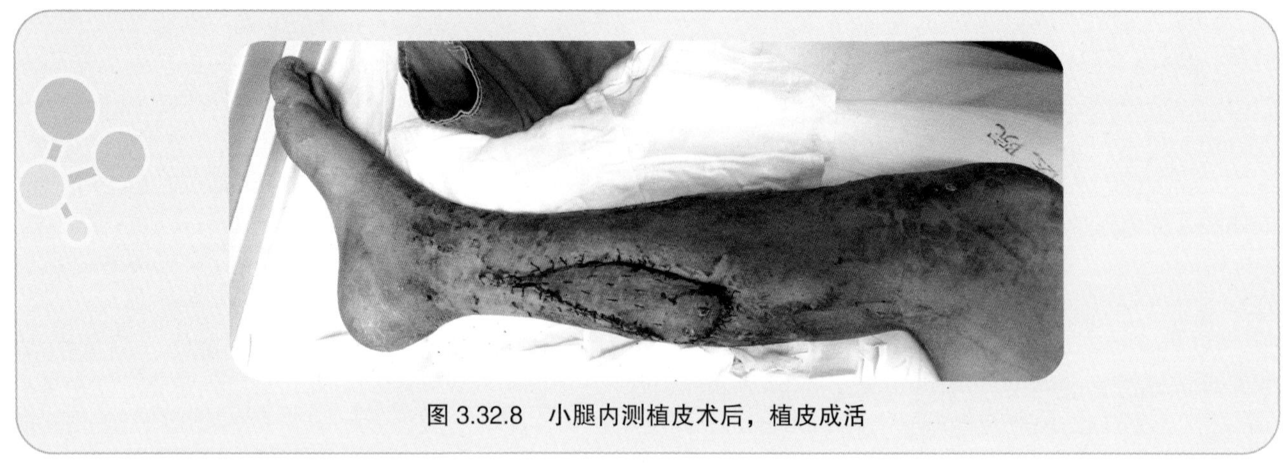

图 3.32.8　小腿内测植皮术后，植皮成活

（陈善亮）

案例三十三　左前踝皮肤缺损

◆ 损伤原因

患者被磨具机摩擦，致左足前踝缺损。

◆ 症状与体征

左前踝剧痛难忍，局部出血不止，肿胀并逐渐加重，活动受限，不能站立行走。左前踝有 6 cm × 5 cm 皮肤软组织缺损，深达距骨，距骨关节面部分外露，足背伸肌腱及血管神经外露，创缘不齐。

◆ 治疗方案

该案例足踝部皮肤软组织缺损，肌腱血管神经骨关节外露，为了保护皮下重要的组织结构，急诊修复创面防止皮下重要组织坏死，外踝上穿支皮瓣是很好的治疗方案之一。

1. 选用腰硬联合麻醉，清创止血，修复皮下血管神经肌腱。

2. 手术过程

2.1 外踝上皮瓣设计：旋转点为外踝上 5 cm 处，胫骨脊与腓骨间为设计线，肌筋膜深层为解剖面，按皮瓣切口设计线，依次切开皮肤至深筋膜，在趾长伸肌与腓骨短肌间隙显露外踝上动脉，保护好腓肠神经，蒂长 3 cm、蒂宽 1.5 cm。

2.2 皮瓣移植：皮瓣解剖结束后，创面喷洒外用重组人碱性成纤维细胞生长因子，促进皮瓣受区愈合。将皮瓣和受区缝合，于左侧大腿前侧切取中厚皮片移植皮瓣供区（图 3.33.1 ～图 3.33.3）。

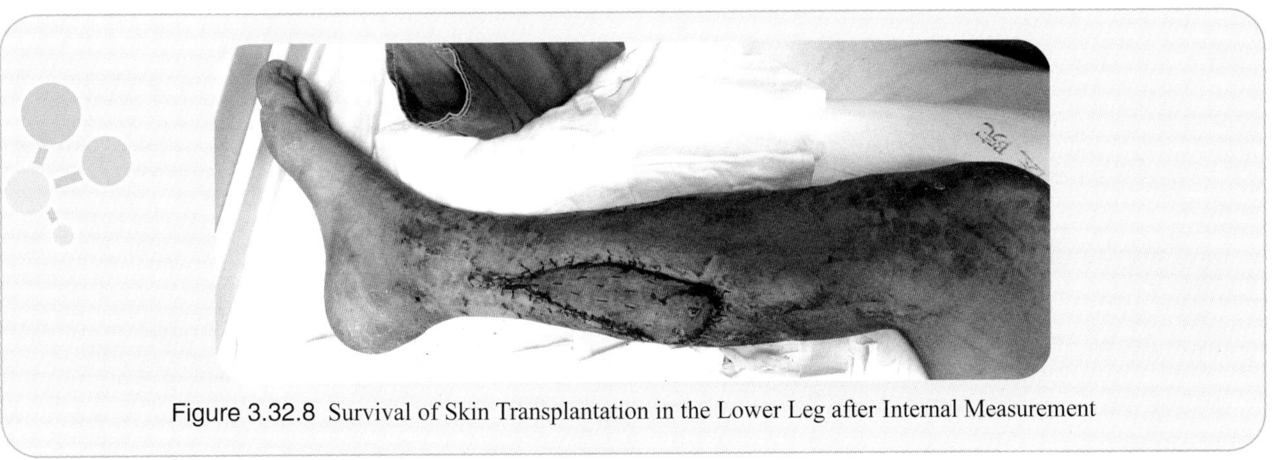

Figure 3.32.8 Survival of Skin Transplantation in the Lower Leg after Internal Measurement

(Chen Shanliang)

Case 33 Left anterior ankle skin defect

◆ Cause of injury

The patient was rubbed by a grinding machine, resulting in a defect in the anterior ankle of the left foot.

◆ Signs and symptoms

Severe pain in the left anterior ankle, persistent local bleeding, swelling that gradually worsens, limited mobility, and inability to stand and walk. There is a 6 cm × 5 cm skin and soft tissue defect in the left anterior ankle, reaching deep into the talus. The joint surface of the talus is partially exposed, and the extensor tendon and vascular nerves of the dorsalis pedis are exposed. The wound margin is uneven.

◆ Treatment plan

In this case, there was a skin and soft tissue defect in the ankle region, with exposed tendons, blood vessels, nerves, and bone joints. In order to protect the important subcutaneous tissue structure, emergency repair of the wound was performed to prevent necrosis of the important subcutaneous tissue. The external ankle perforator flap is one of the good treatment options

1. Use spinal epidural anesthesia, debridement and hemostasis, and repair subcutaneous blood vessels, nerves, and tendons.

2. Surgical process

2.1 Design of the lateral malleolus flap: The rotation point is 5 cm above the lateral malleolus, the design line is between the tibial spine and fibula, and the deep layer of the myofascial layer is the anatomical surface. According to the design line of the flap incision, the skin is cut in sequence to the deep fascia, and the lateral malleolus artery is exposed between the extensor digitorum longus and the peroneal short muscle to protect the peroneal nerve. The pedicle is 3 cm long and 1.5 cm wide.

2.2 Skin flap transplantation: After the dissection of the skin flap is completed, the wound is sprayed with recombinant human basic fibroblast growth factor to promote the healing of the skin flap recipient area. Suture the skin flap and the recipient area, and cut a medium thick skin graft from the anterior side of the left thigh to transplant the skin flap to the donor area (Figure 3.33.1-Figure3.33.3).

3. 术后给予扩容、解痉补充血容量，抗感染治疗，抬高患肢，减轻肿胀。

4. 术后7天进行功能训练，12天拆线，并逐渐负重行走。

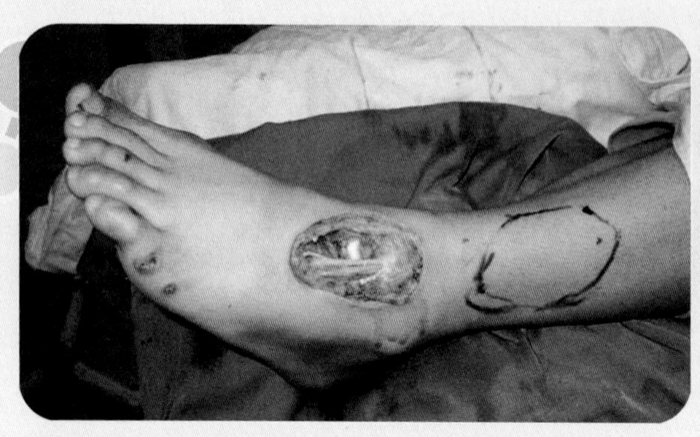

图 3.33.1　左足前踝皮肤缺损，肌腱骨关节面外露，皮瓣设计线

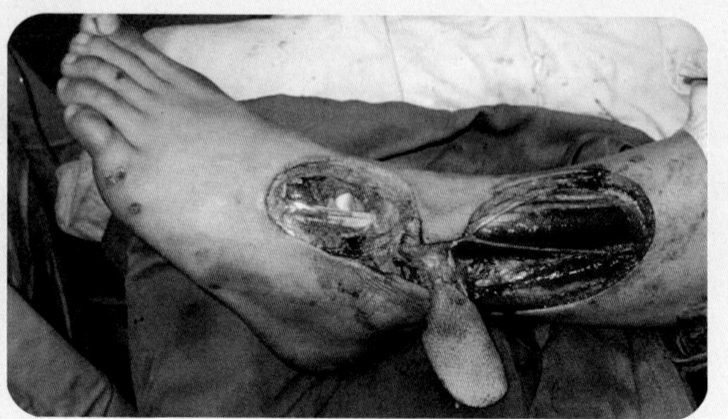

图 3.33.2　外踝上腓动脉穿支皮瓣完全解剖游离

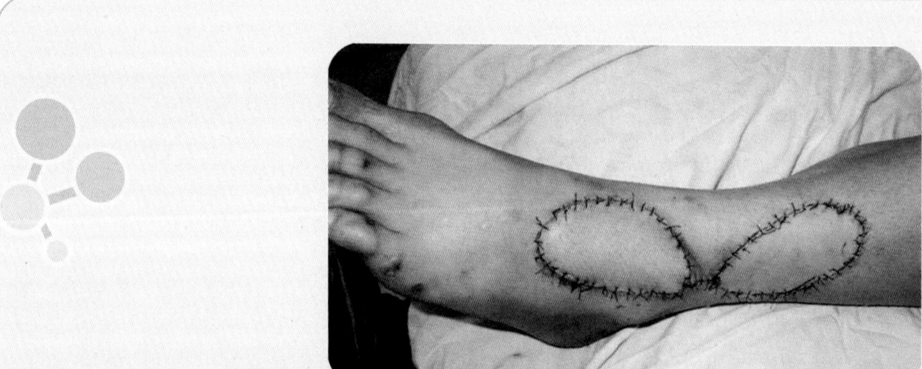

图 3.33.3　外踝上穿支皮瓣行受供区缝合，皮瓣血运良好，供区植皮

（陈善亮）

案例三十四　左足背大面积皮肤软组织缺损

◆ 损伤原因

患者采茶时从高山上滚落、受摩擦，致左足背大面积皮肤软组织缺损。

◆ 症状与体征

左足剧痛，出血不止，肿胀并逐渐加重，不能站立行走。左足前屈畸形，前踝至足背有大面积皮肤软组织缺损，面积8 cm×7 cm，深达距骨及足舟骨，距骨、足舟骨及外侧楔骨骨折，伴摩擦缺损性骨折；足

3. After surgery, provide volume expansion, spasmolysis to supplement blood volume, anti-infection treatment, elevate the affected limb, and reduce swelling.

4. Perform functional training 7 days after surgery, remove stitches 12 days later, and gradually walk with weight-bearing.

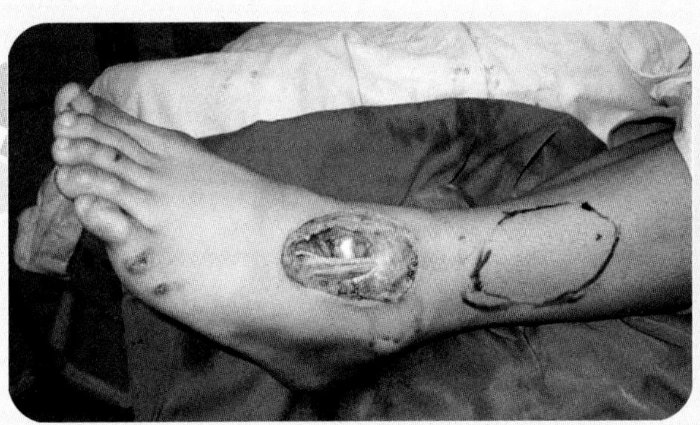

Figure 3.33.1 Left ankle skin defect, exposed tendon bone joint surface, flap design line

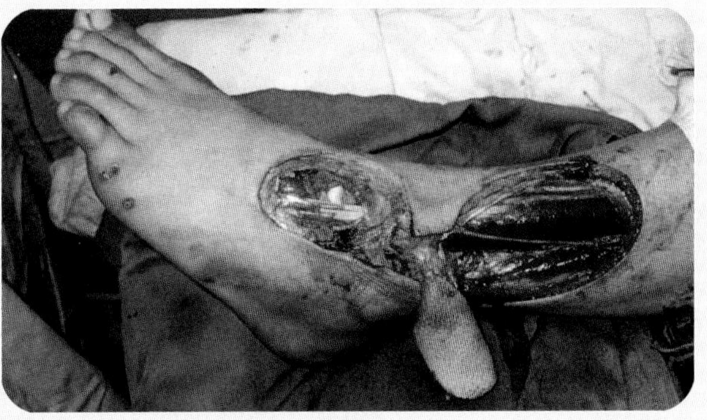

Figure 3.33.2 Complete dissection and free release of the perforator flap of the peroneal artery on the lateral malleolus

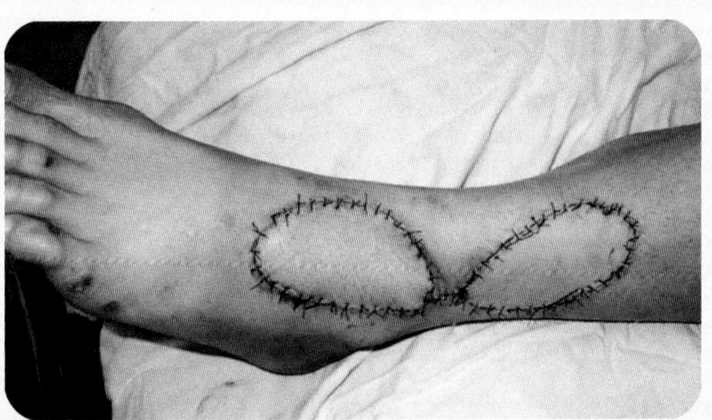

Figure 3.33.3 Suture of the lateral ankle perforator flap at the donor site, with good blood supply to the flap and skin grafting at the donor site

(Chen Shanliang)

Case 34 Large area skin and soft tissue defect on the left dorsum of the foot

◆ Cause of injury

The patient fell from a high mountain and was rubbed during tea picking, resulting in a large area of skin and soft tissue defect on the left foot dorsum.

◆ Signs and symptoms

Severe pain in the left foot, continuous bleeding, swelling that gradually worsens, and inability to stand and walk. Left foot flexion deformity, with a large area of skin and soft tissue defect from the anterior ankle to the dorsum of the foot, measuring 8 cm × 7 cm, reaching deep into the talus and talus bones. Fractures of the talus, talus, and lateral wedge bone are present, accompanied by frictional defect fractures; Defects in the extensor tendons

𧿹趾及第 2 ～ 5 足趾伸肌腱缺损，缺损长度约 6 cm；足背动脉及伴行静脉缺损，缺损长度约 5 cm；伤口污染严重，布满泥沙，关节间隙骨折断端充满泥沙，足𧿹趾及第 2 ～ 5 足趾背伸活动完全受限，足趾屈曲活动良好（图 3.34.1）。足底感觉良好，足背感觉消失，足趾血液反流良好。

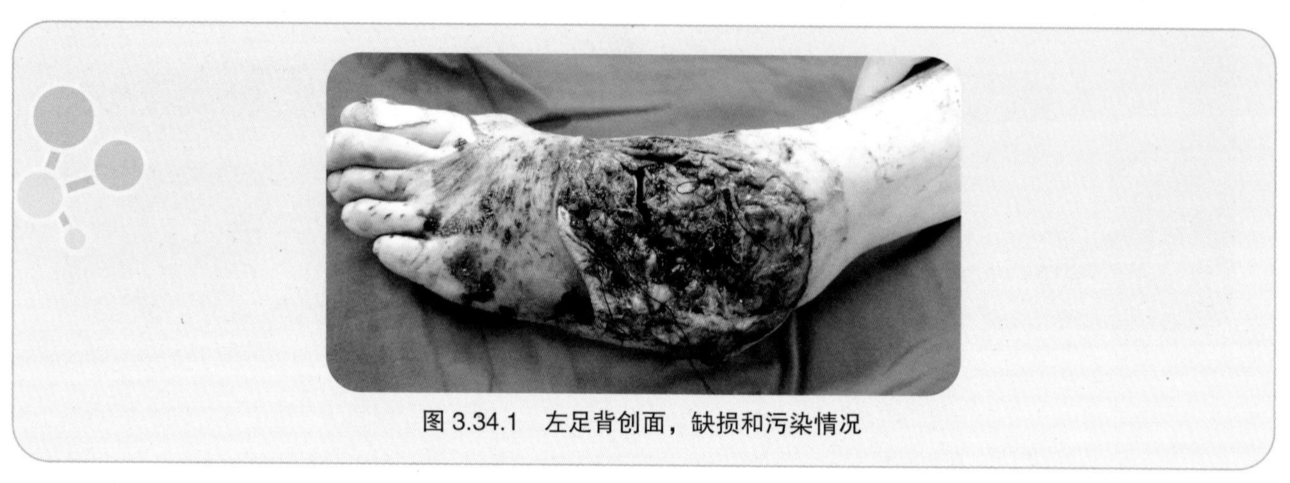

图 3.34.1　左足背创面，缺损和污染情况

◆ 治疗方案

1. 清创，该案例为急性创面，创面污染严重，尽管一期清创较为干净，由于伤口污染严重有感染之可能，故采用一期清创 +VSD+ 外用重组人碱性成纤维细胞生长因子滴注，二期创面新鲜排除感染后，采用腓肠神经营养血管皮瓣移植覆盖创面（图 3.34.2）。

2. 麻醉，选用腰硬联合麻醉。

3. 手术过程

3.1 腓肠神经营养血管支皮瓣设计：外踝与跟腱连线中点上 5 cm 处为皮瓣旋转点，最低点可在外踝尖部上 1 ～ 3 cm 处，旋转点与腓骨小头连线为中轴线，肌筋膜浅层为解剖面，皮瓣蒂长 5 cm、蒂宽 2 cm，皮瓣面积 8 cm × 7 cm（图 3.34.3）。

3.2 皮瓣移植：按皮瓣设计线依次切开皮肤及皮下脂肪达肌筋膜，沿途结扎皮瓣分支，分离腓肠神经加以保护，将小隐静脉包含在皮瓣内。皮瓣解剖结束后，皮瓣血运良好。创面喷洒生长因子，将皮瓣与受区移植并缝合，皮瓣下放置橡皮条引流两枚，供区部分切口缝合，于大腿前侧切取中厚皮片游离移植供区并缝合。包扎并石膏托固定。

4. 术后抬高患肢，严密观察皮瓣血运，日光灯保温，加强换药，术后 48 小时拔出引流条。

5. 扩容、解痉，补充血容量，预防感染，缓解疼痛。

6. 术后 7 天，扶拐下地轻负重，12 天拆线（图 3.34.4、图 3.34.5）。

of the toes and the 2nd to 5th toes, with a length of approximately 6 cm; Defects in the dorsalis pedis artery and accompanying veins, with a length of approximately 5 cm; The wound is heavily contaminated and covered in mud and sand. The fractured end of the joint space is filled with mud and sand, and the dorsiflexion movement of the toes and the 2nd to 5th toes is completely restricted. The flexion movement of the toes is good (Figure 3.34.1). The plantar sensation is good, the dorsum sensation disappears, and the blood reflux in the toes is good.

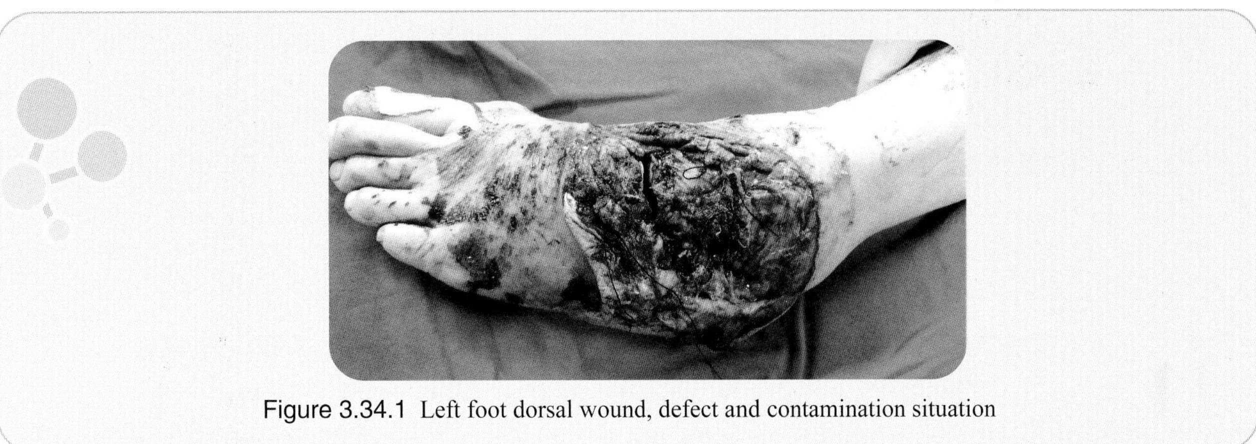

Figure 3.34.1 Left foot dorsal wound, defect and contamination situation

◆ Treatment plan

1. Debridement: This case is an acute wound with severe contamination. Although the first stage of debridement was relatively clean, there was a possibility of infection due to the severe contamination of the wound. Therefore, a combination of first stage debridement, VSD, and topical recombinant human alkaline fibroblast growth factor infusion was used. After fresh elimination of infection from the second stage wound, a sural nerve nutrient vascular skin flap was transplanted to cover the wound (Figure 3.34.2).

2. Anesthesia, using lumbar epidural anesthesia.

3. Surgical process

3.1 Design of Gastrocnemius Neurovascular Branch Flap: The flap rotation point is located 5 cm above the midpoint of the line connecting the lateral malleolus and Achilles tendon, and the lowest point can be located 1-3 cm above the tip of the lateral malleolus. The rotation point is connected to the fibular head as the central axis, and the superficial layer of the myofascial layer is the anatomical surface. The flap pedicle is 5 cm long and 2 cm wide, with a flap area of 8 cm × 7 cm (Figure 3.34.3).

3.2 Skin flap transplantation: Cut open the skin and subcutaneous fat to the fascia according to the design line of the skin flap, ligate the branches of the skin flap along the way, separate the sural nerve for protection, and include the small saphenous vein in the skin flap. After the dissection of the skin flap, the blood supply of the flap is good. Spray growth factor on the wound, transplant and suture the skin flap with the recipient area, place two rubber strips under the skin flap for drainage, suture the incision of the donor area, and cut a medium thick skin graft on the front side of the thigh for free transplantation of the donor area and suture. Wrap and fix with plaster support.

4. After surgery, raise the affected limb, closely observe the blood flow of the skin flap, keep warm with fluorescent lamps, strengthen dressing changes, and remove the drainage strip 48 hours after surgery.

5. Expand capacity, relieve spasms, replenish blood volume, prevent infections, and alleviate pain.

6. After 7 days of surgery, gently load the patient with crutches and remove the stitches 12 days later (Figure 3.34.4, Figure 3.34.5).

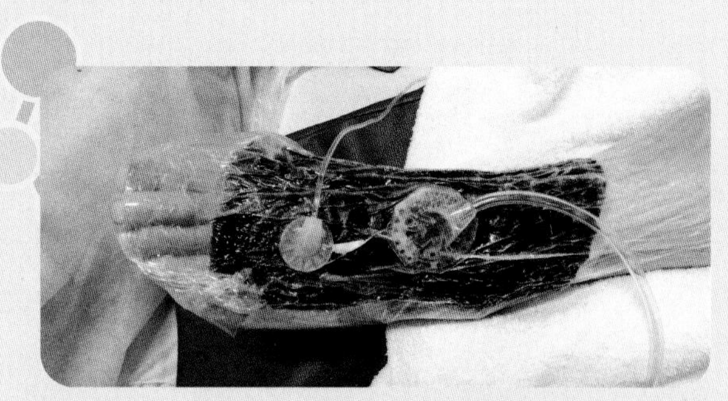

图 3.34.2 清创后，应用 VSD+ 重组人酸性成纤维细胞生长因子滴注冲洗

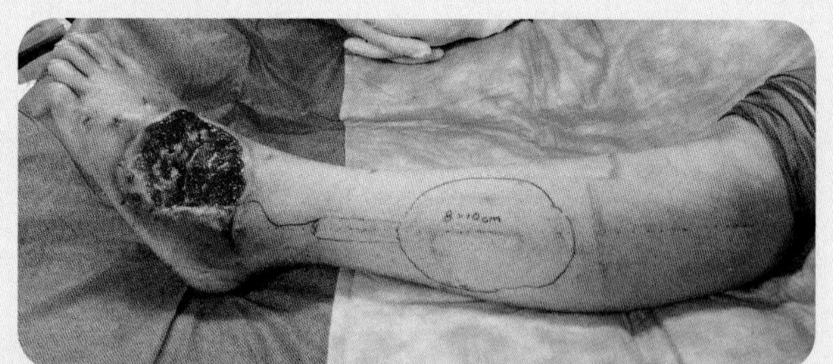

图 3.34.3 经过 VSD+ 重组人酸性成纤维细胞生长因子冲洗治疗，皮瓣移植示意

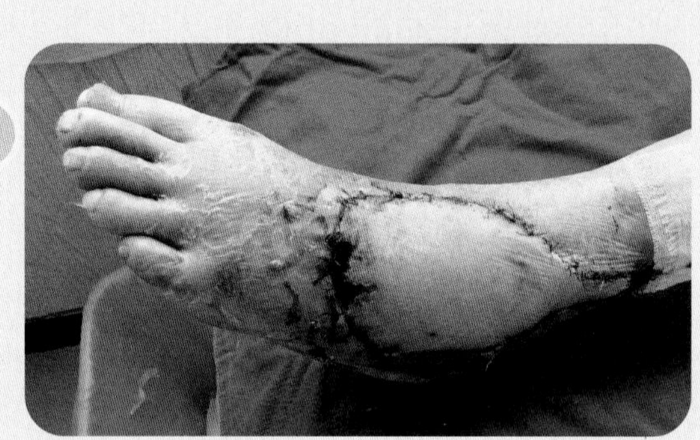

图 3.34.4 术后 9 天，皮瓣成活，远端有少许皮缘坏死

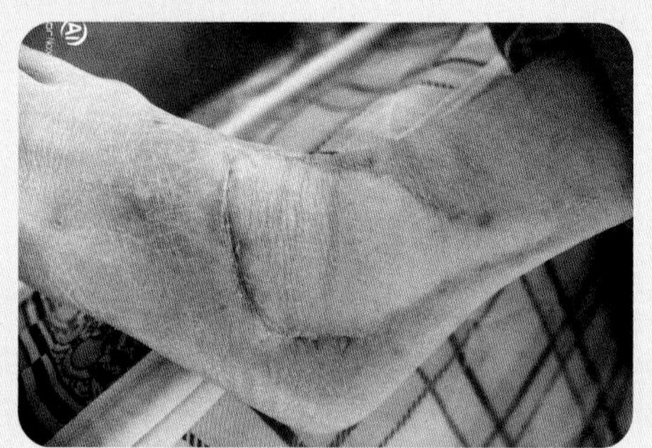

图 3.34.5 皮瓣移植术后 2 个月，皮色外观良好

（陈善亮）

案例三十五 右足足背胫侧皮肤缺损

◆ 损伤原因

患者骑摩托车摔倒，右足受摩擦致右足背胫侧皮肤缺损。

◆ 症状与体征

右足剧痛难忍，出血不止，肿胀并逐渐加重，不能站立行走。右足背内侧有 10 cm × 5 cm 创面，足内侧楔骨和第 1 跖基底部摩擦缺损性缺损，伤口内布满泥沙，皮缘不齐，足䠀趾背伸活动略受限，屈趾活动良好，足内侧感觉消失。足背动脉波动良好，踝关节活动良好。

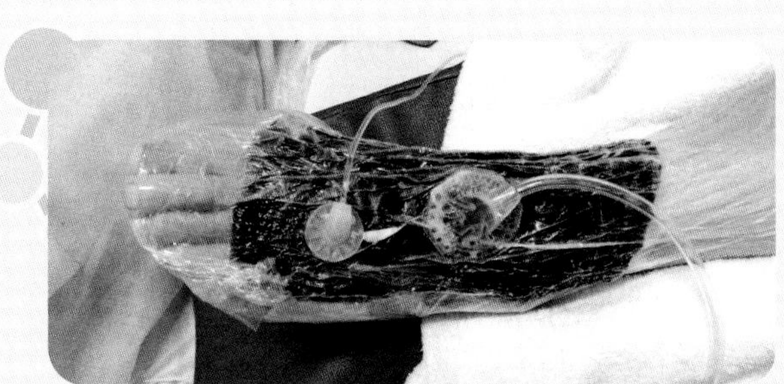

Figure 3.34.2 After debridement, VSD + recombinant human acidic fibroblast growth factor drip irrigation was applied

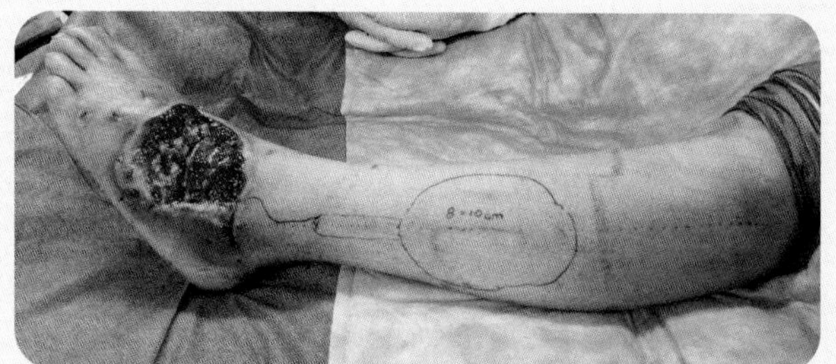

Figure 3.34.3 Schematic diagram of skin flap transplantation after VSD + recombinant human acidic fibroblast growth factor flushing treatment

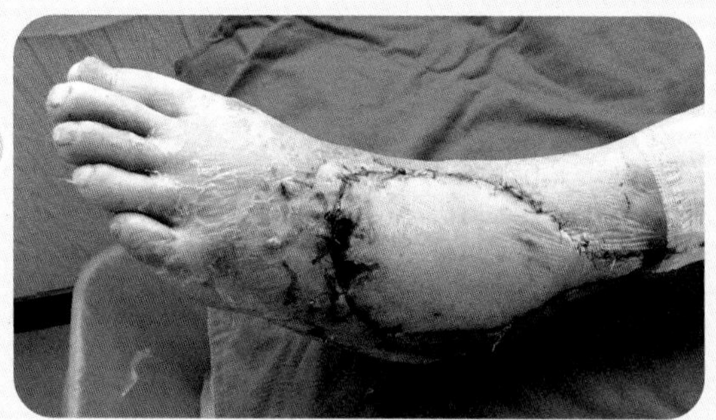

Figure 3.34.4 Nine days after surgery, the skin flap survived with slight necrosis at the distal edge

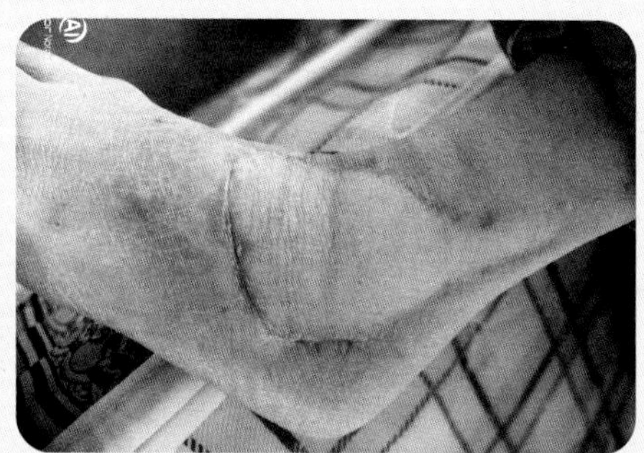

Figure 3.34.5 Two months after skin flap transplantation, the skin color and appearance are good

(Chen Shanliang)

Case 35 Right full back tibial skin defect

◆ Cause of injury

The patient fell while riding a motorcycle and suffered from friction on the right foot, resulting in a skin defect on the dorsal tibial side of the right foot.

◆ Signs and symptoms

The pain in the right foot is unbearable, with continuous bleeding, swelling that gradually worsens, and inability to stand and walk. There is a 10 cm × 5 cm wound on the inner back of the right foot, with a frictional defect between the medial wedge-shaped bone and the base of the first metatarsal. The wound is covered with mud and sand, with uneven skin edges. The dorsiflexion of the toe is slightly restricted, but the flexion of the toe is good, and the sensation on the inner side of the foot disappears. The dorsalis pedis artery fluctuates well and the ankle joint moves well.

◆ 治疗方案

1. 急诊一期清创，VSD+ 外用重组人酸性成纤维细胞生长因子创面滴注冲洗，创面新鲜无感染，择期皮瓣移植手术（图 3.35.1）。

2. 选用腰硬联合麻醉。

3. 手术过程

3.1 内踝上穿支皮瓣设计：以内踝上 4 cm 为旋转点，以内踝和胫骨内侧髁连线为轴线，蒂长为 5 cm，筋膜蒂宽为 3 cm，保留 1 cm 皮蒂，皮瓣面积 10 cm × 5.5 cm，解剖面为深筋膜。

3.2 皮瓣移植：按皮瓣设计线依次切开皮肤达深筋膜，在胫后屈肌、趾长屈肌与跟腱间隙显露胫后动脉的皮瓣穿支，并加以保护。皮瓣完全解剖游离后，将重组人酸性成纤维细胞生长因子喷洒创面，将皮瓣行受供区缝合，皮瓣下放置橡皮条引流两枚，皮瓣供区直接缝合闭合伤口（图 3.35.2、图 3.35.3）。

4. 术后抬高患肢，严密观察皮瓣血运，日光灯保温，加强换药，术后 48 小时拔出引流条。

5. 扩容、解痉，补充血容量，预防感染，缓解疼痛。

6. 术后 7 天，扶拐下地轻负重，12 天拆线（图 3.35.4）。

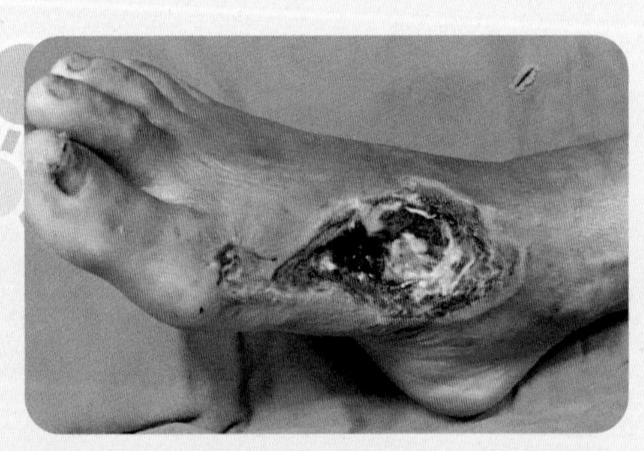

图 3.35.1　伤口肉芽组织新鲜，局部无红肿，待皮瓣移植

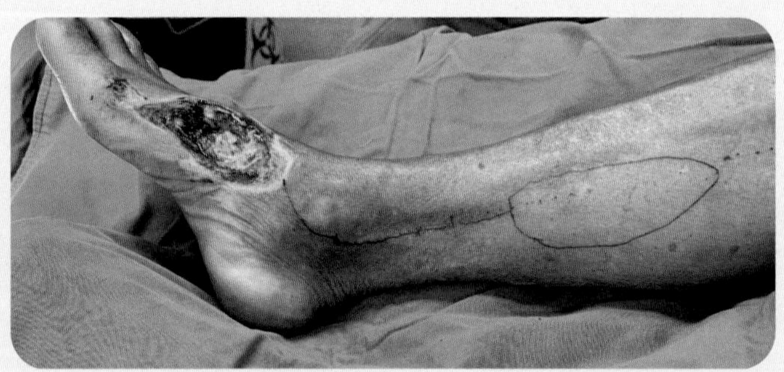

图 3.35.2　内踝上皮瓣设计示意

◆ Treatment plan

1. Emergency first stage debridement, VSD + topical application of recombinant human acidic fibroblast growth factor wound drip irrigation, fresh and infection free wound, elective skin flap transplantation surgery (Figure 3.35.1).

2. Use spinal epidural anesthesia.

3. Surgical process

3.1 Design of the medial malleolus perforator flap: with 4 cm above the medial malleolus as the rotation point, the line connecting the medial malleolus and the medial tibial condyle as the axis, the pedicle length is 5 cm, the fascial pedicle width is 3 cm, and 1 cm of the skin pedicle is retained. The flap area is 10 cm × 5.5 cm, and the anatomical plane is the deep fascia.

3.2 Skin flap transplantation: Cut open the skin to the deep fascia according to the design line of the skin flap, expose the perforating branch of the posterior tibial artery between the flexor tibialis, flexor digitorum longus, and Achilles tendon, and protect it. After the complete dissection and dissociation of the skin flap, the recombinant human acidic fibroblast growth factor was sprayed onto the wound, and the skin flap was sutured in the donor area. Two rubber strips were placed under the skin flap for drainage, and the skin flap donor area was directly sutured to close the wound (Figure 3.35.2, Figure 3.35.3).

4. After surgery, raise the affected limb, closely observe the blood flow of the skin flap, keep warm with fluorescent lamps, strengthen dressing changes, and remove the drainage strip 48 hours after surgery.

5. Expand capacity, relieve spasms, replenish blood volume, prevent infections, and alleviate pain.

6. Seven days after surgery, gently load the patient with crutches and remove the stitches 12 days later (Figure 3.35.4).

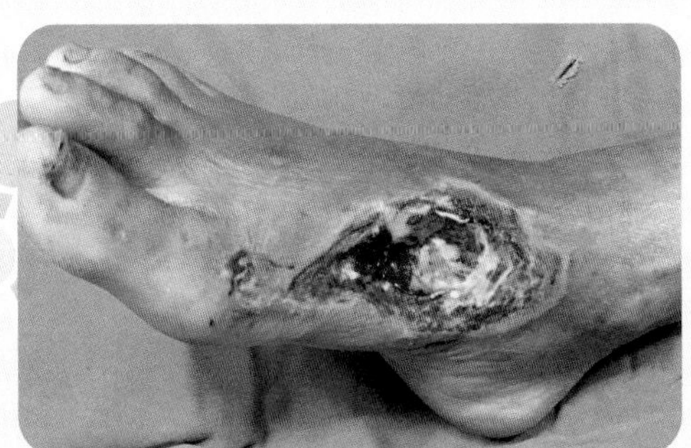

Figure 3.35.1 Fresh granulation tissue from the wound, with no redness or swelling in the local area, awaiting skin flap transplantation

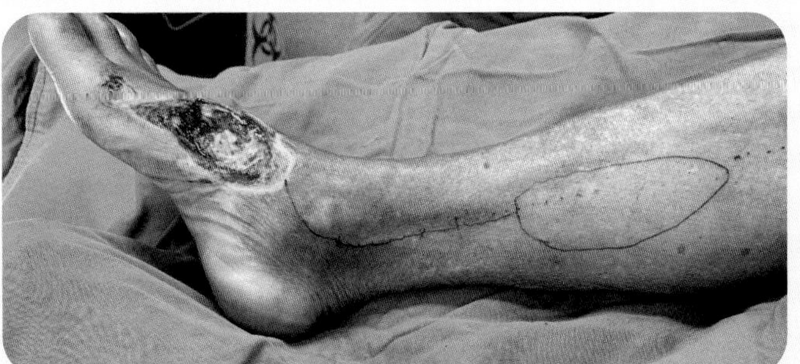

Figure 3.35.2 Schematic design of medial malleolus flap

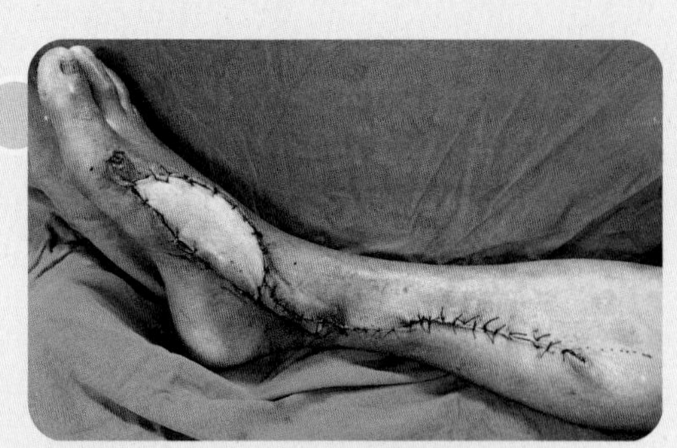

图 3.35.3　内踝上皮瓣移植术后，供区直接缝合

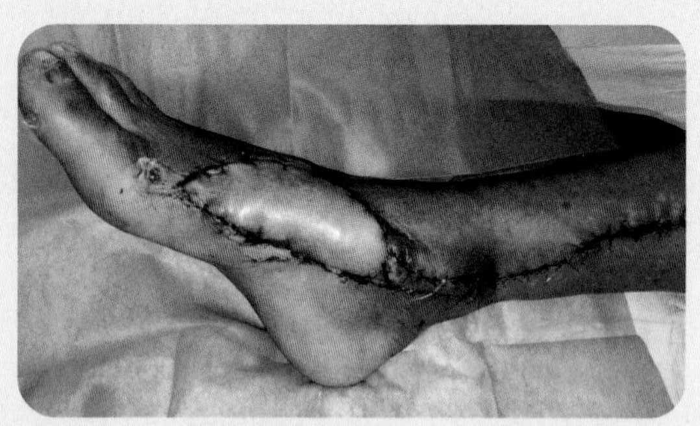

图 3.35.4　皮瓣移植术后 7 天、皮瓣血运良好，轻度肿胀

（陈善亮）

案例三十六　右侧胫骨骨折术后大面积皮肤软组织缺损钢板骨外露

◆ 损伤原因

患者因车祸右腿受挤压，致右侧胫骨骨折伴皮肤软组织缺损，术后出现右小腿大面积皮肤软组织缺损、钢板与胫骨外露。

◆ 症状与体征

车祸后右小腿剧痛，出血不止，不能站立行走，肿胀并逐渐加重，畸形伴反常活动，在当地医院诊断右胫腓骨下段开放粉碎性骨折，伴皮肤软组织缺损。急诊在当地医院行清创、胫腓骨骨折复位钢板内固定术，小腿内侧植皮术，术后 10 天，右小腿皮肤逐渐坏死，并多次进行清创，坏死面积增大，钢板外露，伤口不能愈合，每天伤口流脓水。右侧小腿广泛性肿胀，小腿中下段内侧有大面积皮肤软组织缺损，味恶臭，缺损面积 18 cm × 9 cm，局部有大量炎性渗出。有两枚钢板部分外露，胫骨下段内侧外露，裸露胫骨无骨膜，创面散在部分坏死组织，小腿内侧有不规则瘢痕，创面周围皮肤角化层增厚，皮肤红肿，局部温度增高，足背动脉搏动减弱，足底感觉减退，足趾屈伸活动略受限，左侧腹股沟淋巴结无肿大，膝关节活动良好（图 3.36.1）。

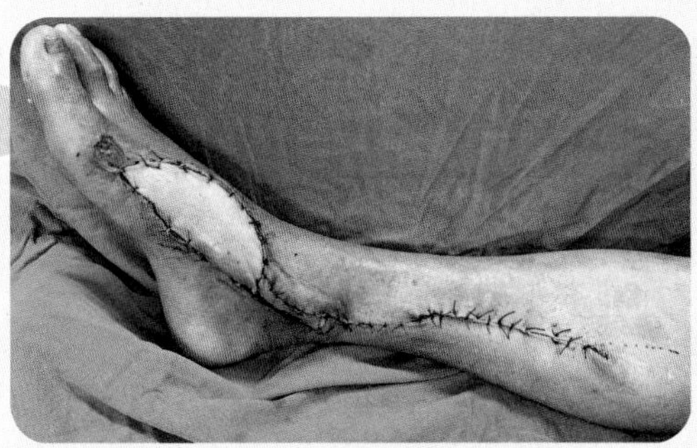

Figure 3.35.3 After internal ankle flap transplantation, the donor site is directly sutured

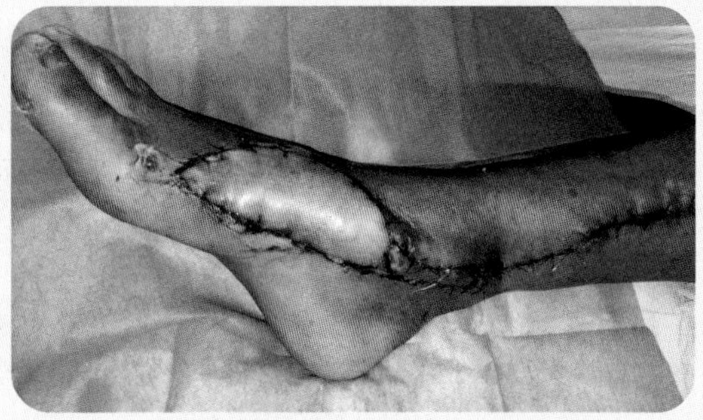

Figure 3.35.4 Seven days after skin flap transplantation, the skin flap has good blood flow and mild swelling

(Chen Shanliang)

Case 36 Large area skin and soft tissue defect with exposed steel plate bone after surgery for right tibial fracture

◆ Cause of injury

The patient's right leg was compressed due to a car accident, resulting in a fracture of the right tibia with skin and soft tissue defects. After surgery, there was a large area of skin and soft tissue defect in the right calf, and the steel plate and tibia were exposed.

◆ Signs and symptoms

After the car accident, there was severe pain in the right calf, continuous bleeding, inability to stand and walk, swelling that gradually worsened, deformity accompanied by abnormal movement. The local hospital diagnosed an open comminuted fracture of the lower segment of the right tibia and fibula, accompanied by skin and soft tissue defects. The emergency department performed debridement, reduction of tibial and fibular fractures with steel plate internal fixation, and skin grafting on the inner side of the lower leg at a local hospital. Ten days after the surgery, the skin on the right lower leg gradually necrotic and underwent multiple debridement procedures. The necrotic area increased, the steel plate was exposed, and the wound could not heal, with pus flowing from the wound every day. There is extensive swelling in the right calf, and there is a large area of skin and soft tissue defect on the inner side of the middle and lower segments of the calf, with a foul odor. The defect area is 18 cm × 9 cm, and there is a large amount of inflammatory exudate in the local area. Two steel plates are partially exposed, the inner side of the lower tibia is exposed, the tibia is exposed without periosteum, the wound is scattered with some necrotic tissue, there are irregular scars on the inner side of the calf, the keratinized layer of the skin around the wound is thickened, the skin is red and swollen, the local temperature is increased, the pulsation of the dorsalis pedis artery is weakened, the plantar sensation is reduced, the flexion and extension of the toes are slightly restricted, the left inguinal lymph nodes are not enlarged, and the knee joint activity is good (Figure 3.36.1).

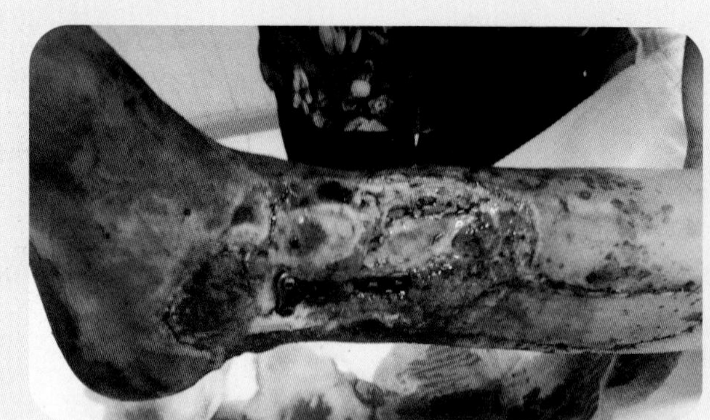

图 3.36.1　右小腿内侧皮肤软组织缺损，钢板和胫骨外露

◆ 治疗方案

该患者为外院转诊来院，外院出诊时已经进行了清创骨折复位钢板内固定，由于皮肤软组织挫伤严重，术后逐渐出现皮肤坏死，钢板外露。

1. 入院后局部细菌培养 + 药物敏感试验，根据敏感菌和药物敏感试验，指导临床规范使用抗菌药物。

2. 加强伤口换药，每天更换敷料 2 次，换药时坏死组织清创，创面外用重组人碱性成纤维细胞生长因子促进伤口肉芽组织新鲜，创口肉芽组织新鲜后，选择皮瓣移植修复创面。

3. 麻醉选择腰硬联合麻醉。

4. 手术过程

4.1 股前外游离皮瓣设计：髂前上棘与髌骨外侧缘连线中点为旋骨外动脉降支的第一肌皮支穿出点（髂髌线），以此点为中心设计皮瓣，髂髌线中点与髂腹股沟韧带中点为连线，该线为旋股外动脉降支走行体表投影线，皮瓣切取面积为 19 cm × 10 cm（图 3.36.2）。

4.2 受区准备：切除创周皮缘和无生机组织，创面缺损 18.5 cm × 9.5 cm。显露胫后动脉儿期两条伴行静脉，胫后动脉断裂伴缺损 5 cm。远近端显露备用，待股前外皮瓣旋骨外动脉桥接（旋股外动脉动静脉桥接修复胫后动脉断裂缺损）。

4.3 皮瓣切取：按切口设计线依次切开皮肤、浅筋膜、深筋膜。在股直肌与股外侧肌间隙进入，于肌间隙中显露旋骨外动脉降支，并保护好进入皮瓣肌皮支，此时皮瓣几乎完全解剖，血管钳夹阻断血运试验，观察皮瓣血供。根据受区血管长度，选择血管切断部位，皮瓣完全游离切取，供区喷洒外用重组人碱性成纤维细胞生长因子，创口直接缝合并包扎。

4.4 皮瓣移植：皮瓣完全切取游离后，受区创面外用重组人碱性成纤维细胞生长因子，将游离皮瓣和

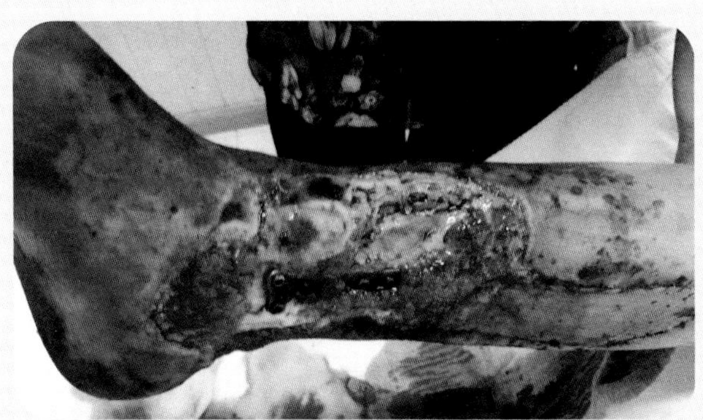

Figure 3.36.1 Skin and soft tissue defect on the inner side of the right calf, with exposed steel plate and tibia

◆ Treatment plan

The patient was referred from an external hospital and underwent debridement, fracture reduction, and steel plate internal fixation during the visit. Due to severe skin and soft tissue contusions, skin necrosis and steel plate exposure gradually occurred after surgery.

1. After admission, local bacterial culture and drug sensitivity test are conducted to guide the standardized use of antibiotics in clinical practice based on sensitive bacteria and drug sensitivity tests.

2. Strengthen wound dressing changes, change dressings twice a day, clean necrotic tissue during dressing changes, apply recombinant human basic fibroblast growth factor externally to the wound to promote fresh granulation tissue. After the granulation tissue is fresh, choose skin flap transplantation to repair the wound.

3. Choose spinal epidural anesthesia for anesthesia.

4. Surgical process

4.1 Design of femoral anterior external free flap: The midpoint of the line connecting the anterior superior iliac spine and the lateral edge of the patella is the exit point of the first musculocutaneous branch of the descending branch of the external circumflex artery (iliac patellar line), and the flap is designed with this point as the center. The midpoint of the iliac patellar line is connected to the midpoint of the ilioinguinal ligament, which is the surface projection line of the descending branch of the external circumflex femoral artery. The area of the flap cut is 19 cm × 10 cm (Figure 3.36.2).

4.2 Preparation for the affected area: Remove the skin margin and non-living tissue around the wound, resulting in a defect of 18.5 cm × 9.5 cm. Two accompanying veins were exposed in several stages of the posterior tibial artery, and the posterior tibial artery was ruptured with a defect of 5 cm. Expose the proximal and distal ends for backup, and wait for the anterior femoral flap to be bridged by the external circumflex femoral artery (to repair the posterior tibial artery rupture defect).

4.3 Skin flap harvesting: Cut the skin, superficial fascia, and deep fascia in sequence according to the incision design line. Enter the gap between the rectus femoris muscle and the lateral thigh muscle, expose the descending branch of the external circumflex artery in the muscle gap, and protect the musculocutaneous branch that enters the skin flap. At this point, the skin flap is almost completely dissected, and a vascular clamp is used to block the blood flow test and observe the blood supply of the skin flap. According to the length of the blood vessels in the receiving area, select the site of vascular incision, completely free the skin flap, spray recombinant human basic fibroblast growth factor externally on the supply area, and directly suture and bandage the wound.

4.4 Skin flap transplantation: After completely cutting and freeing the skin flap, recombinant human basic fibroblast growth factor is applied topically to the wound of the recipient area. The free skin flap is sutured to the

受区缝合，显微镜下修剪胫后动脉及伴行静脉远端和近端吻合口，并上血管夹止血，先行远端血管修复，将皮瓣旋股外动脉及伴行静脉与胫后动脉远端吻合，旋股外动脉及伴行静脉近端与胫后动脉伴行静脉近端吻合。血管吻合结束后放开血管夹，皮瓣血运良好，皮瓣下放置引流管负压引流，完全缝合皮瓣术终（图 3.36.3 ~图 3.36.5）。

5. 术后抬高患肢预防肿胀，严密观察皮瓣四大显微指标，保暖。

6. 扩容、解痉镇痛、抗感染，预防血管痉挛。

7. 每天换药 1 次，创面喷洒外用重组人碱性成纤维细胞生长因子，48 小时拔出橡皮条引流，7 天开始床上练习膝关节，踝关节和足趾各关节活动，12 天拆线，并逐渐下地康复训练。

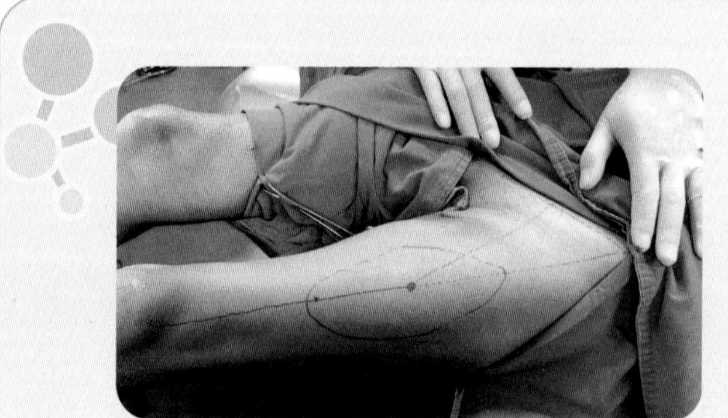

图 3.36.2　左侧股前外游离皮瓣设计示意

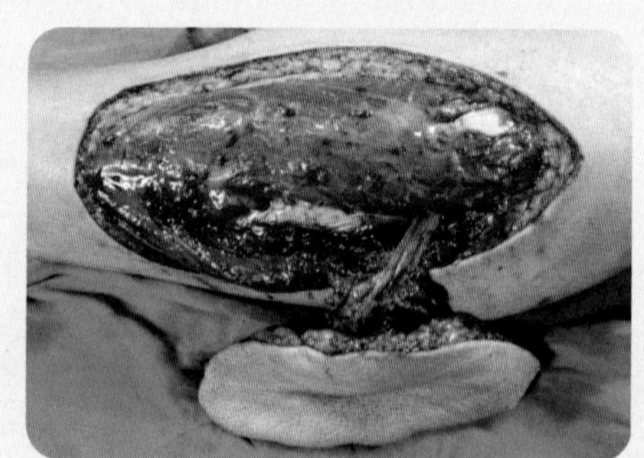

图 3.36.3　股前外皮瓣解剖游离即将血管断蒂

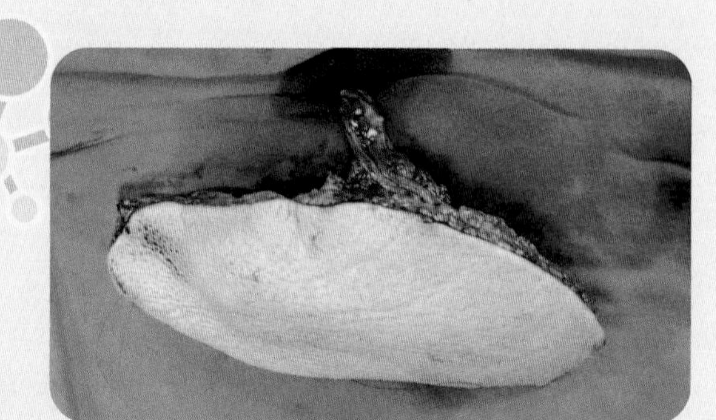

图 3.36.4　股前外皮瓣完全游离

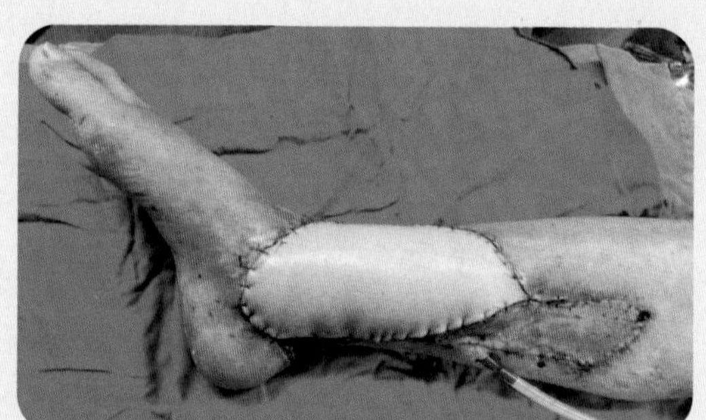

图 3.36.5　股前外皮瓣游离移植术后，皮瓣血运和外观良好

（陈善亮）

recipient area, and the distal and proximal anastomosis of the posterior tibial artery and accompanying vein are trimmed under a microscope. The blood vessels are clamped to stop bleeding, and the distal blood vessels are repaired first. The flap is anastomosed with the distal end of the circumflex femoral artery and accompanying vein, and the proximal end of the circumflex femoral artery and accompanying vein is anastomosed with the proximal end of the tibial artery and accompanying vein. After the vascular anastomosis is completed, the vascular clamp is released, and the blood flow of the skin flap is good. A drainage tube is placed under the skin flap for negative pressure drainage, and the skin flap is completely sutured at the end of the surgery (Figure 3.36.3- Figure 3.36.5).

5. Raise the affected limb after surgery to prevent swelling, closely observe the four major microscopic indicators of the skin flap, and keep warm.

6. Expansion, spasmolysis, analgesia, anti-infection, and prevention of vascular spasm.

7. Change dressing once a day, spray external recombinant human basic fibroblast growth factor on the wound, remove the rubber strip for drainage within 48 hours, start practicing knee joint, ankle joint, and toe joint movements in bed for 7 days, remove stitches for 12 days, and gradually undergo rehabilitation training on the ground.

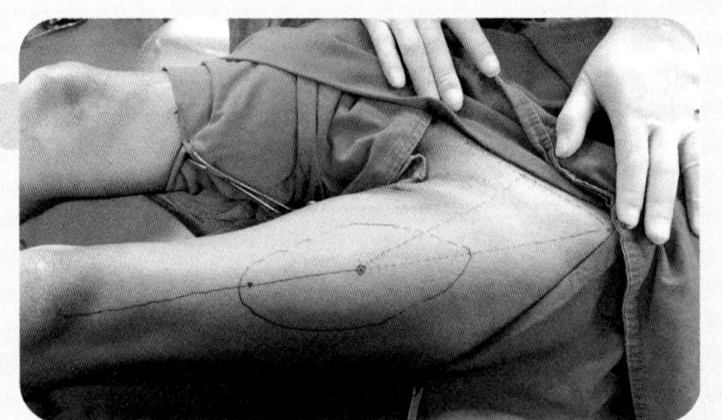

Figure 3.36.2 Schematic Design of Left Anterior Femoral Free Skin Flap

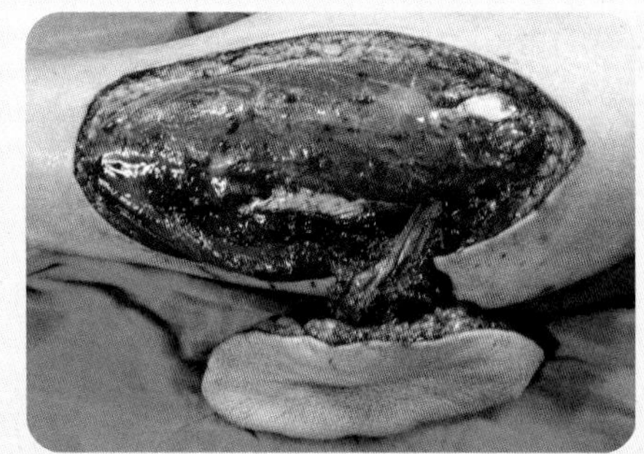

Figure 3.36.3 Dissection and release of anterior femoral skin flap, about to break the vascular pedicle

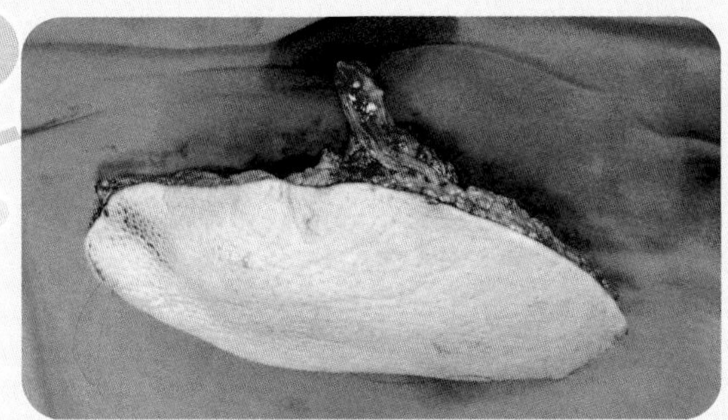

Figure 3.36.4 Complete dissociation of the anterior femoral skin flap

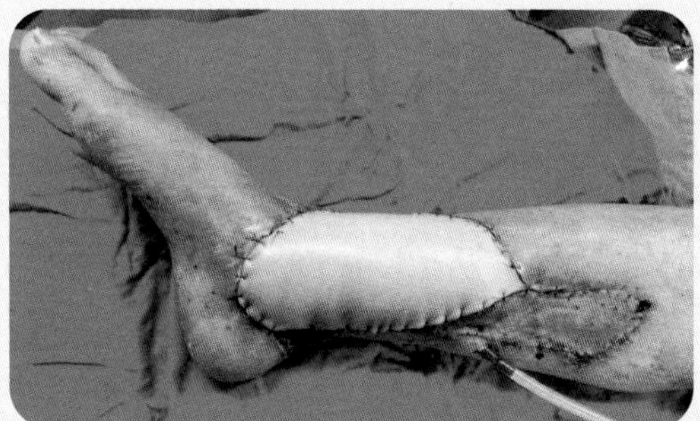

Figure 3.36.5 After free transplantation of the anterior femoral skin flap, the flap has good blood flow and appearance

(Chen Shanliang)

案例三十七　足背逆行撕脱、肌腱血管缺损、骨关节骨折

◆ 损伤原因

患者从高山滚落被石头砸伤，致左足背逆行撕脱、肌腱血管缺损、骨关节骨折。

◆ 症状与体征

左足出血不止，剧痛难忍，畸形，不能站立行走，肿胀并逐渐加重。左足背有大面积逆行撕脱伤口，足背皮肤软组织缺损 9 cm × 8 cm，伤口内布满泥沙，足背伸肌肌腱、足内在肌大部分缺损，第 1 跖骨至第 5 跖骨粉碎性骨折、部分缺损，足背动脉及足背皮神经缺损，足趾伸屈活动受限，足趾血液反流迟缓，足趾感觉减退，足背近端有部分擦皮伤，创缘不齐，足踝以远端广泛性肿胀（图 3.37.1）。

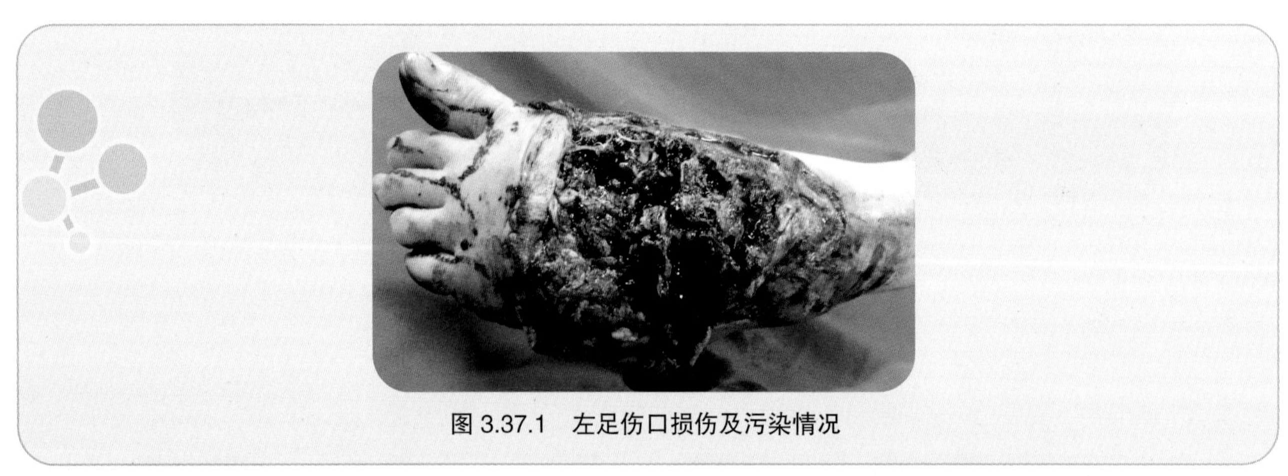
图 3.37.1　左足伤口损伤及污染情况

◆ 治疗方案

该案例由于伤口污染严重，伤口内布满泥沙，一期会增加感染概率，故采用二期皮瓣移植修复创面。

1. 一期清创，骨折复位固定，保留有生机组织，行逆行皮肤原位回植，术后 8 天出现皮肤坏死，局部感染，行坏死皮肤切除和感染灶切除，伤口加强换药治疗，换药时喷洒外用重组人碱性成纤维细胞生长因子，足内侧创面新鲜后，采用游离中厚皮片移植，缩小伤口，减少游离皮瓣供应量（图 3.37.2 ~ 图 3.37.5）。

2. 手术过程

2.1 股前外游离皮瓣设计：髂前上棘与髌骨外侧缘连线中点为旋骨外动脉降支的第一肌皮支穿出点（髂

Case 37 Retrograde avulsion of the dorsum of the foot, tendon and vascular defects, and bone and joint fractures

◆ Cause of injury

The patient fell from a high mountain and was hit by a stone, resulting in retrograde avulsion of the left foot dorsum, tendon and vascular defects, and bone and joint fractures.

◆ Signs and symptoms

The left foot is bleeding continuously, with unbearable pain, deformity, inability to stand and walk, swelling and gradually worsening. There is a large area of retrograde tear off wound on the left dorsum of the foot, with a skin and soft tissue defect of 9 cm × 8 cm on the dorsum of the foot. The wound is covered with mud and sand, and most of the extensor tendons and intrinsic muscles of the dorsum of the foot are missing. The first to fifth metatarsal bones have comminuted fractures and partial defects, and the dorsalis pedis artery and cutaneous nerve of the foot are missing. The extension and flexion of the toes are limited, the blood reflux of the toes is slow, the sensation of the toes is reduced, and there is partial skin abrasion injury at the proximal end of the dorsum of the foot, with uneven wound margins. The ankle is extensively swollen from the distal end (Figure 3.37.1).

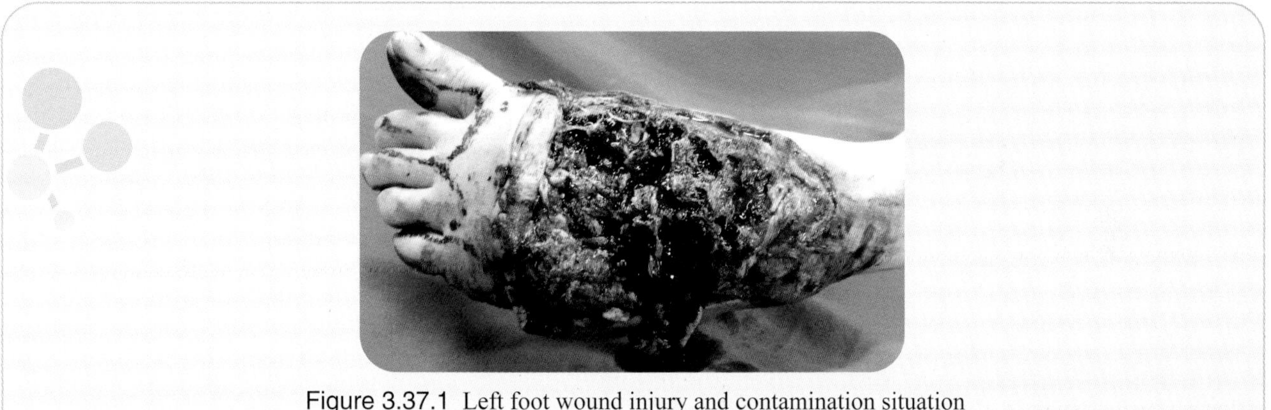

Figure 3.37.1 Left foot wound injury and contamination situation

◆ Treatment plan

Due to severe wound contamination, the wound is covered in mud and sand, which increases the probability of infection in the first stage. Therefore, a second stage skin flap transplantation was used to repair the wound.

1. First stage debridement, fracture reduction and fixation, preservation of viable tissue, retrograde skin in situ transplantation. Skin necrosis and local infection occurred 8 days after surgery. Necrotic skin resection and infection lesion resection were performed, and wound dressing treatment was strengthened. During dressing change, recombinant human alkaline fibroblast growth factor was sprayed topically. After the inner foot wound was fresh, a free medium thick skin graft was transplanted to reduce the wound size and minimize the supply of free skin flaps (Figure 3.37.2- Figure 3.37.5).

2. Surgical process

2.1 Design of femoral anterior external free flap: The midpoint of the line connecting the anterior superior iliac spine and the lateral edge of the patella is the exit point of the first musculocutaneous branch of the descending

髌线），以此点为中心设计皮瓣，髂髌线中点与髂腹股沟韧带中点为连线，该线为旋股外动脉降支走行体表投影线，皮瓣切取面积为 11 cm × 8 cm（图 3.37.6）。

2.2 足背受区准备：于足背近端弧形切口，长约 5 cm，切开皮肤及皮下浅筋膜，显露大隐静脉游离并备用，于趾长伸肌和胫骨长肌间隙显露足背动脉及其伴行静脉并游离并备用，足背创面缺损面积 10.5 cm × 7.5 cm，受区准备结束。

2.3 皮瓣切取：按切口设计线依次切开皮肤、浅筋膜、深筋膜。在股直肌与股外侧肌间隙进入，于肌间隙中显露旋骨外动脉降支，并保护好进入皮瓣肌皮支，此时皮瓣几乎完全解剖，血管钳夹阻断血运试验，观察皮瓣血供。根据受区血管长度保留 4 cm 血管蒂供吻合，皮瓣完全游离切取后，供区喷洒外用重组人碱性成纤维细胞生长因子，创口直接缝合并包扎。

2.4 皮瓣移植：皮瓣完全切取游离后，受区创面喷洒重组人酸性成纤维细胞生长因子，将游离皮瓣和受区缝合，保留血管吻合部分不缝合，显微镜下修剪大隐静脉和胫前动脉及其伴行静脉吻合口并上血管夹，将皮瓣内的旋股外静脉其中粗大分支分离与大隐静脉吻合，另一条分支与胫前动脉伴行静脉吻合，旋股外动脉与胫前动脉吻合，放开血管夹，皮瓣血运良好，皮瓣下放置六枚橡皮条引流，完全闭合伤口，术终（图 3.37.7、图 3.37.8）。

3. 术后抬高患肢预防肿胀，严密观察皮瓣四大显微指标，保暖。

4. 扩容、解痉镇痛、抗感染，预防血管痉挛。

5. 术后 24 小时拔出引流条 3 枚，48 小时将剩余 3 枚引流条完全拔出。

6. 术后 12 天拆线，术后 2 个月拔出克氏针内固定（图 3.37.9）。

branch of the external circumflex artery (iliac patellar line), and the flap is designed with this point as the center. The midpoint of the iliac patellar line is connected to the midpoint of the ilioinguinal ligament, which is the surface projection line of the descending branch of the external circumflex femoral artery. The area of the flap cut is 11 cm × 8 cm (Figure 3.37.6).

2.2 Preparation of dorsalis pedis receptor area: A curved incision of approximately 5 cm is made at the proximal end of the dorsalis pedis to open the skin and subcutaneous superficial fascia, revealing the free great saphenous vein for future use. The dorsalis pedis artery and its accompanying veins are exposed and freed between the extensor digitorum longus and tibialis longus muscles for future use. The defect area of the dorsalis pedis wound is 10.5 cm × 7.5 cm, and the preparation of the receptor area is complete.

2.3 Skin flap harvesting: Cut the skin, superficial fascia, and deep fascia in sequence according to the incision design line. Enter the gap between the rectus femoris muscle and the lateral thigh muscle, expose the descending branch of the external circumflex artery in the muscle gap, and protect the musculocutaneous branch that enters the skin flap. At this point, the skin flap is almost completely dissected, and a vascular clamp is used to block the blood flow test and observe the blood supply of the skin flap. According to the length of the blood vessels in the receiving area, 4 cm of vascular pedicle is reserved for anastomosis. After the skin flap is completely free and cut, the donor area is sprayed with recombinant human basic fibroblast growth factor externally, and the wound is directly sutured and bandaged.

2.4 Skin flap transplantation: After the skin flap is completely cut and freed, recombinant human acidic fibroblast growth factor is sprayed on the wound surface of the recipient area. The free skin flap is sutured to the recipient area, and the vascular anastomosis is retained without suturing. Under the microscope, the great saphenous vein, anterior tibial artery, and their accompanying veins are trimmed and the vascular clip is placed. The large branch of the external circumflex femoral vein inside the skin flap is separated and anastomosed with the great saphenous vein, while the other branch is anastomosed with the anterior tibial artery and its accompanying vein. The external circumflex femoral artery is anastomosed with the anterior tibial artery. The vascular clip is released, and the blood flow of the skin flap is good. Six rubber strips are placed under the skin flap for drainage, and the wound is completely closed. The surgery is completed (Figure 3.37.7,Figure 3.37.8)

3. Raise the affected limb after surgery to prevent swelling, closely observe the four major microscopic indicators of the skin flap, and keep warm.

4. Expand capacity, relieve spasms and pain, resist infections, and prevent vascular spasms.

5. Remove three drainage strips 24 hours after surgery, and completely remove the remaining three drainage strips within 48 hours.

6. The suture was removed 12 days after surgery, and the Kirschner wire was removed for internal fixation 2 months after surgery (Figure 3.37.9).

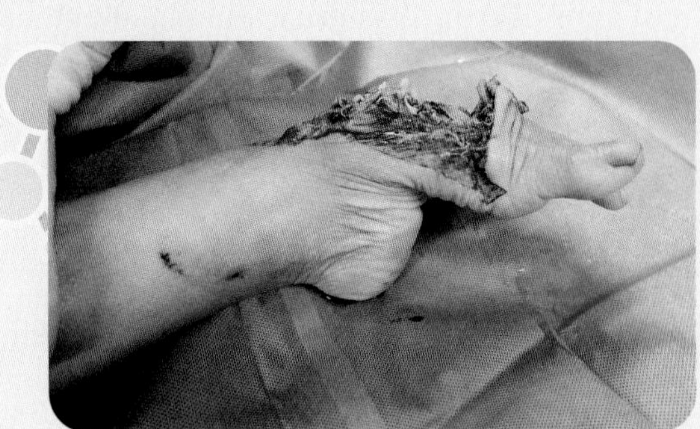

图 3.37.2　清创后有皮肤肌腱缺损，骨关节缺损

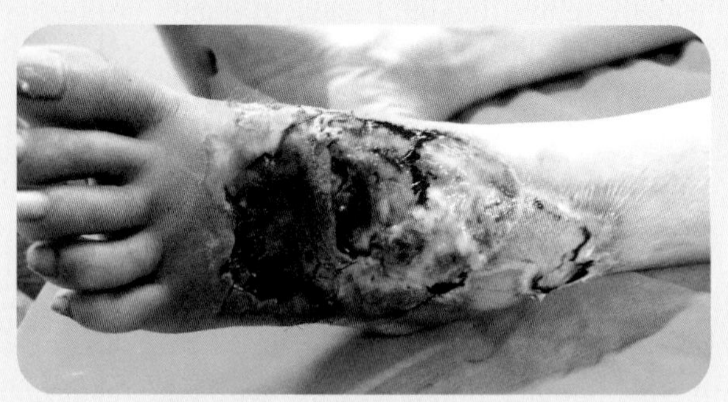

图 3.37.3　清创后骨关节复位克氏针内固定，皮肤原为回植术后，皮肤坏死

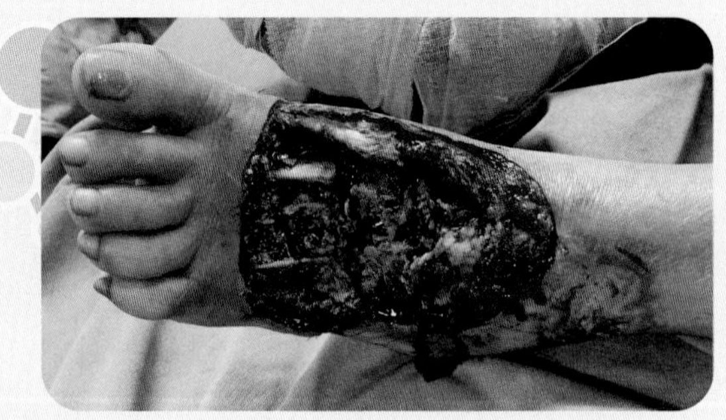

图 3.37.4　经过多次清创和使用生长因子，创面新鲜，待皮瓣移植覆盖创面

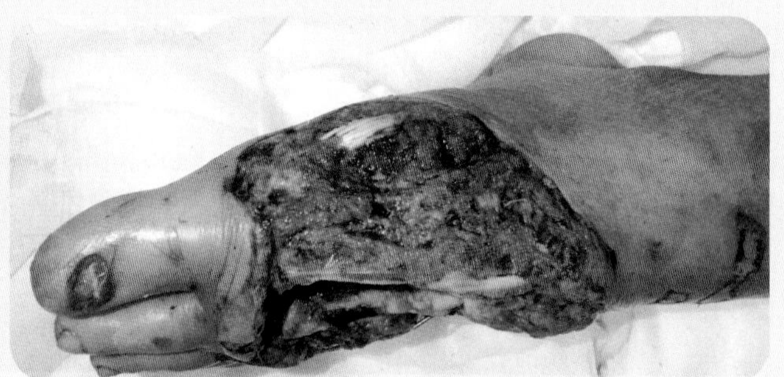

图 3.37.5　足内侧肉芽组织饱满，较新鲜。采用中厚游离皮片移植缩小伤口，减少皮瓣供应量

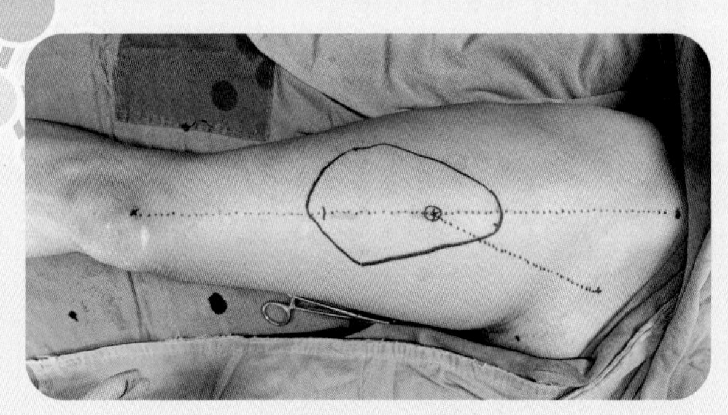

图 3.37.6　右侧股前外游离皮瓣设计示意

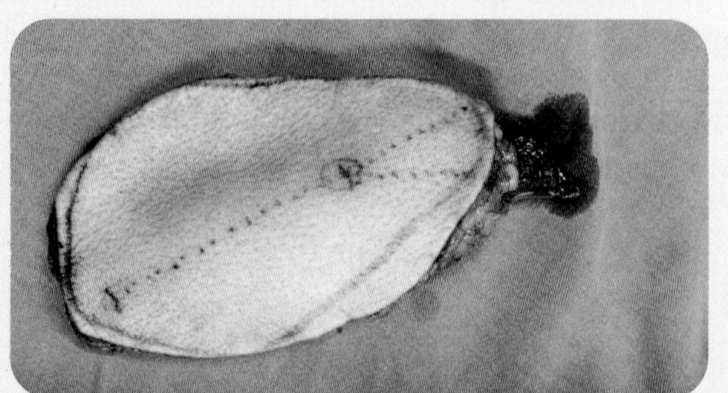

图 3.37.7　股前外皮瓣完全游离

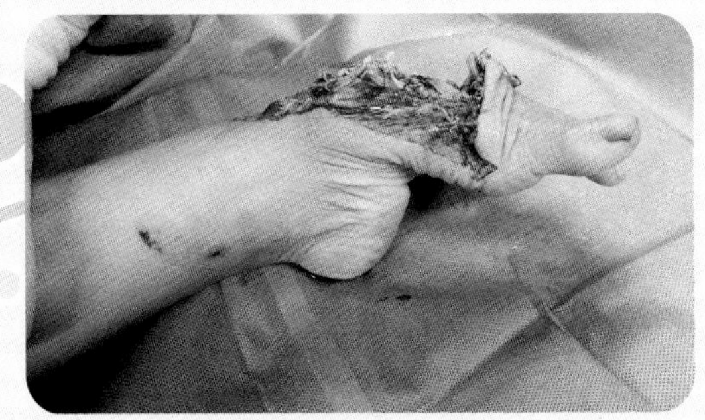

Figure 3.37.2 Skin and tendon defects, bone and joint defects after debridement

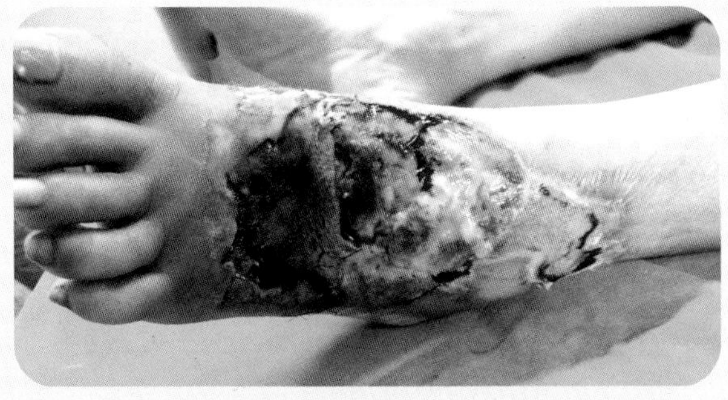

Figure 3.37.3 Reduction of bone and joint after debridement and internal fixation with Kirschner wires. The skin was originally transplanted back after surgery, but the skin died

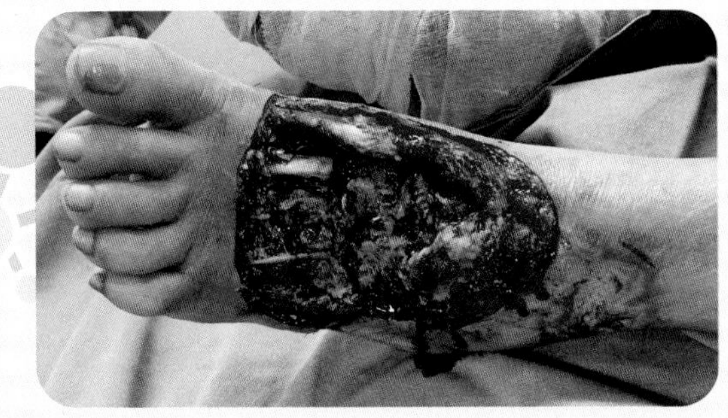

Figure 3.37.4 After multiple debridement and use of growth factors, the wound is fresh and ready for flap transplantation to cover the wound

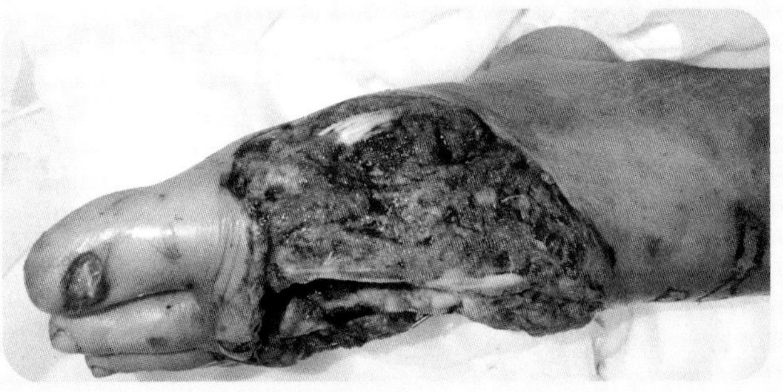

Figure 3.37.5 The granulation tissue on the inner side of the foot is plump and relatively fresh. Using medium thick free skin graft transplantation to reduce wound size and minimize skin flap supply

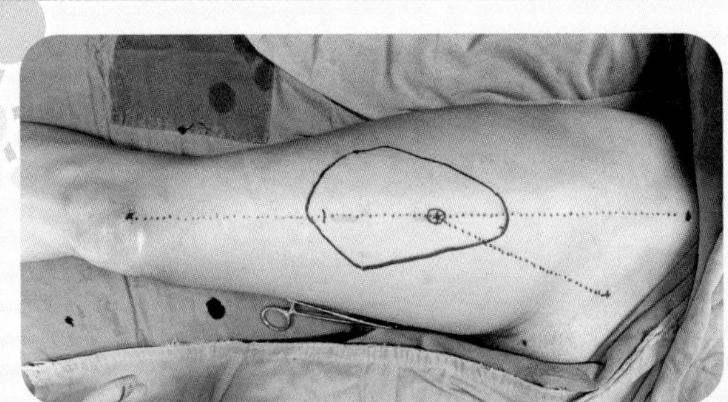

Figure 3.37.6 Schematic Design of Right Anterior Femoral Free Skin Flap

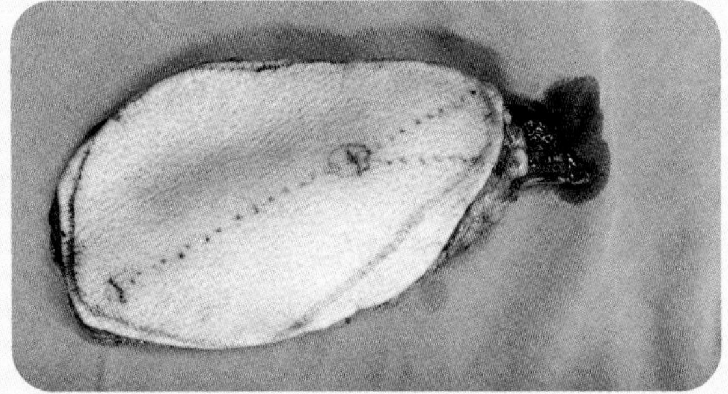

Figure 3.37.7 Complete dissociation of the anterior femoral skin flap

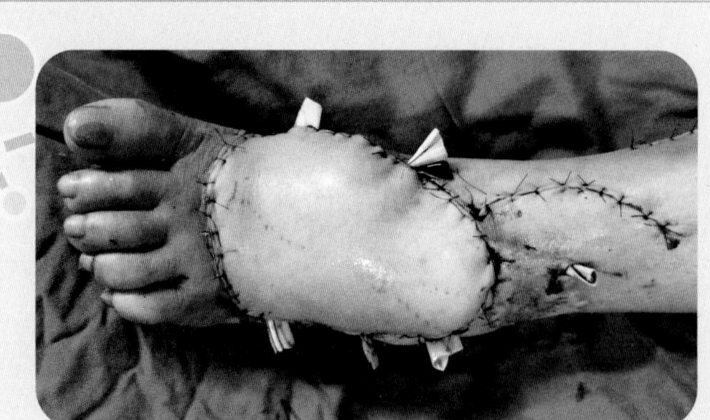

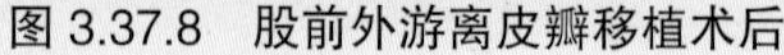

图 3.37.8　股前外游离皮瓣移植术后

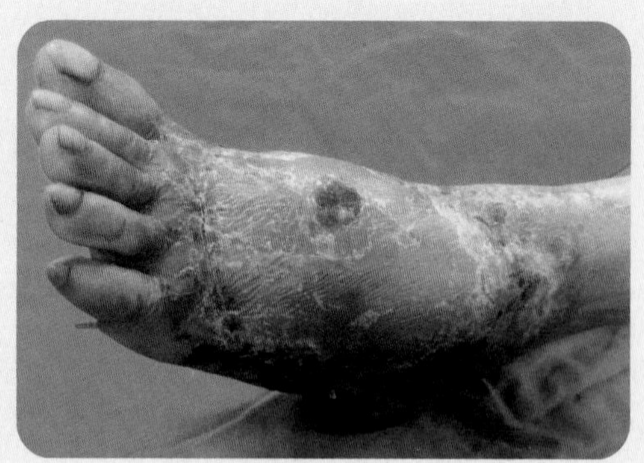

图 3.37.9　股前外皮瓣移植术后 20 天情况

（陈善亮）

案例三十八　示指中指环指离断

◆ 损伤原因

患者因被剪板机切割，致左手示指、中指、环指离断。

◆ 症状与体征

左手示指、中指、环指末节完全离断，断端出血不止，剧痛，伴活动受限，断端整齐，远端苍白无血运，指端冷，局部污染较轻（图 3.38.1）。近节及中指间关节活动良好。

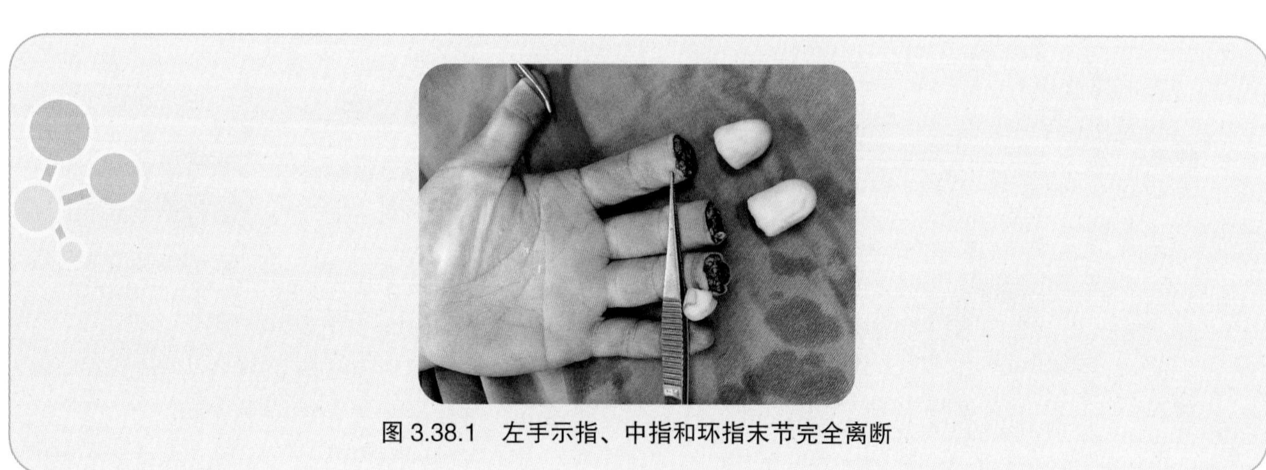

图 3.38.1　左手示指、中指和环指末节完全离断

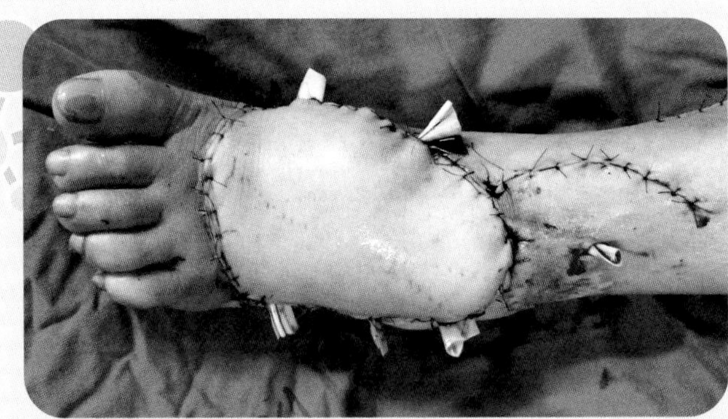

Figure 3.37.8 Postoperative free flap transplantation of anterior and lateral thigh

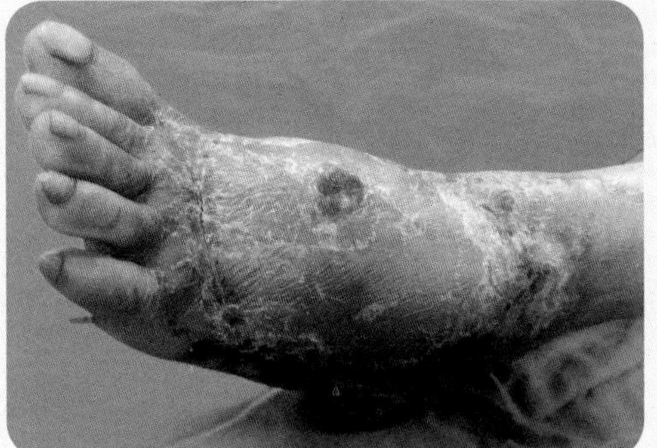

Figure 3.37.9 Postoperatively 20 days after anterior external thigh flap transplantation

(Chen Shanliang)

Case 38 Disconnection of index finger, middle finger and ring finger

◆ Cause of injury

The patient's left index finger, middle finger, and ring finger were severed due to being cut by a shearing machine.

◆ Signs and symptoms

The distal end of the left index finger, middle finger, and ring finger are completely severed, with continuous bleeding and severe pain at the severed end, accompanied by limited mobility. The severed end is neat, and the distal end is pale with no blood flow. The fingertips are cold, and the local contamination is relatively mild (Figure 3.38.1). The joint movement between the proximal and middle fingers is good.

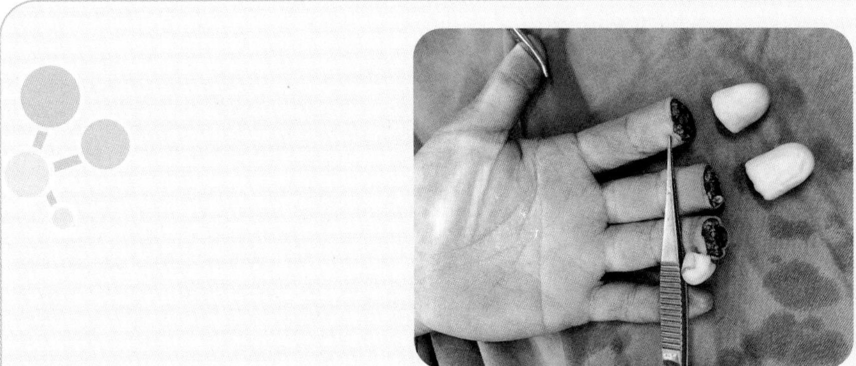

Figure 3.38.1 Left hand index finger, middle finger and ring finger distal end completely disconnected

◆ 治疗方案

1. 急诊包扎伤口减少出血，完善术前准备，预在臂丛麻醉下行清创术，行断指再植术。

2. 手术过程

2.1 清创术：示指、中指末节指间关节面骨折伴关节面缺损，行骨短缩骨关节融合。

2.2 骨支架建立：示指、中指末节关节融合，并采用 1.2 克氏针纵行固定骨折。

2.3 肌腱骨膜修复：示指、中指屈指和伸指肌腱指端缝合，修补腱鞘和骨膜。

2.4 神经修复：显微镜下显露示指、中指和环指两侧指神经，修建断端，应用 10 号显微缝线缝合，每条指神经外膜缝合 4 针。

2.5 血管修复：显微镜下显露示指、中指两侧指动脉，修建血管吻合口外膜，重组人酸性成纤维细胞生长因子冲洗血管管腔，应用 10 号显微针线吻合指动脉，于指腹处显露皮下浅静脉每指两条进行吻合。环指指尖部显露指中央动脉 1 条，修建吻合口外膜，应用 12 号显微针线吻合 4 针。断指端喷洒重组人酸性成纤维细胞生长因子，缝合断指伤口，皮下放置小橡皮条引流，包扎断指，术终（图 3.38.2）。

3. 术后抬高患肢减轻断指肿胀，有利于静脉回流，日光灯照射保温。

4. 常规使用镇痛泵缓解疼痛，减轻因疼痛引发小血管痉挛。

5. 扩容、解痉与抗感染治疗。

6. 术后 2 天拔出橡皮条引流，术后 12 天拆线，1 个月拔出克氏针，并进行功能训练。

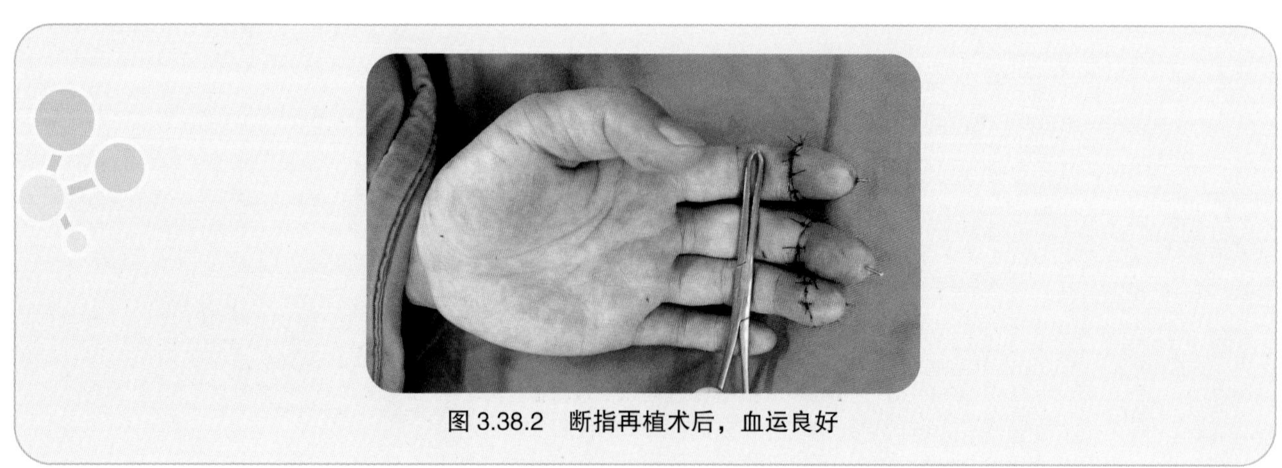

图 3.38.2　断指再植术后，血运良好

（陈善亮）

◆ Treatment plan

1. Emergency dressing of wounds to reduce bleeding, complete preoperative preparation, perform debridement under brachial plexus anesthesia, and perform finger replantation surgery.

2. Surgical process

2.1 Debridement surgery: fracture of the distal interphalangeal joint surface of the index finger and middle finger with joint surface defects, followed by bone shortening and joint fusion.

2.2 Establishment of bone scaffold: fusion of the distal joint of the index finger and middle finger, and longitudinal fixation of the fracture using a 1.2 gram Kirschner wire.

2.3 Tendon and periosteum repair: Suture of the fingertip of the index finger, middle finger, and extensor finger tendons to repair the tendon sheath and periosteum.

2.4 Neural repair: Under a microscope, expose the nerves on both sides of the index finger, middle finger, and ring finger, construct the severed ends, and suture them with 10 gauge microsurgical sutures. Suture the outer membrane of each nerve with 4 stitches.

2.5 Vascular repair: Under the microscope, the arteries on both sides of the index finger and middle finger are exposed, and the outer membrane of the vascular anastomosis is constructed. The vascular lumen is washed with recombinant human acidic fibroblast growth factor, and the finger arteries are anastomosed using a No. 10 microneedle. Two superficial subcutaneous veins are exposed at the fingertip for anastomosis. One central finger artery is exposed at the fingertip of the ring finger, and the outer membrane of the anastomotic site is constructed. Four 12 gauge microneedles are used for anastomosis. Spray recombinant human acidic fibroblast growth factor on the severed finger end, suture the severed finger wound, place a small rubber strip under the skin for drainage, wrap the severed finger, and terminate the surgery(Figure 3.38.2).

3. Postoperative elevation of the affected limb can reduce swelling of the severed finger, facilitate venous return, and provide insulation through exposure to fluorescent lamps.

4. Conventional use of pain pumps to relieve pain and alleviate small vessel spasms caused by pain.

5. Expansion, spasmolysis, and anti-infective treatment.

6. Two days after surgery, remove the rubber strip for drainage. Twelve days after surgery, remove the suture. One month later, remove the Kirschner wire and perform functional training.

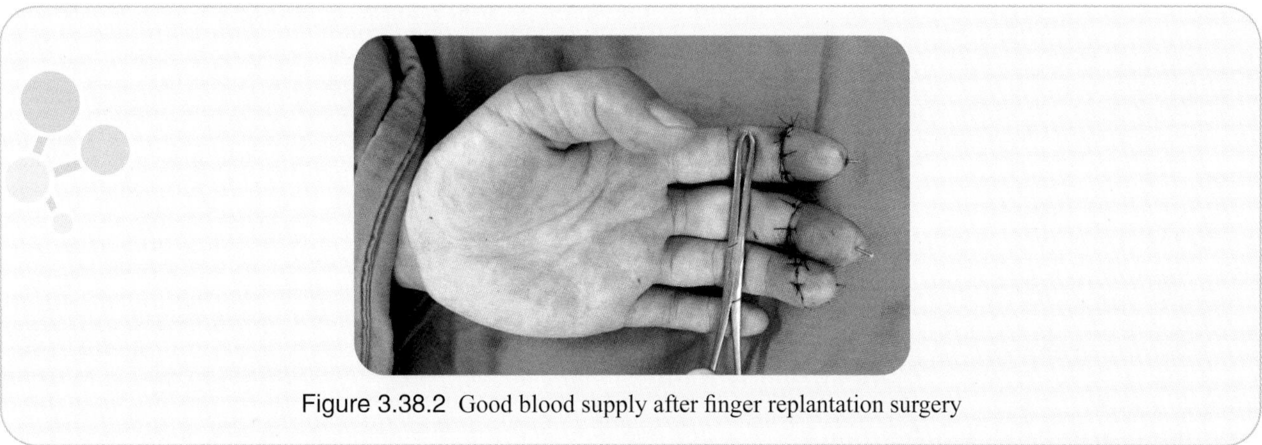

Figure 3.38.2 Good blood supply after finger replantation surgery

(Chen Shanliang)

案例三十九　示指脱套伤离断伤

◆ 损伤原因

患者因机器挤压，致右手示指撕脱性离断，入院时缺血时间 6 小时、脱套皮肤部分风干。

◆ 症状与体征

外伤后右手示指离体落地，示指剧痛难忍，局部出血不止，示指活动受限。右手示指皮肤脱套性撕脱离断，皮肤边缘干燥，远端无血运，指神经抽脱游离 2 cm 并干燥，示指骨架健在，屈伸肌腱腱鞘部分撕脱，肌腱无断裂，指间关节屈伸活动良好，指甲在位无缺损（图 3.39.1）。

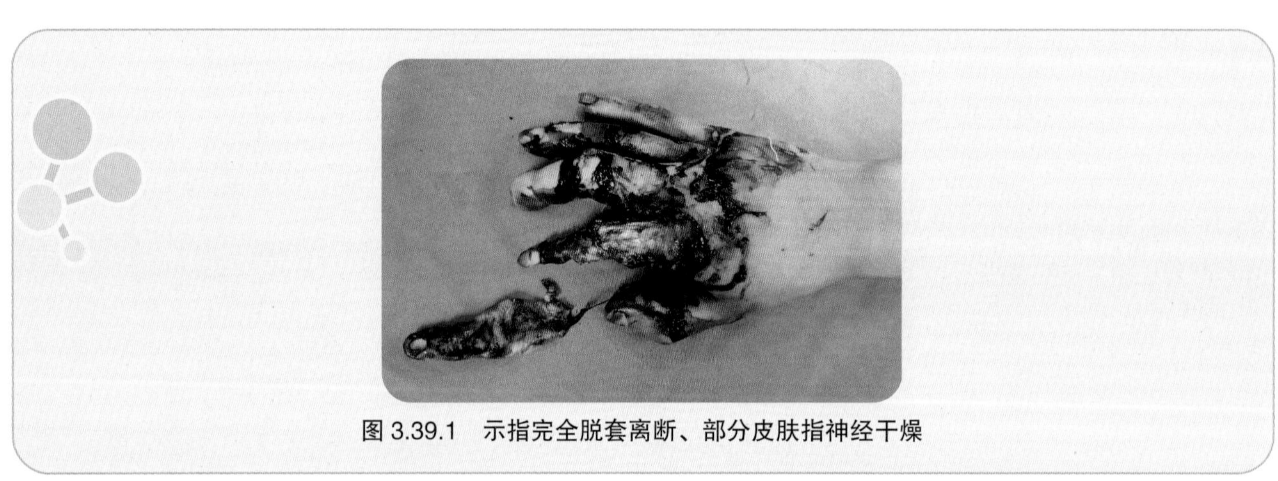

图 3.39.1　示指完全脱套离断、部分皮肤指神经干燥

◆ 治疗方案

1. 右手示指脱套组织离断缺血有 6 小时之久，且皮肤和指神经干燥，入院后立即应用外用重组人碱性成纤维细胞生长因子溶液浸泡离断示指组织块，防止继续干燥坏死（图 3.39.2）。

2. 臂丛麻醉下行示指脱套再植术。

3. 手术过程

3.1 清创术 + 骨支架重建：切除示指脱套挫灭边缘，修剪部分挫灭脂肪，为了血管吻合够长，故将示指末节截除，修补撕裂腱鞘。

3.2 血管神经修复：脱套示指回植后，于指腹处扩大切口 1.5 cm，示指双侧指动脉抽脱 2.0 cm，指动脉卷曲，主干有多条分支撕脱离断，双侧指神经抽脱 2.5 cm，在示指中节远端尺侧找到进入示指进入断指的主干动脉，由于血管抽脱缺损严重，于前臂切取小血管移植倒置吻合示指尺侧指动脉，修复抽脱指神经，缝合示指掌

Case 39 Finger detachment injury and detachment injury

◆ Cause of injury

The patient's right index finger was torn off due to machine compression, and upon admission, there was a 6-hour ischemia time and partial air drying of the detached skin.

◆ Signs and symptoms

After trauma, the index finger of the right hand fell off the body, causing unbearable pain, continuous local bleeding, and limited index finger movement. The skin of the right index finger is detached and broken, with dry skin edges and no blood supply at the distal end. The finger nerve is detached and free by 2 cm and dried. The index finger skeleton is established, and the sheath of the flexor and extensor tendons is partially torn off without tendon rupture. The interphalangeal joint has good flexion and extension activity, and the nail is in place without defects (Figure 3.39.1).

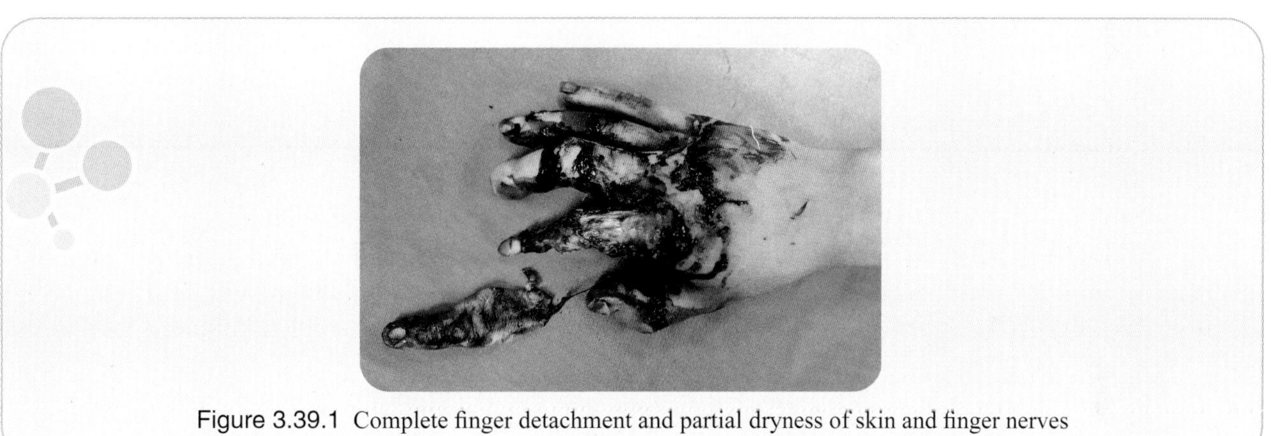

Figure 3.39.1 Complete finger detachment and partial dryness of skin and finger nerves

◆ Treatment plan

1. The right index finger has been detached from the sheath tissue and ischemic for 6 hours, and the skin and finger nerves are dry. After admission, the detached index finger tissue block should be immediately soaked in a solution of recombinant human alkaline fibroblast growth factor for external use to prevent further drying and necrosis (Figure 3.39.2).

2. Under brachial plexus anesthesia, the index finger is detached and replanted.

3. Surgical process

3.1 Debridement surgery + bone stent reconstruction: Remove the edge of the index finger that has been dislodged and bruised, trim some of the bruised fat, and in order to ensure sufficient vascular anastomosis, remove the distal end of the index finger and repair the torn tendon sheath.

3.2 Vascular and nerve repair: After repositioning the index finger, the incision was enlarged by 1.5 cm at the fingertip, and the bilateral digital arteries of the index finger were extracted by 2.0 cm. The digital arteries were curled, and multiple branches of the main trunk were torn off and severed. The bilateral digital nerves were extracted by 2.5 cm. The main artery that entered the index finger into the severed finger was found on the distal ulnar side of the middle segment of the index finger. Due to severe vascular extraction defects, small blood vessels were cut from the forearm and transplanted upside down to anastomose the ulnar digital artery of the index finger. The extracted

侧皮肤掌侧放置橡皮条一枚引流。于示指背侧伤口，显微镜下寻找两条指背静脉，修建血管吻合口，并依次吻合，创面外用重组人碱性成纤维细胞生长因子，缝合伤口，皮下放置橡皮条引流一枚，术终（图 3.39.3）。

4. 术后常规抬高患肢利于减轻肿胀，促进回流，日光灯照射保温。

5. 扩容、解痉镇痛、抗感染，预防血管痉挛。

6. 术后 3 天拔出引流条，12 天拆线。

7. 断指再植成活后即可考虑训练，有利于指间关节松动，减少关节僵硬。

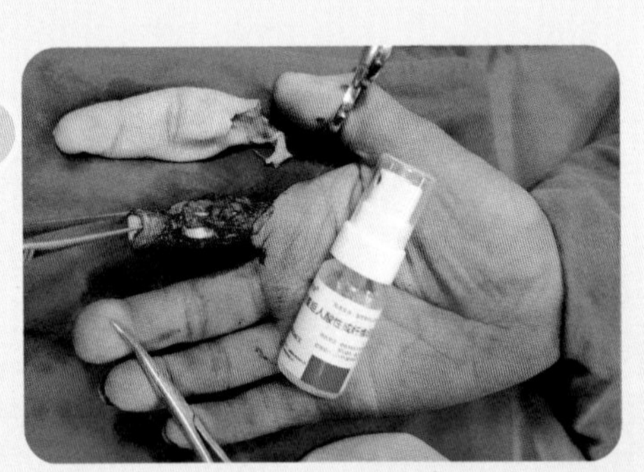

图 3.39.2 清创后，指体短缩，喷洒外用重组人碱性成纤维细胞生长因子

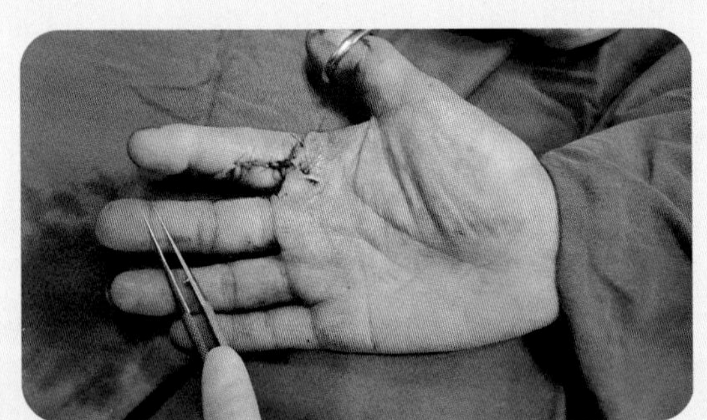

图 3.39.3 示指再植术后，血运良好

（陈善亮）

案例四十 左前臂及腕部开放性创伤

◆ 损伤原因

患者因机器挤压，致左前臂及腕部开放性创伤。

◆ 症状与体征

左前臂及腕部剧痛难忍，伤口出血不止，手指和腕关节活动受限，左前臂掌侧有 12 cm 伤口，腕部有 8 cm 横行伤口，创缘不齐，屈指浅肌和屈指深肌于肌腱移行处抽脱断裂，示指、中指屈指浅肌腱断裂，正中神经有 3 cm 挫伤段，伤口深达尺骨和桡骨，桡动脉及伴行静脉断裂，断端挫伤并形成血栓。尺骨和桡骨无骨折，手掌大鱼际处有 4 cm 伤口，深达大鱼际肌，大鱼际肌有部分撕裂（图 3.40.1、图 3.40.2）。腕掌侧有不规则擦伤，手指桡侧 3 个半指感觉减退，手指屈伸活动受限，腕关节活动受限。

digital nerves were repaired, and a rubber strip was placed on the palmar side of the skin of the index finger for drainage. On the back wound of the index finger, two dorsal veins were found under a microscope, and vascular anastomosis sites were constructed and sequentially anastomosed. Recombinant human basic fibroblast growth factor was applied externally to the wound, and the wound was sutured. A rubber strip was placed subcutaneously to drain the blood, and the surgery was completed (Figure 3.39.3).

4. Routine elevation of the affected limb after surgery is beneficial for reducing swelling, promoting reflux, and providing insulation through exposure to fluorescent lamps.

5. Expand capacity, relieve spasms and pain, resist infections, and prevent vascular spasms.

6. Remove the drainage strip 3 days after surgery and remove the suture 12 days later.

7. After the successful replantation of severed fingers, training can be considered, which is beneficial for loosening the interphalangeal joints and reducing joint stiffness.

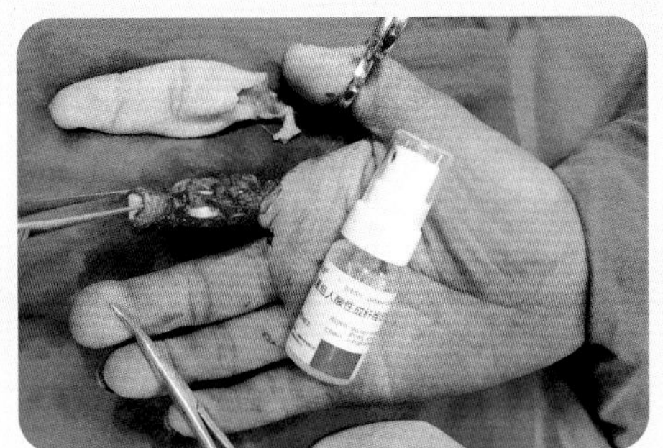

Figure 3.39.2 After debridement, the fingers shorten, and recombinant human basic fibroblast growth factor is sprayed topically

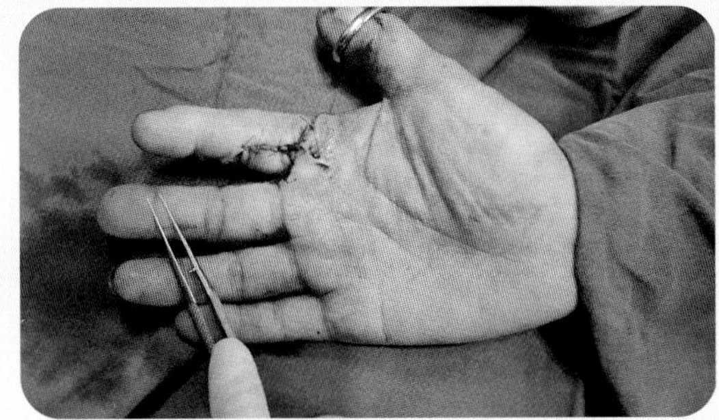

Figure 3.39.3 Good blood supply after finger replantation surgery

(Chen Shanliang)

Case 40 Open trauma of left forearm and wrist

◆ Cause of injury

The patient suffered open trauma to the left forearm and wrist due to machine compression.

◆ Signs and symptoms

Severe pain is unbearable in the left forearm and wrist, with continuous bleeding from the wound and limited movement of the fingers and wrist joints. There is a 12 cm wound on the palmar side of the left forearm and an 8 cm transverse wound on the wrist, with uneven edges. The superficial and deep flexor muscles of the index finger and middle finger have ruptured at the tendon transition site, and the superficial flexor tendons of the index finger and middle finger have ruptured. There is a 3 cm contusion segment of the median nerve, and the wound extends deep to the ulna and radius, with radial artery and accompanying vein ruptures. The severed end is contused and forms a thrombus. There are no fractures in the ulna and radius, but there is a 4cm wound at the great margin of the palm, reaching deep into the great margin muscle, which has partial tearing (Figure 3.40.1, Figure 3.40.2). There are irregular abrasions on the palmar side of the wrist, decreased sensation in three and a half fingers on the radial side of the fingers, restricted finger flexion and extension movement, and restricted wrist joint movement.

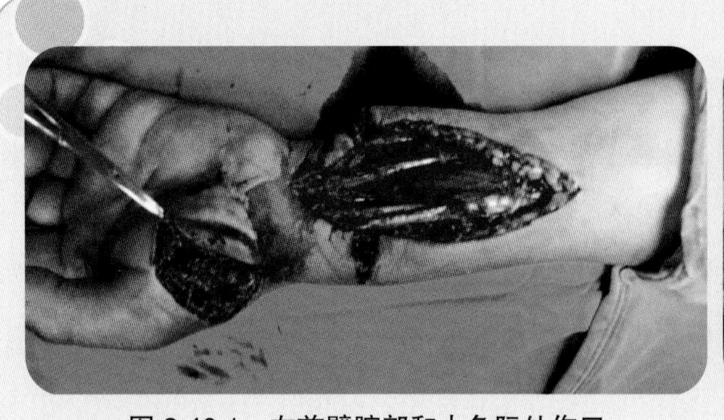

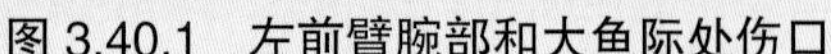

图 3.40.1　左前臂腕部和大鱼际处伤口

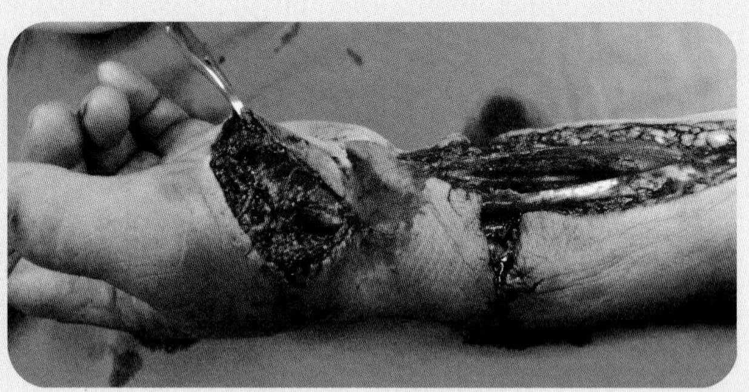

图 3.40.2　桡侧伤口

◆ 治疗方案

1. 急诊入院伤口加压包扎，完善手术前准备，拟在臂丛麻醉下行清创，行血管神经肌肉肌腱修复术。

2. 手术过程

2.1 清创术：由浅入深的剪除皮肤创缘和污染组织，修剪挫灭肌肉组织，结扎活动出血点，生理盐水冲洗伤口。

2.2 肌肉肌腱修复：依次修复断裂肌肉组织，缝合示指和中指浅肌腱，修补撕脱肌筋膜及腱鞘。修补大鱼际肌，缝合大鱼际伤口。

2.3 血管神经修复：显微镜下显露桡动脉及伴行静脉，桡动脉缺损 3 cm，断端形成血栓，修建抽脱血管，显露正常管腔，取生长因子冲洗液冲洗血管管腔。于前臂伤口内切取浅静脉 3.2 cm，倒置后移植于桡动脉缺损段，并进行吻合桡动脉及其两条伴行静脉，放开血管夹，血管通血良好。镜下修补正中神经部分断裂束支和神经外膜。应用外用重组人碱性成纤维细胞生长因子喷洒肌间隙，于伤口深部放置负压引流管，逐层缝合伤口，包扎伤口，石膏固定于屈腕屈指位。

3. 术后抬高患肢有利于减轻肿胀，缓解疼痛，促进静脉回流。

4. 常规扩容、解痉镇痛、抗感染，神经营养。

5. 术后 48 小时拔出引流条，换药时喷洒外用重组人碱性成纤维细胞生长因子促进伤口愈合。

6. 术后 7 天循序渐进进行手指主被动训练，12 天拆线，3 周去石膏进行康复训练。术后 1 个月，伤口愈合良好（图 3.40.3）。

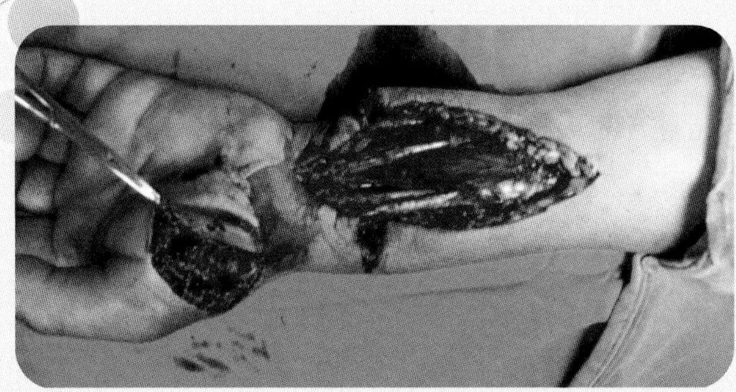

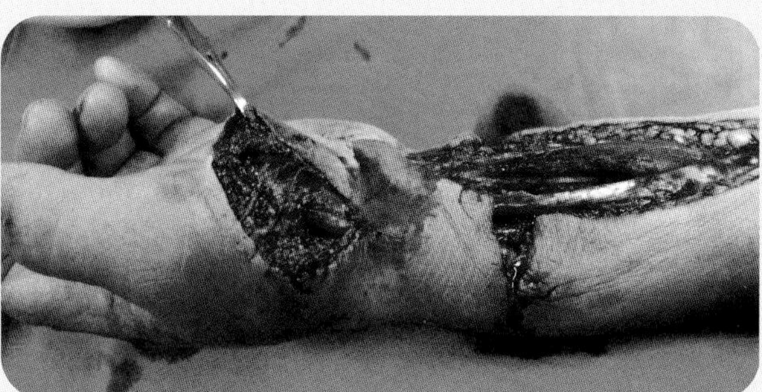

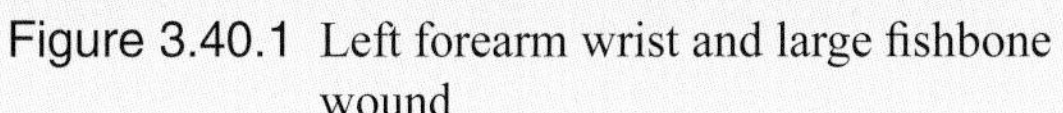

Figure 3.40.1 Left forearm wrist and large fishbone wound

Figure 3.40.2 Radial wound

◆ Treatment plan

1. Apply pressure and bandage to the emergency admission wound, complete preoperative preparation, plan to perform debridement under brachial plexus anesthesia, and perform vascular, nerve, muscle, and tendon repair surgery.

2. Surgical process

2.1 Debridement technique: gradually remove the skin wound margin and contaminated tissue, trim and crush muscle tissue, ligate active bleeding points, and rinse the wound with physiological saline.

2.2 Muscle and tendon repair: sequentially repair the fractured muscle tissue, suture the superficial tendons of the index finger and middle finger, repair the torn muscle fascia and tendon sheath. Repair the interosseous muscle and suture the interosseous wound.

2.3 Vascular and nerve repair: Under the microscope, the radial artery and accompanying veins were exposed. The radial artery defect was 3 cm, and a thrombus was formed at the severed end. The extracted blood vessel was constructed to expose the normal lumen, and growth factor flushing solution was taken to wash the vascular lumen. A superficial vein of 3.2 cm was excised from the forearm wound, inverted, and transplanted into the missing segment of the radial artery. The radial artery and its two accompanying veins were anastomosed, and the vascular clamp was released, resulting in good blood circulation. Repair the ruptured bundle branches and outer membrane of the median nerve under the microscope. Spray recombinant human basic fibroblast growth factor onto the muscle space for external application, place negative pressure drainage tube in the deep part of the wound, suture the wound layer by layer, bandage the wound, and fix it in the wrist and finger flexion position with plaster.

3. Elevating the affected limb after surgery is beneficial for reducing swelling, relieving pain, and promoting venous return.

4. Routine expansion, spasmolysis and analgesia, anti-infection, and nerve nutrition.

5. Remove the drainage strip 48 hours after surgery, and spray external recombinant human basic fibroblast growth factor during dressing change to promote wound healing.

6. After 7 days of surgery, gradually carry out finger active and passive training, remove the stitches on 12 days, and remove the plaster for rehabilitation training at 3 weeks. One month after surgery, the wound healed well (Figure 3.40.3).

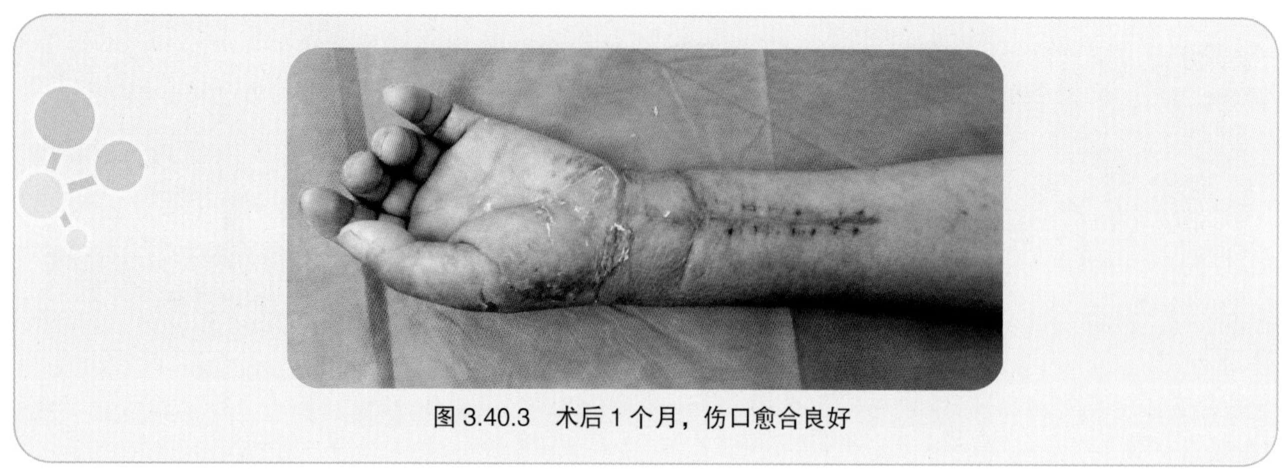

图 3.40.3 术后 1 个月，伤口愈合良好

（陈善亮）

案例四十一 左肘部开放性创伤、肘部血管神经断裂

◆ 损伤原因

患者因电动砂轮片锯伤，致左肘部开放性创伤、肘部血管神经断裂。

◆ 症状与体征

左肘部伤后出血不止，曾喷射状出血，剧痛难忍，肘关节活动受限，手指麻木，伤后工友用毛巾加压包扎送当地医院，当地医院把肘部肱动脉及伴行静脉缝扎，转来我院。左肘部有 8 cm 横行伤口，较深，深达肱骨内侧髁，皮缘不齐有磨损，肘正中静脉断裂。臂内侧皮神经断裂，前臂屈肌屈起点断裂，正中神经断裂，肱动脉及伴行静脉断裂肱二头肌肌腱断裂，肱肌肌腱断裂，肘前关节囊断裂，断裂血管有缝扎线结。伤口渗血活跃。手指屈指活动受限，桡侧三个半手指感觉消失，桡尺动脉波动消失，手指血液反流迟缓，皮温低，苍白。

◆ 治疗方案

1. 入院后立即建立静脉通道，扩充血容量纠正失血性休克，采血备血输血。

2. 伤口钳夹止血，局部加压包扎止血，积极准备急诊手术（图 3.41.1）。

3. 采用臂丛麻醉，麻醉生效后，三角肌下上气囊止血带。

4. 手术过程

4.1 扩大切口：于肘内侧向近端斜行扩大切口 6 cm，依次切开皮肤皮下脂肪，显露肌筋膜，探查伤口

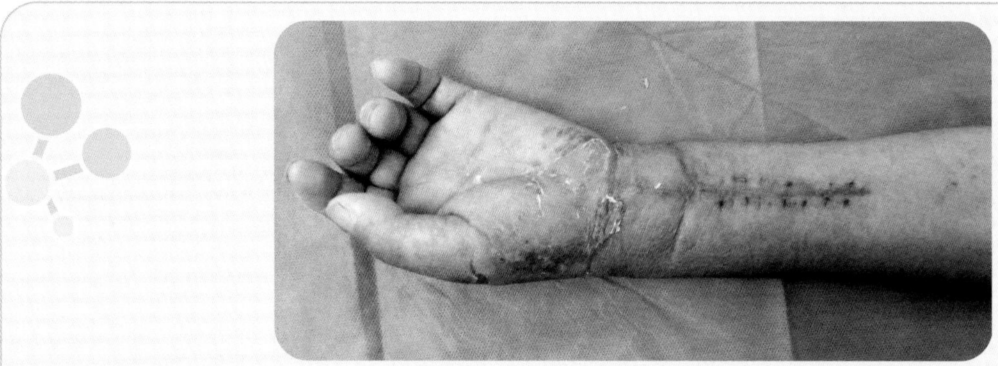

Figure 3.40.3 One month after surgery, the wound healed well

(Chen Shanliang)

Case 41 Left elbow open trauma, elbow vascular and nerve rupture

◆ Cause of injury

The patient suffered an open wound and ruptured blood vessels and nerves in the left elbow due to electric grinding wheel cutting injury.

◆ Signs and symptoms

After the left elbow injury, there was continuous bleeding, with jet like bleeding and unbearable pain. The elbow joint movement was restricted, and the fingers were numb. After the injury, the colleague used a towel to compress and bandage it, and sent it to the local hospital. The local hospital sutured the brachial artery and accompanying vein of the elbow and transferred it to our hospital. There is an 8 cm transverse wound on the left elbow, which is deep and extends to the medial condyle of the humerus. The skin margin is uneven and worn, and the median vein of the elbow is fractured. Fracture of the cutaneous nerve on the inner side of the arm, fracture of the flexor origin of the forearm, fracture of the median nerve, fracture of the brachial artery and accompanying veins, fracture of the biceps tendon, fracture of the humeral tendon, fracture of the anterior elbow joint capsule, and suture knots in the fractured blood vessels. The wound is bleeding actively. Finger flexion activity is restricted, sensation disappears in the three and a half fingers on the radial side, fluctuation of the radial ulnar artery disappears, slow blood reflux in the fingers, low skin temperature, and pallor.

◆ Treatment plan

1. Immediately establish a venous channel upon admission, expand blood volume to correct hemorrhagic shock, and collect blood for preparation and transfusion.

2. Pinch the wound to stop bleeding, apply local pressure and bandage to stop bleeding, and actively prepare for emergency surgery (Figure 3.41.1).

3. Brachial plexus anesthesia is used, and after the anesthesia takes effect, an upper airbag tourniquet is placed under the deltoid muscle.

4. Surgical process

4.1 Enlarged incision: An oblique incision of 6 cm is made on the inner side of the elbow towards the proximal end, and the subcutaneous fat of the skin is sequentially incised to expose the muscle fascia. The wound is explored and found to be deep enough to reach the medial condyle of the humerus, the anterior muscle tendon of the elbow,

见伤口深达肱骨内侧髁，肘前肌肉肌腱及肱动脉肱静脉，正中神经、臂内侧皮神经、肘正中静脉完全断裂，仅肱桡肌相连。断裂血管有结扎线缝合止血。予以清创，剪除皮肤创缘，修剪无生机组织，拆除血管结扎线。生理盐水反复冲洗伤口，结扎细小血管出血点。

4.2 肌肉肌腱韧带修复：依次缝合肘关节前侧关节囊及撕裂韧带，缝合肱肌、桡侧屈腕肌、前臂屈肌群及起点，修补血管神经着床，闭合无效腔。

4.3 神经血管修复：与显微镜下修建正中神经断端，应用 8/0 显微针线外膜缝合正中神经。镜下修建肱动脉及其两条伴行静脉、肘正中静脉吻合口外膜，并结扎其分支，应用外用重组人碱性成纤维细胞生长因子溶液冲洗血管管腔栓子，取 9/0 显微针线依次吻合肱动脉两条伴行静脉→肱动脉→肘正中静脉，放开止血带和血管夹，桡动脉和尺动脉搏动良好，手指红润，血液反流良好。缝合臂内侧皮神经，于伤口深部放负压引流管一条，逐层缝合伤口，包扎伤口，石膏屈肘位制动（图 3.41.2 ~图 3.41.5）。

5. 术后抬高患肢减轻肿胀，有利于静脉回流。

6. 常规扩容、解痉，镇痛泵持续镇痛，神经营养应用。

7. 换药时伤口喷洒生长因子，促进伤口愈合，减轻伤口瘢痕形成。

8. 术后常规进行手指的主被动训练，放置手部关节僵硬，减轻手部肌肉萎缩。

9. 术后 3 天拔引流管，12 天拆线，4 周去石膏，进行肘关节和手功能康复。

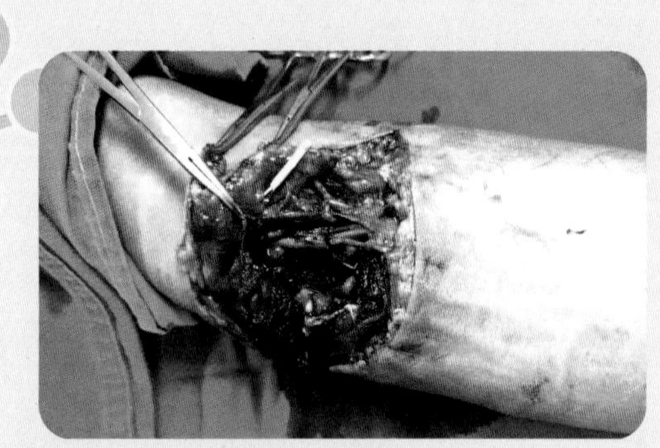

图 3.41.1　左肘伤口，对活动出血点钳夹止血

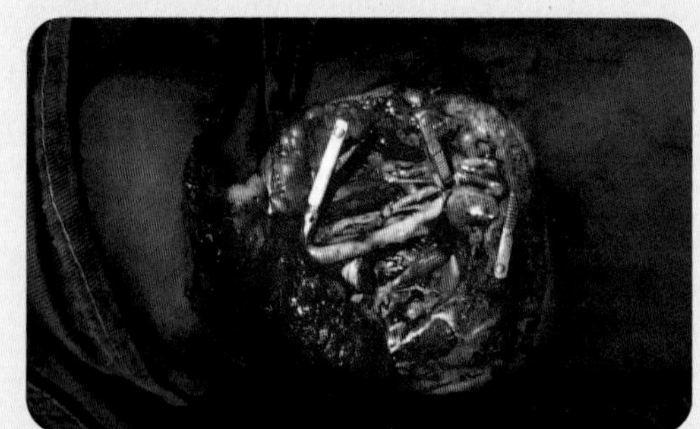

图 3.41.2　显微镜下修复断裂肱动脉及伴行静脉

the brachial artery and vein, the median nerve, the medial cutaneous nerve of the arm, and the median vein of the elbow are completely severed, with only the brachioradialis muscle connected. Broken blood vessels are sutured with ligatures to stop bleeding. Clear the wound, cut off the skin wound margin, trim the lifeless tissue, and remove the vascular ligation line. Repeatedly rinse the wound with physiological saline, ligate small blood vessels and bleeding points.

4.2 Muscle tendon and ligament repair: sequentially suture the anterior joint capsule and torn ligament of the elbow joint, suture the humeral muscle, radial flexor wrist muscle, forearm flexor muscle group and starting point, repair vascular and nerve implantation, and close the ineffective cavity.

4.3 Neurovascular repair: Construct the median nerve stump under a microscope and suture the median nerve with an 8/0 microneedle outer membrane. Under the microscope, the outer membrane of the anastomosis between the brachial artery and its two accompanying veins, as well as the median cubital vein, was constructed, and its branches were ligated. The thrombus in the vascular lumen was washed with a solution of recombinant human alkaline fibroblast growth factor, and a 9/0 microneedle was used to sequentially anastomose the two accompanying veins of the brachial artery, the brachial artery, and the median cubital vein. The tourniquet and vascular clamp were released, and the radial and ulnar arteries pulsated well, with red fingers and good blood reflux. Suture the medial cutaneous nerve of the arm, place a negative pressure drainage tube in the deep part of the wound, suture the wound layer by layer, bandage the wound, and apply plaster to the elbow flexion position (Figure 3.41.2- Figure 3.41.5).

5. Elevating the affected limb after surgery can reduce swelling and facilitate venous return.

6. Routine expansion, spasmolysis, continuous analgesia with an analgesic pump, and application of neurotrophic therapy.

7. When changing dressing, spray growth factors on the wound to promote wound healing and reduce scar formation.

8. Routine finger active and passive training is performed after surgery, with stiff hand joints placed to alleviate hand muscle atrophy.

9. Remove the drainage tube 3 days after surgery, remove the stitches 12 days later, and remove the plaster at 4 weeks for elbow joint and hand function rehabilitation.

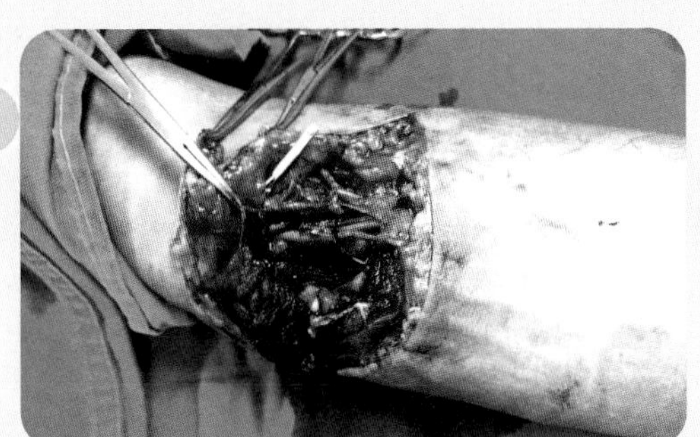

Figure 3.41.1 Left elbow wound, clamp and stop bleeding at the active bleeding point

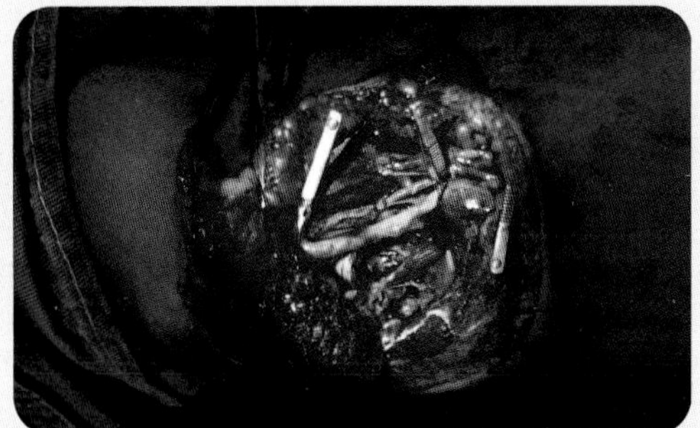

Figure 3.41.2 Microscopic repair of ruptured brachial artery and accompanying veins

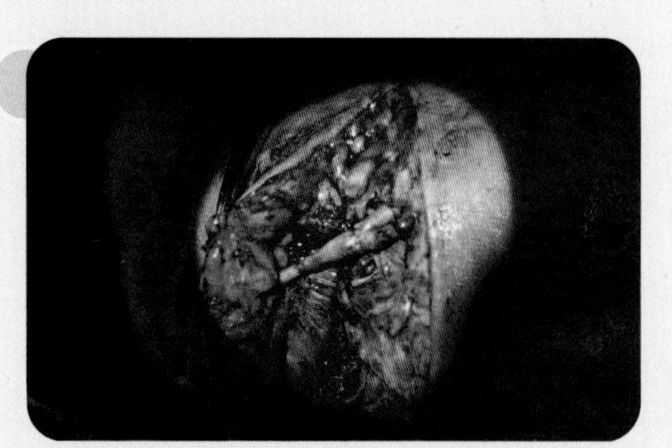

图 3.41.3　修复肘正中静脉

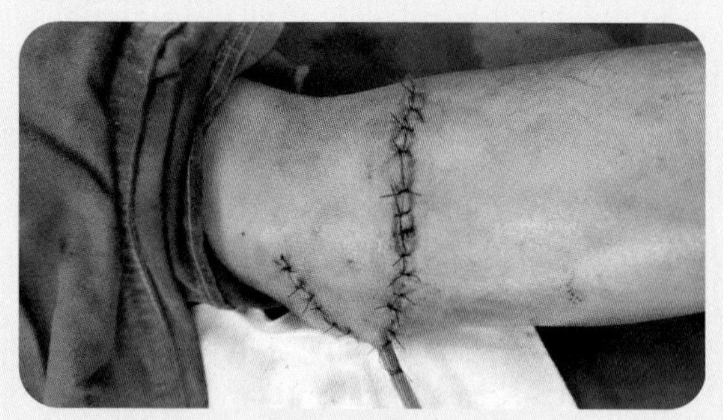

图 3.41.4　肌肉血管神经修复术后，肘部伤口缝合

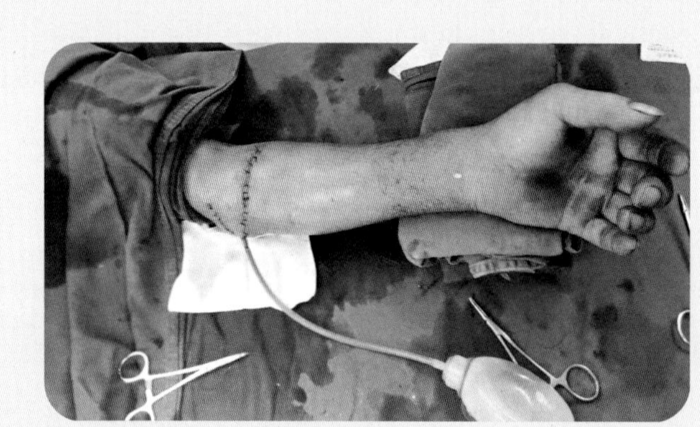

图 3.41.5　手术结束，伤口深部放置负压引流，放止深部血肿形成

（陈善亮）

案例四十二　腕部纵行开放性创伤

◆ 损伤原因

患者因电锯割伤，致左手腕部纵行开放性创伤。

◆ 症状与体征

电锯伤后伤口出血不止，剧痛难忍，腕手伸屈活动受限。左手腕部有 11 cm，斜行伤口，深达掌侧，第 2 掌骨基底部骨折月骨、豌豆骨、头状骨、钩状骨骨折，桡骨远端和尺骨小头骨折。拇长伸肌腱、示指伸肌腱、中指伸肌腱和环指伸肌腱断裂，桡动脉鼻咽窝支断裂，桡神经浅支断裂，腕关节伸腕伸指功能完全受限（图 3.42.1）。

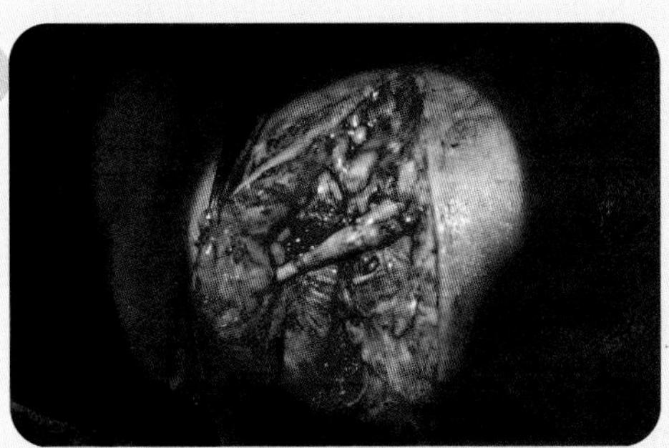

Figure 3.41.3 Repairing the median cubital vein

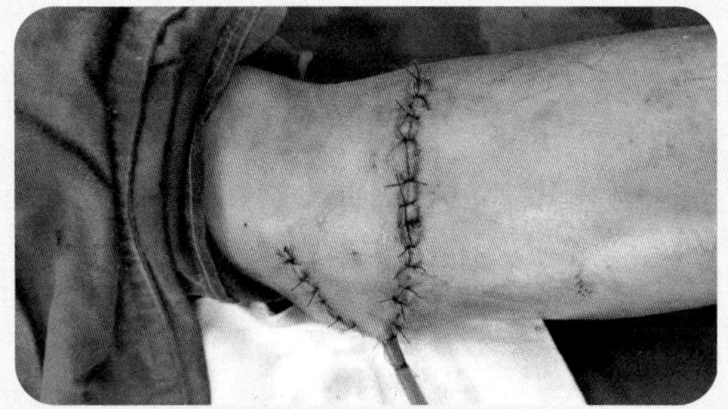

Figure 3.41.4 Suture of elbow wound after muscle vascular and nerve repair surgery

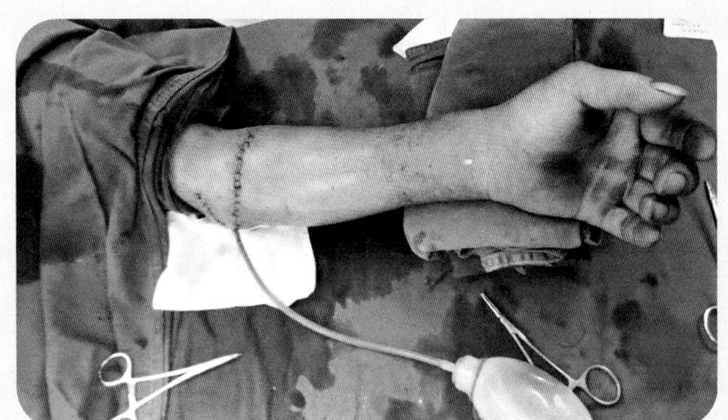

Figure 3.41.5 After the surgery is completed, negative pressure drainage is placed in the deep part of the wound to stop the formation of deep hematoma

(Chen Shanliang)

Case 42 Longitudinal open trauma of wrist

◆ Cause of injury

The patient suffered a longitudinal open wound on the left wrist due to a chainsaw cut.

◆ Signs and symptoms

After the electric saw injury, the wound continued to bleed and the pain was unbearable. The wrist and hand movements were restricted. There is an 11 cm oblique wound on the left wrist, reaching deep into the palmar side. There are fractures in the basal part of the second metacarpal bone, including the Moon bone, Pea bone, Head bone, and Hook bone, as well as fractures in the distal radius and ulnar small head. The extensor pollicis longus, extensor digitorum, extensor middle finger, and extensor ring finger tendons were ruptured, the nasopharyngeal branch of the radial artery was ruptured, the superficial branch of the radial nerve was ruptured, and the wrist and finger extension function was completely restricted (Figure 3.42.1).

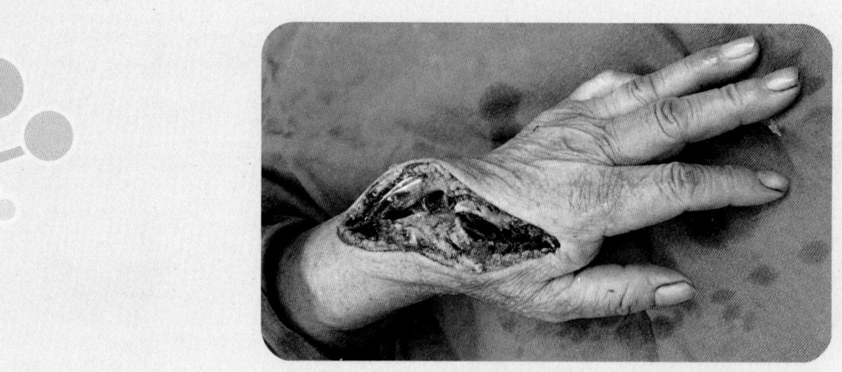

图 3.42.1　左腕背部伤口，显露断裂骨折和肌腱

◆ 治疗方案

1. 入院后立即加压包扎止血，完善术前检查后行骨折复位肌腱血管神经修复术。

2. 臂丛神经阻滞麻醉。

3. 手术过程

3.1 清创术：首先切除皮肤创缘及无生机组织，结扎活动出血点，取出关节内游离粉碎骨折片（图 3.42.2）。

3.2 骨折复位内固定术：依次将桡骨远端、尺骨小头、豌豆骨、头状骨、钩状骨和第 2 掌骨钳夹复位，并用 1.2 ~ 1.5 克氏针逐一固定，修补骨膜和断裂韧带。

3.3 肌腱修复：修剪肌腱断端，依次缝合拇长伸肌腱、示指伸肌腱、中环指伸指肌腱，缝合腱鞘。

3.4 神经血管修复：显微镜下显露桡神经鼻咽窝支和尺神经手背支断端，修建整齐后，应用 9/0 显微针线行外膜缝合。显露桡动脉鼻咽窝支，修剪血管管吻合口外膜，外用重组人碱性成纤维细胞生长因子冲洗液冲洗管腔，应用 10/0 显微针线吻合桡动脉，放开血管夹，吻合的桡动脉通血良好，取外用重组人碱性成纤维细胞生长因子喷洒创面和肌间隙，逐层缝合伤口，术终，石膏托固定功能位（图 3.42.3）。

4. 手术后常规抬高患肢，局部冰敷，减轻肿胀。

5. 术后 12 天拆线，4 周去石膏托固定。

6. 术后 1.5 个月取出克氏针，并循序渐进进行康复训练。

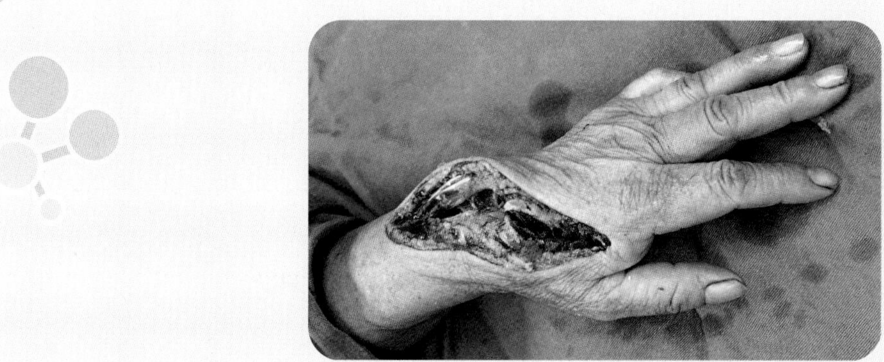

Figure 3.42.1 Left wrist back wound, revealing fractured bones and tendons

◆ Treatment plan

1. Immediately apply pressure and bandage to stop bleeding after admission, complete preoperative examination, and perform fracture reduction, tendon vascular nerve repair surgery.

2. Brachial plexus block anesthesia.

3. Surgical process

3.1 Debridement surgery: First, remove the skin wound margin and lifeless tissue, ligate the active bleeding point, and remove the free comminuted fracture fragment within the joint (Figure 3.42.2).

3.2 Fracture reduction and internal fixation surgery: The distal radius, ulnar head, pea bone, cranial bone, hooked bone, and second metacarpal bone are clamped and reduced in sequence, and fixed one by one with a 1.2-1.5 Kirschner wire to repair the periosteum and fractured ligament.

3.3 Tendon repair: Trim the tendon stump, sequentially suture the extensor hallucis longus tendon, extensor digitorum longus tendon, extensor digitorum medians tendon, and suture the tendon sheath.

3.4 Neurovascular repair: Under a microscope, the severed ends of the radial nerve nasopharyngeal fossa branch and ulnar nerve dorsal branch are exposed, and after being neatly constructed, the outer membrane is sutured using a 9/0 microneedle. Expose the nasopharyngeal fossa branch of the radial artery, trim the outer membrane of the vascular tube anastomosis, rinse the lumen with recombinant human alkaline fibroblast growth factor flushing solution, use a 10/0 microneedle to anastomose the radial artery, release the vascular clamp, and ensure good blood circulation of the anastomosed radial artery. Spray the wound and muscle space with recombinant human alkaline fibroblast growth factor, suture the wound layer by layer, and fix the functional position with a plaster cast at the end of the operation (Figure 3.42.3).

4. After surgery, raise the affected limb and apply local ice to reduce swelling.

5. The stitches were removed 12 days after surgery, and the plaster cast was removed and fixed 4 weeks later.

6. Remove the Kirschner wire 1.5 months after surgery and gradually undergo rehabilitation training.

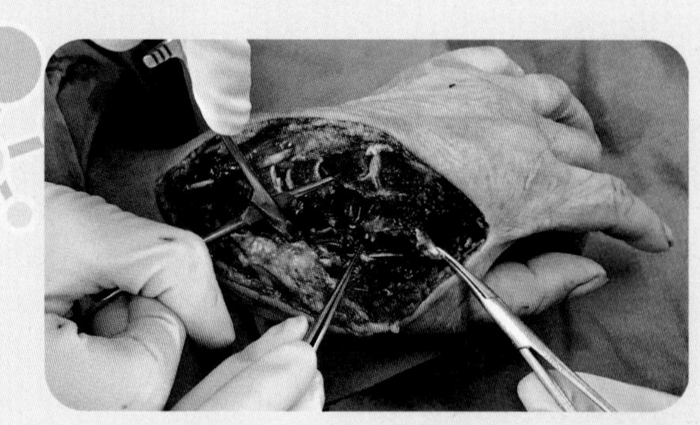

图 3.42.2　清创后，见示指中指和环指屈指深肌腱断裂

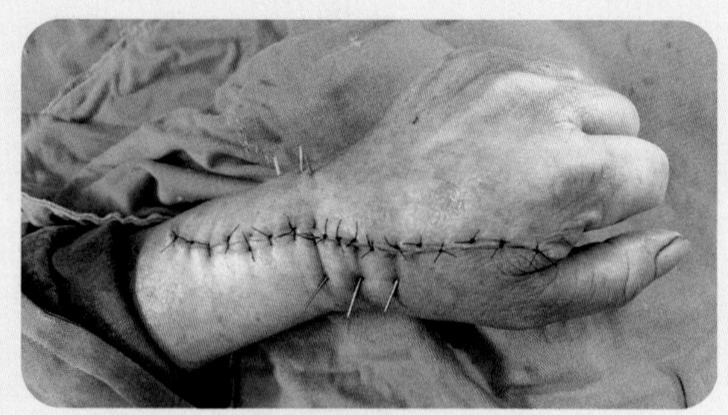

图 3.42.3　骨折复位血管神经修复术后

（陈善亮）

案例四十三　右前臂开放性创伤，肌腱、血管神经断裂

◆ 损伤原因

患者因电锯切割伤，致右前臂开放性创伤，肌腱、血管神经断裂。

◆ 症状与体征

电锯伤后右前臂出血不止，曾喷射状出血，剧痛难忍，肿胀并逐渐加重，右腕关节和拇指、示指活动受限。右前臂桡侧有 18 cm 纵行伤口，深达桡骨，桡骨有 3 cm 纵行锯痕，桡骨无断离，肱桡肌、桡侧伸腕肌、桡侧屈腕肌、拇长伸肌腱断裂，肌腱移行断裂；桡神经浅支断裂，桡动脉及伴行静脉断裂，头静脉断裂，肌腱断端参差不齐，断端回缩（图 3.43.1）。拇指背伸活动受限，腕关节背伸桡偏活动受限，桡动脉远端波动消失，腕背及虎口区感觉消失。

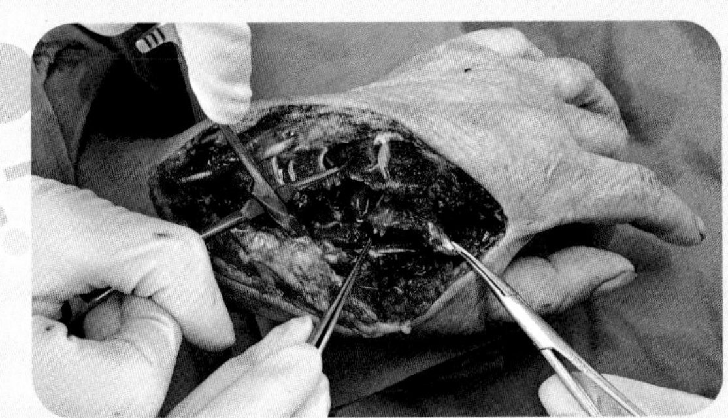

Figure 3.42.2 After debridement, rupture of the deep flexor tendon in the middle finger and ring finger of the index finger is observed

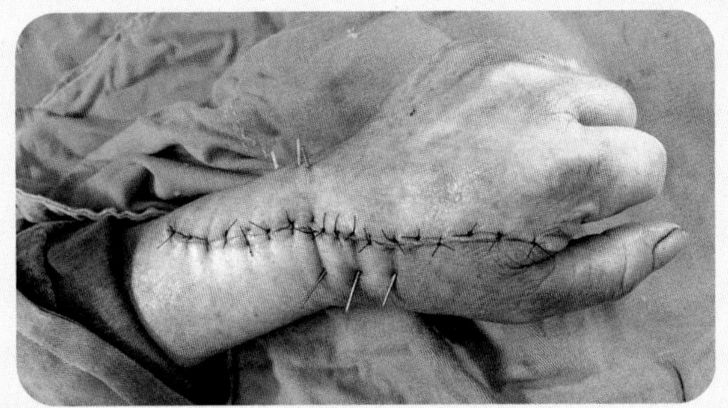

Figure 3.42.3 After fracture reduction and vascular nerve repair surgery

(Chen Shanliang)

Case 43 Open trauma of the right forearm, tendon, vascular and nerve rupture

◆ Cause of injury

The patient suffered an open injury to the right forearm due to electric saw cutting, resulting in tendon and vascular nerve rupture.

◆ Signs and symptoms

After the electric saw injury, there was continuous bleeding in the right forearm, with occasional jet like bleeding. The pain was unbearable, and the swelling gradually worsened. The movement of the right wrist joint, thumb, and index finger was restricted. There is an 18 cm longitudinal wound on the radial side of the right forearm, reaching deep into the radius. There is a 3 cm longitudinal saw mark on the radius, and there is no detachment of the radius. The brachioradialis muscle, radial extensor carpi muscle, radial flexor carpi muscle, and extensor pollicis longus tendon are all ruptured, and the tendon has migrated and ruptured; Fracture of the superficial branch of the radial nerve, rupture of the radial artery and accompanying veins, rupture of the cephalic vein, uneven tendon ends, and retraction of the ends (Figure 3.43.1). The back extension of the thumb is restricted, the back extension and radial deviation of the wrist joint are restricted, the distal fluctuation of the radial artery disappears, and the sensation in the wrist back and tiger mouth area disappears.

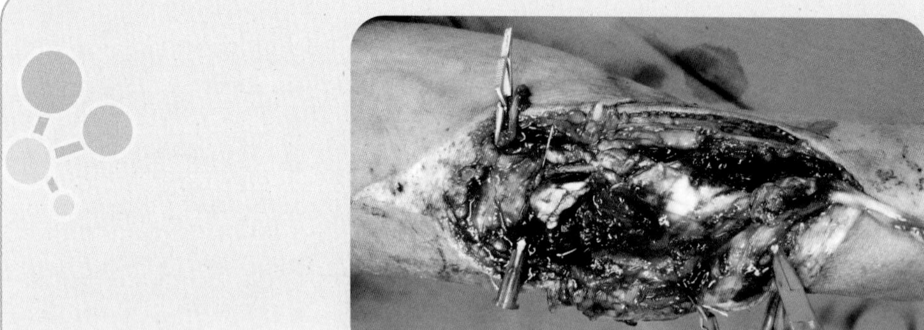

图 3.43.1　右前臂有巨大伤口，肌腱血管神经断裂

◆ 治疗方案

1. 入院后加压包扎止血，建立静脉通道补充血容量，完善术前准备。

2. 臂丛神经阻滞麻醉。

3. 手术过程

3.1 臂丛神经麻醉生效后，清创，切除创缘及污染组织，结扎血管分支止血，修剪肌腱断端，游离显露桡动脉及伴静脉，血管两端上血管夹。待显微镜下修建吻合口。清创时保护好桡神经浅支两断端。

3.2 肌腱修复：依次缝合肱桡肌、桡侧屈腕肌、桡侧伸腕肌及拇长伸肌腱，缝合肌筋膜（图 3.43.2）。

3.3 血管神经修复：显微镜下显露桡动脉及伴行静脉、头静脉及桡神经浅支，显露血管两断端，修建血管吻合口外膜，结扎血管主干分支，外用重组人碱性成纤维细胞生长因子冲洗液冲洗血管吻合口，取 9/0 显微针线，依次吻合头静脉→桡动脉→头静脉→桡神经浅支。

3.4 肌间隙及创面外用重组人碱性成纤维细胞生长因子，伤口深部放橡皮条一枚引流，逐层缝合伤口，包扎伤口，石膏固定于功能位。

4. 术后抬高患肢，冰敷伤口，减轻肿胀。

5. 扩容、解痉镇痛、抗感染治疗。

6. 术后 3 天拔出橡皮条引流，12 天拆线，3 周拆石膏并进行康复训练（图 3.43.3）。

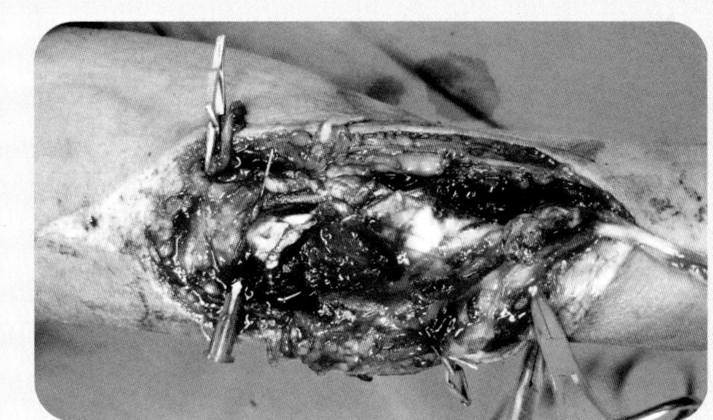

Figure 3.43.1 There is a huge wound on the right forearm, with ruptured tendons, blood vessels, and nerves

◆ Treatment plan

1. After admission, apply pressure and bandage to stop bleeding, establish a venous channel to supplement blood volume, and improve preoperative preparation.

2. Brachial plexus block anesthesia.

3. Surgical process

3.1 After the brachial plexus anesthesia takes effect, debridement is performed, the wound margin and contaminated tissue are removed, the blood vessel branches are ligated to stop bleeding, the tendon ends are trimmed, the radial artery and accompanying veins are freely exposed, and the blood vessels are clamped at both ends. Construct the anastomosis under the microscope. Protect the two severed ends of the superficial branch of the radial nerve during debridement.

3.2 Tendon repair: Suture the brachioradialis muscle, radial flexor wrist muscle, radial extensor wrist muscle, and extensor hallucis longus tendon in sequence, and suture the myofascia (Figure 3.43.2).

3.3 Vascular and nerve repair: Under a microscope, expose the radial artery, accompanying veins, cephalic vein, and superficial branches of the radial nerve, expose the two ends of the blood vessels, construct the outer membrane of the vascular anastomosis site, ligate the main branches of the blood vessels, apply recombinant human alkaline fibroblast growth factor flushing solution to wash the vascular anastomosis site, take 9/0 microneedle, and sequentially anastomose the cephalic vein → radial artery → cephalic vein → superficial branches of the radial nerve.

3.4 Recombinant human alkaline fibroblast growth factor is applied topically to the muscle gap and wound. A rubber strip is placed deep in the wound for drainage, and the wound is sutured layer by layer, wrapped, and fixed in a functional position with plaster.

4. Raise the affected limb after surgery, apply ice to the wound, and reduce swelling.

5. Expansion, spasmolysis, analgesia, and anti-infection treatment.

6. Remove the rubber strip for drainage 3 days after surgery, remove the stitches 12 days later, remove the plaster and conduct rehabilitation training 3 weeks later (Figure 3.43.3).

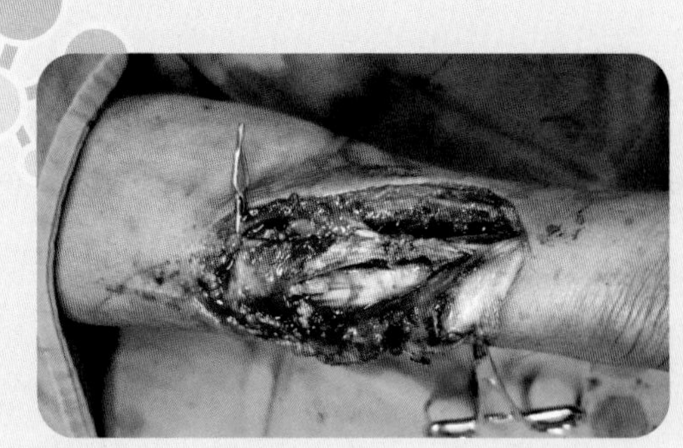

图 3.43.2　肌腱修复术后，待修复血管神经

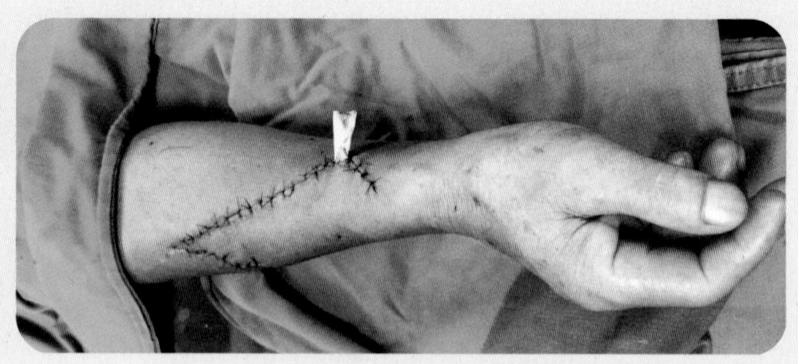

图 3.43.3　术后第 2 天，引流待拔出

（陈善亮）

案例四十四　臀部皮肤缺损

◆ 损伤原因

患者因滑倒臀部不慎坐在除草机上，致臀部皮肤缺损。

◆ 症状与体征

伤后臀部出血不止，衣裤迅速被血液浸透打湿，剧痛难忍，不能站立行走。肿胀并逐渐加重。左侧臀部有 13 cm × 11 cm 创面，皮肤大面积缺损，臀部脂肪垫外露皮缘不齐，伤口距肛门仅 3 cm，局部出血活跃；右侧臀部有 10 cm × 7 cm 伤口，伤口中间有多条皮肤组织间桥，伤口参差不齐；双侧臀部伤口布满碎草削，局部肿胀明显，压痛明显（图 3.44.1）。双下肢感觉运动自如。

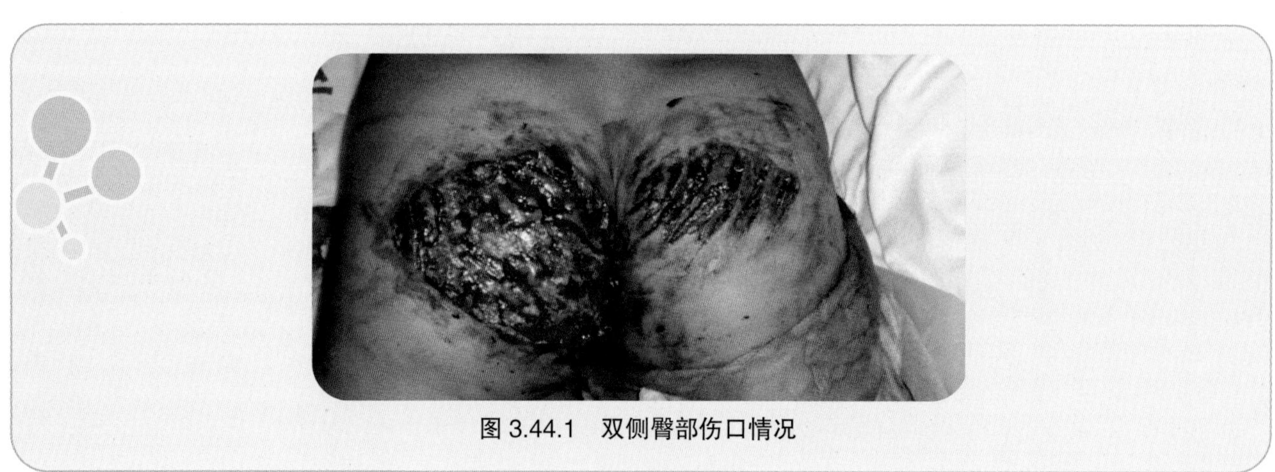

图 3.44.1　双侧臀部伤口情况

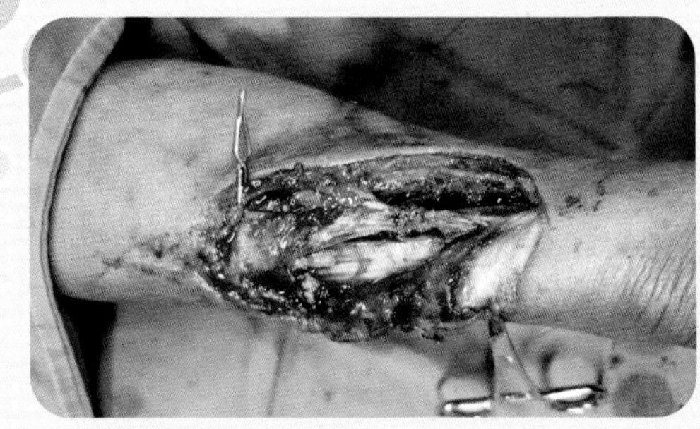
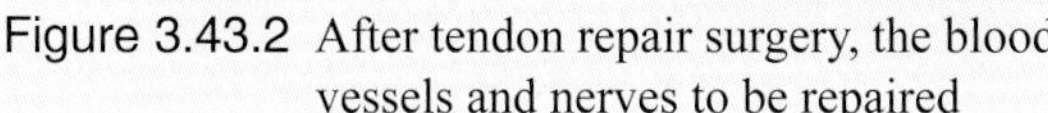

Figure 3.43.2 After tendon repair surgery, the blood vessels and nerves to be repaired

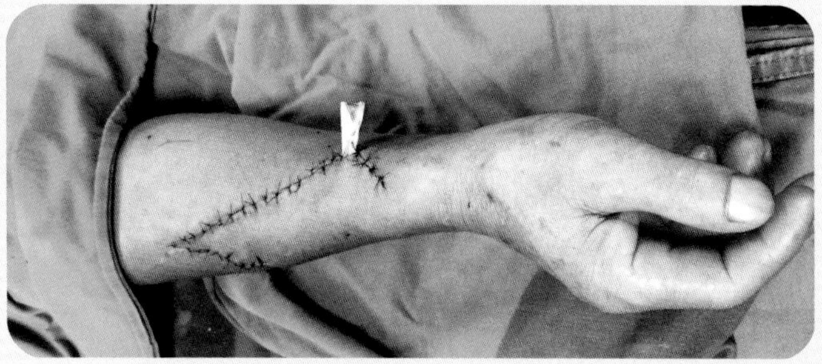

Figure 3.43.3 On the second day after surgery, drainage is to be removed

(Chen Shanliang)

Case 44 Skin defect on the hip

◆ Cause of injury

The patient slipped and accidentally sat on the lawnmower, resulting in skin defects on the buttocks.

◆ Signs and symptoms

After the injury, the buttocks were bleeding continuously, and the clothes and pants were quickly soaked and soaked in blood, causing unbearable pain and making it impossible to stand and walk. Swelling and gradually worsening. There is a 13 cm × 11 cm wound on the left buttocks, with a large area of skin defect. The fat pad on the buttocks is exposed with uneven skin edges, and the wound is only 3 cm away from the anus. Local bleeding is active; There is a 10 cm × 7 cm wound on the right buttocks, with multiple skin tissue bridges in the middle of the wound, and the wound is uneven; The wounds on both buttocks are covered in broken grass and have obvious local swelling and tenderness (Figure 3.44.1). Both lower limbs feel free to move.

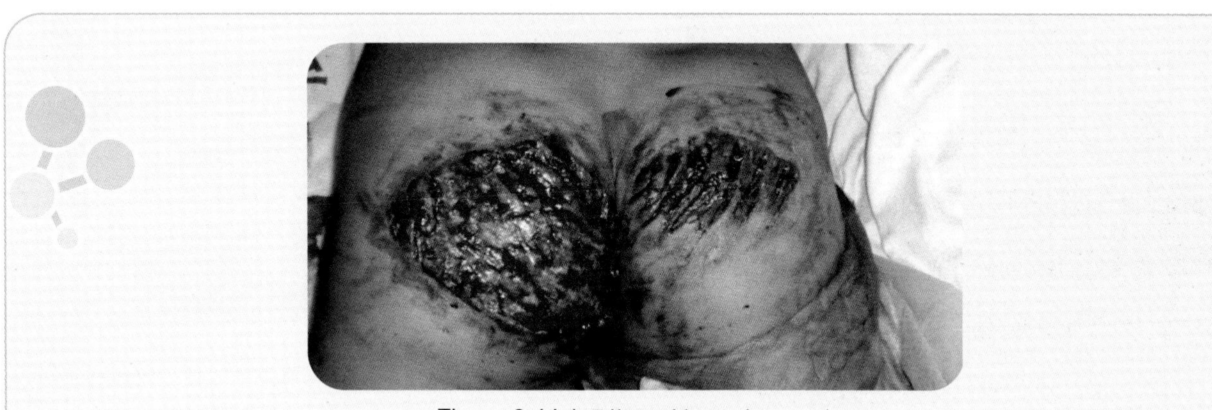

Figure 3.44.1 Bilateral buttock wounds

◆ 治疗方案

1. 患者入院后立即包扎伤口，减少出血，建立静脉通道，完善术前准备。

2. 麻醉选择腰硬联合麻醉，麻醉生效后，采用俯卧位。

3. 手术过程

3.1 清创术：切除伤口创缘及挫伤无生机组织，清洗污染物，结扎伤口活动出血点，清创后左侧臀部创面为 13 cm × 13.5 cm，右侧臀部伤口直接缝合（图 3.44.2）。

3.2 左侧臀部皮瓣设计：于左侧臀部设计臀上筋膜皮瓣，皮瓣蒂长 14 cm、蒂宽 7 cm，解剖面臀肌筋膜浅层。臀下筋膜皮瓣，皮瓣蒂长 14 cm、蒂宽 8 cm，解剖面为臀肌筋膜浅层。

3.3 皮瓣移植：依次切开皮肤及皮下脂肪达肌筋膜浅层，电凝活动出血点。解剖创面喷洒外用重组人碱性成纤维细胞生长因子，行皮瓣缝合，皮瓣下放置橡皮条引流。皮瓣移植术后，外形饱满，皮瓣血运良好，包扎伤口，术终（图 3.44.3 ~ 图 3.44.5）。

4. 术后采用侧卧位，即左侧卧位、右侧卧位交替卧位，避免平卧位压迫臀部皮瓣影响血运。

5. 由于创面巨大，术后渗出较多，应加强换药，每天更换敷料 2 次，根据创面渗出情况减少换药次数。

6. 术后 7 天内全流食或半流食，减少食物残渣饮食，减少排便次数，防止污染切口，预防伤口感染。

7. 常规给予扩容、抗感染药物。

8. 术后 7 天起床下地行走，术后 12 天拆线，并逐渐坐卧康复训练。

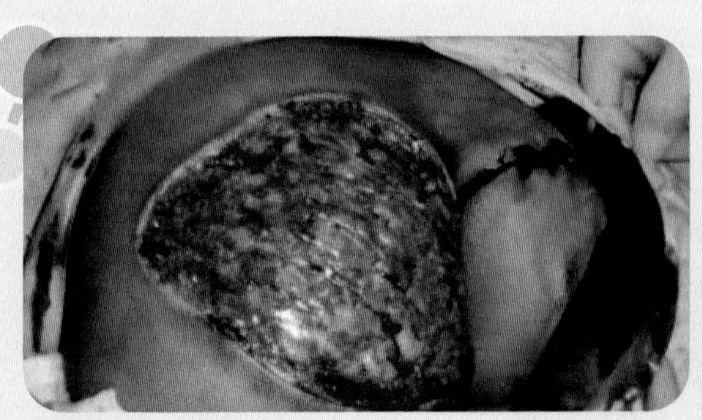

图 3.44.2 左侧清创后创面巨大，右侧臀部清创后缝合

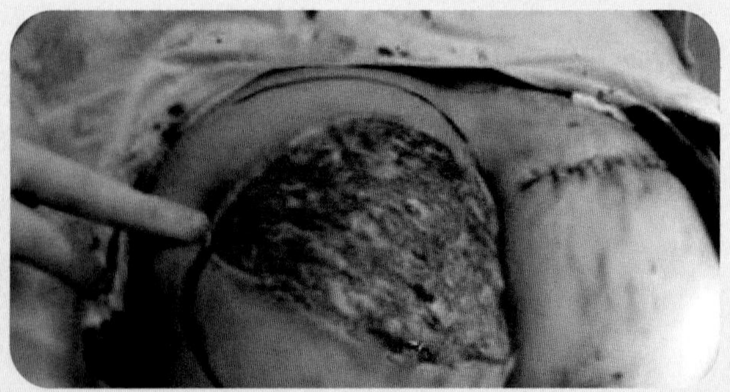

图 3.44.3 左侧创面行臀上臀下筋膜皮瓣移植，切口设计线示意

◆ Treatment plan

1. After admission, the patient immediately bandages the wound to reduce bleeding, establishes a venous channel, and improves preoperative preparation.

2. The anesthesia should be a combination of lumbar and hard anesthesia. After the anesthesia takes effect, the prone position should be used.

3. Surgical process

3.1 Debridement surgery: Remove the wound margin and non-viable tissue from the contusion, clean the contaminants, ligate the active bleeding point of the wound. After debridement, the left hip wound is 13 cm × 13.5 cm, and the right hip wound is directly sutured (Figure 3.44.2).

3.2 Left buttock flap design: A fascia flap is designed on the left buttock, with a pedicle length of 14 cm and a pedicle width of 7 cm, dissecting the superficial layer of the gluteal muscle fascia. The inferior gluteal fascia flap has a pedicle length of 14 cm and a pedicle width of 8 cm, with the anatomical surface being the superficial layer of the gluteal fascia.

3.3 Skin flap transplantation: Cut open the skin and subcutaneous fat in sequence to reach the superficial layer of the fascia, and electrocoagulate the bleeding point. Dissect the wound and spray external recombinant human basic fibroblast growth factor, suture the skin flap, and place a rubber strip under the skin flap for drainage. After the skin flap transplantation, the appearance was plump, the blood supply of the skin flap was good, the wound was bandaged, and the surgery was completed (Figure 3.44.3- Figure 3.44.5).

4. After surgery, adopt a lateral position, alternating between left and right lateral positions, to avoid compression of the hip skin flap and affecting blood flow in the supine position.

5. Due to the large size of the wound and significant postoperative exudation, dressing changes should be strengthened by changing dressings twice a day and reducing the frequency of dressing changes based on the extent of wound exudation.

6. Within 7 days after surgery, consume whole or semi liquid food, reduce food residue, decrease bowel movements, prevent contamination of the incision, and prevent wound infection.

7. Routine administration of expansion and anti-infective drugs.

8. Wake up and walk on the ground 7 days after surgery, remove the stitches 12 days after surgery, and gradually perform sit and lie rehabilitation training.

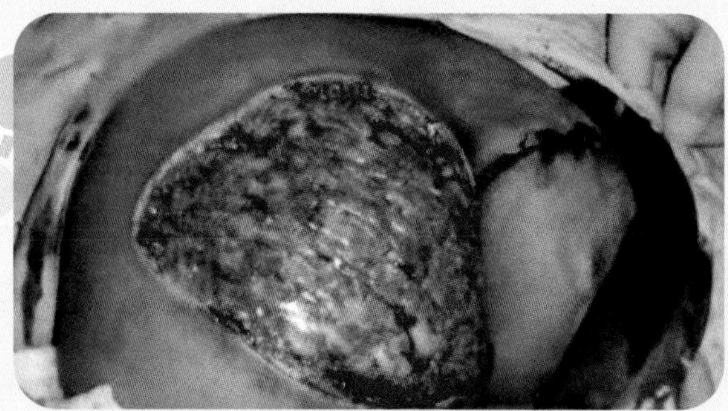

Figure 3.44.2 The wound on the left side is huge after debridement, and the wound on the right hip is sutured after debridement

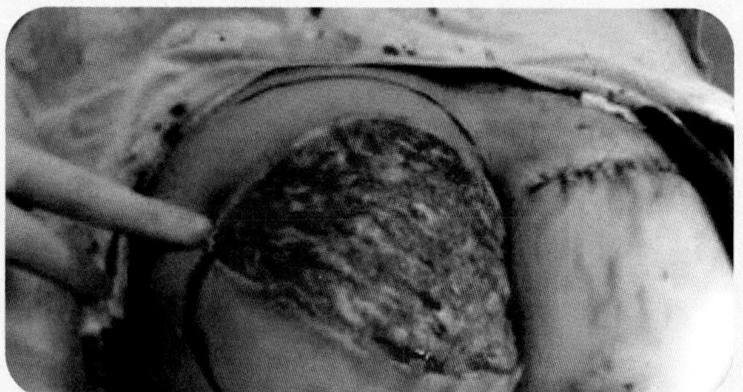

Figure 3.44.3 Left wound underwent upper and lower gluteal fascia flap transplantation, with a schematic diagram of the incision design line

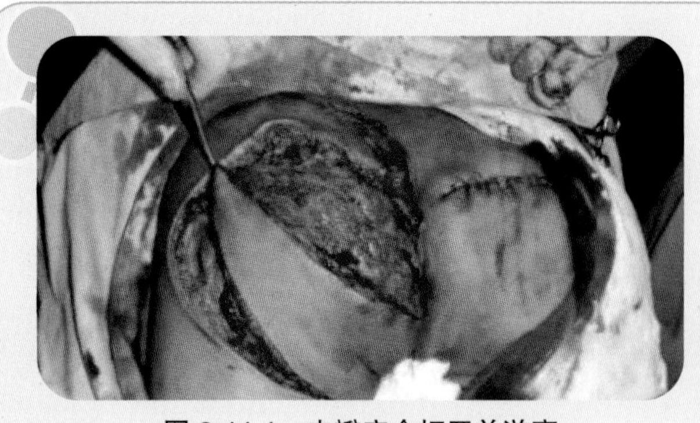

图 3.44.4　皮瓣完全切开并游离

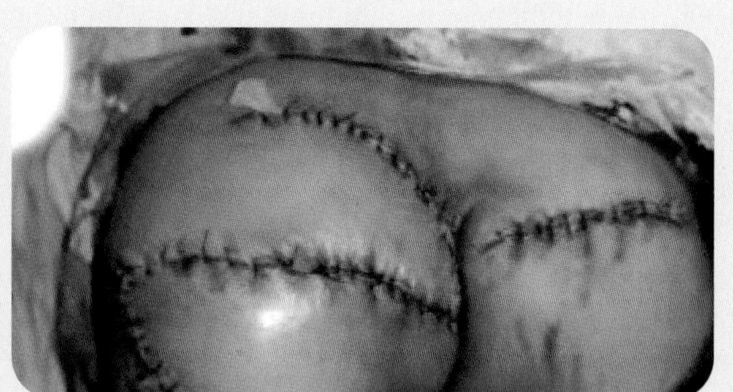

图 3.44.5　皮瓣移植缝合术后，外形良好

（陈善亮）

案例四十五　手掌多发贯通伤

◆ 损伤原因

患者因在笔厂被制笔磨具压伤左手，致左手掌多发贯通伤创面。

◆ 症状与体征

左手掌剧痛难忍，出血不止，肿胀并逐渐加重，手指不能屈伸活动，手指麻木。左手掌散在 18 个空洞创面，贯穿手掌，孔洞皮缘整齐，污染不重，部分肌肉组织溢处皮肤外，手掌背侧孔洞皮肤圆形缺损，示指、中指伸指功能受限，中指、环指指端感觉减退，屈指功能良好，指端血运良好，第 2 掌骨骨擦感、骨擦音阳性，每个圆形伤口约 0.8 cm × 0.8 cm，掌侧每个孔洞皮肤有皮蒂相连，形成的皮瓣血运欠佳（图 3.45.1、图 3.45.2）。

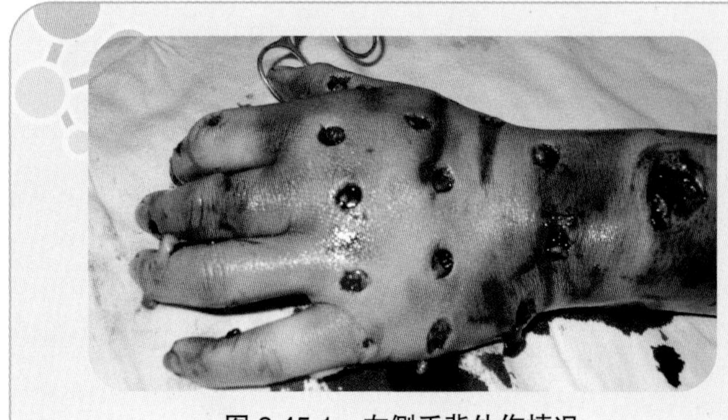

图 3.45.1　左侧手背外伤情况

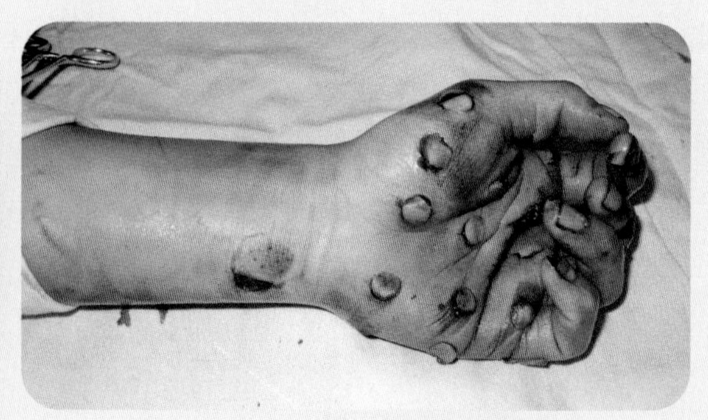

图 3.45.2　左侧手掌外伤情况

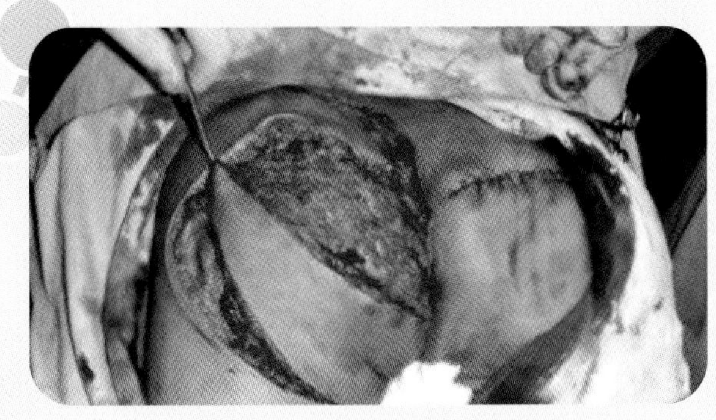

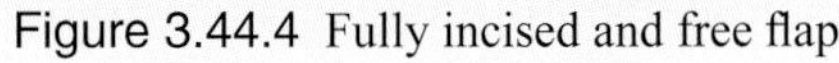

Figure 3.44.4 Fully incised and free flap

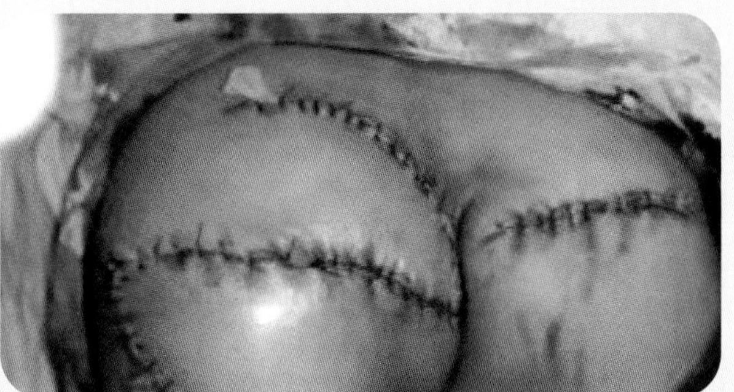

Figure 3.44.5 Good appearance after flap transplantation and suturing surgery

(Chen Shanliang)

Case 45 Multiple penetrating injuries to the palm

◆ Cause of injury

The patient's left hand was injured by pressure from a pen grinding tool at the pen factory, resulting in multiple penetrating wounds on the left palm.

◆ Signs and symptoms

The pain in the left palm is unbearable, with continuous bleeding, swelling that gradually worsens, inability to bend and stretch the fingers, and numbness in the fingers. There are 18 hollow wounds scattered in the left palm, which run through the palm. The skin edges of the holes are neat and the pollution is not heavy. Some muscle tissue overflows outside the skin. The skin of the holes on the back of the palm is circular and defective. The extension function of the index finger and middle finger is limited, and the sensation of the middle finger and ring finger ends is reduced. The flexion function is good, and the blood supply of the finger ends is good. The bone rubbing sensation and bone rubbing sound of the second palm are positive. Each circular wound is about 0.8 cm × 0.8 cm. The skin of each hole on the palm side is connected by a skin pedicle, and the blood supply of the formed skin flap is poor (Figure 3.45.1, Figure 3.45.2).

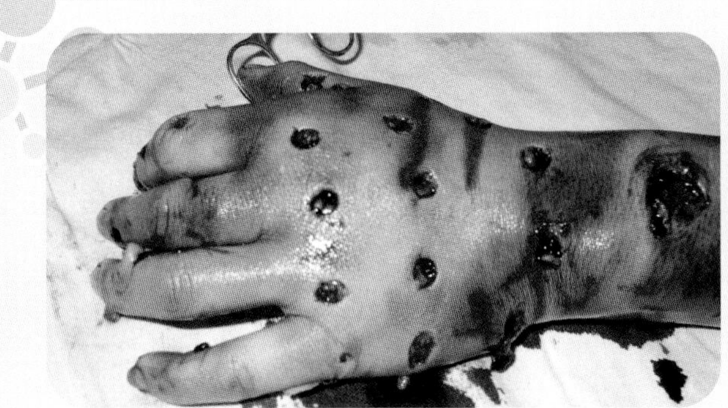

Figure 3.45.1 Left Hand Back Trauma Situation

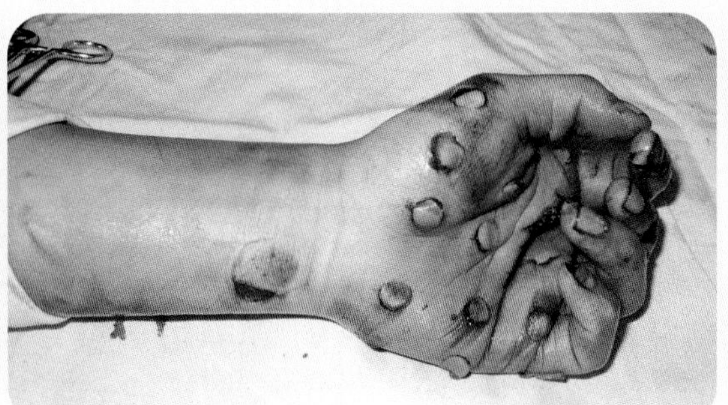

Figure 3.45.2 Left Palm Trauma Situation

◆ 治疗方案

1. 入院后立即包扎伤口减少出血，完善手术前准备，拍片确定骨折损伤情况。

2. 采用臂丛神经阻滞麻醉。

3. 第 2 掌骨骨折采用 2.0 克氏针纵行闭合固定。

4. 深部碘伏擦拭消毒，预防深部感染。由于手掌手背多发贯穿伤口，皮肤扩创容易形成不规则瘢痕。伸肌腱二次修复。

5. 利用外伤形成自然伤口，在多个伤口深部放置橡皮条引流，利于深部渗出，放置血肿和脓肿形成。

6. 采用 5.0 丝线缝合掌侧伤口，手背伤口不缝合，采用异种脱细胞真皮基质敷料外用，待手背伤口自然愈合，人工缝合容易出现皮肤挛缩。

7. 术后 2 天拔出橡皮条引流。

8. 术后 2 周去掉异种脱细胞真皮基质敷料，伤口完全愈合，手掌侧皮肤拆线，甲级愈合，并进行训练。1.5 个月后拔出克氏针，并二期修复示指伸肌腱（图 3.45.3、图 3.45.4）。

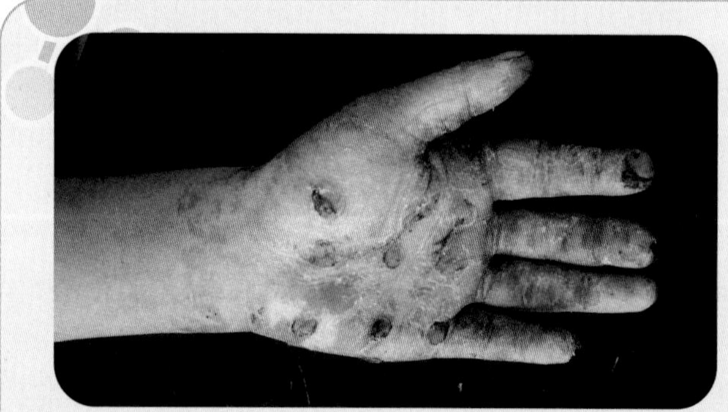

图 3.45.3　左手掌伤口愈合情况

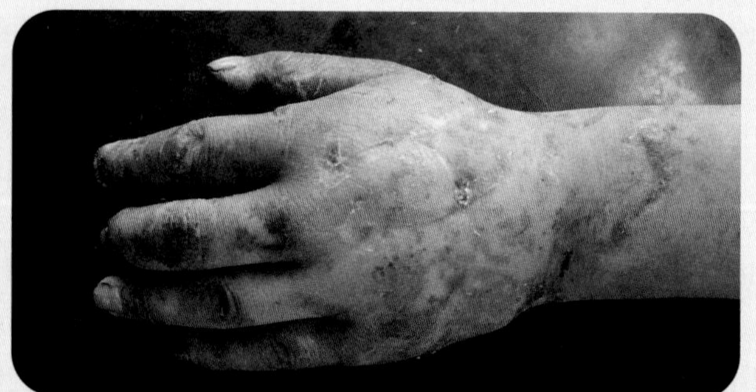

图 3.45.4　左手背愈合情况

（陈善亮）

◆ Treatment plan

1. Immediately bandage the wound after admission to reduce bleeding, improve preoperative preparation, and take X-rays to determine the extent of the fracture injury.

2. Use brachial plexus block anesthesia.

3. The fracture of the second metacarpal bone was fixed using a 2.0 Kirschner wire for longitudinal closure.

4. Wipe and disinfect deep areas with iodine to prevent deep infections. Due to multiple incisions on the palms and backs of the hands, skin expansion can easily lead to irregular scars. Secondary repair of extensor tendon.

5. Utilize trauma to form natural wounds, and place rubber strips in the deep parts of multiple wounds for drainage, which facilitates deep exudation and the formation of hematomas and abscesses.

6. Use 5.0 silk thread to suture the palmar wound, without suturing the wound on the back of the hand. Apply a heterologous decellularized dermal matrix dressing externally, and wait for the wound on the back of the hand to heal naturally. Artificial suturing can easily cause skin contractures.

7. Two days after surgery, remove the rubber strip for drainage.

8. Two weeks after surgery, the heterologous decellularized dermal matrix dressing was removed, and the wound fully healed. The skin on the palm side was sutured, achieving Grade A healing, and training was conducted. After 1.5 months, the Kirschner wire was removed and the extensor tendon of the index finger was repaired in two stages (Figure 3.45.3, Figure 3.45.4).

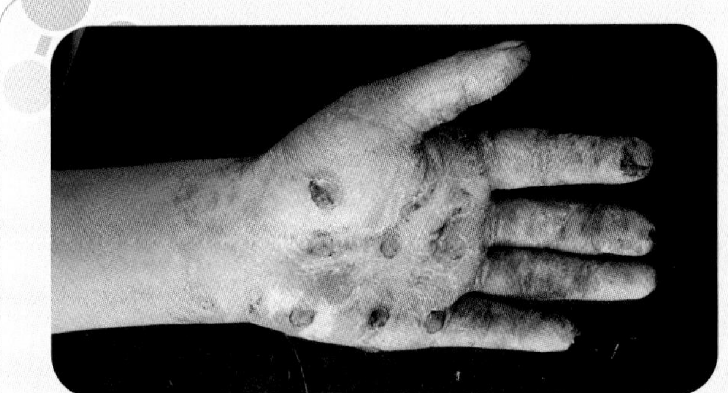

Figure 3.45.3 Healing of Left Palm Wound

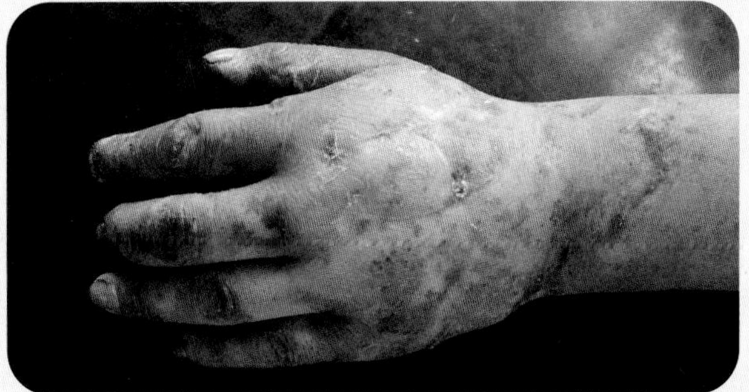

Figure 3.45.4 Left Hand Back Healing Status

(Chen Shanliang)

第 4 章
Chapter 4

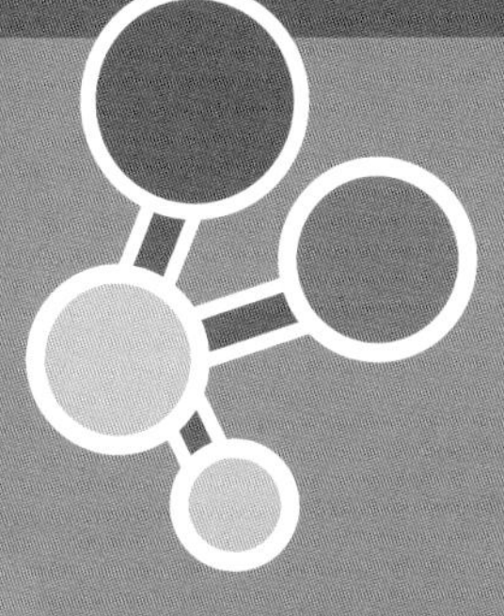

压力性创面修复
Repair of Pressure Wounds

案例一　腰骶尾部压疮

◆ 致病原因

患者因高血压脑出血致骶尾部压疮，曾2次手术行局部转移皮瓣修复创面，均失败，在家自用草药外用，创面逐渐增大。

◆ 症状与体征

骶尾部创面长期流脓，红肿热痛，查体见骶尾部有9 cm × 11 cm巨大创面，创面较深，深达尾骨，第5腰椎横突和棘突外露，局部肉芽组织老化，创口周围硬化，并有不规则切口瘢痕，伤口内污染严重，有粪便污染伤口，伤口有大量炎性渗出，散在白色脓苔，局部皮温较高，创缘于皮下潜行，双下肢肌力2级，双下肢曾痉挛瘫，关节屈曲僵硬。双侧足跟有较深压疮，深达跟骨，跟骨坏死疏松，左足跟创面5 cm × 3 cm，皮缘内陷，创面肉芽组织污秽不清，右侧足跟创面6 cm × 4 cm，皮缘内陷硬化，肉芽组织老化，骶尾部创面和双足创面味恶臭（图4.1.1 ~ 图4.1.3）。

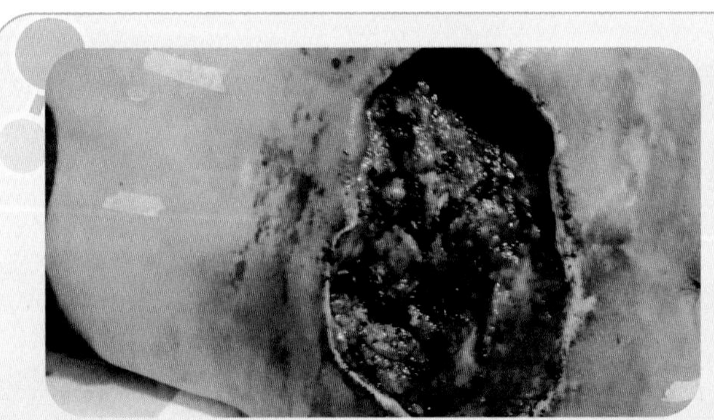

图4.1.1　骶尾部巨大创面，创面粪便污染严重

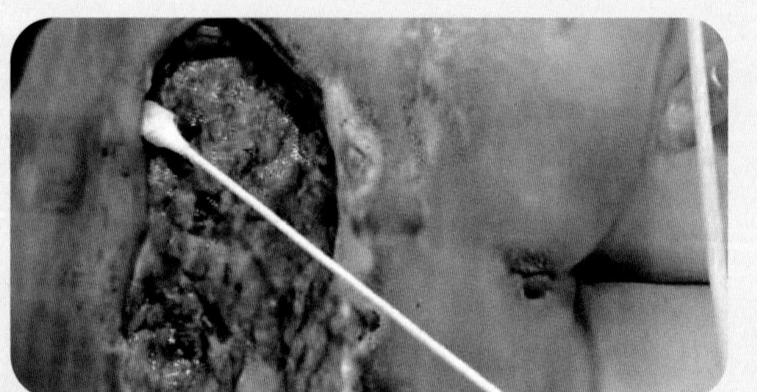

图4.1.2　压力性创面肉芽组织增生，污秽不清

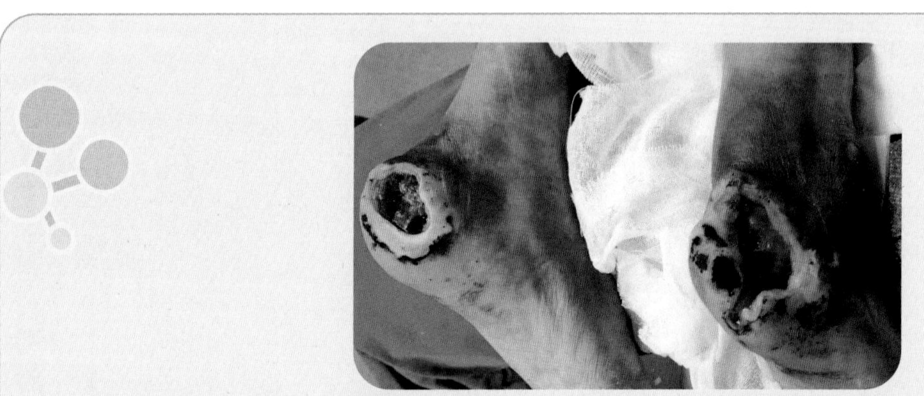

图4.1.3　双侧足后跟凹陷创面，跟骨外露，并有跟骨坏死

Case 1 Lumbosacral and coccygeal pressure ulcers

◆ Cause of illness

The patient suffered from sacrococcygeal pressure ulcers due to hypertensive cerebral hemorrhage. Two surgeries were performed to repair the wound with local transfer skin flaps, but both failed. The wound gradually grew larger after using herbal medicine at home.

◆ Signs and symptoms

The wound on the coccyx has been oozing pus for a long time, with redness, swelling, and pain. Physical examination showed a huge wound of 9 cm × 11 cm on the coccyx, which is deep and extends to the coccyx. The transverse and spinous processes of the fifth lumbar vertebra are exposed, and local granulation tissue is aging. The wound is hardened around the wound and has irregular incision scars. The wound is heavily contaminated, with feces contaminating the wound. There is a large amount of inflammatory exudate, scattered white pus coating, and high local skin temperature. The wound is caused by subcutaneous infiltration. The muscle strength of both lower limbs is level 2, and both lower limbs have spasmed and paralyzed, with stiff joint flexion. There are deep pressure ulcers on both heels, reaching as deep as the calcaneus bone. The calcaneus bone is necrotic and loose, and the wound on the left heel is 5 cm × 3 cm, with a sunken skin edge and unclear granulation tissue. The wound on the right heel is 6 cm × 4 cm, with a hardened skin edge, aging granulation tissue, and a foul odor on the sacrococcygeal and bilateral foot wounds (Figure 4.1.1 - Figure 4.1.3).

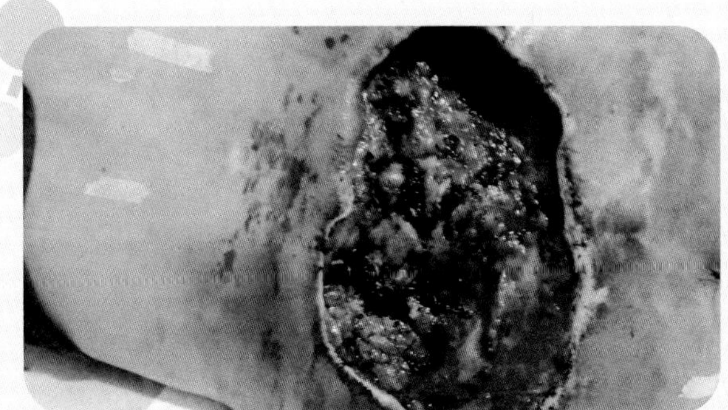

Figure 4.1.1 A huge wound on the coccyx with severe fecal contamination

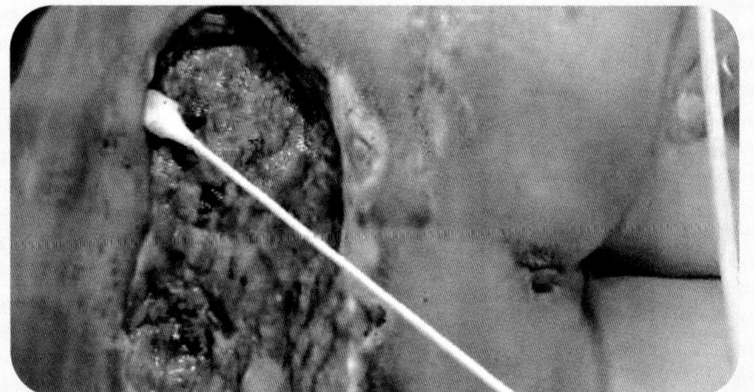

Figure 4.1.2 granulation tissue proliferation and uncleanliness in pressure wound

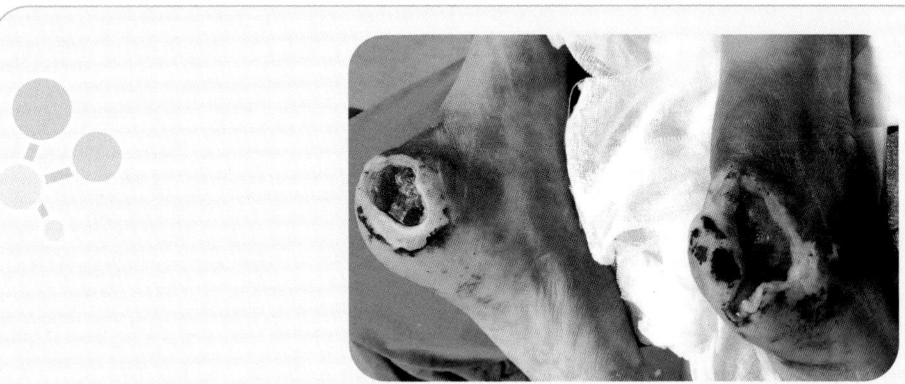

Figure 4.1.3 Bilateral heel depression wounds with exposed calcaneus and calcaneus necrosis

◆ 治疗方案

该患者为中风多年，中风后骶尾部和双足跟出现巨大压疮，曾在本地医院 2 次行局部皮瓣转移手术，术后皮瓣坏死，致使骶尾部压疮越来越大而不能愈合，骶尾部创面棘突和横突骨外露，由于创面较深面积较大自行愈合十分困难。

1. 入院后增加换药次数，每次换药刮出无生机组织和老化肉芽组织，喷洒重组人碱性成纤维细胞生长因子，加强基础护理防止骶尾部和双侧足跟继续受压。局部红外线理疗，每天 3 次，局部按摩促进血液循环，四肢各个关节松动，防止关节继续挛缩。

2. 入院 7 天后，行局部大清创，因骶尾部无痛觉，无须麻醉；行 VSD+ 重组人碱性成纤维细胞生长因子滴注创面冲洗，促进创面新鲜，为创面植皮提供时机。VSD 负压 + 重组人碱性成纤维细胞生长因子冲洗治疗 5 天，拆除 VSD 装置，创面新鲜可以手术植皮（图 4.1.4）。

3. 手术过程

3.1 俯卧位，手术区域碘伏常规消毒，铺无菌巾单，使用电动取皮刀调制超薄皮片厚度，根据创面大小，于右侧大腿外侧切取相应面积游离皮片，将皮片修剪成邮票大小，移植于骶尾部创面，局部包扎固定，防止游离皮片滑脱，5 天后换药时植皮成活一半，另一半坏死，考虑翻身时皮片滑动而坏死，但创面明显缩小。未愈合创面继续换药喷洒生长因子。足跟创面经过清创换药和喷洒重组人碱性成纤维细胞生长因子，双侧足跟压疮于入院后 30 天完全愈合（图 4.1.5、图 4.1.6）。

3.2 骶尾部创面二次植皮，侧卧位，手术区域常规消毒，铺无菌巾单，使用电动取皮刀调制超薄皮片厚度，于左侧大腿外侧切取相应面积游离皮片，将皮片修剪成邮票大小，移植于骶尾部剩余创面，局部包扎固定（图 4.1.7、图 4.1.8）。

4. 术后加强翻身护理，防止因翻身不当引发植皮滑动移位，影响植皮成活率，骶尾部植皮手术护理十分重要，术后常规侧卧位，左侧卧位和右侧卧位交替翻身，使用气垫床，肢体气垫防止肢体重叠压迫引起的新的压疮。

5. 二次植皮手术后 5 天，游离植皮全部成活，骶尾部和双足跟压疮完全治愈出院（图 4.1.9、图 4.1.10）。

◆ Treatment plan

The patient has been suffering from a stroke for many years. After the stroke, there were huge pressure ulcers on the coccyx and both heels. Two local flap transfer surgeries were performed at the local hospital, but the flaps died after the surgery, causing the pressure ulcers on the coccyx to become larger and unable to heal. The spinous and transverse process bones of the coccyx wound were exposed, and it was very difficult for them to heal on their own due to the deep and large area of the wound.

1. Increase the frequency of dressing changes after admission, scrape out lifeless tissue and aged granulation tissue during each dressing change, spray recombinant human basic fibroblast growth factor, and strengthen basic care to prevent further compression of the coccyx and bilateral heels. Local infrared therapy, 3 times a day, local massage promotes blood circulation, loosens various joints in the limbs, and prevents joint contraction.

2. 7 days after admission, a local debridement was performed, but anesthesia was not necessary as there was no pain sensation in the sacrococcygeal region; VSD + recombinant human basic fibroblast growth factor infusion for wound flushing promotes wound freshness and provides an opportunity for wound skin grafting. VSD negative pressure + recombinant human basic fibroblast growth factor flushing treatment for 5 days, removal of VSD device, fresh wound can be treated with surgical skin grafting (Figure 4.1.4).

3. Surgical process

3.1 Prone position, routine iodine disinfection in the surgical area, laying sterile drapes, using an electric skin knife to adjust the thickness of ultra-thin skin patches, cutting the corresponding area of free skin patches on the outer side of the right thigh according to the size of the wound, trimming the skin patches to the size of stamps, transplanting them onto the wound at the coccyx, locally wrapping and fixing them to prevent the free skin patches from slipping. When changing dressing 5 days later, half of the skin grafts survived, while the other half died. It is considered that the skin patches may slide and die when turning over, but the wound size is significantly reduced. Continue to change dressing and spray growth factors on unhealed wounds. After debridement, dressing change, and spraying of recombinant human basic fibroblast growth factor on the heel wound, the bilateral heel pressure ulcers fully healed within 30 days after admission (Figure 4.1.5, Figure 4.1.6).

3.2 Secondary skin grafting on the sacrococcygeal wound, lying on the side, routine disinfection of the surgical area, laying sterile drapes, using an electric skin knife to adjust the thickness of ultra-thin skin, cutting a corresponding area of free skin on the outer side of the left thigh, trimming the skin into the size of a postage stamp, transplanting it onto the remaining wound on the sacrococcygeal region, and locally bandaging and fixing it (Figure 4.1.7, Figure 4.1.8).

4. Strengthen postoperative turning care to prevent skin graft sliding and displacement caused by improper turning, which affects the survival rate of skin grafting. Nursing care for sacrococcygeal skin grafting surgery is very important. After surgery, it is common to turn over in a lateral position, alternating between left and right lateral positions, using an air cushion bed and limb air cushion to prevent new pressure ulcers caused by limb weight compression.

5. Five days after the second skin grafting surgery, all free skin grafts survived, and the sacrococcygeal and heel pressure ulcers were completely cured and discharged (Figure 4.1.9, Figure 4.1.10).

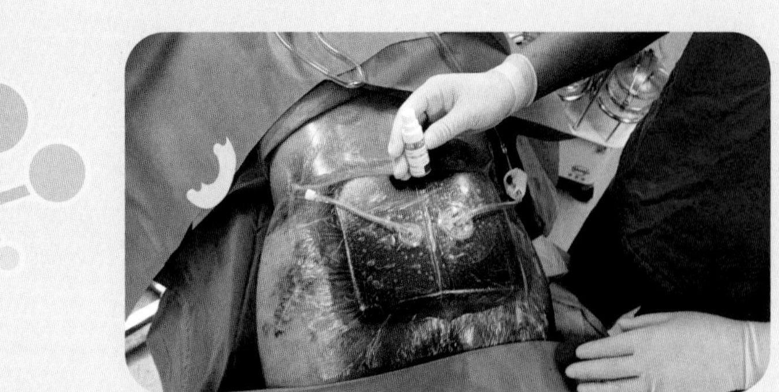

图 4.1.4　清创术 +VSD+ 重组人碱性成纤维细胞生长因子，促进创面新鲜，为植皮提供时间窗

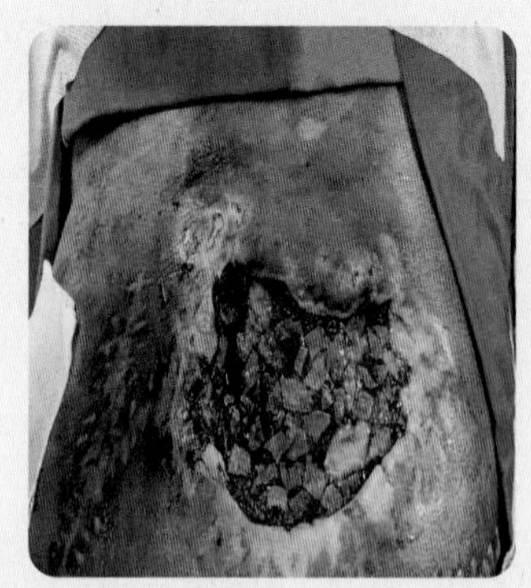

图 4.1.5　创面新鲜，第一次邮票点状植皮

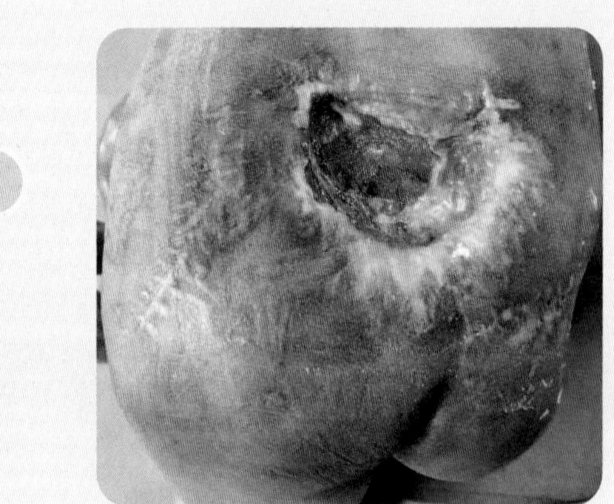

图 4.1.6　第一次植皮有部分成活，创面逐渐缩小

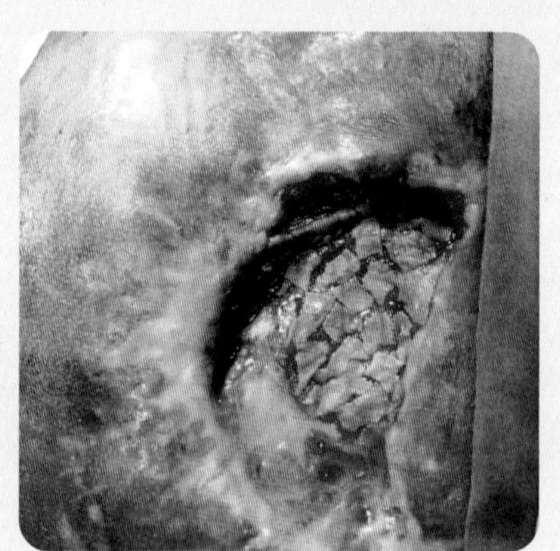

图 4.1.7　第二次邮票点状植皮

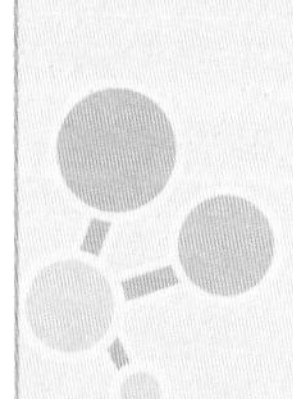

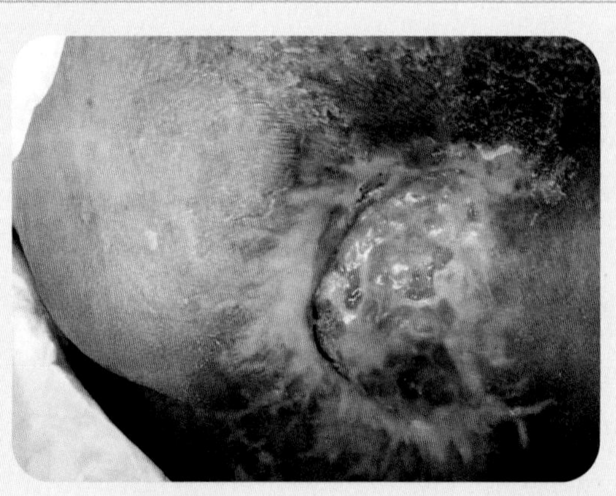

图 4.1.8　第二次植皮，植皮全部成活，创面基本痊愈

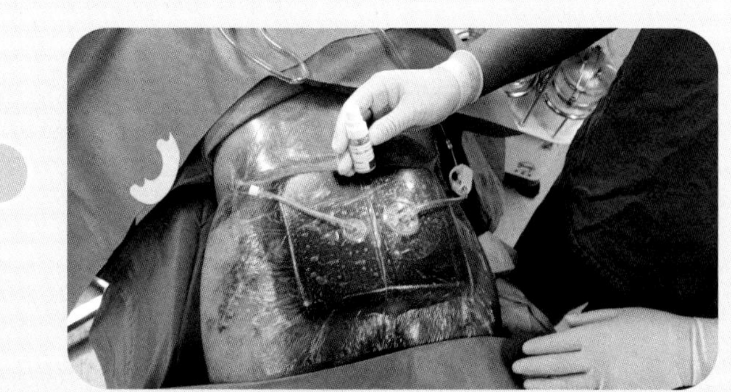

Figure 4.1.4 Debridement +VSD+ recombinant human basic fibroblast growth factor promotes wound freshness and provides a time window for skin grafting

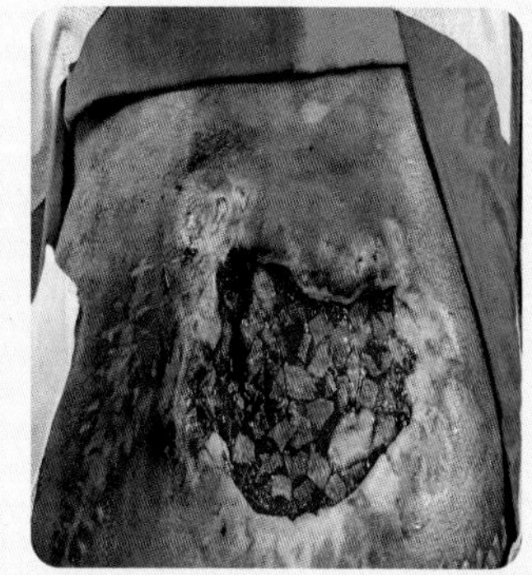

Figure 4.1.5 Fresh wound, first stamp like skin graft

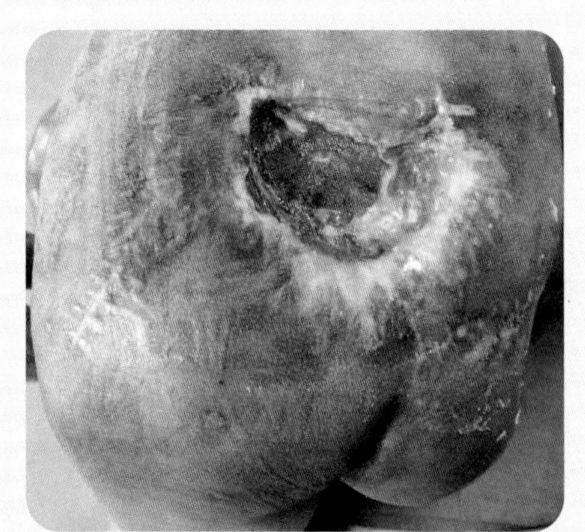

Figure 4.1.6 Partial survival of the first skin graft, with the wound gradually shrinking

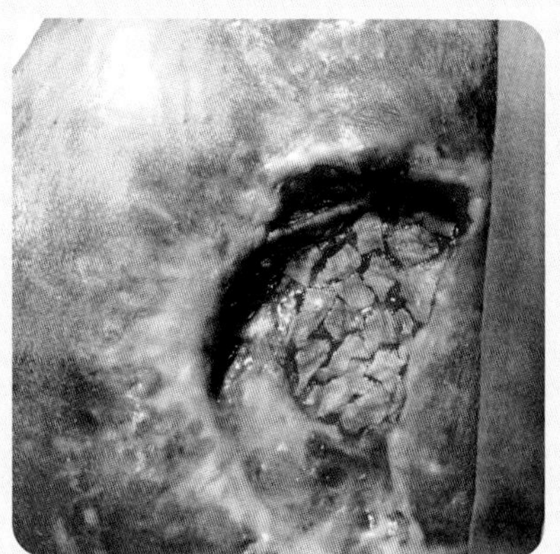

Figure 4.1.7 Second Stamp Spot Skin Transplantation

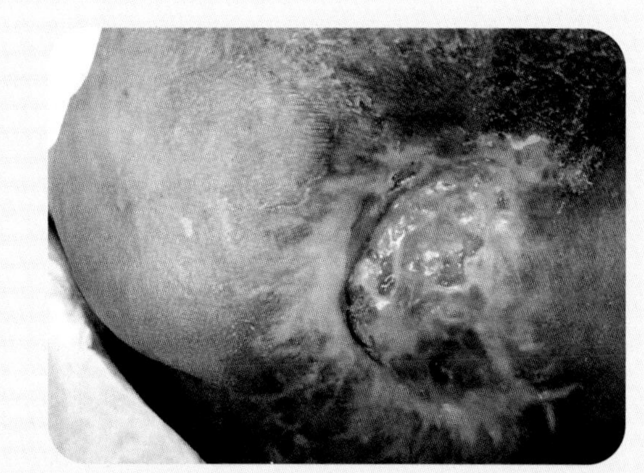

Figure 4.1.8 Second skin grafting, all skin grafts survived, and the wound was basically healed

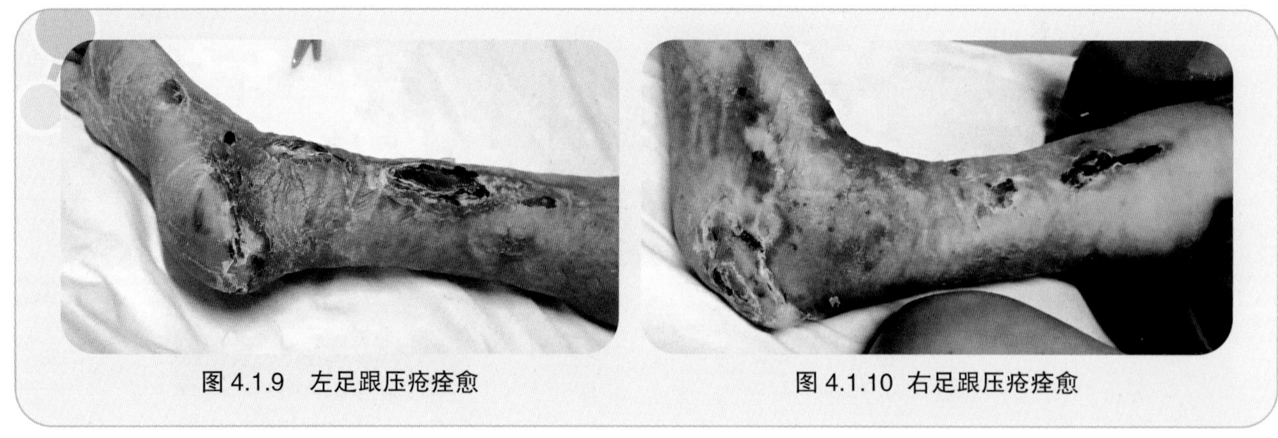

图 4.1.9　左足跟压疮痊愈　　图 4.1.10　右足跟压疮痊愈

（陈善亮）

案例二　右髋压疮合并坏死性肌筋膜炎

◆ 致病原因

患者为 42 岁中年男性，因车祸致胸椎骨折高位截瘫，致右侧髋部压疮髋部坏死性筋膜炎 25 年。

◆ 症状与体征

右侧髋部大粗隆有 6 cm × 4 cm 溃疡，创腔较深且潜行，股骨大粗隆筋膜坏死，混合白色脓液溢出，皮下脂肪液化，局部皮缘内陷，瘢痕硬化，下肢肌肉严重萎缩，髋关节膝关节足踝关节弯曲僵硬，平脐以下感觉运动缺失，足背动脉搏动减弱，胸背正中有 15 cm 纵行切口瘢痕，局部反复破溃流脓，味恶臭。

◆ 治疗方案

1. 入院完善全身情况评估，细菌培养 + 药物敏感试验，使用敏感抗菌药物。

2. 一期，清创 +VSD+ 重组人碱性成纤维细胞生长因子冲洗（图 4.2.1）。

3. 二期，设计臀上筋膜皮瓣，坏死筋膜和筋膜腔彻底切除，利用臀大肌皮瓣填塞无效腔，然后皮瓣覆盖创面，深部创腔放置负压引流管（图 4.2.2 ~ 图 4.2.7）。

4. 术后 3 天后拔出引流管，15 天拆线。

5. 术后多鼓励患者俯卧位，避免骶尾部和皮瓣受压，防止形成新的压疮。

6. 由于骶尾部压疮，贴近肛门、尿道（女性患者增加了阴道部位），应增加高蛋白、高维生素、易于消化的食物，减少食物残渣排泄，以免污染术后切口。

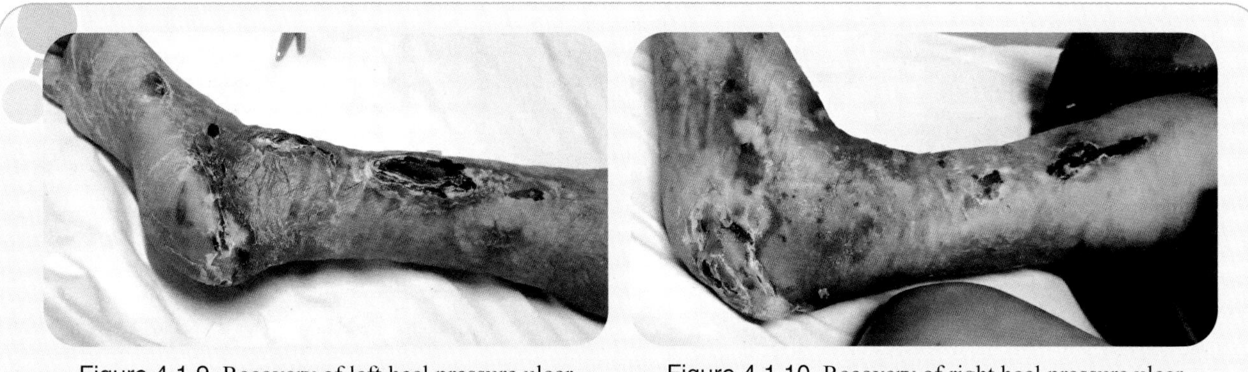

Figure 4.1.9 Recovery of left heel pressure ulcer　　Figure 4.1.10 Recovery of right heel pressure ulcer

(Chen Shanliang)

Case 2 Right hip pressure ulcer combined with necrotizing fasciitis

◆ Cause of illness

The patient is a 42-year-old middle-aged male who suffered a thoracic vertebral fracture and high paraplegia due to a car accident, resulting in a pressure ulcer on the right hip and necrotizing fasciitis of the hip for 25 years.

◆ Signs and symptoms

There is a 6 cm × 4 cm ulcer on the right hip's greater trochanter, with a deep and insidious wound cavity. The fascia of the femur's greater trochanter is necrotic, mixed with white pus overflow, subcutaneous fat liquefaction, local skin margin invagination, scar hardening, severe muscle atrophy in the lower limbs, hip joint, knee joint, ankle joint bending and stiffness, sensory and motor loss below the navel, weakened dorsalis pedis artery pulsation, and a 15 cm longitudinal incision scar in the center of the chest and back. The local area repeatedly ruptures and flows pus, with a foul odor.

◆ Treatment plan

1. Complete a comprehensive assessment of the overall condition upon admission, including bacterial culture and drug sensitivity testing, and use of sensitive antibiotics.
2. Phase 1, debridement + VSD + recombinant human basic fibroblast growth factor washing (Figure 4.2.1).
3. In the second phase, design a fascial flap on the buttocks, completely remove the necrotic fascia and fascial cavity, use the gluteus maximus flap to fill the ineffective cavity, then cover the wound with the flap, and place a negative pressure drainage tube in the deep wound cavity (Figure 4.2.2-Figure 4.2.7).
4. Remove the drainage tube 3 days after surgery and remove the suture 15 days later.
5. Encourage patients to lie prone after surgery to avoid compression of the sacrococcygeal region and skin flaps, and prevent the formation of new pressure ulcers.
6. Due to sacrococcygeal pressure ulcers, which are close to the anus and urethra (female patients have an increased vaginal area), high protein, high vitamin, and easily digestible foods should be added to reduce food residue excretion and avoid contaminating the postoperative incision.

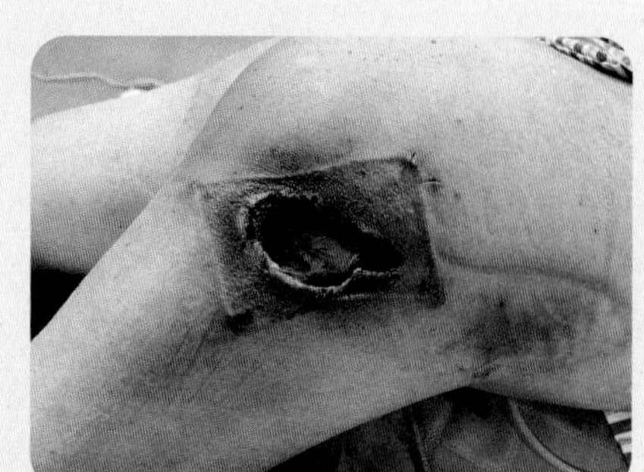

图 4.2.1　右侧髋部大粗隆处可见较深溃疡（已经过 VSD 治疗 1 次，创腔基本干净）

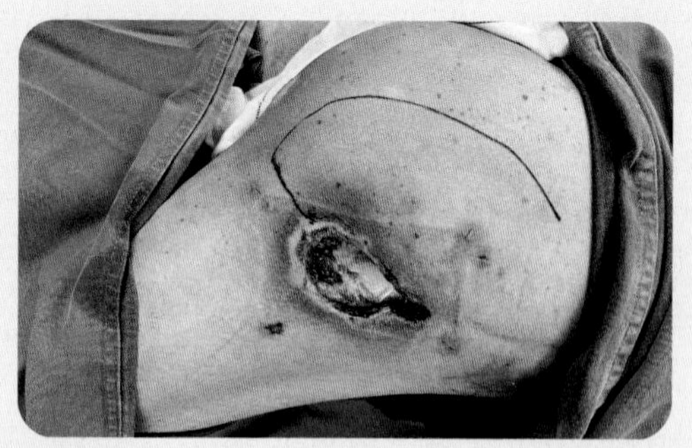

图 4.2.2　于臀部设计臀上筋膜蒂皮瓣示意

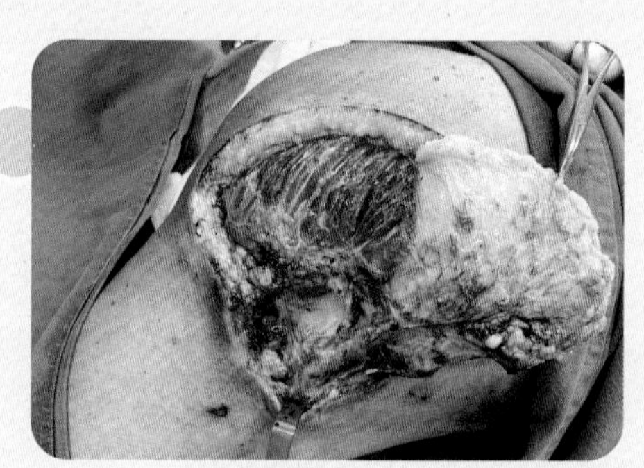

图 4.2.3　手术掀起皮瓣，显露深部较大筋膜腔和坏死滑膜，缺血韧带

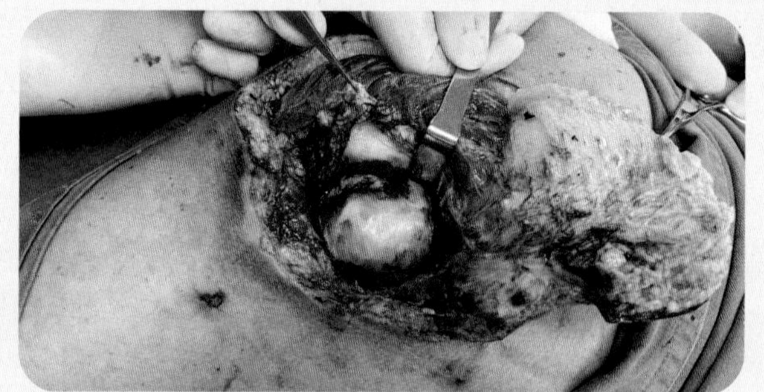

图 4.2.4　掀起臀大肌部分，显露股骨粗隆深部滑膜腔，充满淡黄色炎性液体

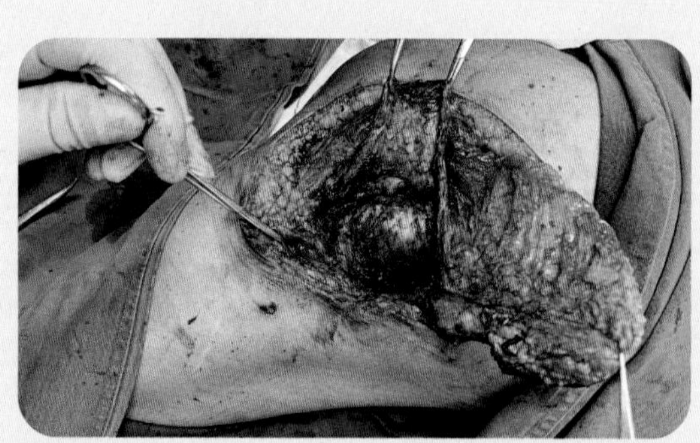

图 4.2.5　彻底切除滑膜组织和滑膜腔、待闭合伤口

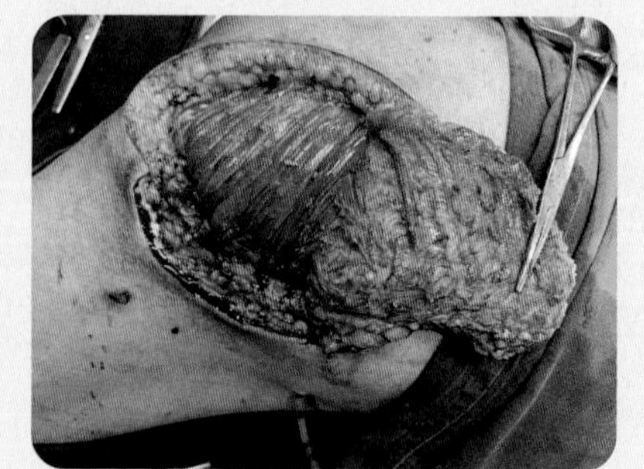

图 4.2.6　滑膜腔清创结束后，将臀大肌皮瓣填塞无效腔，深部放置引流管

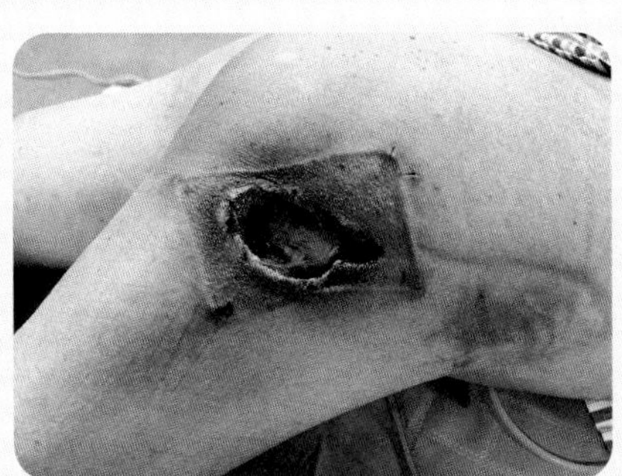

Figure 4.2.1 Deep ulcer can be seen at the large trochanter of the right hip (already treated with VSD once, the wound cavity is basically clean)

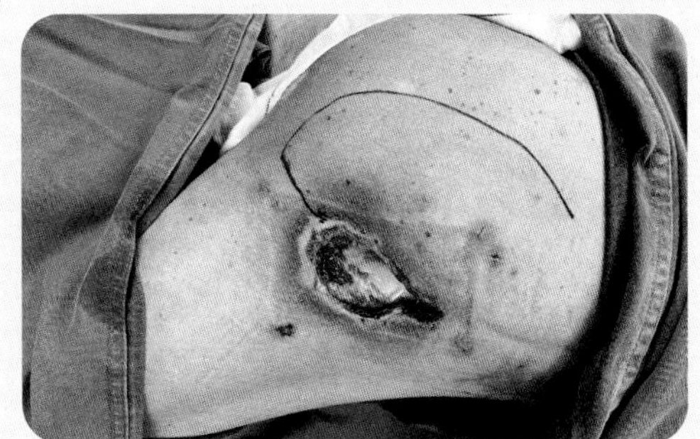

Figure 4.2.2 Schematic diagram of the design of the fascia pedicle flap on the buttocks

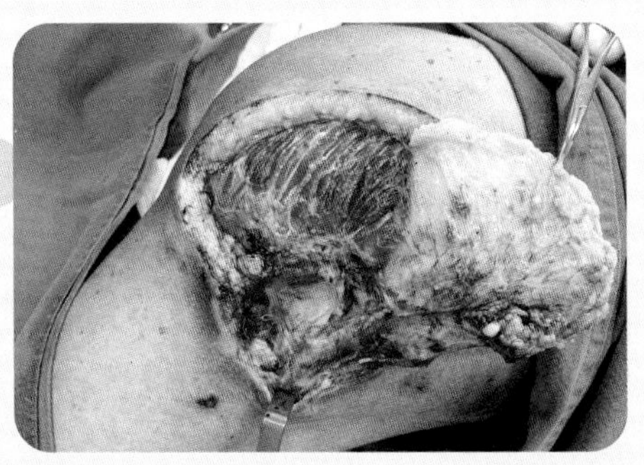

Figure 4.2.3 Surgical lifting of the skin flap reveals a large deep fascial cavity and necrotic synovium, as well as ischemic ligaments

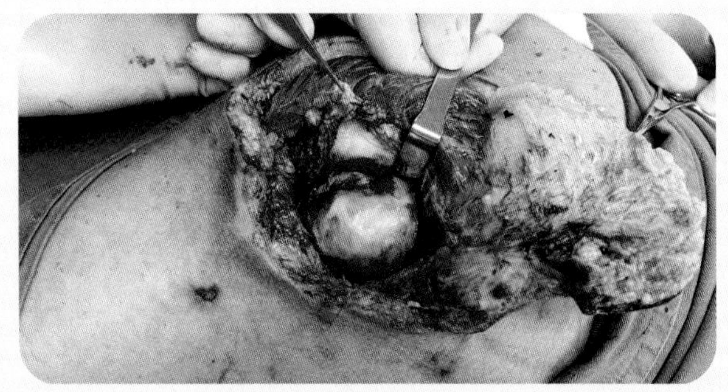

Figure 4.2.4 Lift up the gluteus maximus muscle to expose the deep synovial cavity of the femur trochanter, which is filled with pale yellow inflammatory fluid

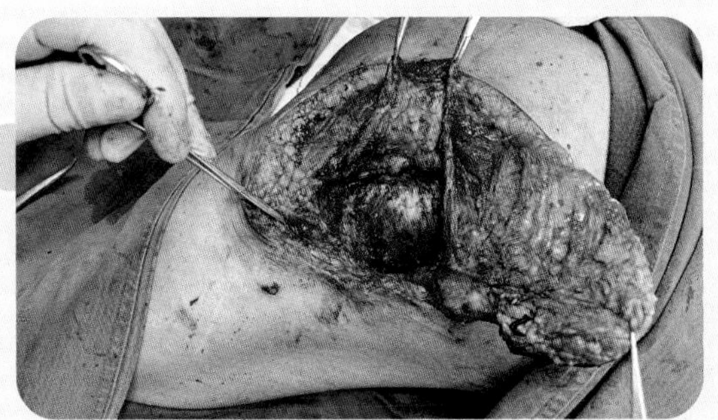

Figure 4.2.5 Thoroughly remove synovial tissue and synovial cavity, and open wound to be closed

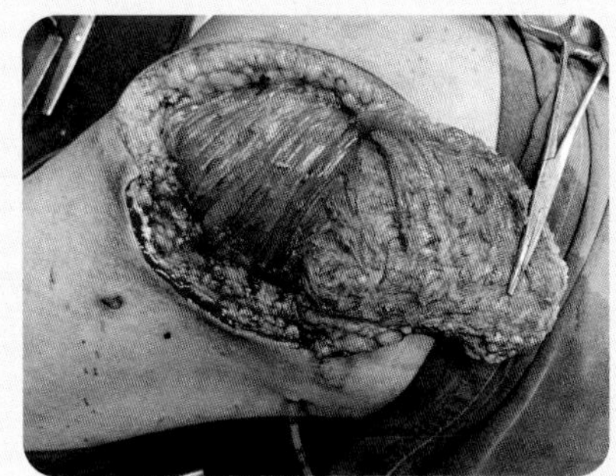

Figure 4.2.6 After the synovial cavity debridement is completed, fill the ineffective cavity with the gluteus maximus skin flap and place a drainage tube in the deep part

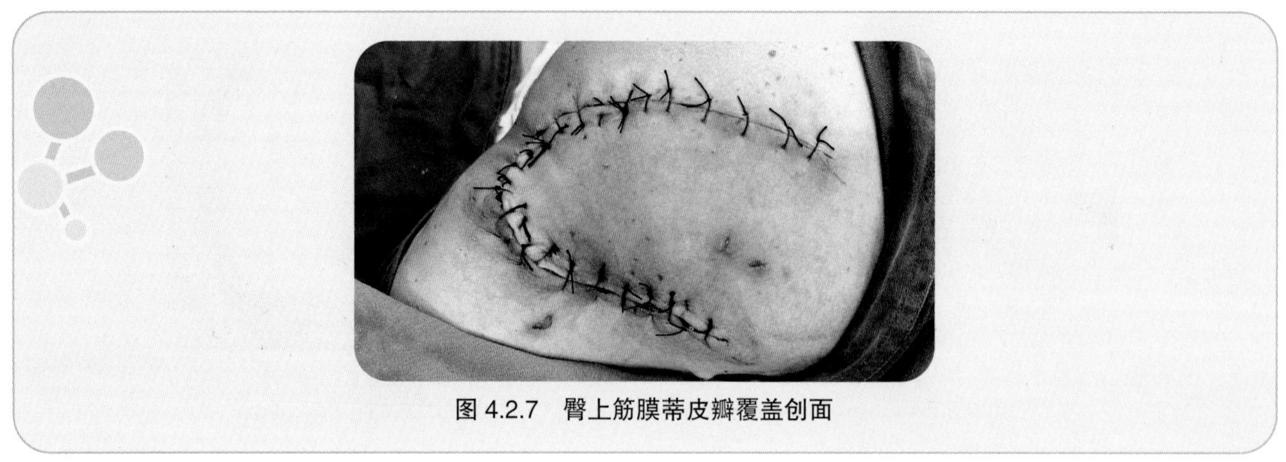

图 4.2.7 臀上筋膜蒂皮瓣覆盖创面

（陈善亮）

案例三 左侧髋关节化脓性感染伴压疮

◆ 致病原因

患者，男性，56 岁，因车祸致颈椎骨折颈髓损伤伴高位截瘫 11 年，左髋关节化脓性感染伴压疮。

◆ 症状与体征

患者颈椎骨折脊髓损伤伴高位截瘫 11 年，骶尾部压破左髋反复破溃流脓 9 年。颈后侧有 7 cm 纵行切口瘢痕，平乳头以下感觉运动消失，下肢严重萎缩，髋关节、膝关节、足踝关节僵硬，足背动脉搏动减弱，足趾感觉运动消失。骶尾部有 2 cm × 2 cm 压疮；左侧坐骨结节有 1 cm × 1 cm 压疮，较浅表，周边皮肤有较硬瘢痕；左侧髋部大粗隆处有 4 cm × 5 cm 压疮，有较深腔隙，深达大粗隆和关节间隙中，可触及增生滑膜组织，有较多炎性渗出，可触及股骨大粗隆虫食样变（图 4.3.1）。

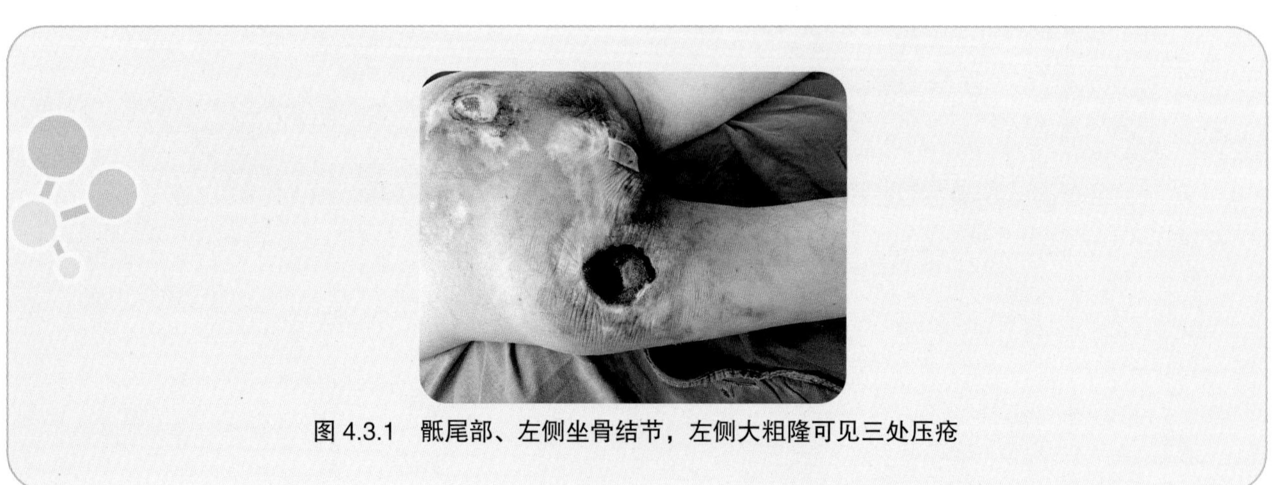

图 4.3.1 骶尾部、左侧坐骨结节，左侧大粗隆可见三处压疮

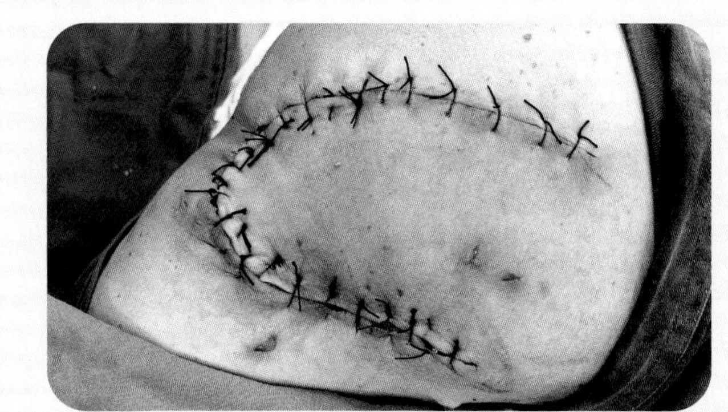

Figure 4.2.7 Covering the wound with the fascial flap of the superior gluteal fascia

(Chen Shanliang)

Case 3 Purulent infection with pressure ulcers in the left hip joint

◆ Cause of illness

The patient, a 56-year-old male, suffered from cervical spine fracture and spinal cord injury with high paraplegia due to a car accident for 11 years. He also had purulent infection of the left hip joint with pressure ulcers.

◆ Signs and symptoms

The patient suffered from cervical spine fracture and spinal cord injury accompanied by high paraplegia for 11 years, and repeated rupture and pus discharge from the left hip due to sacrococcygeal compression for 9 years. There is a 7-cm longitudinal incision scar on the back of the neck, and the sensation and movement below the nipple disappear. The lower limbs are severely atrophied, and the hip, knee, and ankle joints are stiff. The pulsation of the dorsalis pedis artery is weakened, and the sensation and movement of the toes disappear. There are 2 cm × 2 cm pressure ulcers in the coccyx; There is a 1 cm × 1 cm pressure ulcer on the left ischial tuberosity, which is relatively superficial and has hard scars on the surrounding skin; There is a 4 cm × 5 cm pressure ulcer at the left hip's greater trochanter, with deep cavities reaching into the greater trochanter and joint space. Hypertrophic synovial tissue can be felt, and there is a lot of inflammatory exudate. Insect like changes can be felt in the femur's greater trochanter (Figure 4.3.1).

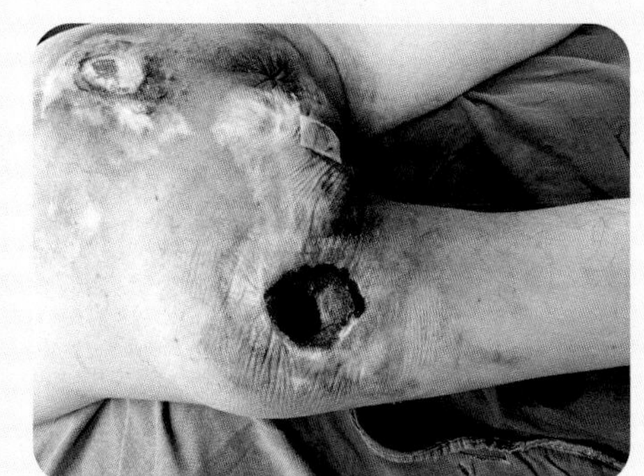

Figure 4.3.1 Sacral coccyx, left ischial tuberosity, and three pressure ulcers visible on the left greater trochanter

◆ 治疗方案

1. 入院后训练俯卧位，减少平卧继续受压次数。

2. 细菌培养 + 药物敏感试验，使用敏感抗菌药物，加强换药。

3. 一期，清创 +VSD+ 重组人碱性成纤维细胞生长因子冲洗。

4. 二期，亚加蓝颜色扩创，坏死筋膜、感染骨切除，局部皮瓣覆盖（图 4.3.2 ～图 4.3.5）。

5. 引流少于 10 mL 拔出，拔出引流条前，局部超声检查，确定是否有深部积液。

6. 术后 2 周拆线，持续训练俯卧位休息。

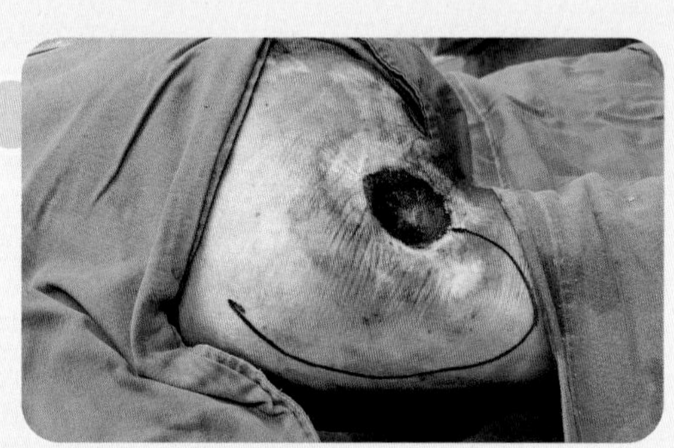

图 4.3.2　深部滑膜腔注入亚加蓝颜色，局部设计切口线

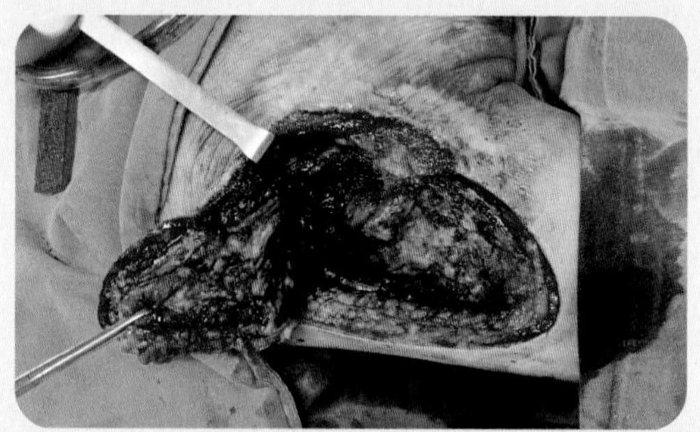

图 4.3.3　按切口线逐层进入，并显露亚加蓝颜色组织

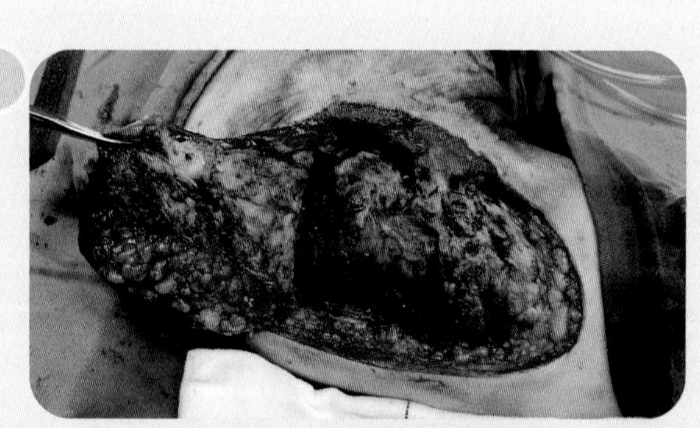

图 4.3.4　亚加蓝颜色组织彻底切除并止血

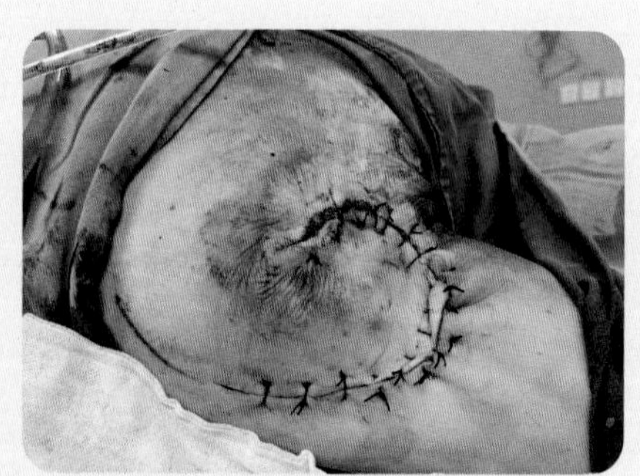

图 4.3.5　臀部皮瓣覆盖创面

（陈善亮）

◆ Treatment plan

1. After admission, train in a prone position to reduce the number of times one continues to be under pressure while lying flat.

2. Bacterial culture + drug sensitivity test, use sensitive antibiotics, and strengthen dressing changes.

3. Phase one, debridement +VSD+ recombinant human basic fibroblast growth factor washing.

4. In the second stage, methylene blue color expansion was performed, necrotic fascia and infected bone were removed, and local skin flaps were used for coverage (Figure 4.3.2 - Figure 4.3.5).

5. If the drainage volume is less than 10 mL, remove it. Before removing the drainage strip, perform a local ultrasound examination to determine if there is any deep fluid accumulation.

6. Remove the stitches 2 weeks after surgery and continue training in a prone position for rest.

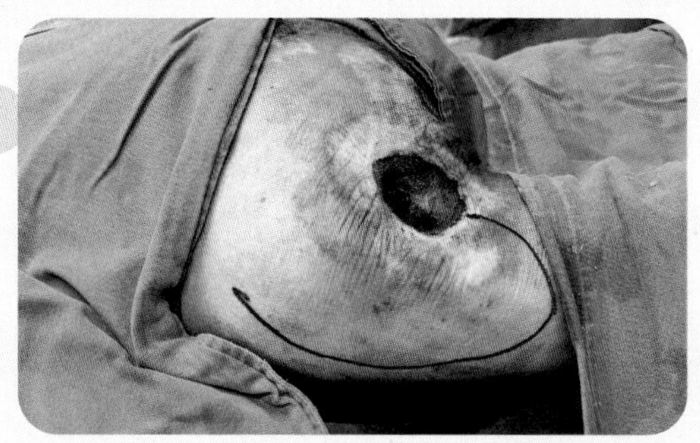

Figure 4.3.2 Deep synovial cavity injection with methylene blue color, locally designed incision line

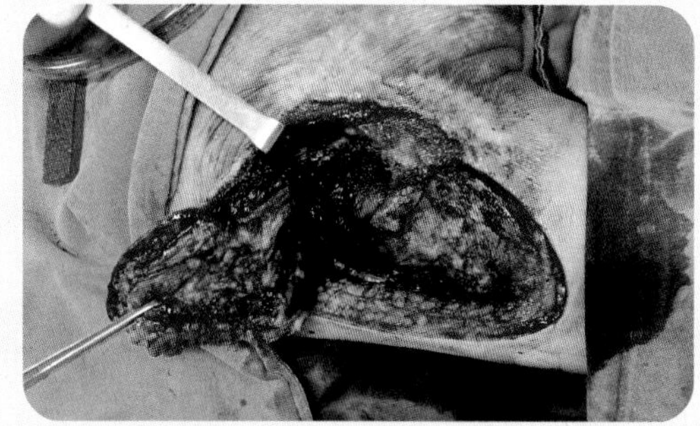

Figure 4.3.3 Enter layer by layer according to the incision line and expose the methylene blue colored tissue

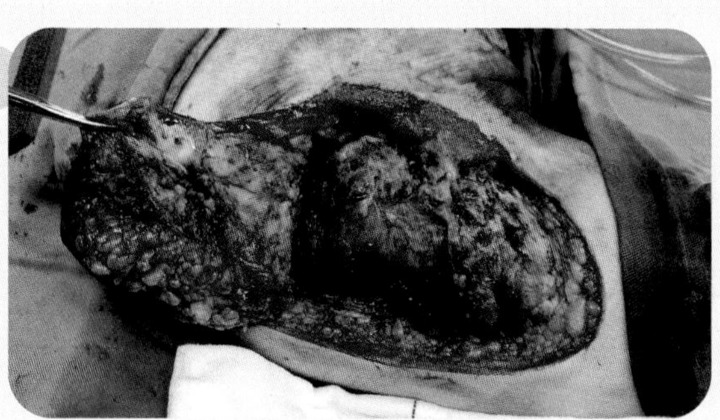

Figure 4.3.4 Complete resection and hemostasis of methylene blue colored tissue

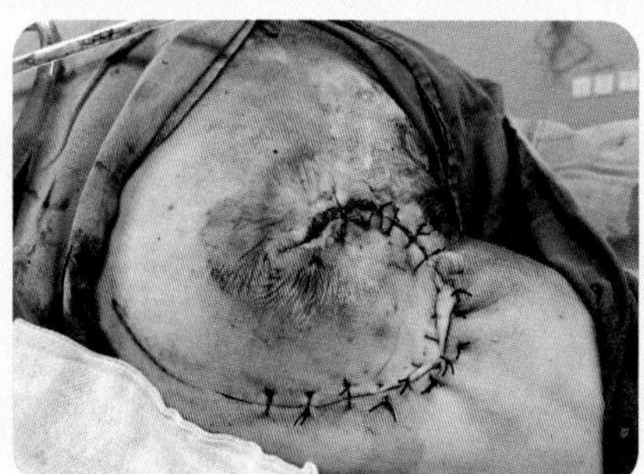

Figure 4.3.5 Hip skin flap covering wound

(Chen Shanliang)

案例四　舞蹈症失能伴骶尾部压疮

◆ 致病原因

患者，女性，62 岁，患舞蹈症 5 年，失能而卧床，骶尾部出现压疮。

◆ 症状与体征

患者体态消瘦，严重营养不良，神志不清，牙齿咬合摩擦不停，头颈及四肢不自主抽动，口唇及齿龈苍白重度，指甲苍白。骶尾部有 6 cm × 7 cm 创面，创面内陷似火山口，肉芽组织污秽不清、水肿，创面中间有坏死组织间桥相连，骶骨外露，皮缘下方潜行，创面有大量炎性渗出，味恶臭（图 4.4.1）。

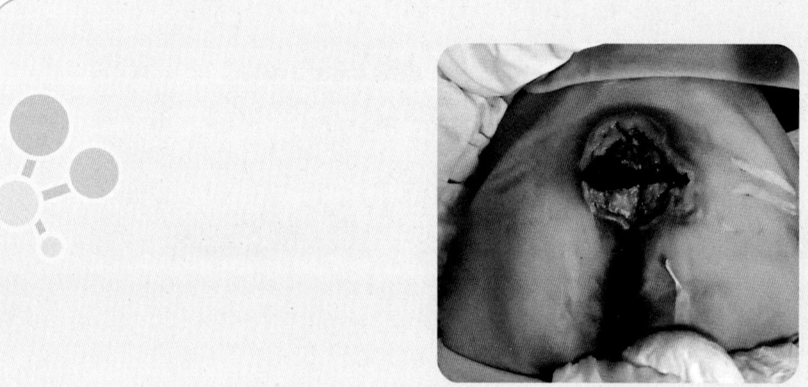

图 4.4.1　骶尾部有 6 cm × 7 cm 压疮，压疮中心有坏死组织间桥

◆ 治疗方案

1. 局部细菌培养 + 药物敏感试验，选用敏感抗菌药物。

2. 加强基础护理，定时翻身，防止继续受压。

3. 加强关节松动，防止关节痉挛强直。

4. 创面清创局部换药，换药时创面喷洒重组人碱性成纤维细胞生长因子，促进创面肉芽组织新鲜。由于创面有大量炎性渗出，每天增加换药次数。

5. 经过半个月换药，创面逐渐新鲜，肉芽组织饱满，采用臀上筋膜蒂皮瓣移植。

6. 手术过程

6.1 麻醉选择：气管插管全身麻醉。

6.2 麻醉生效后，采用俯卧位，手术区域碘伏常规消毒，铺无菌巾单。

6.3 皮瓣设计：于左侧臀部设计臀上筋膜蒂皮瓣，皮瓣蒂宽 5.5 cm，皮瓣长 12 cm，解剖面为肌筋膜层。修剪创缘并刮出增生肉芽组织，压迫创面渗血（图 4.4.2）。

Case 4 Dysfunction of chorea with sacrococcygeal pressure ulcers

◆ Cause of illness

Patient, female, 62 years old, has been suffering from chorea for 5 years, is bedridden due to disability, and has pressure ulcers in the coccyx.

◆ Signs and symptoms

The patient has a thin body, severe malnutrition, confusion, constant friction between teeth, involuntary twitching of the head, neck, and limbs, severe pale lips and gums, and pale nails. There is a 6 cm × 7 cm wound on the coccyx, which is sunken like a volcano. The granulation tissue is dirty and swollen, and there is a bridge connecting necrotic tissue in the middle of the wound. The sacrum is exposed, and the skin edge is hidden below. There is a large amount of inflammatory exudate and a foul odor on the wound (Figure 4.4.1).

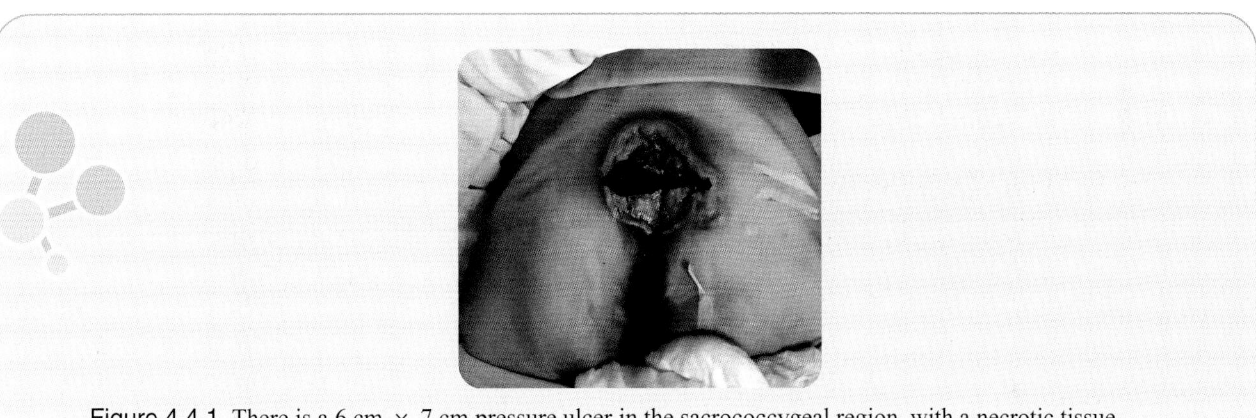

Figure 4.4.1 There is a 6 cm × 7 cm pressure ulcer in the sacrococcygeal region, with a necrotic tissue bridge at the center of the ulcer

◆ Treatment plan

1. Local bacterial culture + drug sensitivity test, using sensitive antibiotics.

2. Strengthen basic care, regularly turn over, and prevent further pressure.

3. Strengthen joint looseness to prevent joint spasms and rigidity.

4. Local dressing change for wound debridement, spraying recombinant human basic fibroblast growth factor on the wound during dressing change to promote fresh granulation tissue. Due to the large amount of inflammatory exudate from the wound, increase the frequency of dressing changes daily.

5. After half a month of dressing change, the wound gradually became fresh and the granulation tissue was plump. A buttock fascia pedicle flap was used for transplantation.

6. Surgical process

6.1 Anesthesia selection: General anesthesia with tracheal intubation.

6.2 After the anesthesia takes effect, the patient is placed in a prone position, disinfected with iodine in the surgical area, and a sterile drape is laid.

6.3 Skin flap design: A fascial pedicle skin flap with a width of 5.5 cm and a length of 12 cm is designed on the left buttock, and the anatomical surface is the myofascial layer. Trim the wound margin and scrape out the proliferating granulation tissue, compressing the wound and causing bleeding (Figure 4.4.2).

6.4 皮瓣移植：依次切开皮瓣皮肤皮下脂肪直达臀上筋膜层，将皮瓣游离掀起，结扎活动出血点，创面喷洒重组人碱性成纤维细胞生长因子，皮瓣与受区移植并缝合，供区创口直接缝合，皮瓣下放置橡皮条引流。包扎伤口，术终（图 4.4.3）。

7. 术后加强控制舞蹈症用药，以减轻全身不自主抽搐，防止皮瓣缝线拉脱。多采用侧卧位避免皮瓣受压。

8. 加强换药，换药时喷洒重组人碱性成纤维细胞生长因子，术后 3 天拔出橡皮条，术后 12 天拆线。

9. 骶尾部压疮患者，大多数为失能人群，这样人群对护理依赖要求很高，术后加强护理十分重要。

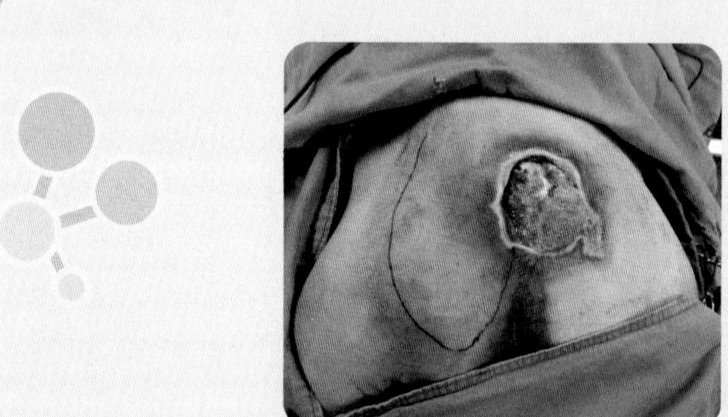

图 4.4.2　经过清创、换药、喷洒重组人碱性成纤维细胞生长因子，创面新鲜，臀上筋膜蒂皮瓣设计示意

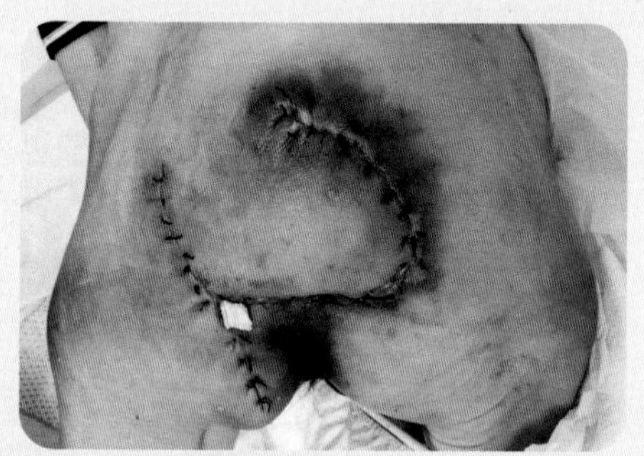

图 4.4.3　皮瓣移植后 3 天，皮瓣血运和外形良好

（陈善亮）

案例五　人工股骨头置换术后骶尾部巨大压疮

◆ 致病原因

患者，女性，78 岁，左侧股骨头骨折人工股骨头置换术后，卧床骶尾部压破，经久不愈合 6 月余。

◆ 症状与体征

患者卧床状态，不能下地自理，下肢各关节弯曲畸形，膝关节屈曲挛缩，下肢肌肉萎缩，足背动脉搏动良好，感觉正常，轻度贫血貌，骶尾部有 12 cm × 9 cm 较深凹陷行压疮，深达尾骨棘突和横突，骶尾部有坏死筋膜，并有稀薄黄白色脓液溢出，味臭，溃疡周边皮肤潜行游离，左侧髋关节触及脱位状态（图 4.5.1）。局部触痛明显。

6.4 Skin flap transplantation: sequentially cut open the subcutaneous fat of the skin flap to reach the fascia layer above the buttocks, lift the skin flap free, ligate the active bleeding point, spray recombinant human basic fibroblast growth factor on the wound, transplant and suture the skin flap to the recipient area, directly suture the donor site wound, and place a rubber strip under the skin flap for drainage. Wrap the wound and perform the surgery (Figure 4.4.3).

7. Strengthen postoperative medication control for chorea to alleviate involuntary convulsions throughout the body and prevent flap suture detachment. Use a lateral position to avoid pressure on the skin flap.

8. Strengthen dressing changes, spray recombinant human basic fibroblast growth factor during dressing changes, remove the rubber strip 3 days after surgery, and remove the stitches 12 days after surgery.

9. Most patients with sacrococcygeal pressure ulcers are disabled individuals, who have a high demand for nursing care. Therefore, it is important to strengthen postoperative nursing care.

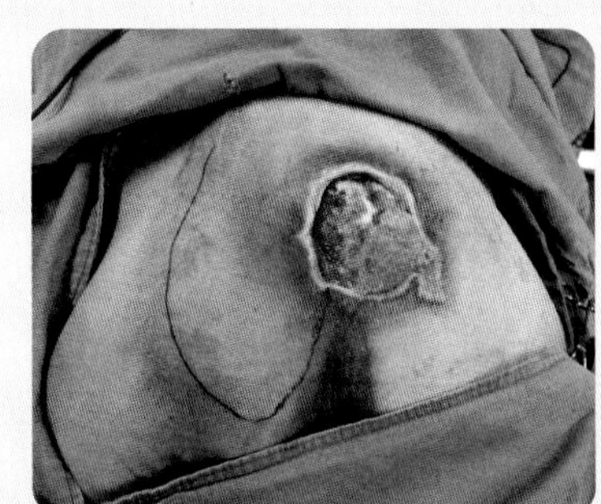

Figure 4.4.2 After debridement, dressing change, and spraying of recombinant human basic fibroblast growth factor, the wound is fresh, and the design of the gluteal fascia flap is illustrated

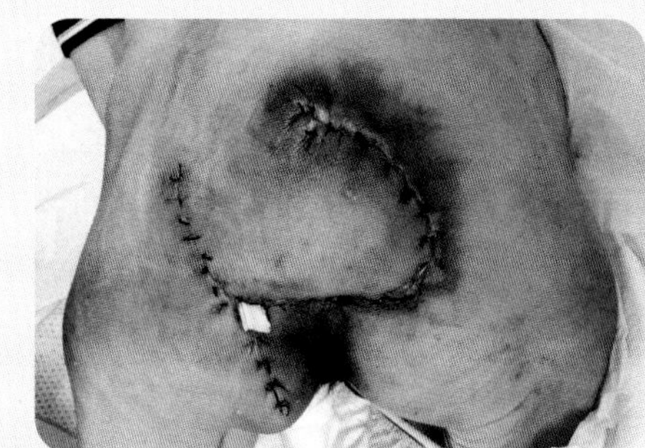

Figure 4.4.3 Three days after skin flap transplantation, the blood supply and appearance of the skin flap are good

(Chen Shanliang)

Case 5 Individuals with massive pressure ulcers in the sacrococcygeal region after femoral head replacement surgery

◆ Cause of illness

The patient, a 78-year-old female, had a left femoral head fracture and underwent artificial femoral head replacement surgery. She was bedridden with a coccygeal compression and did not heal for more than 6 months.

◆ Signs and symptoms

The patient is bedridden and unable to take care of themselves. The joints of the lower limbs are bent and deformed, the knee joint is flexed and contracted, the lower limb muscles are atrophied, and the dorsalis pedis artery has good pulsation and feels normal. The patient has a mild anemia appearance. There is a 12 cm × 9 cm deep depression and pressure ulcer in the coccyx, which extends to the spinous and transverse processes of the coccyx. There is necrotic fascia in the coccyx and coccyx, and there is thin yellow white pus overflow with a foul odor. The skin around the ulcer is free and the left hip joint is dislocated (Figure 4.5.1). Local tenderness is obvious.

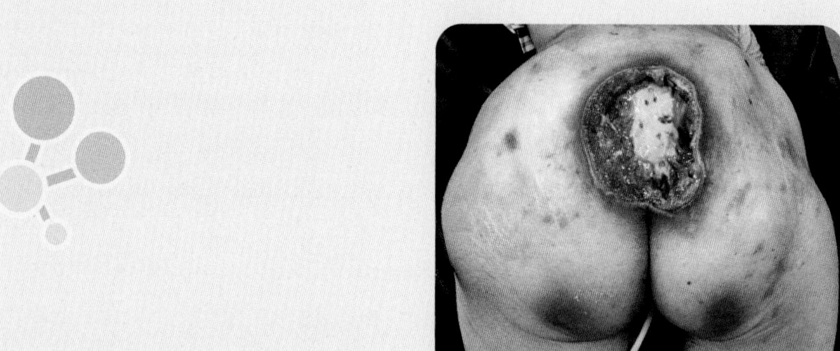

图 4.5.1 骶尾部见巨大创面，筋膜缺血坏死，肉芽组织灰白

◆ 治疗方案

由于患者年龄较大，骶尾部感染消耗，类似案例大多数伴有贫血低蛋白，合并肺部和尿路感染，入院时积极纠正基础疾病，否则创面很难愈合。

1. 局部细菌培养 + 药物敏感试验，给予敏感抗菌药物。

2. 加强创面换药，初始渗出较多，每天更换 2 次敷料，并及时清创坏死组织，凡坏死组织必须及时清除，不能等待自行脱落。

3. 加强翻身训练，既左侧卧位、右侧卧位、平卧位，避免骶尾部骨隆突处受压，增加患者卧位适应度。

4. 局部清创 +VSD+ 外用重组人碱性成纤维细胞生长因子，这样治疗可以减少换药次数，可以有效促进局部肉芽组织新鲜，改善局部血液循环，缩短治疗周期，为皮瓣移植争取时间窗。

5. 通过综合治疗后，全身基本情况得到明显改善，局部创面新鲜。给予左侧臀大肌肌皮瓣移植，移植于骶尾部溃疡，臀大肌可以有效填塞深部无效腔，由于臀大肌血运丰富，可以改善局部血运循环，促进创面愈合，但有增加局部受压度、放置骶尾部再次受压坏死、二次复发等缺点（图 4.5.2 ～图 4.5.5）。

6. 术后加强基础护理，加强换药，保持引流通畅，防止皮瓣下血肿形成和皮瓣下感染，术后 3 天拔出引流条。术后 2 周拆线，皮瓣成活，创面消灭，康复出院（图 4.5.6）。

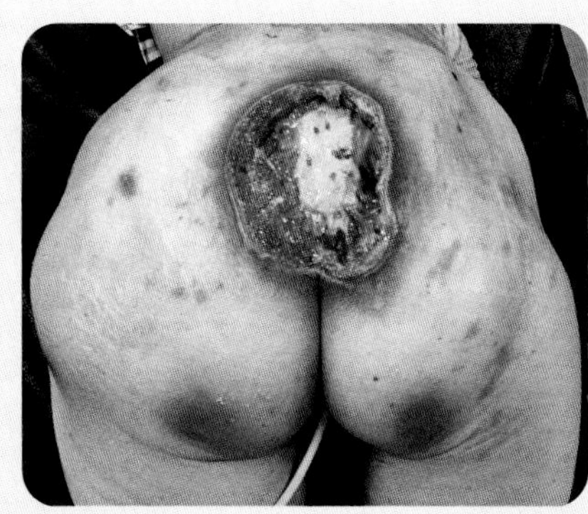

Figure 4.5.1 A huge wound is seen in the coccyx, with fascia ischemic necrosis and gray white granulation tissue

◆ Treatment plan

Due to the older age of the patients and the consumption of sacrococcygeal infections, most similar cases are accompanied by anemia and low protein, combined with pulmonary and urinary tract infections. It is important to actively correct underlying diseases upon admission, otherwise the wound will be difficult to heal.

1. Local bacterial culture + drug sensitivity test, administering sensitive antibiotics.

2. Strengthen wound dressing changes. If there is initial exudation, change the dressing twice a day and promptly remove necrotic tissue. Any necrotic tissue must be removed in a timely manner and cannot wait to fall off on its own.

3. Strengthen turning training, including left lateral position, right lateral position, and supine position, to avoid compression at the sacral and coccygeal bone prominence and increase the patient's adaptability to lying position.

4. Local debridement + VSD + topical application of recombinant human basic fibroblast growth factor can reduce dressing changes, effectively promote local granulation tissue freshness, improve local blood circulation, shorten the treatment period, and provide a time window for skin flap transplantation.

5. After comprehensive treatment, the overall basic condition of the body was significantly improved, and the local wounds were fresh. Transplantation of the left gluteus maximus muscle flap was performed on the ulcer of the coccyx. The gluteus maximus muscle can effectively fill the deep ineffective cavity. Due to the abundant blood supply of the gluteus maximus muscle, it can improve local blood circulation and promote wound healing. However, it has disadvantages such as increased local compression, re compression and necrosis of the coccyx, and secondary recurrence (Figure 4.5.2-Figure 4.5.5).

6. Strengthen basic nursing after surgery, enhance dressing changes, maintain smooth drainage, prevent hematoma formation and infection under the skin flap, and remove the drainage strip 3 days after surgery. Two weeks after surgery, the stitches were removed, the skin flap survived, the wound was eliminated, and the patient recovered and was discharged (Figure 4.5.6).

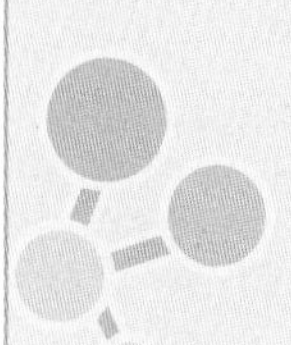

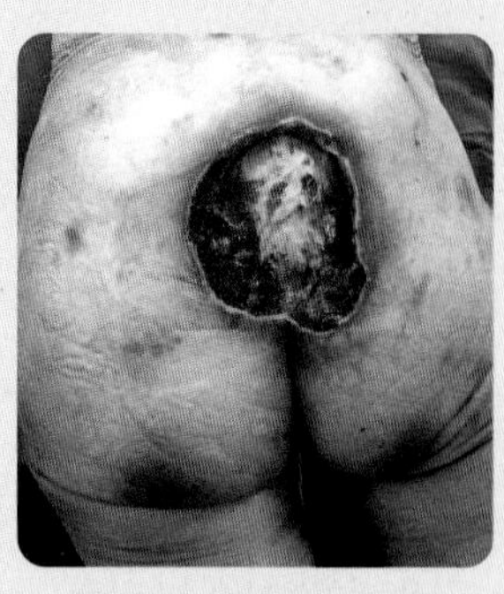

图 4.5.2　经过 1 次清创 +VSD+ 外用重组人碱性成纤维细胞生长因子治疗，创面逐渐新鲜

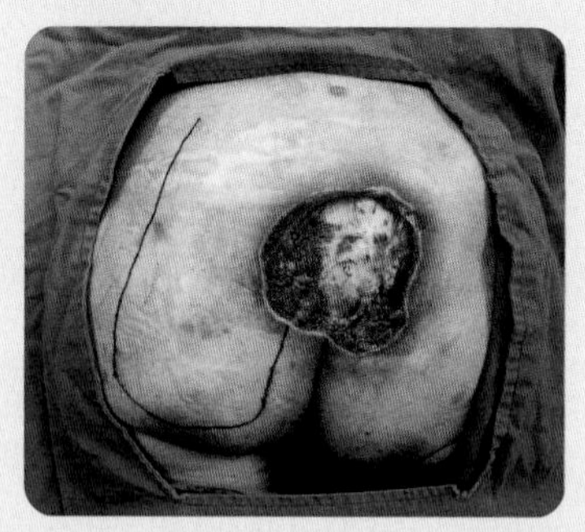

图 4.5.3　创面基本新鲜，没有继续坏死迹象、臀部皮瓣设计线

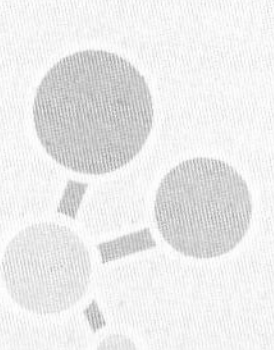

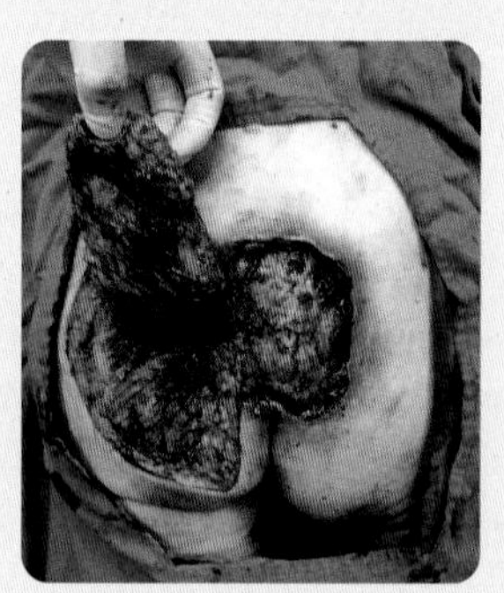

图 4.5.4　坏死筋膜彻底切除，臀部皮瓣游离并携带部分臀大肌组织填塞深腔

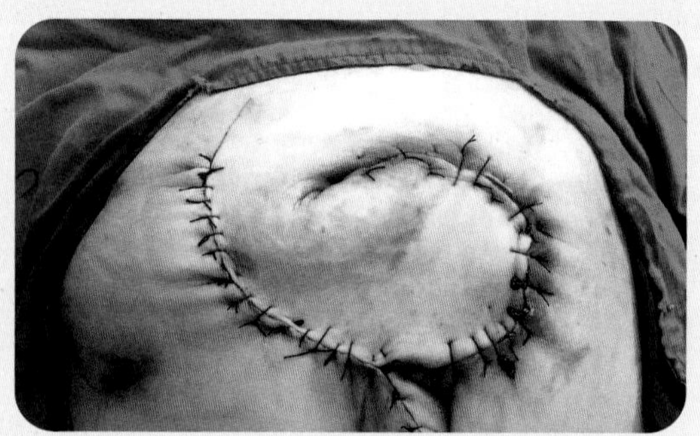

图 4.5.5　臀部皮瓣游离后覆盖巨大创面

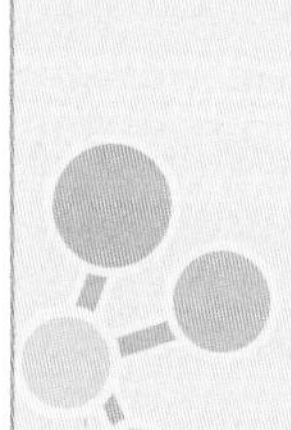

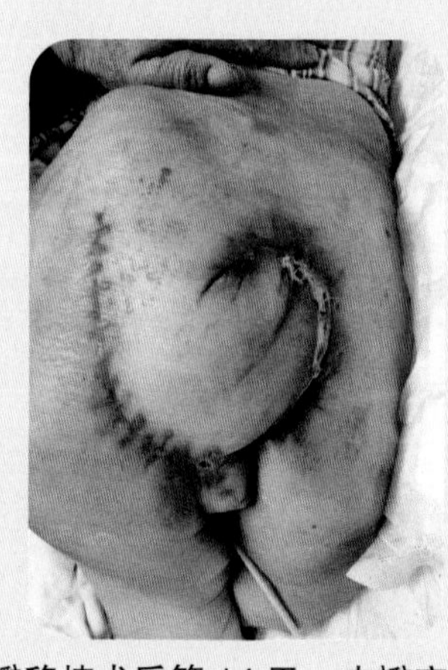

图 4.5.6　臀部皮瓣移植术后第 14 天，皮瓣完全成活并消灭创面

（陈善亮　李正英）

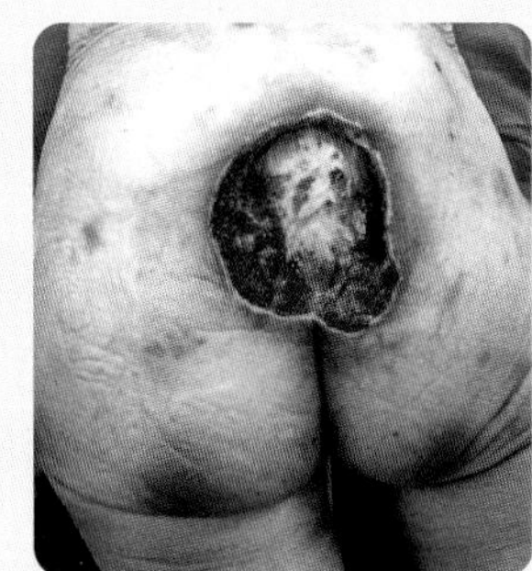

Figure 4.5.2 After one session of debridement + VSD + topical treatment with recombinant human basic fibroblast growth factor, the wound gradually becomes fresh

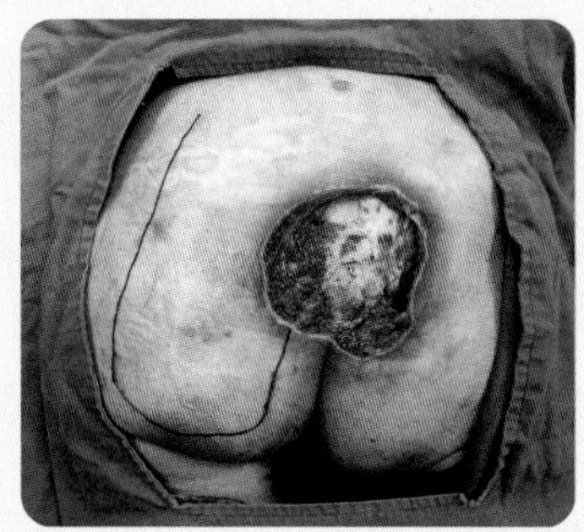

Figure 4.5.3 The wound is basically fresh, with no further signs of necrosis and the design line of the hip flap

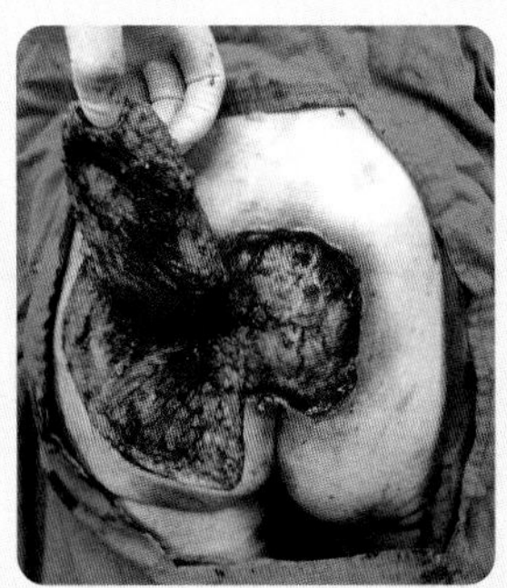

Figure 4.5.4 Complete removal of necrotic fascia, free hip skin flap and partial filling of dccp cavity with gluteus maximus muscle tissue

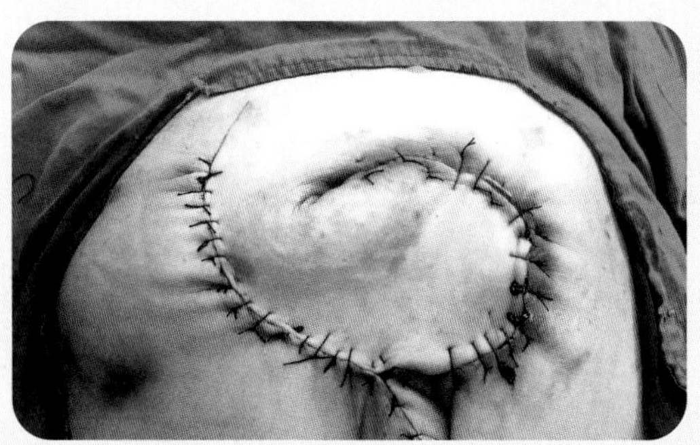

Figure 4.5.5 Covering a huge wound with a free hip skin flap

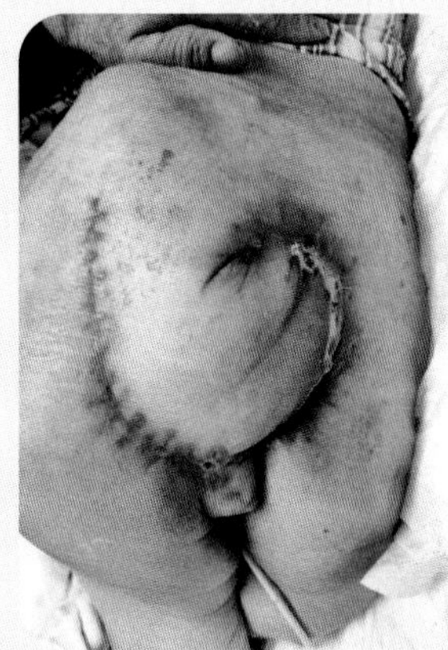

Figure 4.5.6 On the 14th day after the hip flap transplantation, the flap completely survived and eliminated the wound

(Chen Shanliang, Li Zhengying)

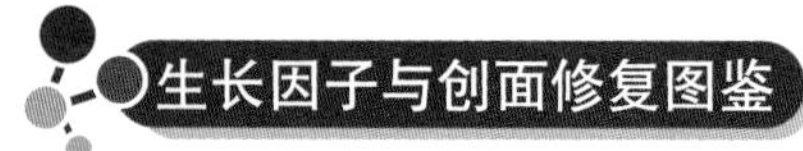

案例六　重度颅脑损伤偏瘫性骶尾部压疮

◆ 致病原因

患者，男性，72 岁，在工地被重物砸伤头部，致重度颅脑损伤，行开颅血肿清除术，术后偏瘫失语、尿便失禁、失能、骶尾部破损流脓流水并逐渐增大 5 年余。骶尾部多次住院手术史。

◆ 症状与体征

右侧颞顶部有巨大颅骨缺损，局部凹陷，有弧形切口瘢痕，左侧肢体偏瘫，肌力 0 级，四肢关节僵硬强直，仅右侧上肢腕手部关节肌力 3 级。骶尾部有 18 cm × 12 cm 凹陷压疮，局部有大量炎性渗出，皮缘硬化纤维板增厚，皮缘色沉，质地较硬，创面肉芽组织水肿，苍白（图 4.6.1）。污秽不清，触之不出血，局部味臭。

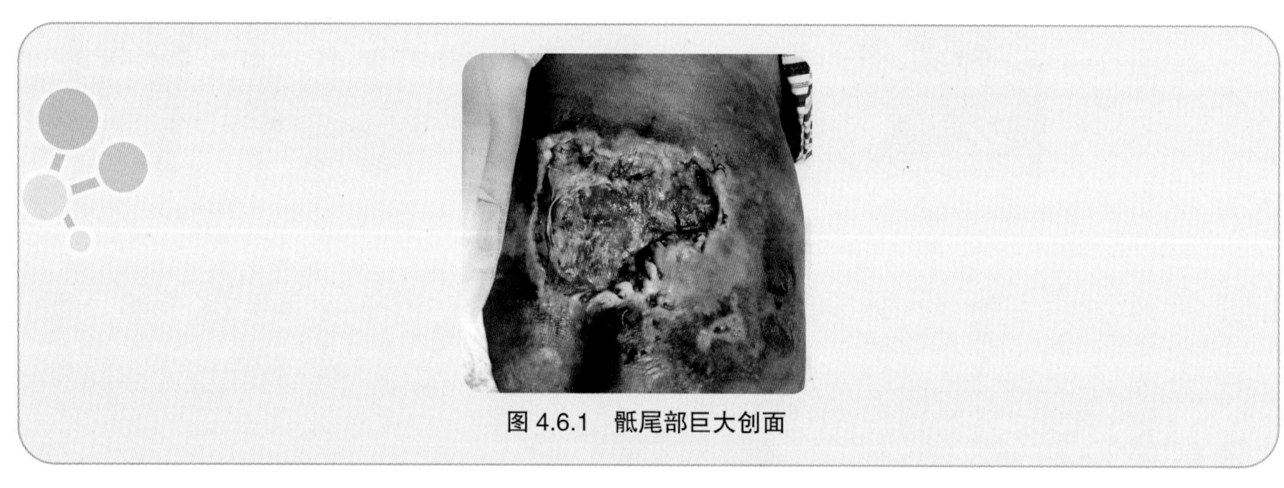
图 4.6.1　骶尾部巨大创面

◆ 治疗方案

1. 积极治疗基础疾病，纠正贫血、低蛋白血症。

2. 细菌培养 + 药物敏感试验，给予敏感抗菌药物。

3. 加强换药，机械性的刮除增生肉芽组织和坏死组织，创面每天更换敷料 2 次，并喷洒重组人碱性成纤维细胞生长因子，促进肉芽组织新鲜（图 4.6.2、图 4.6.3）。

4. 锻炼俯卧位休息姿势，避免平卧，减少臀部继续受压，下肢骨隆突处放置肢体垫，气垫圈，常规使用气垫床，加强翻身。

5. 增加高蛋白食物，减少食物残渣类饮食，多饮水，导尿留置定时开放导尿夹闭。

6. 创面完全新鲜后，局部行植皮手术，于左侧臀部切取中厚皮肤，并将游离皮肤修剪成 0.5 cm × 0.5 cm

Case 6 Hemiplegic sacrococcygeal pressure ulcer caused by severe traumatic brain injury 

◆ Cause of illness

The patient, a 72-year-old male, suffered a severe head injury due to being hit by a heavy object at a construction site. He underwent craniotomy for hematoma removal surgery, and after the surgery, he became hemiplegic, aphasia, urinary and fecal incontinence, disability, and had pus discharge from the sacrococcygeal region, which gradually increased for more than 5 years. History of multiple hospitalizations and surgeries for the sacrococcygeal region.

◆ Signs and symptoms

There is a huge skull defect and local depression at the top of the right temporal lobe, with arc-shaped incision scars. The left limb is hemiplegic with muscle strength grade 0, and the limb joints are stiff and rigid. Only the wrist hand joint muscle strength of the right upper limb is grade 3. There are 18 cm × 12 cm concave pressure sores in the coccyx, with a large amount of inflammatory exudate in the local area. The skin edge is hardened, the fibrous plate is thickened, the skin edge is dark in color, the texture is hard, and the granulation tissue of the wound is swollen and pale (Figure 4.6.1). Unclear dirt, no bleeding when touched, local odor.

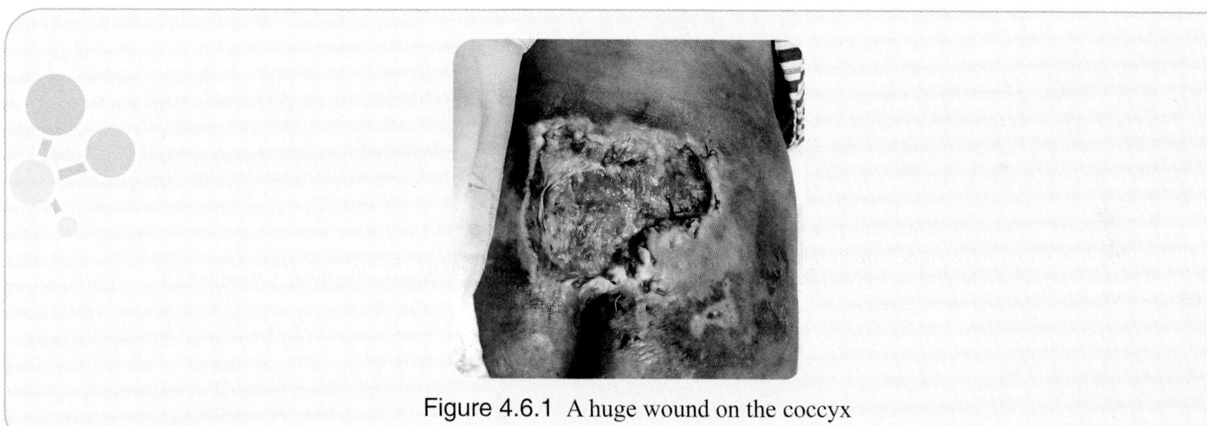

Figure 4.6.1 A huge wound on the coccyx

◆ Treatment plan

1. Actively treat underlying diseases, correct anemia and hypoalbuminemia.

2. Bacterial culture + drug sensitivity test, administering sensitive antibiotics.

3. Strengthen dressing changes, mechanically scrape off hypertrophic granulation tissue and necrotic tissue, change dressings twice a day on wounds, and spray recombinant human basic fibroblast growth factor to promote fresh granulation tissue (Figure 4.6.2, Figure 4.6.3).

4. Exercise the prone position for rest, avoid lying flat, reduce further pressure on the buttocks, place limb cushions and air cushion rings at the bone prominence of the lower limbs, regularly use an air cushion bed, and strengthen turning over.

5. Increase high protein foods, reduce food residue diets, drink more water, and keep the catheterization clip open and closed at regular intervals.

6. After the wound is completely fresh, local skin grafting surgery is performed. Medium thick skin is cut from

大小，分别游离移植于骶尾部创面，均匀的平铺在凹陷创面之中，外用重组人碱性成纤维细胞生长因子喷洒创面，取双层人工真皮修复材料覆盖植皮创面中，厚棉垫覆盖伤口粘贴包扎固定敷料，供皮敷贴凡士林油纱覆盖包扎。

7. 由于创面较大，为了观察植皮是否移动滑脱，术后 3 天，打开伤口观察植皮成活情况，将所有覆盖材料轻轻去除，放置因植入材料和植皮粘贴紧密，将皮肤撕下，用生理盐水浸润后再更换取下敷料，见植皮大部分成活，邮票植皮没有滚动和移位。局部凡士林包扎固定（图 4.6.4、图 4.6.5）。

8. 每隔 1 天换药 1 次，见植皮成活逐渐牢固并和每个植皮间融合愈合，并连接愈合成片。植皮手术后 10 天，植皮完全愈合并上皮化，供皮区也完全愈合，康复出院（图 4.6.6 ~ 图 4.6.8）。

9. 出院后定期随访，指导康复训练，预防压疮再次复发。

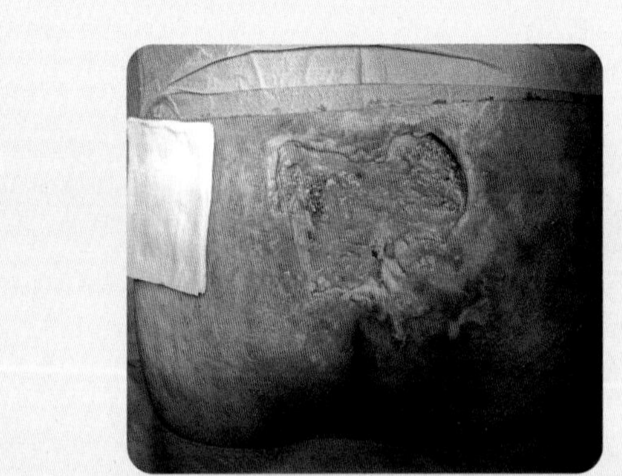

图 4.6.2　局部清创后，加强换药，创面逐渐新鲜

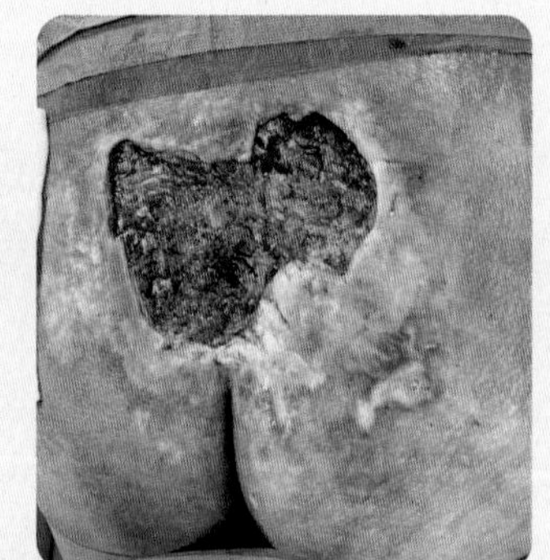

图 4.6.3　经过 9 天换药，创面新鲜

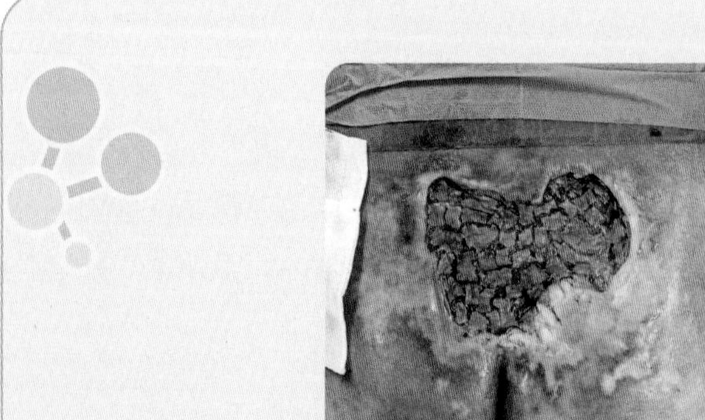

图 4.6.4　中厚皮片，邮票状植皮

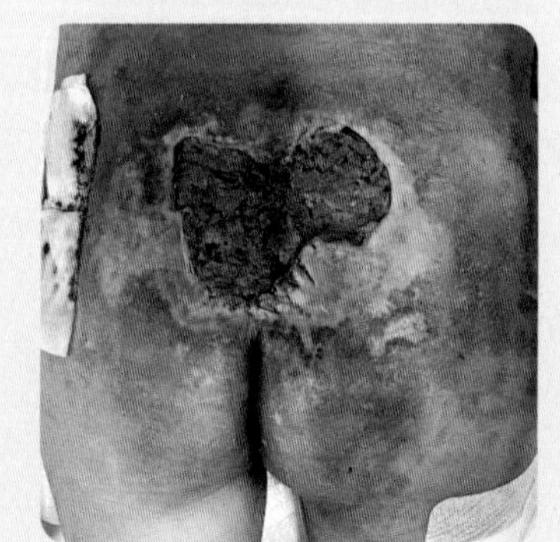

图 4.6.5　植皮术后 3 天、植皮逐渐红润，有成活迹象

the left buttock, and the free skin is trimmed to a size of 0.5 cm × 0.5 cm. It is then freely transplanted onto the sacrococcygeal wound and evenly spread in the concave wound. The wound is sprayed with recombinant human alkaline fibroblast growth factor, and a double-layer artificial leather repair material is taken to cover the skin grafting wound. A thick cotton pad is used to cover the wound, and a fixed dressing is applied. Vaseline gauze is applied to cover the skin for dressing.

7. Due to the large size of the wound, in order to observe whether the skin graft moves and slips, 3 days after surgery, the wound was opened to observe the survival of the skin graft. All covering materials were gently removed, and the skin was torn off due to the tight adhesion between the implant material and the skin graft. After soaking in physiological saline, the dressing was replaced and removed. It was found that most of the skin graft survived, and the stamp skin graft did not roll or shift. Localized Vaseline dressing and fixation (Figure 4.6.4, Figure 4.6.5).

8. Change the dressing once every day, and observe that the skin graft gradually solidifies and fuses with each skin graft, and connects to form a healing patch. Ten days after the skin grafting surgery, the skin graft completely healed and epithelialized, and the donor site also fully healed. The patient recovered and was discharged from the hospital (Figure 4.6.6 - Figure 4.6.8).

9. Regular follow-up after discharge, guidance on rehabilitation training, and prevention of pressure ulcer recurrence.

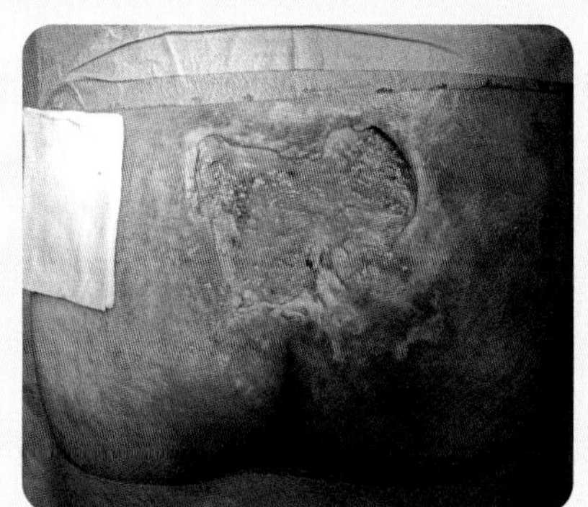

Figure 4.6.2 After local debridement, strengthen dressing changes and gradually make the wound fresh

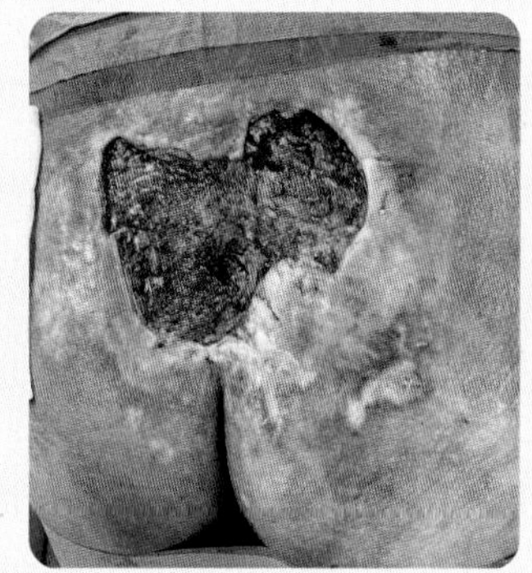

Figure 4.6.3 After 9 days of dressing change, the wound is fresh

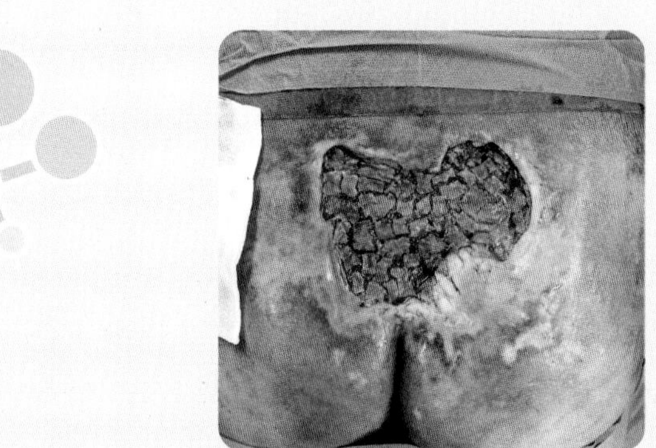

Figure 4.6.4 Medium thick skin graft, stamp shaped skin graft

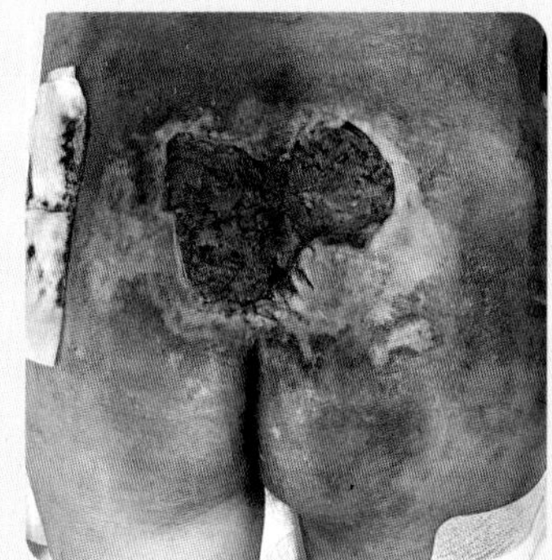

Figure 4.6.5 Three days after skin grafting, the skin gradually turns red and shows signs of survival

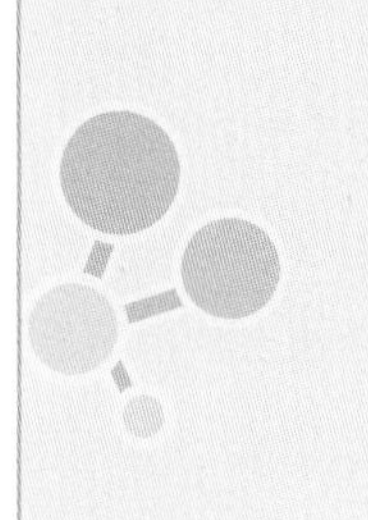

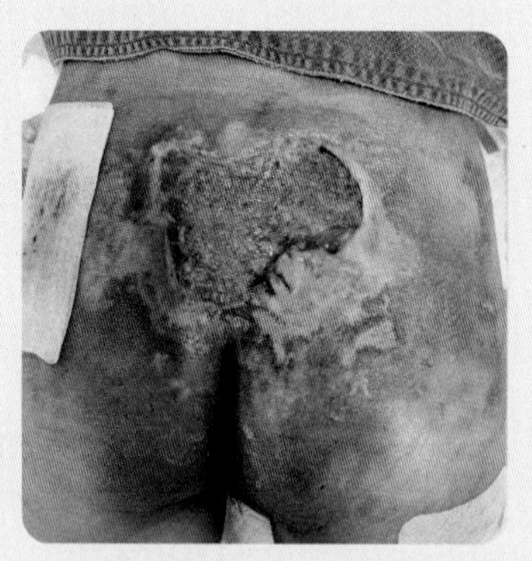

图 4.6.6　植皮术后 5 天，显示基本成活，皮岛间愈合相连成片

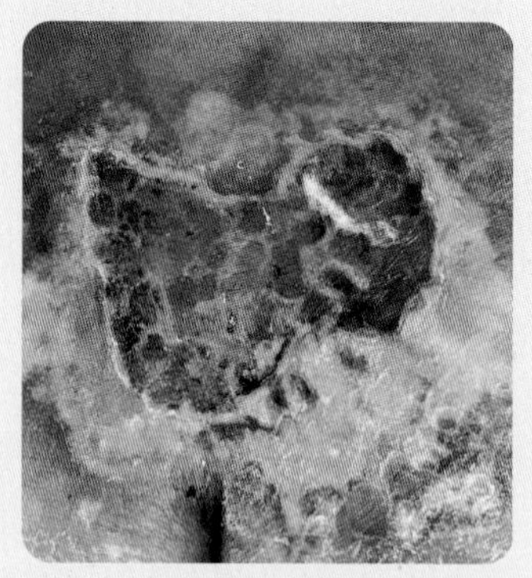

图 4.6.7　术后 7 天，植皮完全成活，仅部分皮岛间未愈合

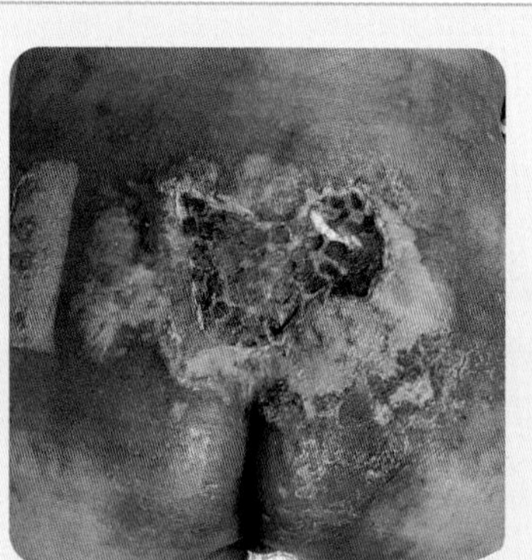

图 4.6.8　植皮术后 10 天，皮岛间连成一片，完全愈合

（陈善亮　曹　丽）

案例七　骶尾部Ⅳ期巨大压疮

◆ 致病原因

患者长期卧床，压力性损伤致骶尾部Ⅳ期巨大压疮。

◆ 症状与体征

慢性病容，骶尾部可及约 10 cm × 10 cm 大小皮肤破溃，深达骶尾骨，基底为黄白色坏死组织，呈拉丝样改变，表面及大量脓性分泌物，周缘红肿明显（图 4.7.1）。

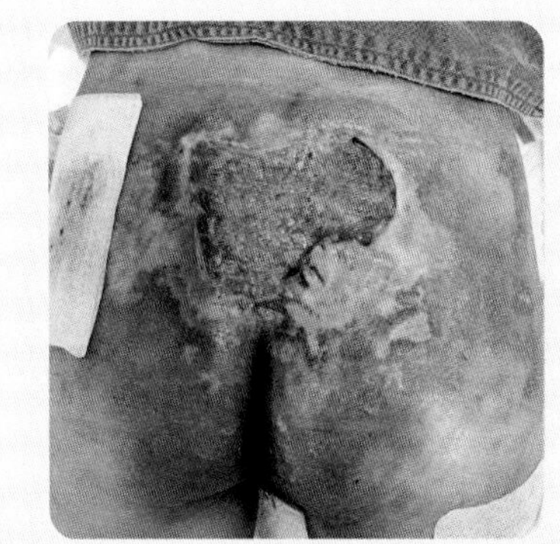

Figure 4.6.6 After 5 days of skin grafting, it shows basic survival, and the skin islands are healed and connected into patches

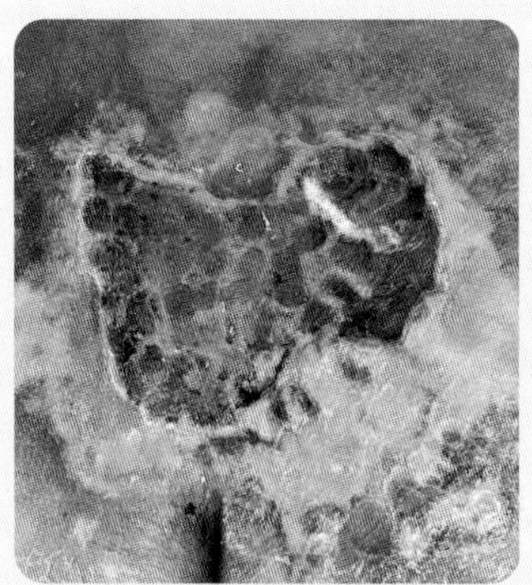

Figure 4.6.7 Seven days after surgery, the skin graft completely survived, with only a portion of the skin islands remaining unhealed

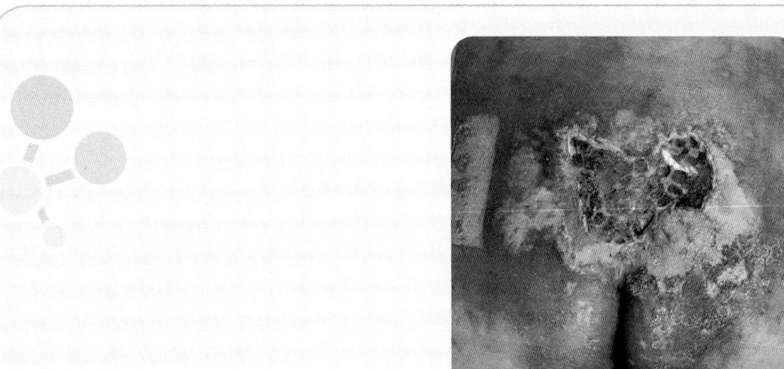

Figure 4.6.8 Ten days after skin grafting, the skin islands are connected and completely healed

(Chen Shanliang, Cao Li)

Case 7 Stage 4 giant pressure ulcer in the sacral tail

◆ Cause of illness

The patient has been bedridden for a long time, and pressure injuries have caused stage IV giant pressure ulcers in the sacrococcygeal region.

◆ Signs and symptoms

Chronic appearance, skin ulceration of approximately 10 cm × 10 cm size can be seen in the coccyx, reaching deep into the coccyx bone. The base is yellow white necrotic tissue with a brushed appearance, with a large amount of purulent discharge on the surface and obvious redness and swelling around the periphery (Figure 4.7.1).

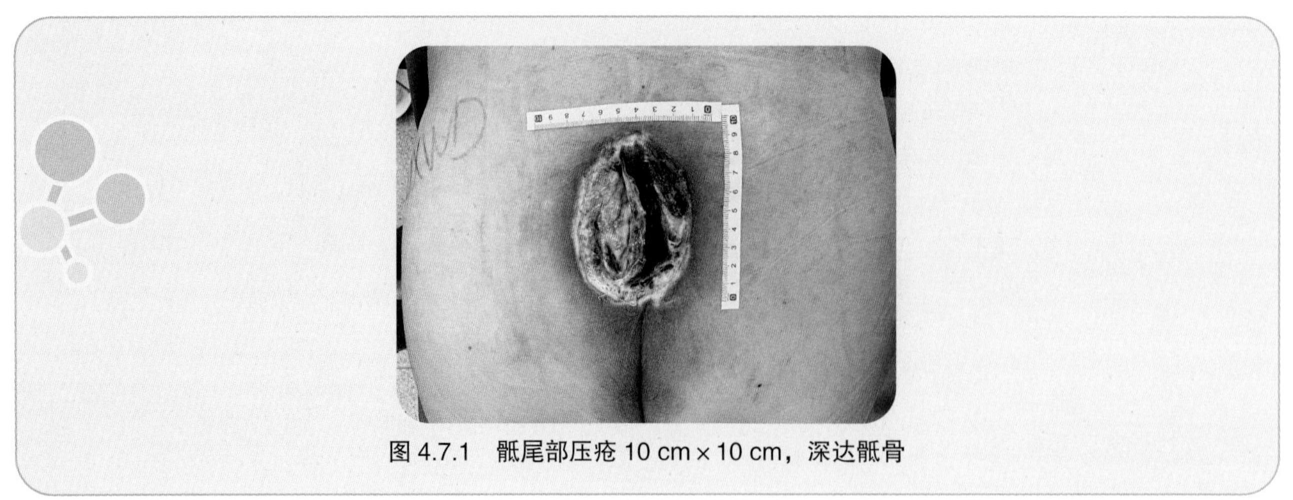

图 4.7.1　骶尾部压疮 10 cm × 10 cm，深达骶骨

◆ 治疗方案

1. 完善各项检查，明确诊断，纠正负氮平衡、贫血、低蛋白血症。给予抗感染、加强营养等对症支持治疗，全程辅以生长因子外用促进创面肉芽组织生长，流体悬浮床对创面施行减压等综合治疗。

2. 积极术前准备，排除手术禁忌。

3. 全麻下进行第一次手术，沿创缘外侧 1 cm，完整切除骶尾部褥疮创面坏死组织，术中发现创面累及骶骨，部分骶骨晦暗，予咬除部分骶骨骨皮质，局部细胞生长因子喷洒；术后继续生长因子每日冲洗，至第二次手术前，可见骶尾部创面新鲜肉芽组织生长（图 4.7.2、图 4.7.3）。第二次手术，骶尾部扩创 + 臀大肌旋转肌皮瓣，生长因子喷洒伤口，沿髂后上嵴与股骨大转子连线中上 1/3，设计肌皮瓣，显露臀上动脉浅支，逐层缝合，留置引流管；皮瓣成活（图 4.7.4 ～图 4.7.7）。

4. 术后加强护理、减压、避免二便污染伤口等。

5. 骶尾部压疮受周缘皮瓣弹性受限等因素，因此相较于其他部位的压疮更难修复，术后常因皮瓣张力大、护理不当、大便污染等因素，出现皮瓣远端坏死或开裂。采用臀大肌肌皮瓣修复，除了能有效避免上述风险，还能提供更为饱满的软组织，降低骶尾部压疮的远期复发率。

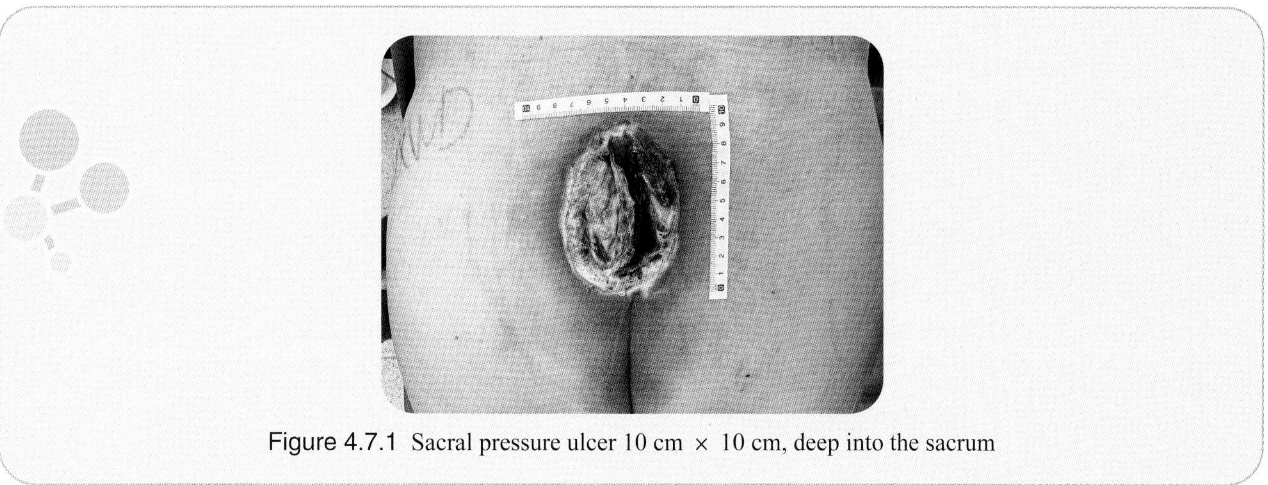

Figure 4.7.1 Sacral pressure ulcer 10 cm × 10 cm, deep into the sacrum

◆ Treatment plan

1. Improve various examinations, clarify diagnosis, correct negative nitrogen balance, anemia, and hypoalbuminemia. Provide symptomatic supportive treatment such as anti-infection and enhanced nutrition, supplemented with external application of growth factors to promote granulation tissue growth in the wound, and comprehensive treatment such as decompression of the wound using a fluid suspension bed.

2. Actively prepare before surgery and eliminate surgical contraindications.

3. The first surgery was performed under general anesthesia, and the necrotic tissue of the sacral and coccygeal pressure ulcer wound was completely removed along the outer 1 cm of the wound edge. During the surgery, it was found that the wound involved the sacrum, and some of the sacrum was dull. Part of the sacrum cortex was bitten off and local cell growth factor was sprayed; After surgery, the growth factor was continued to be washed daily until the second surgery, and fresh granulation tissue growth was observed in the sacrococcygeal wound (Figure 4.7.2, Figure 4.7.3). The second surgery involved expanding the sacrococcygeal region and using a gluteus maximus rotating myocutaneous flap. Growth factor was sprayed onto the wound, and a myocutaneous flap was designed along the upper one-third of the line connecting the posterior iliac crest and the greater trochanter of the femur. The superficial branch of the superior gluteal artery was exposed, and the flap was sutured layer by layer with a drainage tube inserted; The skin flap survived (Figure 4.7.4- Figure 4.7.7).

4. Strengthen postoperative care, relieve stress, and avoid contamination of the wound by fecal matter.

5. Sacral and caudal pressure ulcers are more difficult to repair compared to pressure ulcers in other areas due to factors such as limited elasticity of the peripheral skin flap. After surgery, distal necrosis or cracking of the skin flap often occurs due to factors such as high skin flap tension, improper care, and fecal contamination. The use of gluteus maximus myocutaneous flap for repair not only effectively avoids the aforementioned risks, but also provides fuller soft tissue, reducing the long-term recurrence rate of sacrococcygeal pressure ulcers.

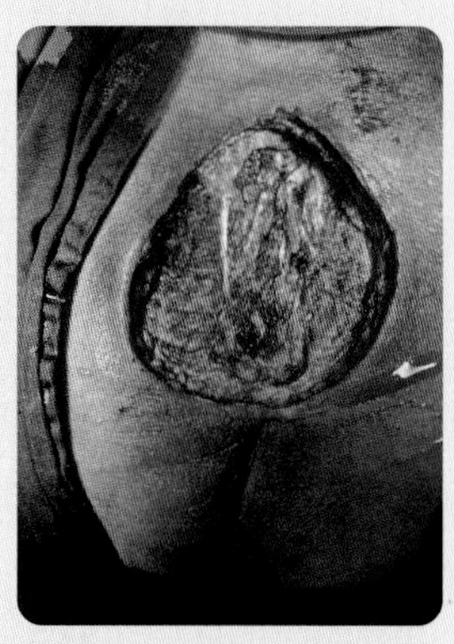

图 4.7.2　第一次手术前

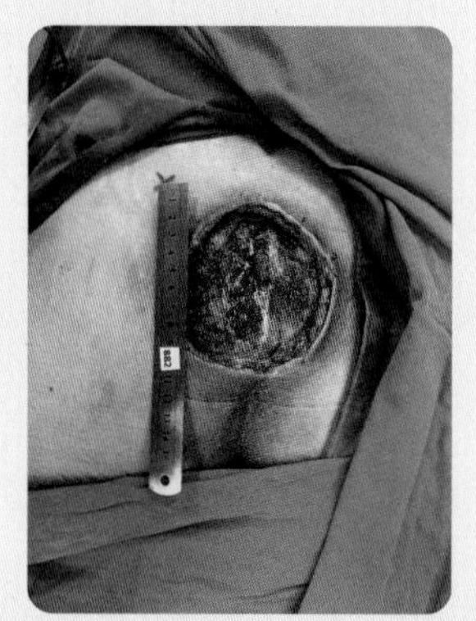

图 4.7.3　第二次手术前，可见骶尾部创面新鲜肉芽组织生长

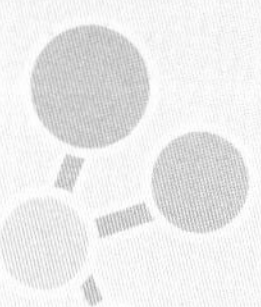

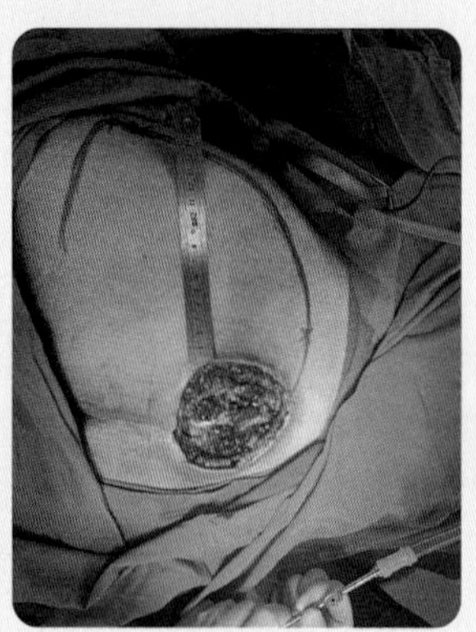

图 4.7.4　肌皮瓣设计示意

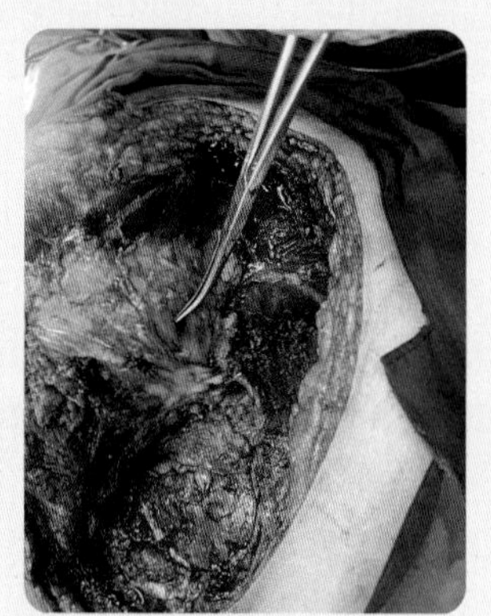

图 4.7.5　显露臀上动脉浅支

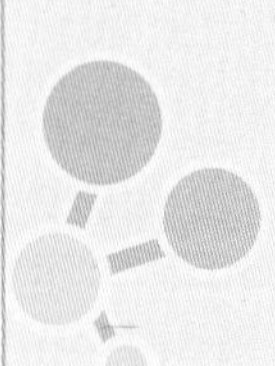

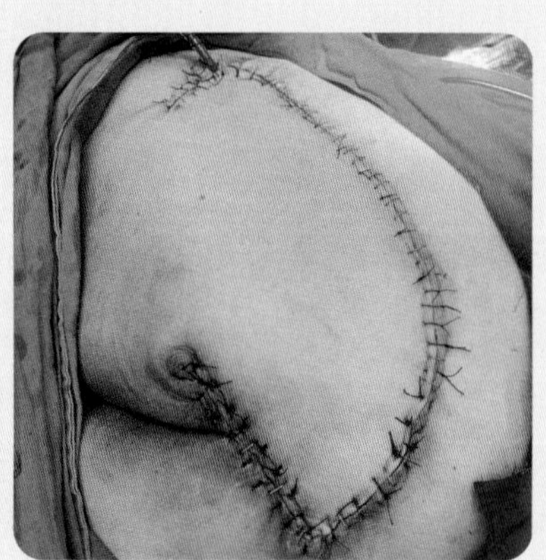

图 4.7.6　逐层缝合，留置引流管

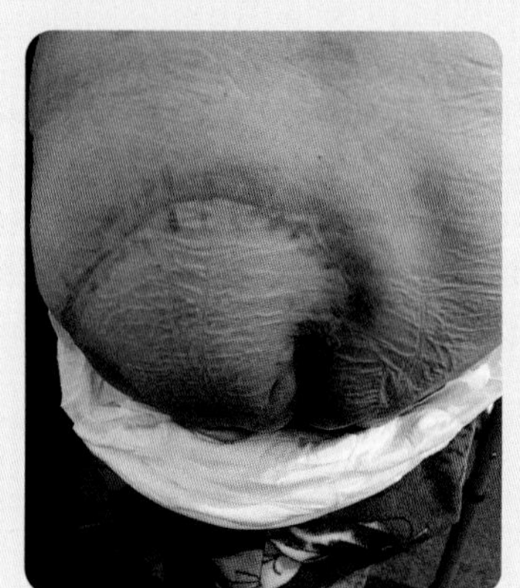

图 4.7.7　皮瓣成活

（夏卫东　林　才）

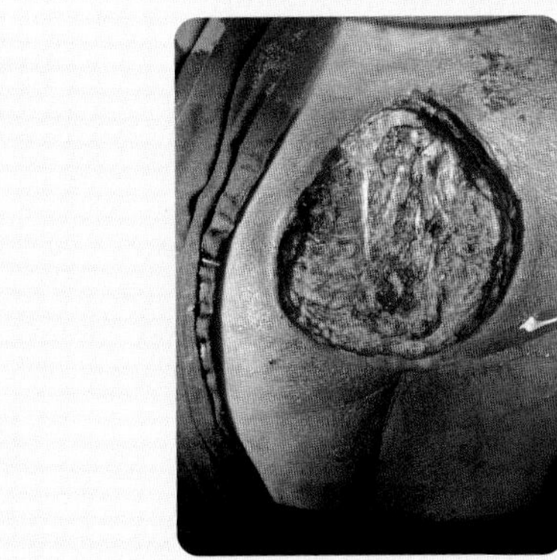

Figure 4.7.2 Before the first surgery

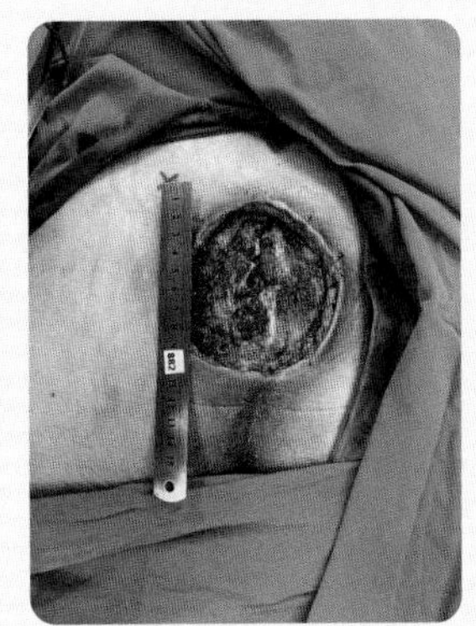

Figure 4.7.3 Before the second surgery, fresh granulation tissue growth can be seen on the wound surface of the sacrococcygeal region

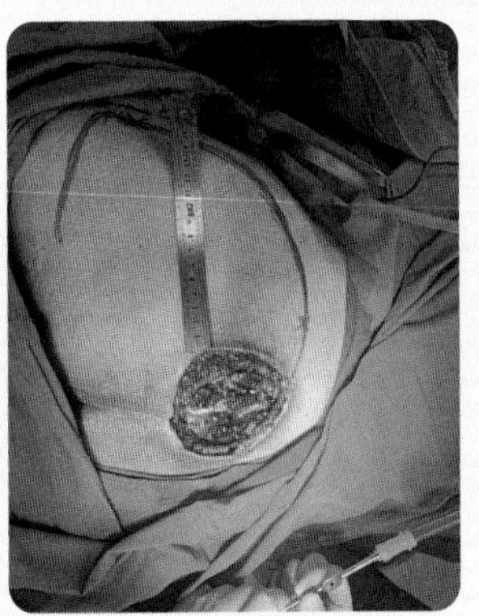

Figure 4.7.4 Schematic diagram of muscle flap design

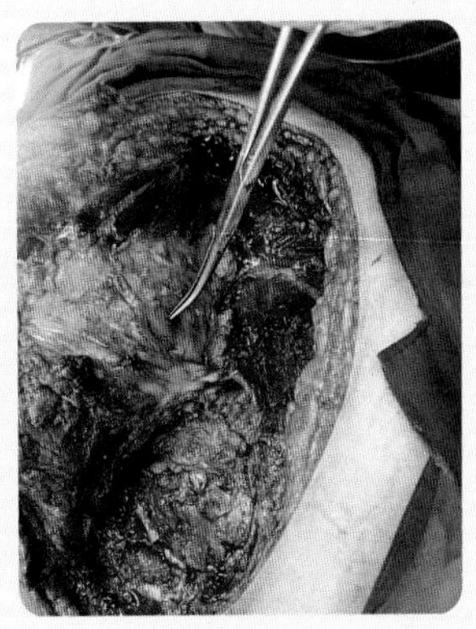

Figure 4.7.5 Revealing the superficial branch of the superior gluteal artery

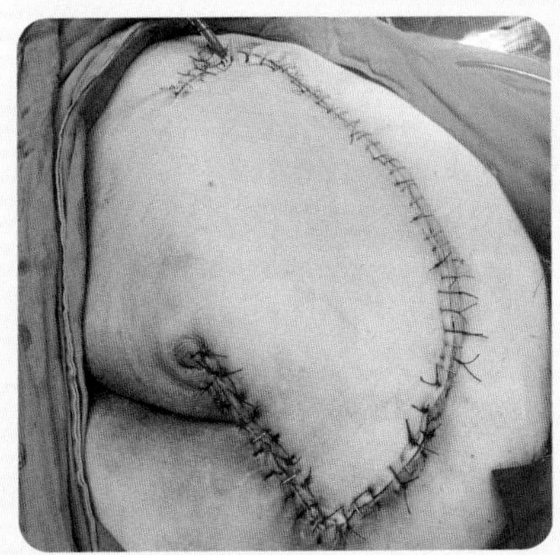

Figure 4.7.6 Stitching layer by layer and placing drainage tube

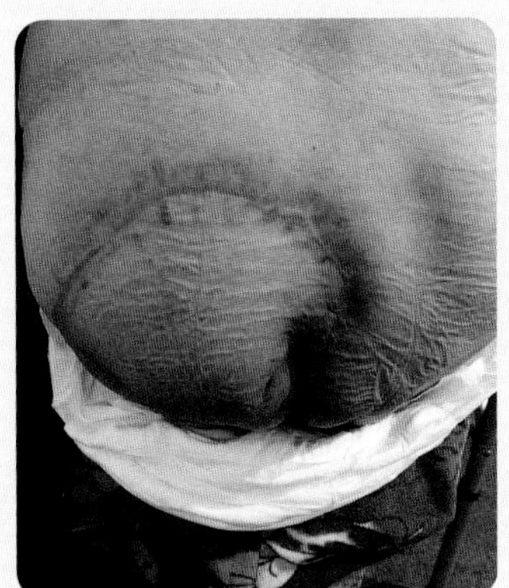

Figure 4.7.7 Survival of skin flap

(Xia Weidong, Lin Cai)

案例八　慢性再生障碍性贫血合并硬膜下血肿的压力性损伤（多处）

◆ 致病原因

患者因慢性再生障碍性贫血病史，长期卧床，致压力性损伤。

◆ 症状与体征

慢性病容，全身皮肤黏膜青紫，多处擦伤。血红蛋白 58 g/L，白细胞计数 2.6×10^9/L，血小板 40×10^9/L。尾骶部压力性创面（不可分期）5.8 cm × 5.5 cm，左足外踝压力性创面Ⅲ期 4.5 cm × 2 cm × 0.2 cm，脊柱正中压力性损伤Ⅲ期 11 cm × 2 cm（图 4.8.1）。

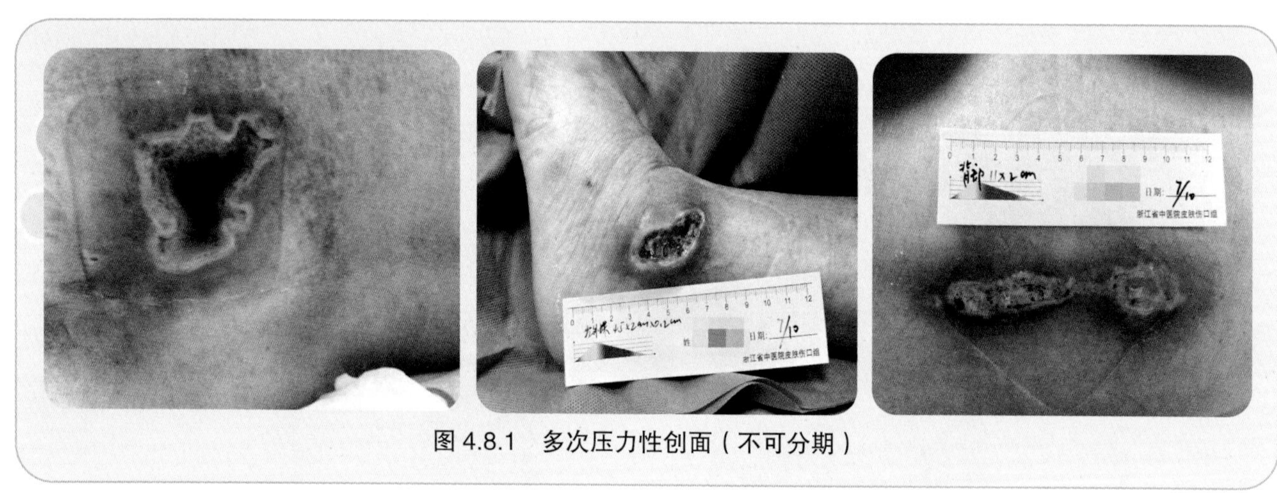

图 4.8.1　多次压力性创面（不可分期）

◆ 治疗方案

1. 患者白细胞、红细胞和血小板数量均低于正常范围，基础疾病阻碍创面修复，给予营养支持及出血的风险评估。

2. 清创：开始采用机械 + 自溶清创，创面感染机械清创。尾骶部压疮Ⅳ期，创面腐臭，清创胶 + 亲水纤维银填塞 + 泡沫。1 周后创面用清创胶 + 生长因子促进肉芽组织生长。

3. 每日换药，创面新鲜后，喷洒生长因子促进肉芽组织生长。左足外踝及脊柱正中创面 1 周后范围缩小，脊柱正中创面 28 天后愈合；尾骶部肉芽组织生长停止，给予输血浆及红细胞营养支持，生长因子 + 藻酸盐促进肉芽组织生长 + 泡沫保护。左足外踝 1 个月后愈合。尾骶部创面红色新鲜肉芽组织，触之易出血，创面用云南白药 + 藻酸盐 + 泡沫敷料，尾骶部 3 月余愈合（图 4.8.2 ～图 4.8.5）。

4. 换药时主动了解患者的顾虑，告知患者创面恢复情况，使其积极配合治疗与护理。

Case 8 Pressure injury in chronic aplastic anemia with subdural hematoma (multiple locations)

◆ Cause of illness

The patient has a history of chronic aplastic anemia and has been bedridden for a long time, resulting in pressure injuries.

◆ Signs and symptoms

Chronic appearance, with bruises on the skin and mucous membranes throughout the body, and multiple abrasions. Hemoglobin 58 g/L, white blood cell count 2.6×10^9/L, platelet count 40×10^9/L. The pressure wound in the coccyx (non-staged) is 5.8 cm × 5.5 cm, the pressure wound in the lateral malleolus of the left foot is stage III 4.5 cm × 2 cm × 0.2 cm, and the pressure injury in the midline of the spine is stage III 11 cm × 2 cm (Figure 4.8.1).

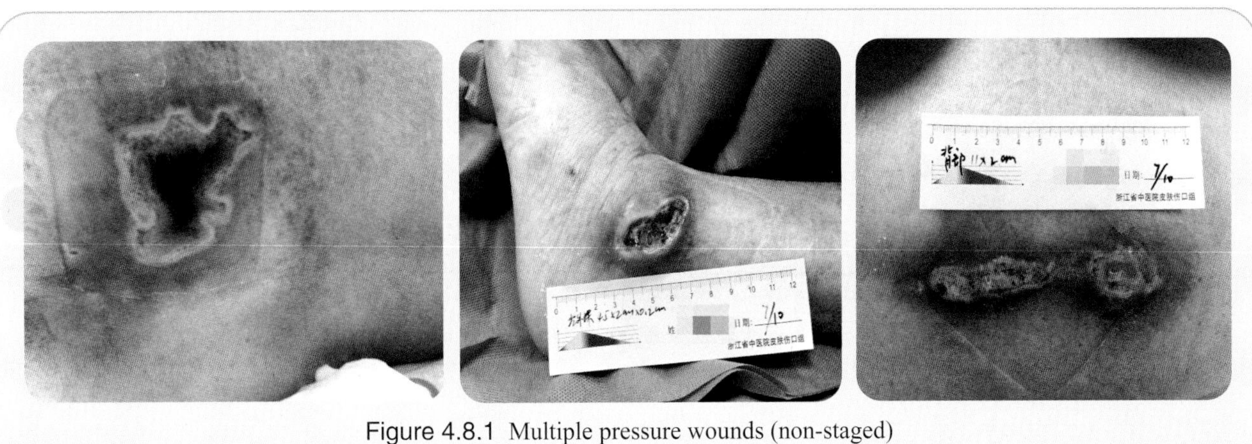

Figure 4.8.1 Multiple pressure wounds (non-staged)

◆ Treatment plan

1. The patient's white blood cell, red blood cell, and platelet counts are all below the normal range, and the underlying disease hinders wound repair. Nutritional support and risk assessment of bleeding should be provided.

2. Debridement: Start using mechanical + autolysis debridement, and perform mechanical debridement on infected wounds. Stage IV coccosacral pressure sore, wound putrid, debridement gel + hydrophilic fiber silver tamponade + foam. One week later, the wound was treated with debridement glue and growth factor to promote granulation tissue growth.

3. Change dressing daily and spray growth factors to promote granulation tissue growth after the wound is fresh. After one week, the extent of the left ankle and spinal midline wound decreased, and the spinal midline wound healed after 28 days; The growth of granulation tissue in the caudal region was stopped. Plasma transfusion and erythrocyte nutrition support were given. Growth factor + alginate promoted the growth of granulation tissue + foam protection. The left ankle healed after one month. The red fresh granulation tissue on the wound of the caudal region is easy to bleed when touched. The wound was treated with Yunnan Baiyao + alginate + foam dressing, and the caudal region healed for more than three months (Figure 4.8.2-Figure4.8.5).

4. Proactively understand the patient's concerns when changing dressing, inform them of the wound recovery situation, and encourage them to actively cooperate with treatment and nursing.

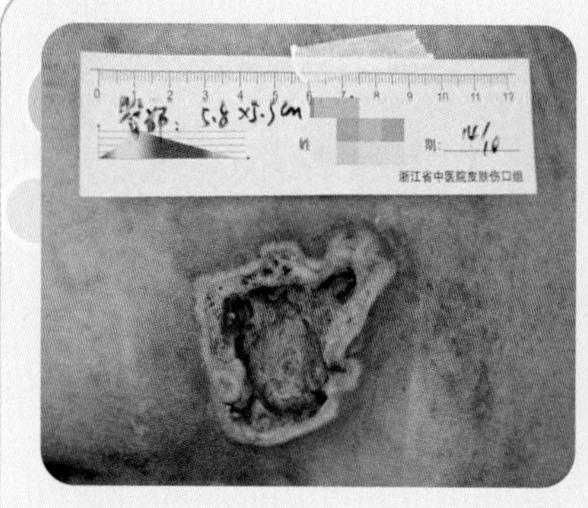
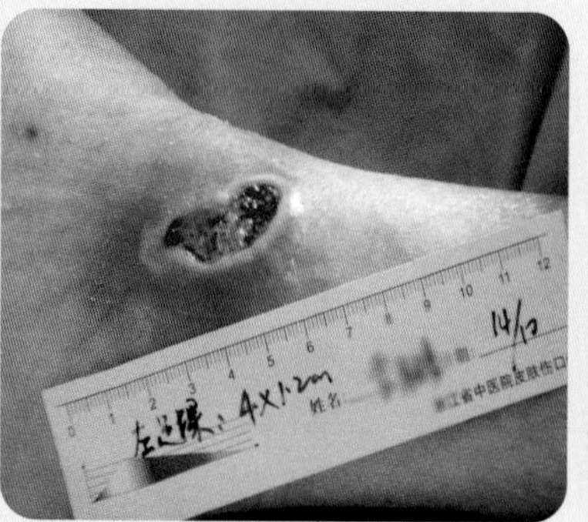
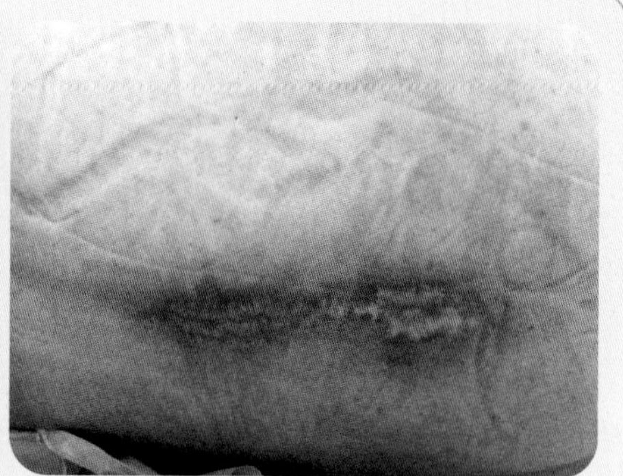

图 4.8.2　创面用清创胶 + 生长因子后情况

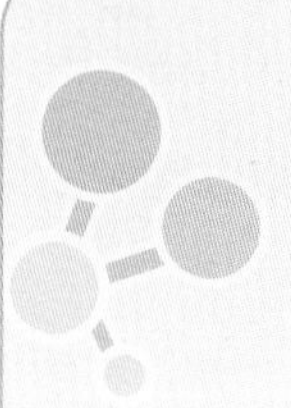
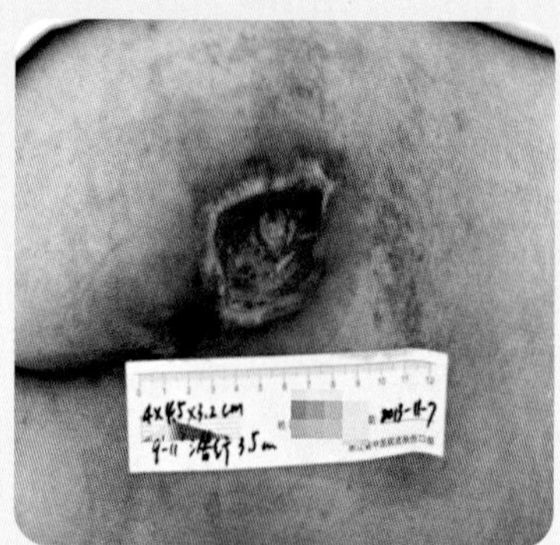
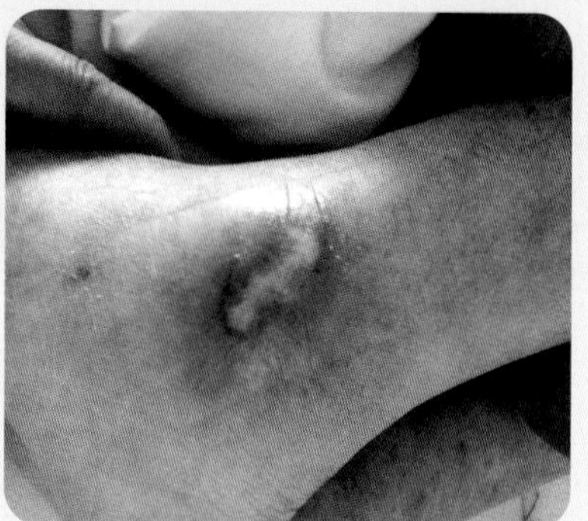

图 4.8.3　创面用生长因子 + 藻酸盐促进肉芽组织生长 + 泡沫保护后情况

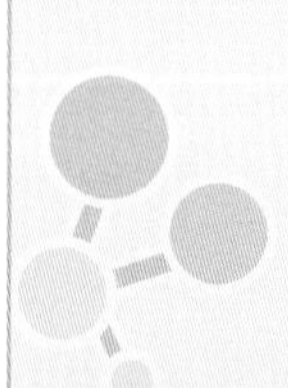
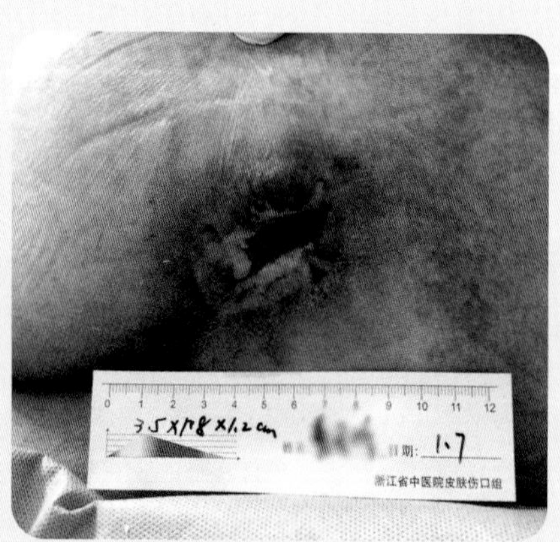

图 4.8.4　创面用云南白药 + 藻酸盐 + 泡沫敷料后情况

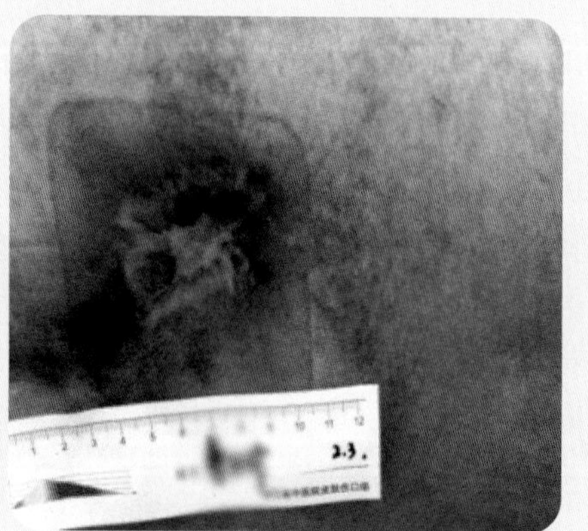

图 4.8.5　尾骶部愈合情况

（倪斐琳　王永高）

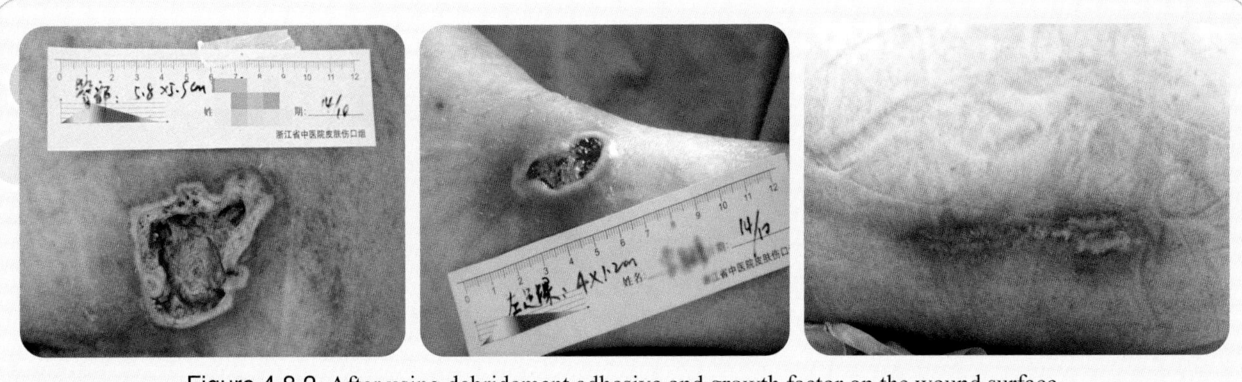

Figure 4.8.2 After using debridement adhesive and growth factor on the wound surface

Figure 4.8.3 After wound growth factor + alginate promoting granulation tissue growth + foam protection

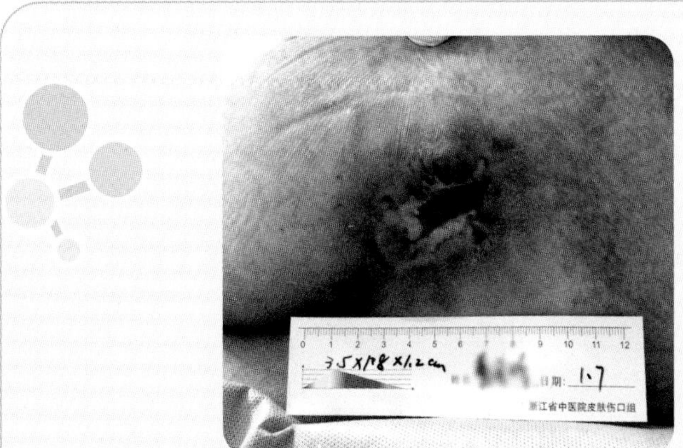

Figure 4.8.4 Condition of wound after applying Yunnan Baiyao + alginate + foam dressing

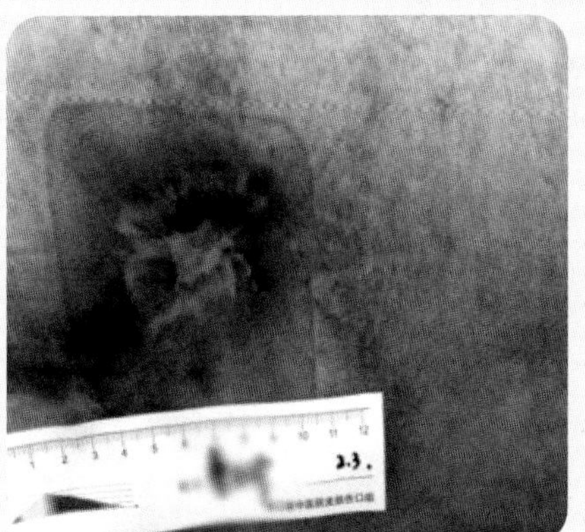

Figure 4.8.5 Tailosacral Healing Status

(Ni Feilin, Wang Yonggao)

案例九　儿童 4 期压力性损伤

◆ 致病原因

患儿卧床 4 月余、大小便失禁 1 月余，骶尾部皮肤长期受压、潮湿，致压力性损伤。

◆ 症状与体征

患儿诊断为一氧化碳中毒性脑病，意识障碍，气管切开状态，躯体活动障碍，长期卧床，大小便失禁，骶尾部 3 cm × 3 cm × 1 cm 压力性损伤 4 期，中央见一皮肤溃疡口，直径 1 cm，可见皮下大片组织空虚，组织及筋膜坏死，少许渗出（图 4.9.1）。伤口分泌物培养结果为鲍曼不动杆菌（++）。

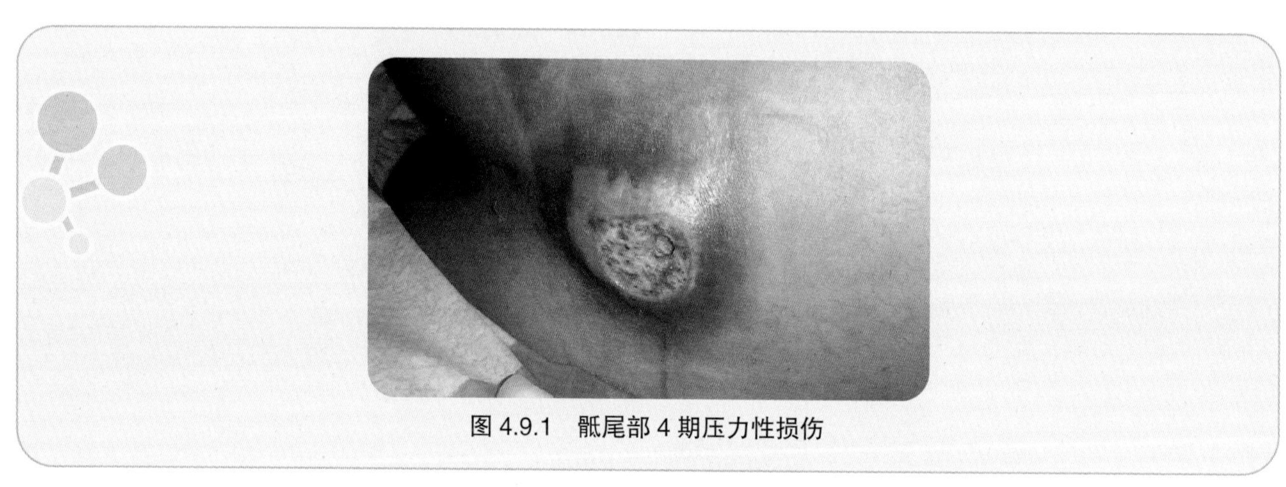

图 4.9.1　骶尾部 4 期压力性损伤

◆ 治疗方案

1. 扩创，清除坏死组织，行 VSD 持续引流术。

2. 加强翻身，骶尾部避免受压；留置尿管，避免尿液污染创面；留置胃管，鼻饲肠内营养粉剂加强营养，促进肉芽组织生长。

3. 静脉用药控制感染。

4. 行 4 次 VSD 后，骶尾部 3 cm × 3 cm × 1 cm 压力性损伤 4 期，可见皮下组织及筋膜，创面愈合不佳，改行富血小板血浆（PRP）治疗。采集患儿自体血，分离出富血小板血浆，伤口清创、消毒，将富血小板血浆注射于伤口周围，给予吸收性明胶海绵浸透富血小板血浆后平铺于伤口上方，再予无菌手术敷料覆盖伤口（图 4.9.2、图 4.9.3）。

5. 行 8 次 PRP 治疗后，创面基本愈合（图 4.9.4）。

6. 此例儿童 4 期压力性损伤因伴有鲍曼不动杆菌感染，且受损部位为骶尾部，易受尿液污染，愈合较为困难，治疗周期较长。

Case 9 Stage 4 stress injury in children

◆ Cause of illness

The child has been bedridden for more than 4 months and has been experiencing urinary and fecal incontinence for more than 1 month. The skin at the coccyx and coccyx has been under long-term pressure and dampness, resulting in stress injury.

◆ Signs and symptoms

The child was diagnosed with carbon monoxide toxic encephalopathy, consciousness disorders, tracheotomy status, physical activity disorders, long-term bed rest, urinary and fecal incontinence, stage 4 pressure injury of 3 cm × 3 cm × 1 cm in the sacrococcygeal region, and a central skin ulcer with a diameter of 1 cm. A large area of subcutaneous tissue was found to be empty, with tissue and fascia necrosis and slight exudation (Figure 4.9.1). The result of wound secretion culture is Acinetobacter baumannii (++).

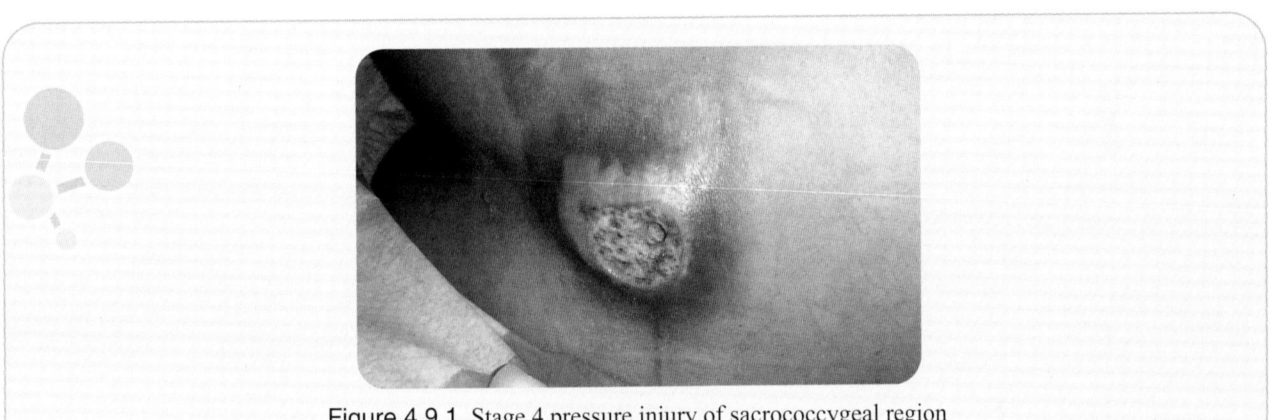

Figure 4.9.1 Stage 4 pressure injury of sacrococcygeal region

◆ Treatment plan

1. Expand the wound, remove necrotic tissue, and perform VSD continuous drainage surgery.

2. Strengthen turning over and avoid pressure on the sacrum and coccyx; Indwelling a urinary catheter to avoid urine contamination of the wound; Retain a gastric tube and administer enteral nutrition powder through nasal feeding to enhance nutrition and promote granulation tissue growth.

3. Intravenous medication is used to control infections.

4. After four VSDs, there were four stages of pressure injury in the sacrococcygeal region, with visible subcutaneous tissue and fascia. The wound healing was poor, and treatment with platelet rich plasma (PRP) was switched. Collect autologous blood from the patient, isolate platelet rich plasma, clean and disinfect the wound, inject platelet rich plasma around the wound, apply absorbent gelatin sponge soaked in platelet rich plasma and spread it flat on top of the wound, and then cover the wound with sterile surgical dressing (Figure 4.9.2, Figure 4.9.3).

5. After 8 rounds of PRP treatment, the wound healed basically (Figure 4.9.4).

6. In this case, the fourth stage pressure injury in a child was accompanied by Acinetobacter baumannii infection, and the damaged area was in the sacrococcygeal region, which was easily contaminated by urine and difficult to heal, resulting in a longer treatment period.

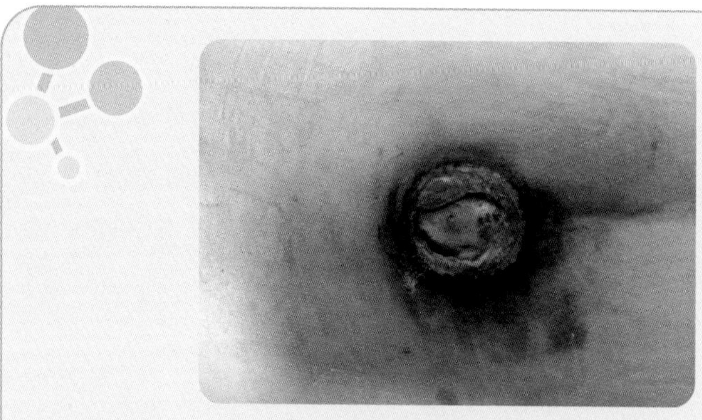

图 4.9.2　4 次 VSD 后，伤口愈合不佳

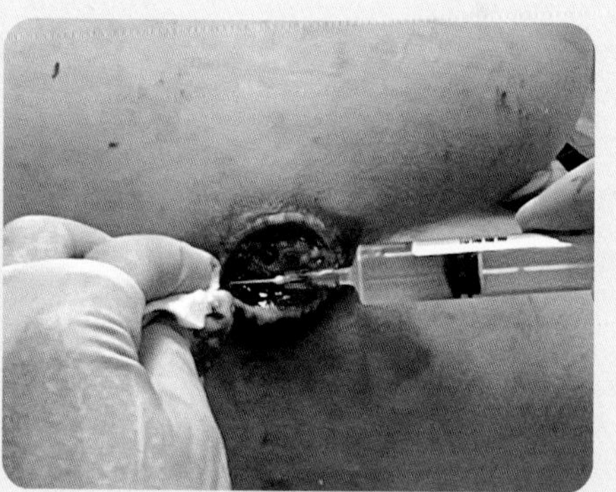

图 4.9.3　PRP 治疗中

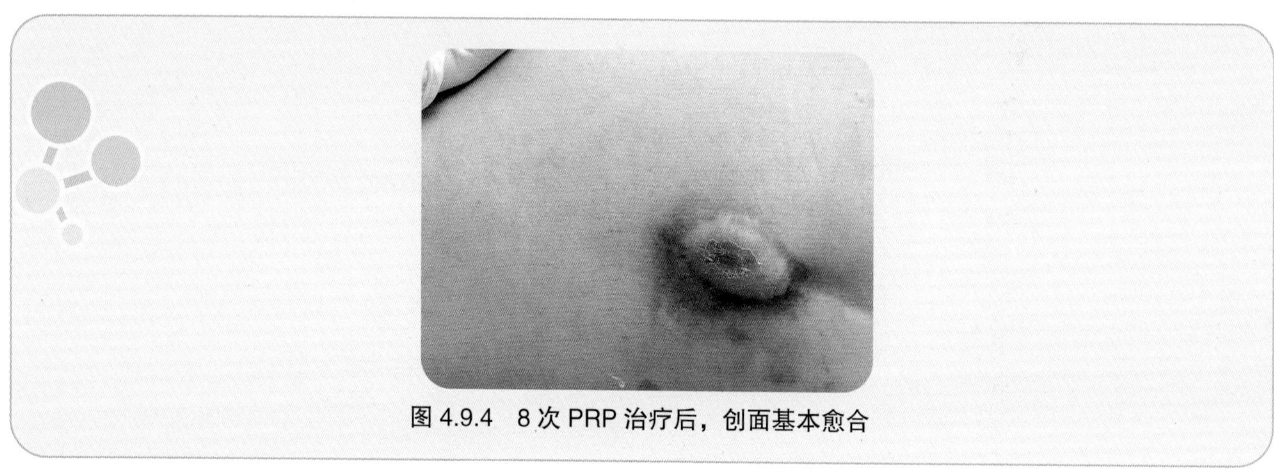

图 4.9.4　8 次 PRP 治疗后，创面基本愈合

（沈玲明　郑雅婷）

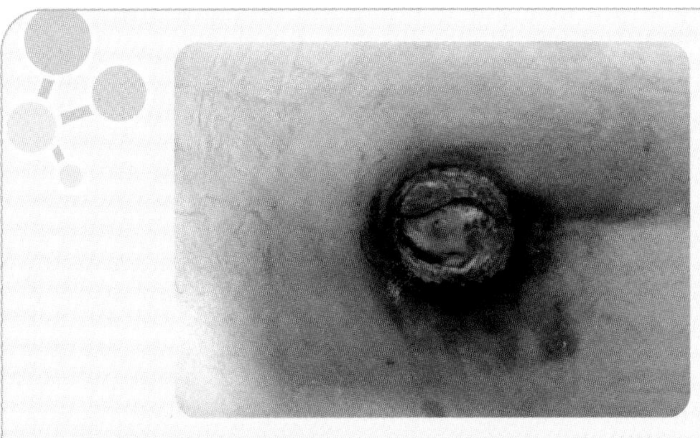

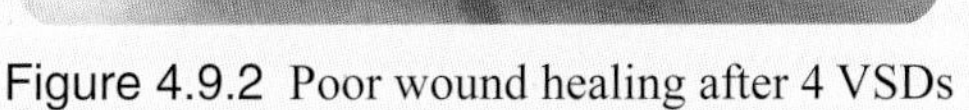

Figure 4.9.2 Poor wound healing after 4 VSDs

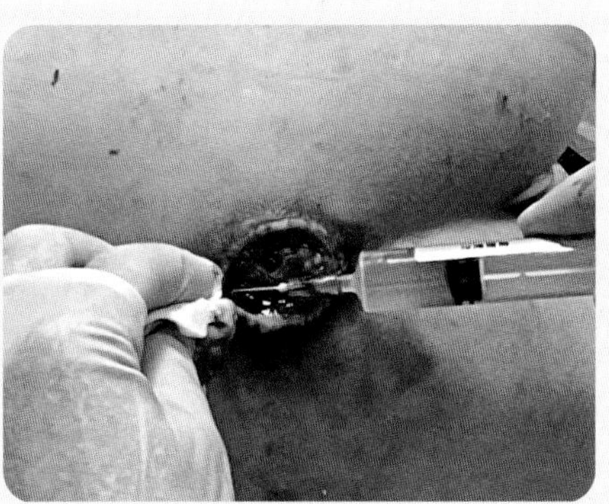

Figure 4.9.3 During PRP treatment

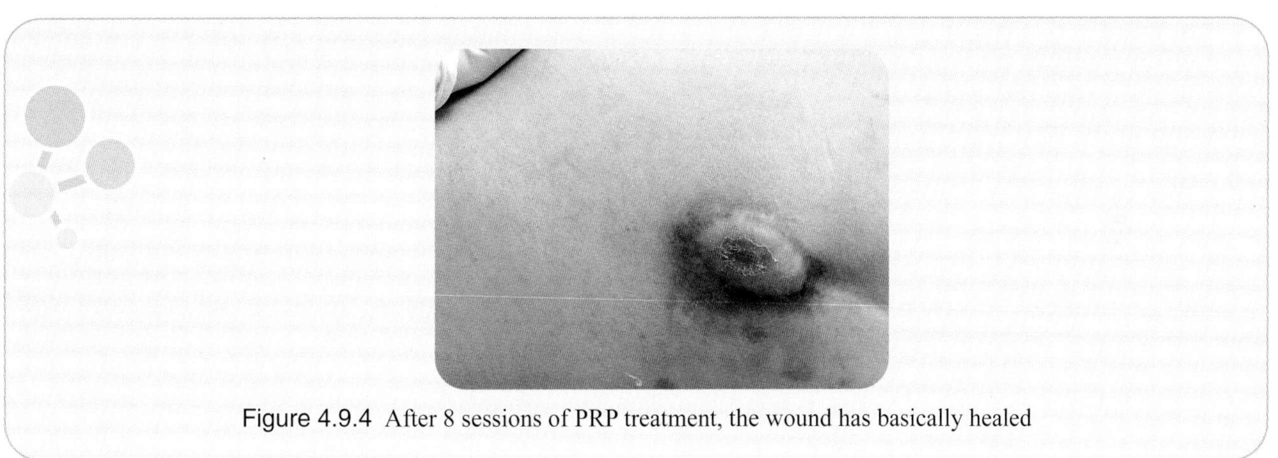

Figure 4.9.4 After 8 sessions of PRP treatment, the wound has basically healed

(Shen Lingming, Zheng Yating)

第 5 章
Chapter 5

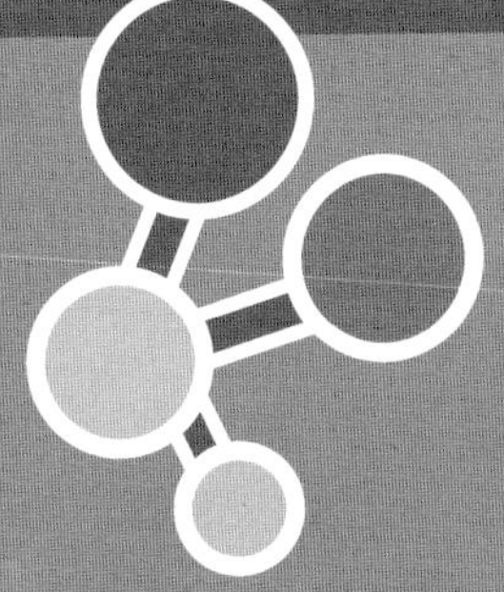

感染性创面修复
Repair of Infectious Wounds

案例一 双小腿慢性溃疡

◆ 致病原因

患者，58 岁，男性，智力障碍，左小腿碰伤后经久不愈合 48 年，右小腿碰伤经久不愈合 12 年，既往患有肝硬化腹水、门静脉高压，脾大 22 年。

◆ 症状与体征

走路跛行，口唇齿龈中度苍白，指甲及皮肤黏膜中度苍白，左小腿可见巨大环形皮肤缺损，创面缺损面积约 22 cm × 24 cm，环绕小腿缺损，中间有部分皮岛，小腿皮肤广泛性色素沉着，皮缘内陷，瘢痕硬化，前踝瘢痕挛缩，踝关节前屈受限，创面肉芽组织老化且苍白水肿，创面有大量炎性渗出，味臭，有白色脓性分泌物，足背动脉和胫后动脉波动减弱，足趾活动良好，足底感觉正常。右侧内踝区有 3 cm × 3 cm 创面，皮缘内陷，创面肉芽组织污秽不清，水肿，创缘皮肤瘢痕老化，创缘周边皮肤色素沉着，踝关节活动良好，足背动脉和胫后动脉波动良好，足趾活动良好，足底感觉正常（图 5.1.1）。

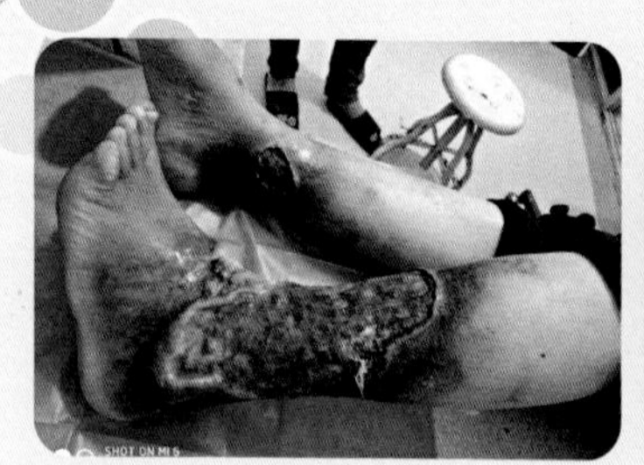
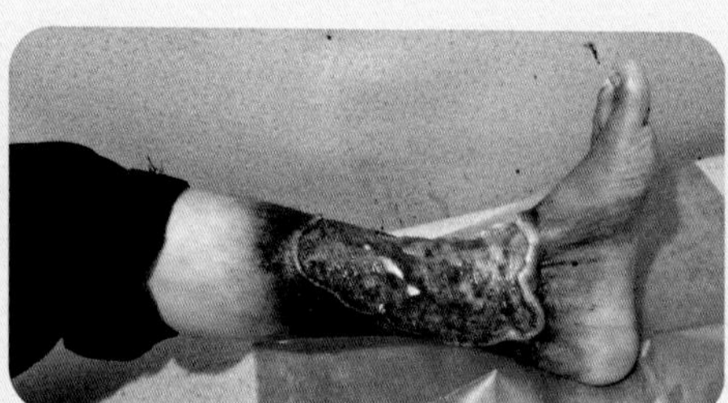
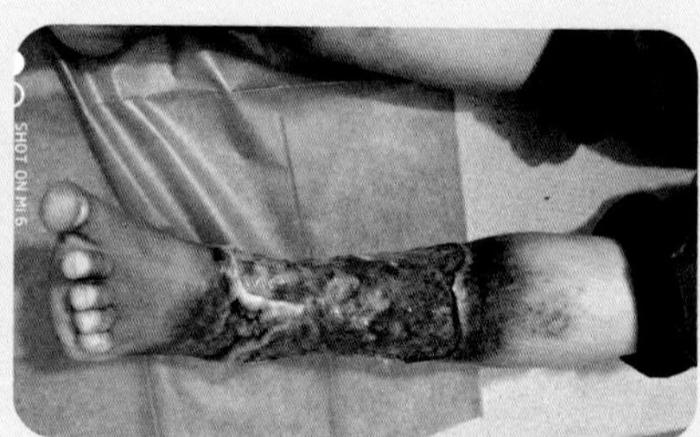

图 5.1.1 左小腿巨大环形创面，右侧内踝区创面

◆ 治疗方案

该患者为智力障碍人士，全身基础疾病多，如严重的肝硬化腹水、脾大、门静脉高压、贫血、低蛋白血症。左小腿溃疡没有规范治疗等综合原因，造成左小腿和右小腿溃疡经久不愈合。

1. 入院后积极治疗原发病，纠正肝硬化腹水，输血、冰冻血浆和白蛋白，快速纠正贫血和低蛋白血症。根据细菌培养给予敏感抗菌药物控制感染。

2. 换药时用刮匙刮出污秽不清污染组织和老化肉芽组织，双氧水浸泡消毒，生理盐水反复冲洗，每天换药 2 次，局部喷洒重组人碱性成纤维细胞生长因子。双侧小腿红外线，微波理疗促进瘢痕软化，改善局部血液循环。

3. 贫血和低蛋白纠正后，在腰硬联合麻醉下行双侧小腿清创 +VSD+ 重组人碱性成纤维细胞生长因子滴注冲洗，促进肉芽组织生长新鲜，为植皮提供时间窗（图 5.1.2）。

4. VSD+ 重组人碱性成纤维细胞生长因子创面滴注治疗 5 天，拆除 VSD 装置，可见双小腿创面红润新鲜、

Case 1 Chronic ulcers in the lower legs

◆ Cause of illness

The patient is 58 years old, male, with intellectual disability. The left calf injury has not healed for 48 years, and the right calf injury has not healed for 12 years. He has a history of liver cirrhosis ascites, portal hypertension, and splenomegaly for 22 years.

◆ Signs and symptoms

Walking limp, lips and gums moderately pale, nails and skin mucosa moderately pale, a huge circular skin defect can be seen on the left calf, with a wound defect area of about 22 cm × 24 cm, surrounding the calf defect, with some skin islands in the middle. The calf skin is extensively pigmented, the skin edge is sunken, the scar is hardened, the anterior ankle scar is contracted, the ankle joint is limited in forward flexion, the granulation tissue on the wound is aging and pale and swollen, there is a large amount of inflammatory exudate on the wound, a foul odor, and white purulent secretion. The fluctuation of the dorsalis pedis artery and posterior tibial artery is weakened, the toe movement is good, and the plantar sensation is normal. There is a 3 cm × 3 cm wound in the right medial malleolus area, with an inward retraction of the skin edge, unclear granulation tissue contamination, edema, aging scar tissue around the wound edge, pigmentation around the wound edge, good ankle joint movement, good fluctuation of the dorsal and posterior tibial arteries, good toe movement, and normal plantar sensation (Figure 5.1.1).

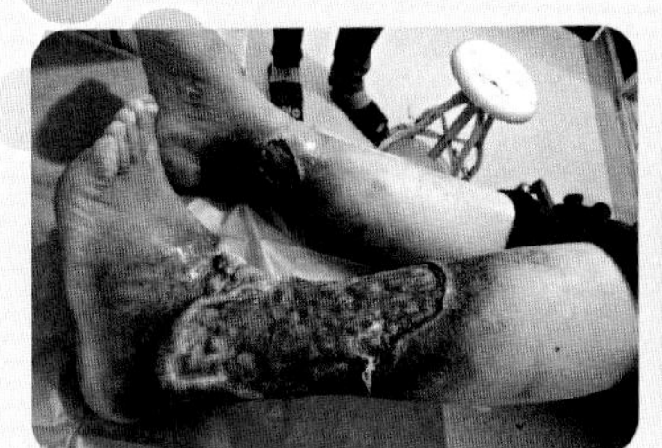
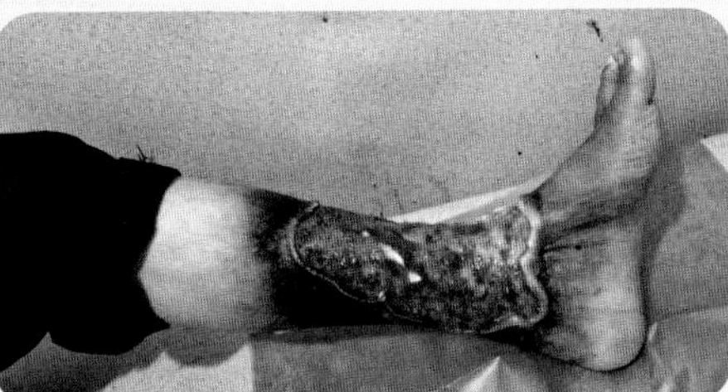
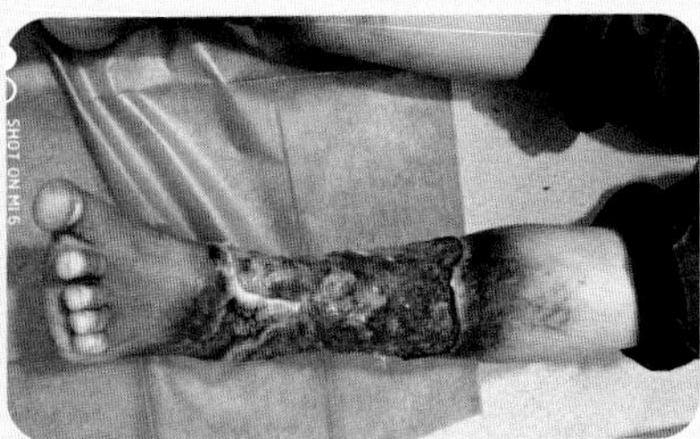

Figure 5.1.1 Large circular wound on the left calf and wound on the right medial malleolus area

◆ Treatment plan

The patient is an intellectual disability with multiple underlying systemic diseases, such as severe liver cirrhosis, ascites, splenomegaly, portal hypertension, anemia, and hypoalbuminemia. Due to comprehensive reasons such as lack of standardized treatment for left calf ulcers, the ulcers in the left and right calves have not healed for a long time.

1. Actively treat the primary disease after admission, correct liver cirrhosis ascites, transfusion, frozen plasma and albumin, and quickly correct anemia and hypoalbuminemia. Administer sensitive antibiotics based on bacterial culture to control infections.

2. When changing the dressing, use a scraper to scrape off the contaminated and aged granulation tissue, soak in hydrogen peroxide for disinfection, rinse repeatedly with physiological saline, change the dressing twice a day, and locally spray recombinant human alkaline fibroblast growth factor. Bilateral calf infrared and microwave therapy promote scar softening and improve local blood circulation.

3. After correcting anemia and low protein, bilateral calf debridement + VSD + recombinant human basic fibroblast growth factor drip irrigation was performed under lumbar epidural anesthesia to promote fresh granulation tissue growth and provide a time window for skin grafting (Figure 5.1.2).

4. VSD + recombinant human basic fibroblast growth factor wound infusion therapy for 5 days. After removing the VSD device, it was observed that the wounds on both calves were red and fresh, with active bleeding and full

渗血活跃，肉芽组织饱满（图 5.1.3）。在腰硬联合麻醉下行中厚游离皮片移植术，根据创面大小，使用电动取皮刀调节中厚皮片厚度，于大腿前侧切取中厚大张皮片，移植于双侧小腿受区，移植前创面喷洒重组人碱性成纤维细胞生长因子，皮缘缝合，局部加压包扎。

5. 植皮术后抬高患肢，冰敷 3 天，3 天后局部红外线理疗，床上训练关节活动，预防深静脉血栓（静脉气压泵治疗）。继续巩固治疗原发病。

6. 术后 10 天，植皮区拆线，植皮全部成活，双下肢创面完全愈合（图 5.1.4）。

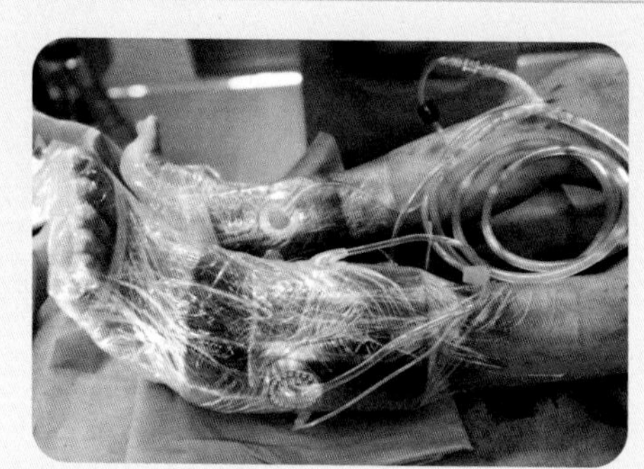

图 5.1.2　VSD+ 重组人碱性成纤维细胞生长因子滴注冲洗

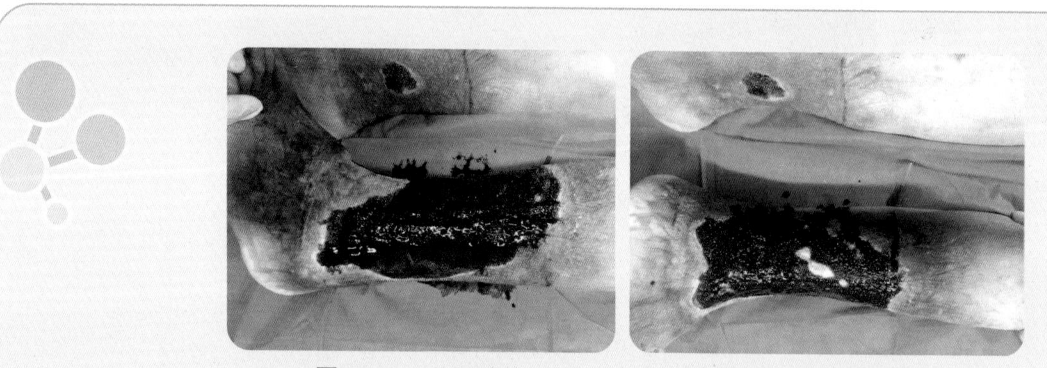

图 5.1.3　VSD 治疗 5 天，创面饱满新鲜、创面渗血活跃

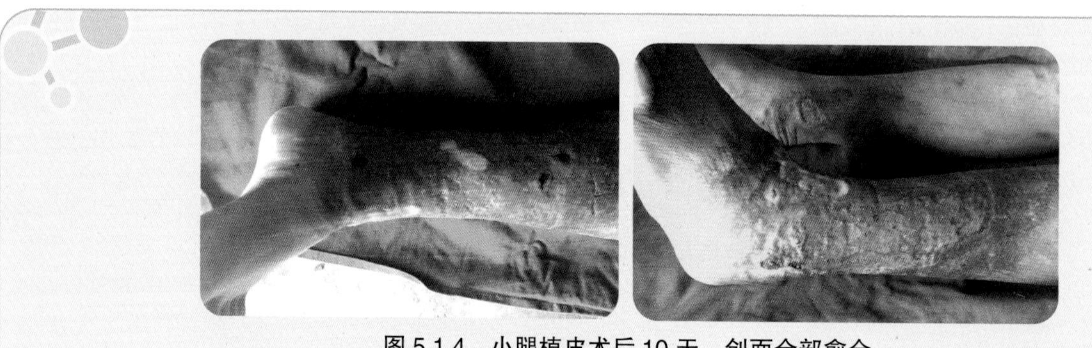

图 5.1.4　小腿植皮术后 10 天，创面全部愈合

（陈善亮）

granulation tissue (Figure 5.1.3). Under spinal epidural anesthesia, medium thick free skin graft transplantation is performed. According to the size of the wound, an electric skin knife is used to adjust the thickness of the medium thick skin graft. A large medium thick skin graft is cut from the front of the thigh and transplanted into the recipient areas of both calves. Before transplantation, the wound is sprayed with recombinant human basic fibroblast growth factor, the skin edge is sutured, and local pressure bandaging is applied.

5. After skin grafting, raise the affected limb and apply ice for 3 days. After 3 days, perform local infrared therapy, train joint movement in bed, and prevent deep vein thrombosis (treated with venous pressure pump). Continue to consolidate the treatment of the primary disease.

6.10 days after surgery, the stitches in the skin graft area were removed, and all skin grafts survived. The wounds on both lower limbs were completely healed (Figure 5.1.4).

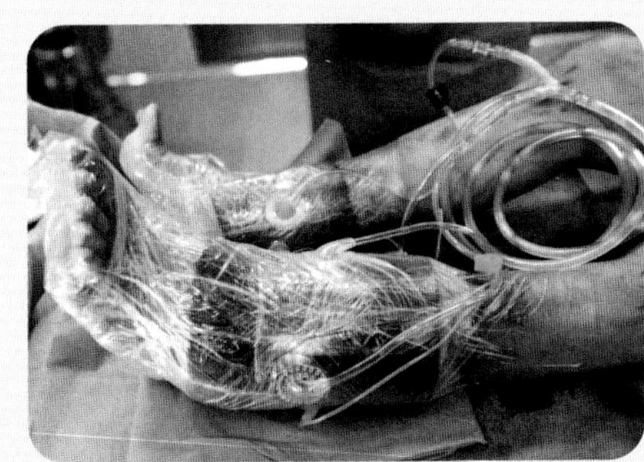

Figure 5.1.2 VSD+ recombinant human basic fibroblast growth factor drip irrigation

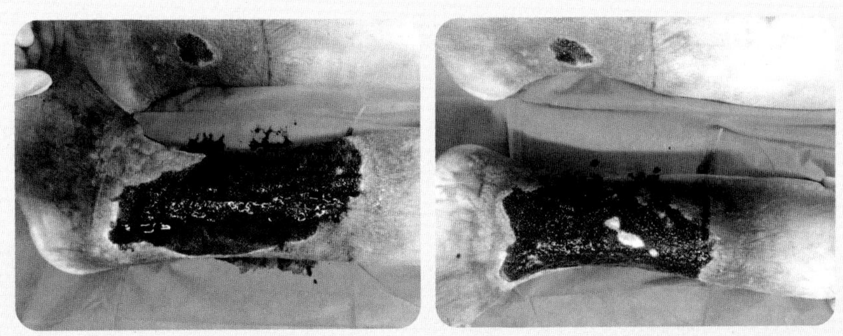

Figure 5.1.3 After 5 days of VSD treatment, the wound is full and fresh, with active bleeding from the wound

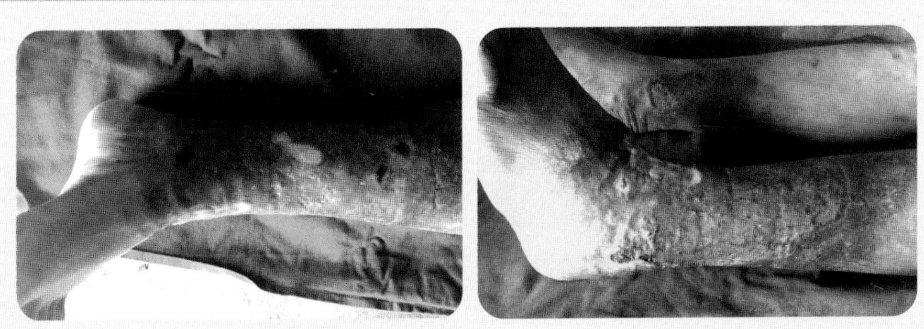

Figure 5.1.4 10 days after calf skin grafting, all wounds healed

(Chen Shanliang)

案例二　左小腿内侧溃疡

◆ 致病原因

患者，男性，80 岁，左小腿反复破溃流脓 56 年。56 年前不慎被巨石砸伤双侧小腿，致双小腿巨大伤口，住院治疗 5 天后回家用土制草药外敷，伤口反复溃烂不能愈合，右小腿 12 年后自行愈合，左小腿内侧留有巨大伤口未愈合至今，曾有蛆虫生长，反复流脓水，每天在家自用碎布草药包扎。

◆ 症状与体征

扶拐行走、跛行，左小腿溃疡持续性疼痛。左小腿内侧至足踝区有不规则溃疡，面积 12 cm × 5 cm，肉芽组织污秽不清，肉芽组织水肿且老化，皮缘内陷，有炎性渗出，味臭。小腿中下段至足踝区有大面积硬化皮肤瘢痕，色素沉着，皮肤纤维化，足背动脉波较弱，足底感觉正常，膝关节活动良好，踝关节僵硬，足趾活动良好，腹股沟淋巴结无肿大（图 5.2.1）。右小腿前侧和内踝前侧有大面积瘢痕，局部皮肤曾纤维化，局部皮肤角化增厚，无弹性，膝关节活动良好，右踝关节略僵硬，活动略受限，足趾活动良好，足背动脉胫后动脉波动良好，足底感觉正常。

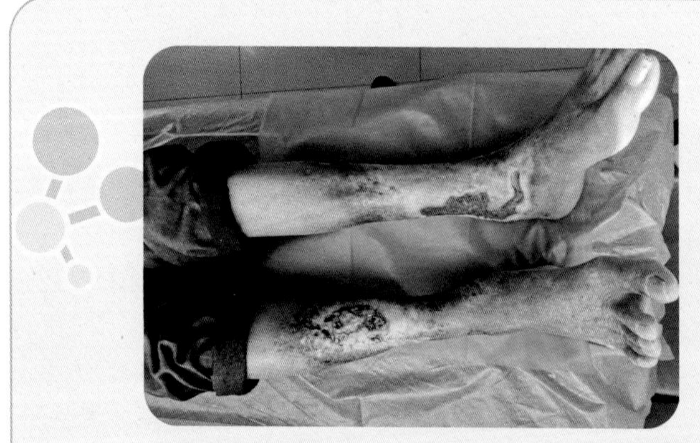

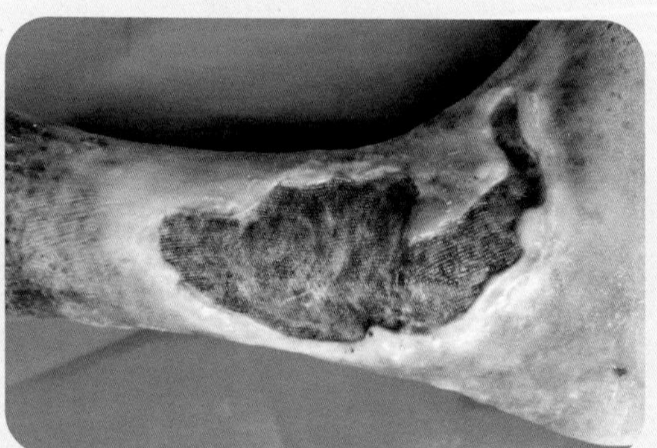

图 5.2.1　左小腿内侧至内踝区有不规则溃疡，皮缘内陷、肉芽组织老化

◆ 治疗方案

该患者左小腿溃疡长达 56 年未愈合，究其原因：①个人卫生差，自用草药外敷，增加感染概率；②未去医院规范治疗；③局部长期感染，伤口未能愈合，造成营养不良性贫血；④创面瘢痕化，皮肤无生长爬行能力。

1. 积极治疗原发病，纠正贫血，改善局部血液循环，给予敏感抗菌药物，清创，增加换药次数，局部应用生长因子促进肉芽组织新鲜。

Case 2 Ulcer on the inner side of the left calf

◆ Cause of illness

Patient, male, 80 years old, with recurrent rupture and pus discharge from the left calf for 56 years. 56 years ago, I was accidentally hit by a giant rock on both sides of my calves, causing huge wounds. After being hospitalized for 5 days, I went home and applied homemade herbs externally, but the wounds repeatedly ulcerated and could not heal. After 12 years, my right calf healed on its own, but there is a huge wound on the inner side of my left calf that has not yet healed. There have been maggots growing and pus flowing repeatedly. I use crushed cloth and herbs to bandage my legs at home every day.

◆ Signs and symptoms

Walking with crutches, limping, and persistent pain in the left calf ulcer. There is an irregular ulcer on the inner side of the left calf to the ankle area, with an area of 12 cm × 5 cm. The granulation tissue is dirty and unclear, with swelling and aging of the granulation tissue, inward retraction of the skin margin, inflammatory exudation, and a foul odor. There are large areas of hardened skin scars, pigmentation, skin fibrosis, weak dorsal artery waves, normal plantar sensation, good knee joint movement, ankle joint stiffness, good toe movement, and no swelling of inguinal lymph nodes in the middle and lower leg to ankle area (Figure 5.2.1). There are large areas of scars on the anterior side of the right calf and the anterior side of the medial malleolus. The local skin has been fibrotic, with keratinized and thickened skin that is inelastic. The knee joint has good mobility, while the right ankle joint is slightly stiff with limited mobility. The toes have good mobility, and the posterior tibial artery of the dorsalis pedis has good fluctuations. The plantar sensation is normal.

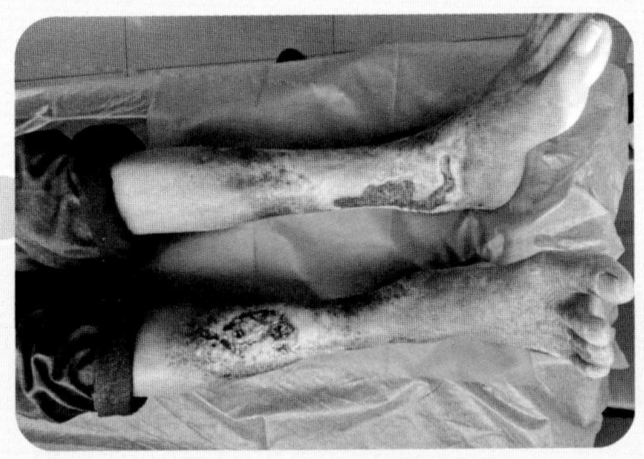
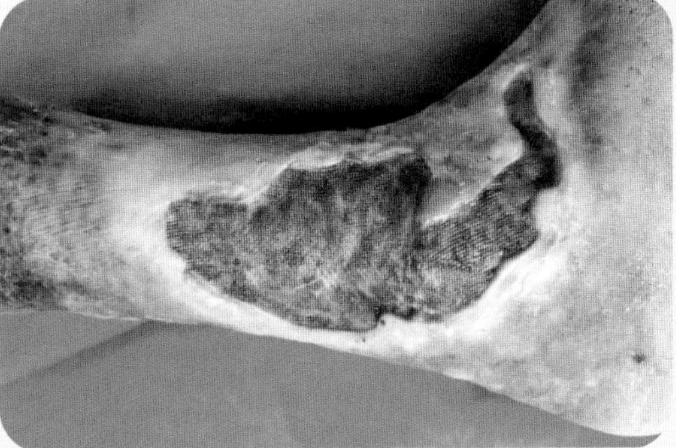

Figure 5.2.1 Irregular ulcer, inward retraction of skin margin, and aging of granulation tissue in the inner ankle area of the left calf

◆ Treatment plan

The patient's left calf ulcer has not healed for 56 years. The reasons for this are: ① Poor personal hygiene, self use of herbal medicine for external application, increasing the probability of infection; ② Not seeking standardized treatment at the hospital; ③ Local long-term infection, failure of wound healing, resulting in malnutrition anemia; ④ Scaring of the wound and lack of skin growth and crawling ability.

1. Actively treat the primary disease, correct anemia, improve local blood circulation, administer sensitive antibiotics, clear wounds, increase dressing changes, and locally apply growth factors to promote fresh granulation tissue.

2. 贫血纠正后，局部应用VSD+重组人碱性成纤维细胞生长因子创面滴注综合治疗，促进肉芽组织新鲜，为植皮提供时间窗（图 5.2.2）。

3. VSD+ 重组人碱性成纤维细胞生长因子创面滴注综合治疗 7 天，拆除 VSD 装置，于腰硬联合麻醉下，行中厚游离皮片移植，并喷洒重组人碱性成纤维细胞生长因子，促进植皮成活。植皮缝合固定，加压包扎（图 5.2.3 ~ 图 5.2.5）。

4. 术后抬高患肢，局部冰敷减少创面渗血，防止植皮浮起。术后局部红外线、微波理疗，改善局部血液循环。床上训练下肢关节活动，防止深静脉血栓。

5. 术后 10 天拆线，植皮成活，创面完全愈合，康复出院（图 5.2.6）。

6. 出院后继续保护好皮肤，防止二次破溃。

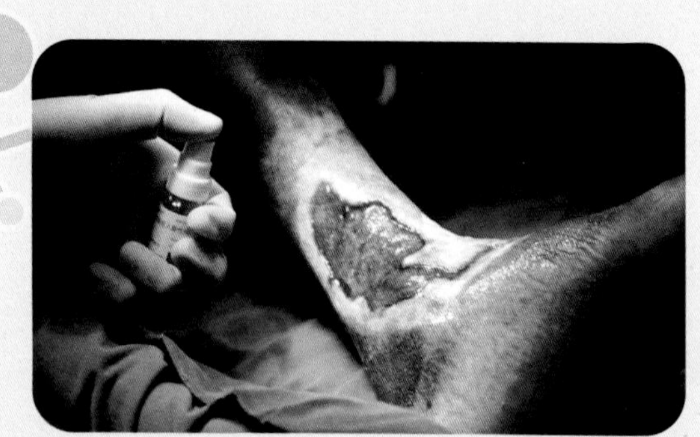

图 5.2.2　清创、换药、喷洒生长因子，肉芽组织渐新鲜

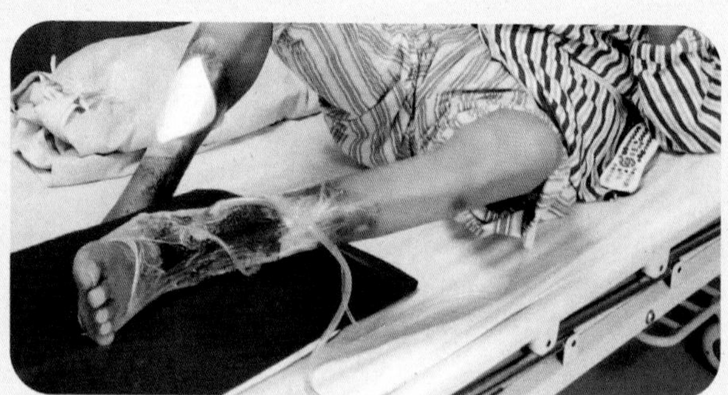

图 5.2.3　VSD+ 生长因子创面滴注冲洗治疗

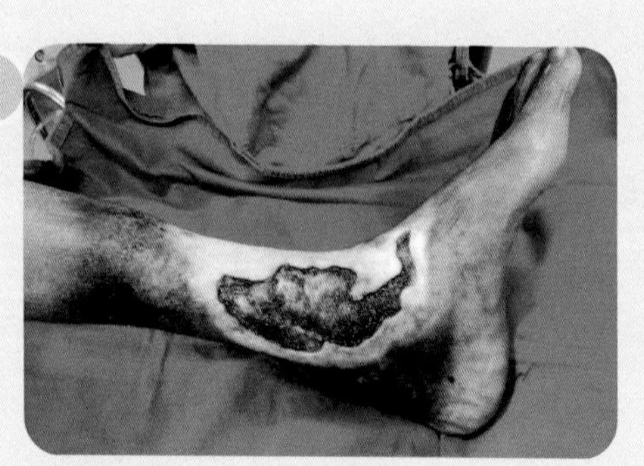

图 5.2.4　VSD 治疗后，创面新鲜

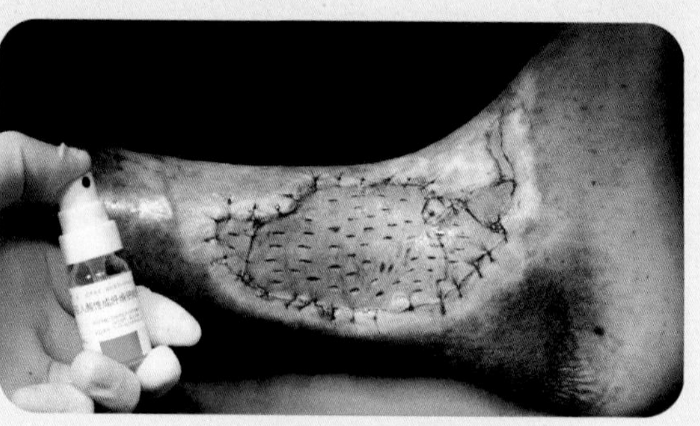

图 5.2.5　创面行中厚游离皮片移植

2. After correcting anemia, local application of VSD + recombinant human basic fibroblast growth factor wound infusion comprehensive treatment promotes fresh granulation tissue and provides a time window for skin grafting (Figure 5.2.2).

3. Comprehensive treatment of VSD + recombinant human alkaline fibroblast growth factor wound infusion for 7 days. The VSD device was removed, and under spinal epidural anesthesia, medium thick free skin grafts were transplanted and recombinant human alkaline fibroblast growth factor was sprayed to promote skin graft survival. Skin grafting, suturing and fixation, and pressure bandaging (Figure 5.2.3 - Figure 5.2.5).

4. After surgery, elevate the affected limb and apply local ice to reduce wound bleeding and prevent skin grafting from floating. Postoperative local infrared and microwave therapy to improve local blood circulation. Training lower limb joint movements in bed to prevent deep vein thrombosis.

5. 10 days after surgery, the stitches were removed, the skin graft survived, the wound healed completely, and the patient recovered and was discharged (Figure 5.2.6).

6. Continue to protect the skin after discharge to prevent secondary rupture.

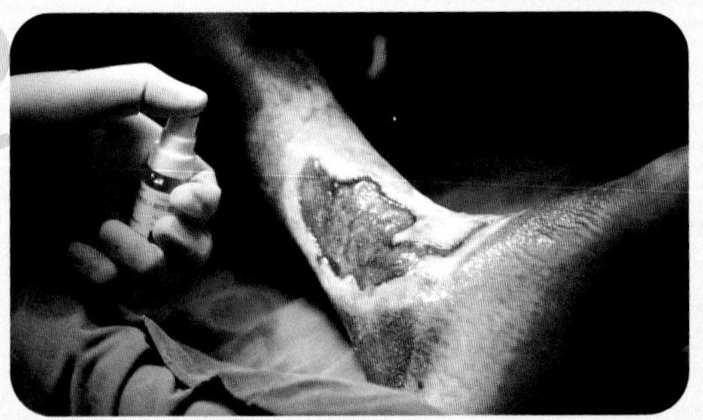

Figure 5.2.2 Debridement, dressing change, and spraying of growth factors result in the gradual freshness of granulation tissue

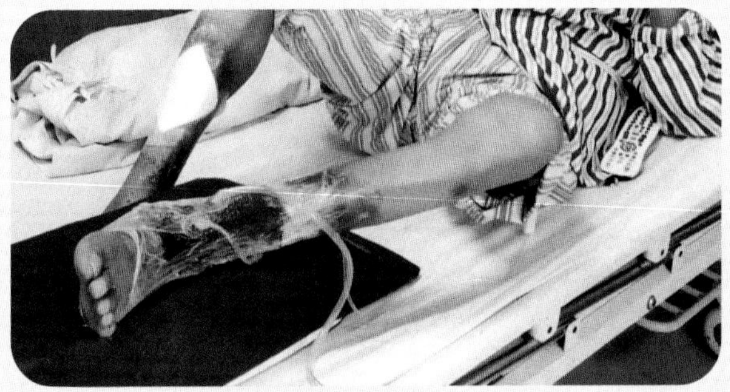

Figure 5.2.3 VSD + growth factor wound drip irrigation treatment

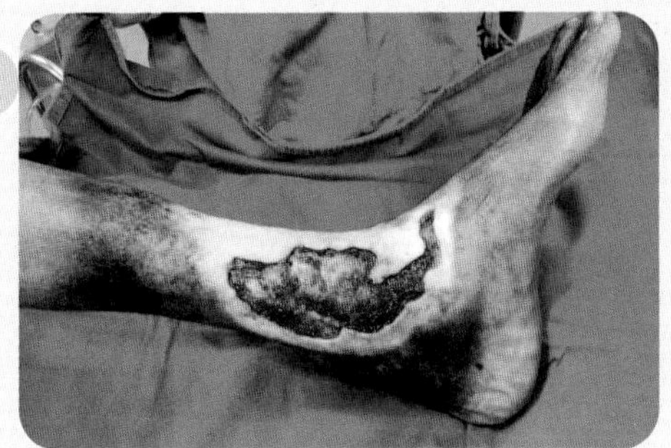

Figure 5.2.4 Fresh wound after VSD treatment

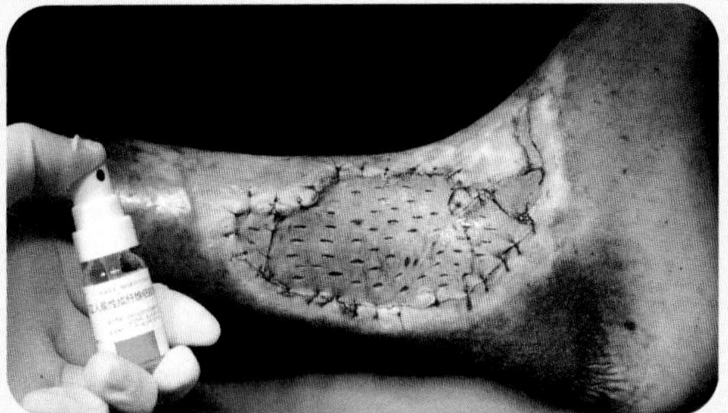

Figure 5.2.5 Transplantation of medium thick free skin graft on the wound surface

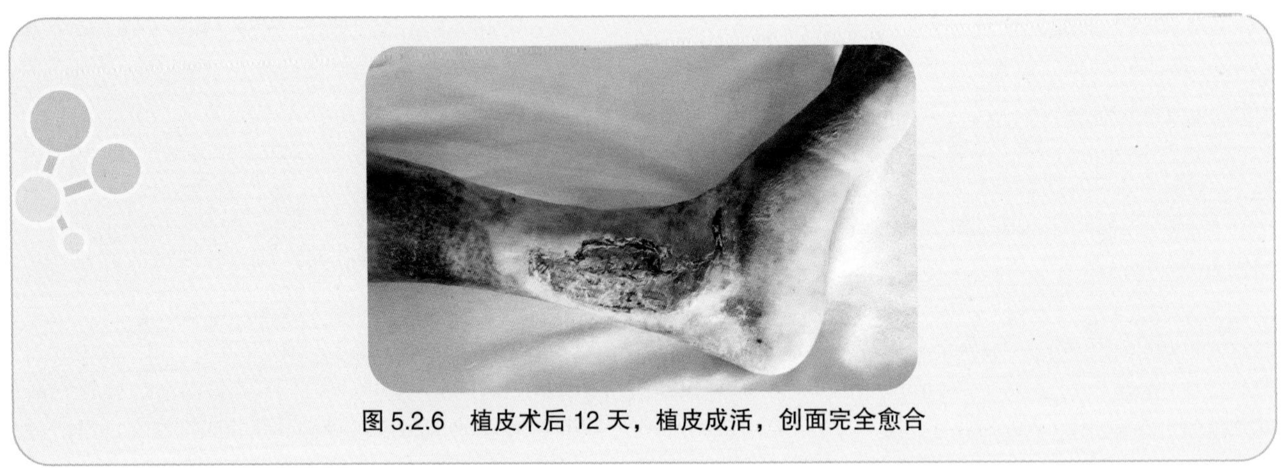

图 5.2.6 植皮术后 12 天，植皮成活，创面完全愈合

（陈善亮）

案例三 会阴部多发溃疡

◆ 致病原因

患者，男性，69 岁，孤寡老人，阴囊、肛门周边、两侧大腿根部剧痛，溃疡破溃经久不愈合 4 年。未去医院规范治疗，在家自用马应龙痔疮膏涂抹，不见好转，溃疡逐渐增大。

◆ 症状与体征

会阴部曾持续性剧痛，彻夜不眠，口服散利痛等镇痛药物不缓解，流脓水，走路跛行。会阴部、肛门周边髂腹股沟和大腿根部内侧有大面积红肿区域，触痛敏感，散在五处不规则创面，阴囊处有 4 cm × 4 cm 溃疡，睾丸外露，两侧大腿内侧各有两处 5 cm × 3 cm 溃疡，肛门右侧有 2 cm × 3 cm 创面，局部有大量炎性渗出，创面有稀薄白色脓性分泌物，红肿区皮肤散在米粒大小水疱（图 5.3.1）。

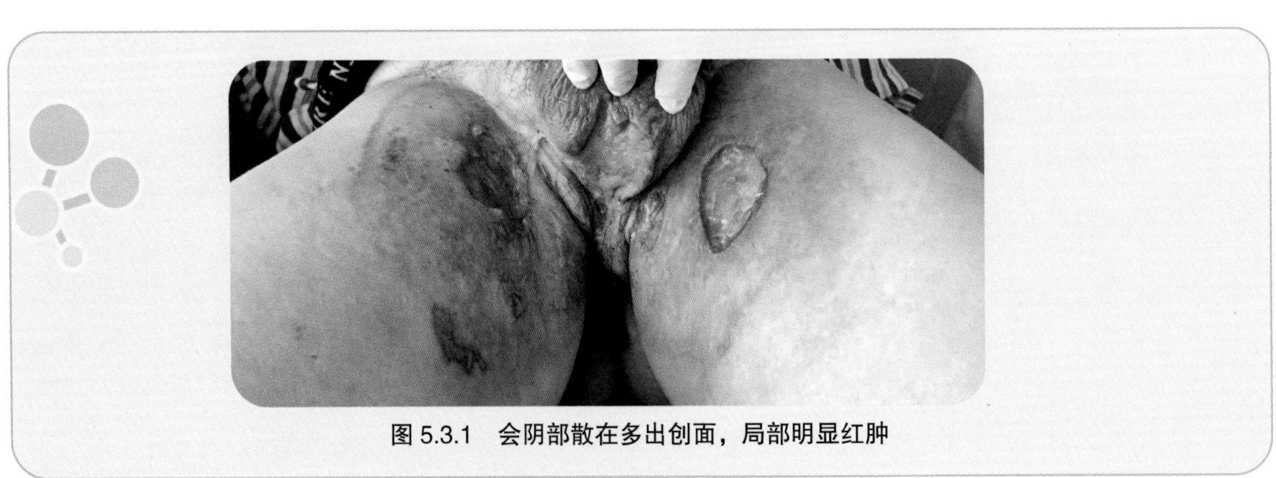

图 5.3.1 会阴部散在多出创面，局部明显红肿

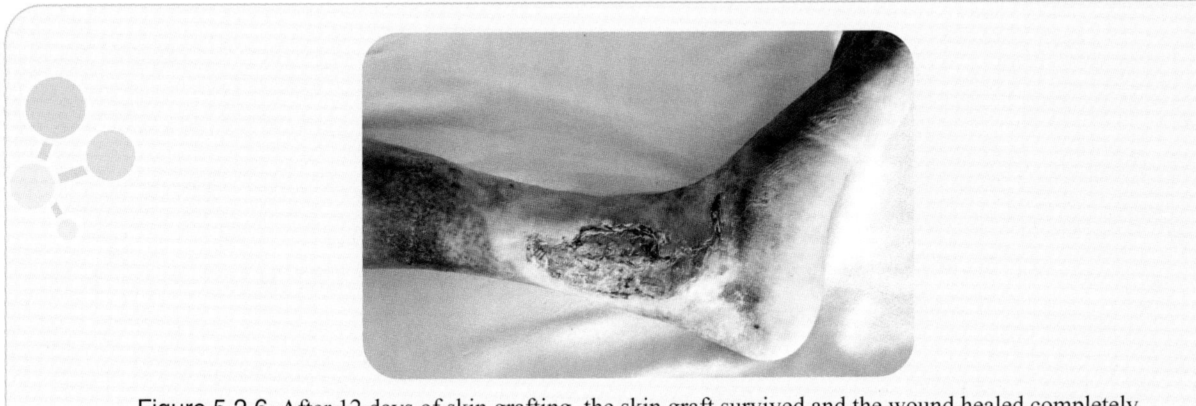

Figure 5.2.6 After 12 days of skin grafting, the skin graft survived and the wound healed completely

(Chen Shanliang)

Case 3 Multiple ulcers in the perineum

◆ Cause of illness

The patient, a 69-year-old male, is a solitary elderly person with severe pain in the scrotum, perianal area, and root of both thighs. Ulcers have been ulcerated for 4 years without healing. I did not seek standardized treatment at the hospital and applied Ma Yinglong Hemorrhoids Cream at home, but there was no improvement and the ulcer gradually increased.

◆ Signs and symptoms

Persistent severe pain in the perineum, staying up all night, taking painkillers such as San Li Tong orally without relief, experiencing pus discharge, and walking with a limp. There are large areas of redness and swelling in the perineum, the iliac inguinal region around the anus, and the inner side of the thigh root, which are sensitive to pain and scattered in five irregular wounds. There are 4 cm × 4 cm ulcers in the scrotum, exposed testicles, and two 5 cm × 3 cm ulcers on each side of the inner thigh. There is a 2 cm × 3 cm wound on the right side of the anus, with a large amount of inflammatory exudate locally. The wound has thin white purulent discharge, and the skin in the redness and swelling area is scattered with rice sized blisters (Figure 5.3.1).

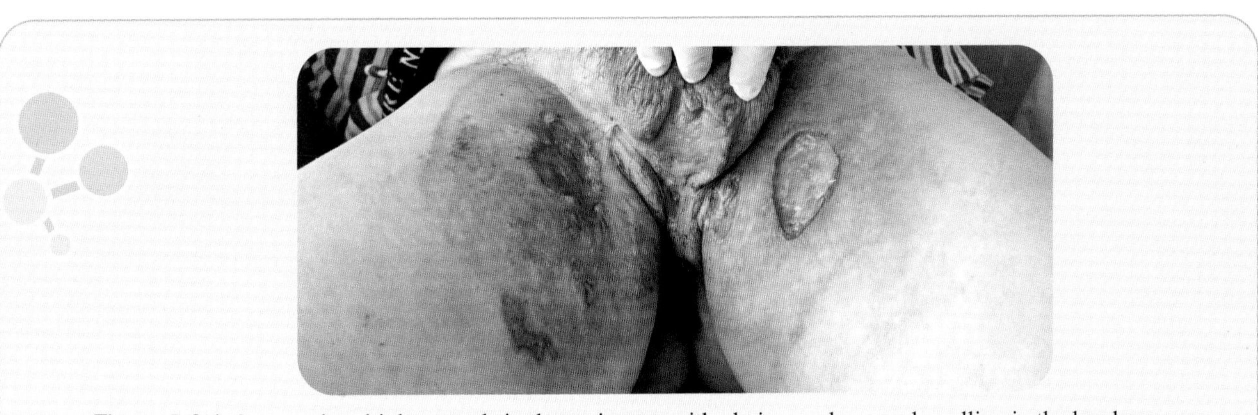

Figure 5.3.1 Scattered multiple wounds in the perineum, with obvious redness and swelling in the local area

◆ 治疗方案

1. 该案例和其他慢性创面有所不同，即创面曾持续性剧痛，给予镇痛药物不能缓解，创面周围大面积红肿，触痛敏感，考虑是细菌和病毒混合感染，抗病毒联合抗菌药物治疗有效。

2. 局部红肿消退后，进行清创缝合，由于皮肤组织脆性增加，术后 3 天缝线逐渐滑脱，伤口逐渐裂开，于 1 周后再次缝合，伤口缝线又再次裂开，考虑缝合不能闭合创面，故改用换药加植皮，溃疡面喷洒重组人碱性成纤维细胞生长因子，致使创面完全愈合（图 5.3.2 ～图 5.3.5）。

3. 患者每天数次涂抹偏方中草药，加上局部排尿排便排气致使伤口污染严重，出院宣教，明确告知局部卫生管理十分重要，否则局部溃疡会再次复发。

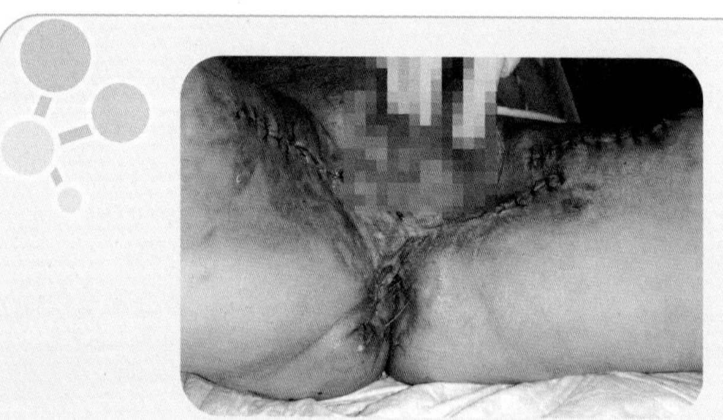

图 5.3.2　第一次清创缝合

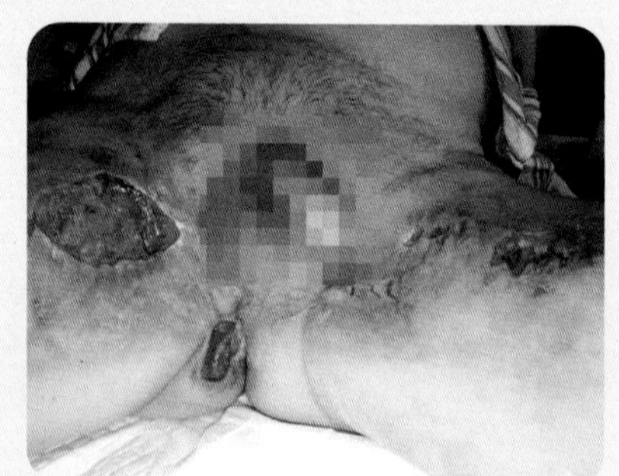

图 5.3.3　术后 7 天，部分伤口裂开

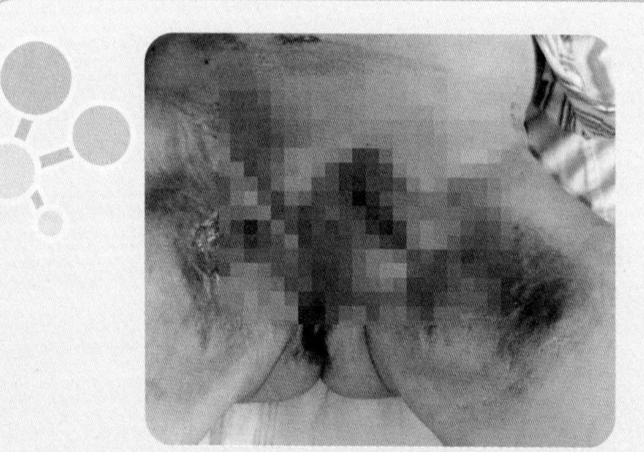

图 5.3.4　经过换药阴囊和左侧大腿内侧愈合

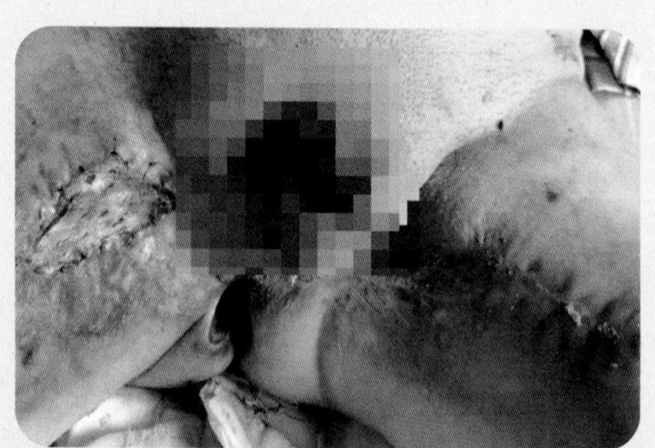

图 5.3.5　右侧大腿创面植皮

（陈善亮）

◆ Treatment plan

1. This case is different from other chronic wounds in that the wound had persistent severe pain that could not be relieved by painkillers, and there was extensive redness and swelling around the wound, making it sensitive to touch. It is considered to be a mixed infection of bacteria and viruses, and antiviral combined with antibacterial treatment is effective.

2. After the local redness and swelling subsided, debridement and suturing were performed. Due to the increased fragility of the skin tissue, the suture gradually slipped and the wound gradually opened three days after surgery. After one week, it was sutured again, but the wound suture opened again. Considering that suturing could not close the wound, dressing change and skin grafting were used. Recombinant human alkaline fibroblast growth factor was sprayed on the ulcer surface, resulting in complete wound healing (Figure 5.3.2 - Figure 5.3.5).

3. The patient applies traditional Chinese herbal medicine several times a day, and combined with local urination, defecation, and exhaust, the wound is severely contaminated. Discharge education should clearly inform the importance of local hygiene management, otherwise the local ulcer will recur.

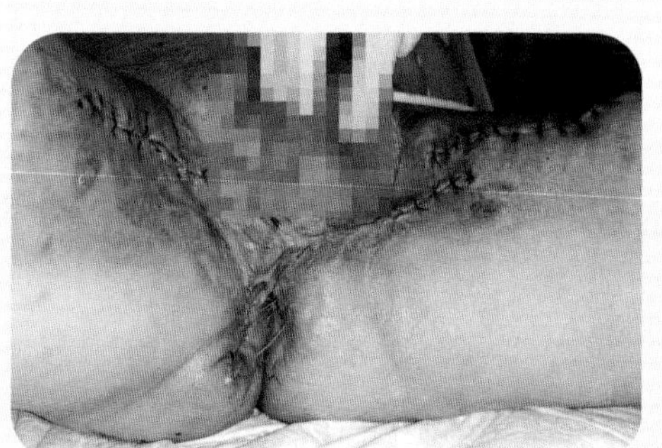

Figure 5.3.2 First debridement and suturing

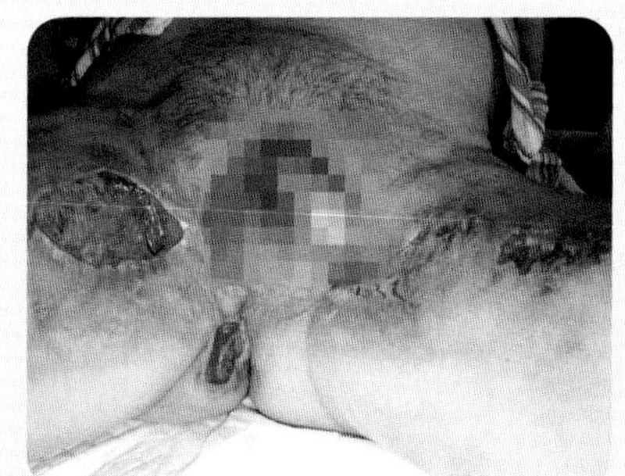

Figure 5.3.3 Seven days after surgery, some wounds split open

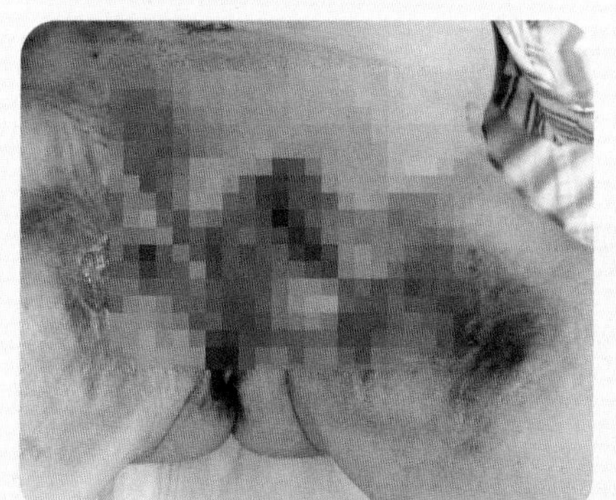

Figure 5.3.4 Healing of scrotum and left inner thigh after dressing change

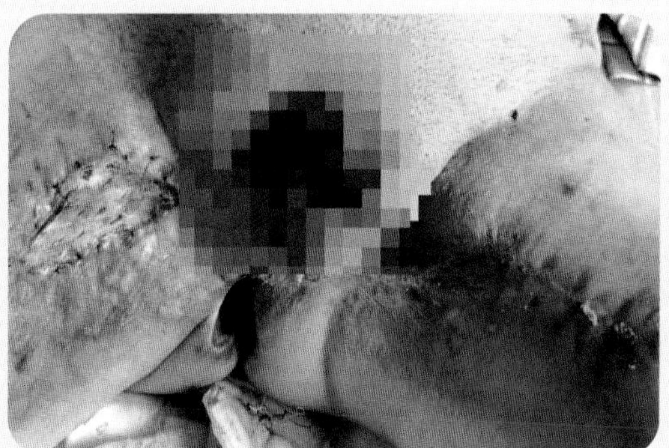

Figure 5.3.5 Right thigh wound skin graft

(Chen Shanliang)

案例四 抽脂术后继发严重腹壁感染坏死

◆ 致病原因

患者腹壁行抽脂术时误穿原切口疝处，导致肠穿孔后腹壁广泛严重感染，腹壁抽脂手术后切口感染、严重腹壁感染、肠穿孔肠梗阻。曾有阑尾炎手术史、剖宫产手术史。

◆ 症状与体征

患者因腹部抽脂术后出现疼痛、呕吐、发热等症状，急诊入院。神志清，全腹膨隆，下腹部可见一陈旧性刀疤，下腹部皮肤红肿，全腹部压痛，皮下组织可触及捻发感（图 5.4.1）。术前急诊 CT 检查，示右下腹壁疝、肠梗阻、多发腹壁皮下大量积气及渗出（图 5.4.2）。

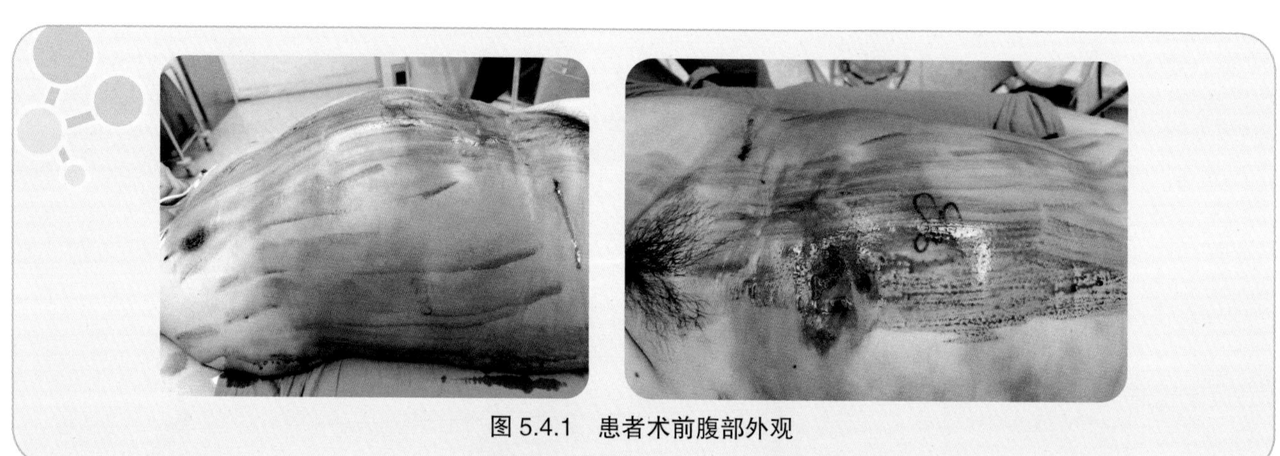

图 5.4.1 患者术前腹部外观

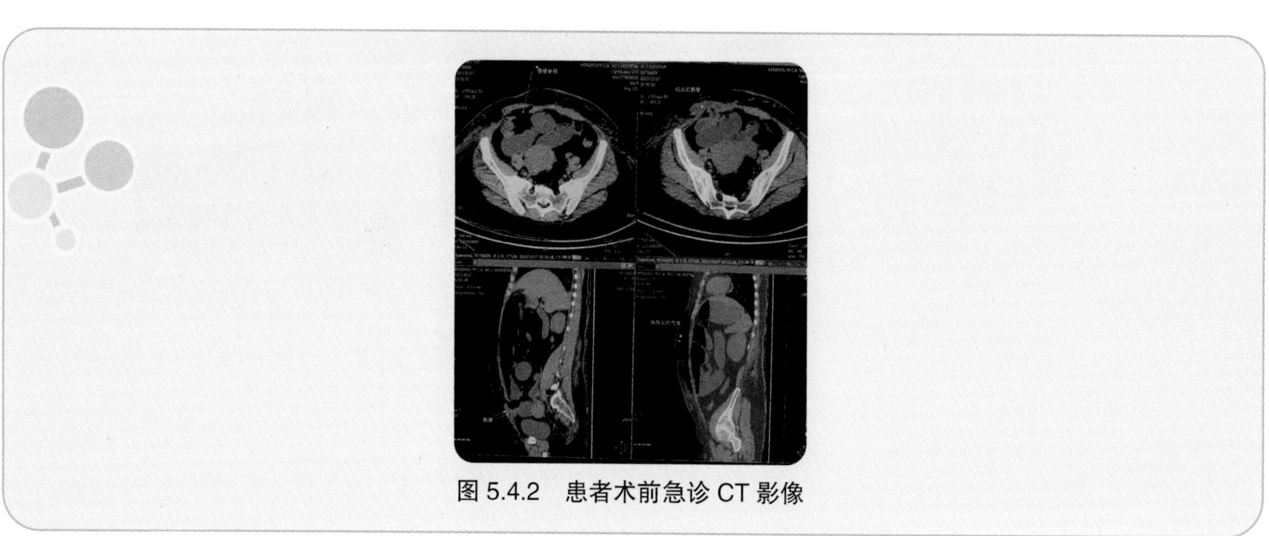

图 5.4.2 患者术前急诊 CT 影像

Case 4 Severe abdominal wall infection and necrosis secondary to liposuction surgery

◆ Cause of illness

During the abdominal wall liposuction surgery, the patient accidentally punctured the hernia site of the original incision, resulting in widespread and severe infection of the abdominal wall after intestinal perforation. After the abdominal wall liposuction surgery, the incision was infected, severe abdominal wall infection occurred, and intestinal perforation caused intestinal obstruction. Has a history of appendicitis surgery and cesarean section surgery.

◆ Signs and symptoms

The patient was admitted to the emergency department due to symptoms such as pain, vomiting, and fever after abdominal liposuction surgery. Clear consciousness, bulging entire abdomen, with an old scar visible in the lower abdomen. The skin in the lower abdomen is red and swollen, with tenderness throughout the abdomen. The subcutaneous tissue can feel a twisting sensation (Figure 5.4.1). Preoperative emergency CT scan showed right lower abdominal hernia, intestinal obstruction, multiple subcutaneous gas accumulation and exudation in the abdominal wall (Figure 5.4.2).

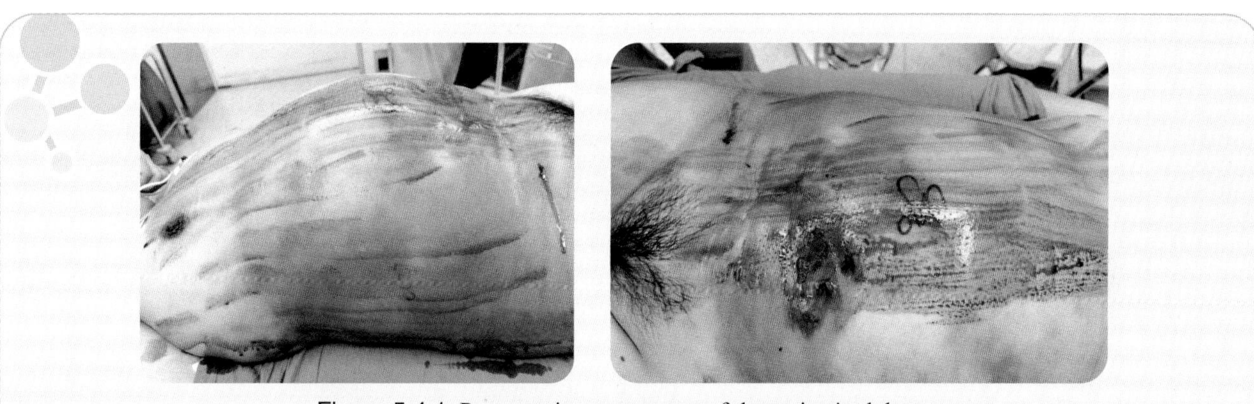

Figure 5.4.1 Preoperative appearance of the patient's abdomen

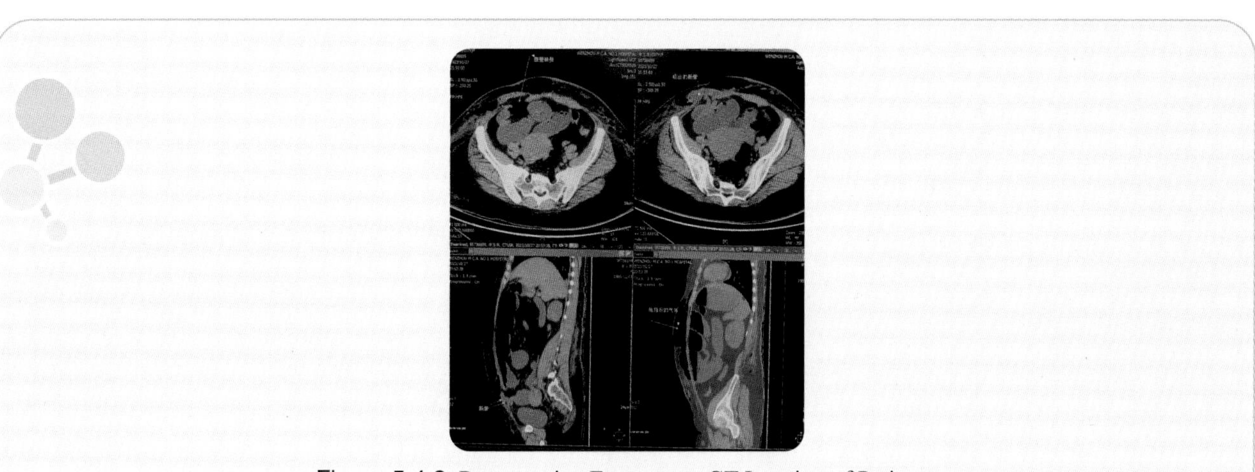

Figure 5.4.2 Preoperative Emergency CT Imaging of Patients

◆ 治疗方案

1. 急诊处理，初步评估和稳定病情。

2. 手术治疗，分离肠壁与腹壁的粘连，并对梗阻肠管进行减压，离断了肠穿孔的坏死肠管，进行回肠侧侧吻合，修复肠穿孔。术中发现腹壁、胸壁、背部广泛浸润的脓性粪性渗出，右下腹腹壁缺损，范围约 6 cm × 5 cm，回肠疝出于皮下，肠壁可见数处破口（图 5.4.3）。再行腹壁感染创口清创术，多切口探查，引流。

3. 使用 VSD 材料覆盖创口，充分引流，对小肠外露处进行异体皮覆盖，保护小肠。

4. 多次清创，右侧腹腔放置 2 根引流管。形成约 7 cm × 8 cm 腹壁缺损创面，VSD 治疗，部分小肠外露处覆盖异体皮保护，其余创面外用成纤维细胞生长因子换药，促进创面肉芽组织生长，加速创面愈合（图 5.4.4）。

5. 设计邻位带蒂旋转皮瓣，修复腹壁缺损，覆盖小肠外露，残余创面，继续生长因子外用，促进愈合（图 5.4.5）。

6. 患者出院后残余小创面继续门诊换药，功能锻炼康复。

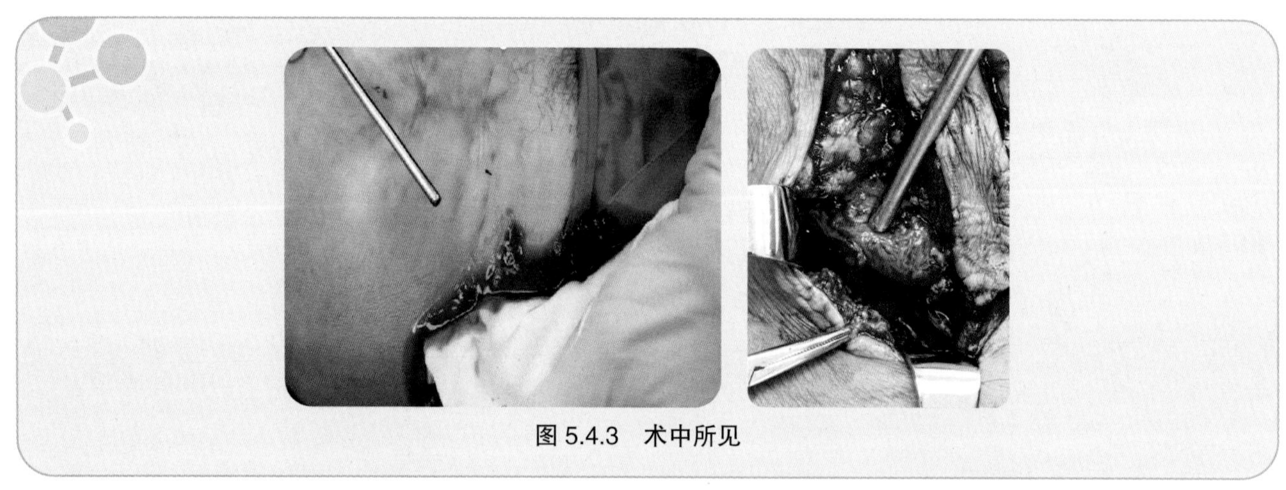

图 5.4.3　术中所见

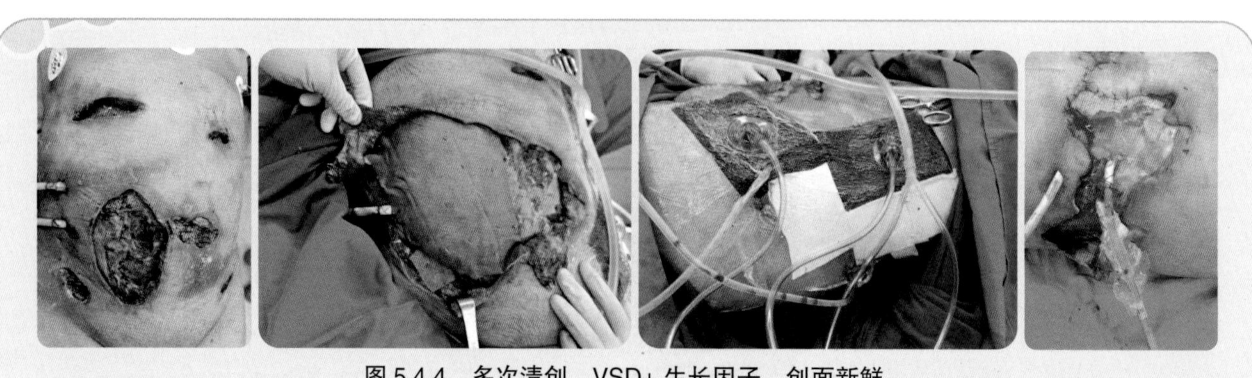

图 5.4.4　多次清创，VSD+ 生长因子，创面新鲜

◆ Treatment plan

1. Emergency treatment, preliminary assessment, and stabilization of the condition.

2. Surgical treatment involves separating the adhesions between the intestinal wall and abdominal wall, and reducing the pressure on the obstructed intestinal tube. The necrotic intestinal tube of the intestinal perforation is severed, and a lateral anastomosis of the ileum is performed to repair the intestinal perforation. During the operation, purulent fecal exudate was found extensively infiltrating the abdominal wall, chest wall, and back. There was a defect in the right lower abdominal wall, measuring approximately 6 cm × 5 cm. The ileal hernia was located subcutaneously, and several incisions were visible in the intestinal wall (Figure 5.4.3). Perform abdominal wall infection wound debridement, multiple incision exploration, and drainage.

3. Cover the wound with VSD material, fully drain, and cover the exposed small intestine with allogeneic skin to protect the small intestine.

4. Multiple debridement and placement of 2 drainage tubes in the right abdominal cavity. A 7 cm × 8 cm abdominal wall defect wound was formed, treated with VSD, and partially covered with allogeneic skin for protection. The remaining wounds were treated with fibroblast growth factor dressing to promote granulation tissue growth and accelerate wound healing (Figure 5.4.4).

5. Design an adjacent pedicle rotary skin flap to repair abdominal wall defects, cover exposed small intestine and residual wounds, and continue to apply growth factors externally to promote healing (Figure 5.4.5).

6. After the patient is discharged, residual small wounds will continue to be treated with dressing changes and functional exercise rehabilitation in the outpatient department.

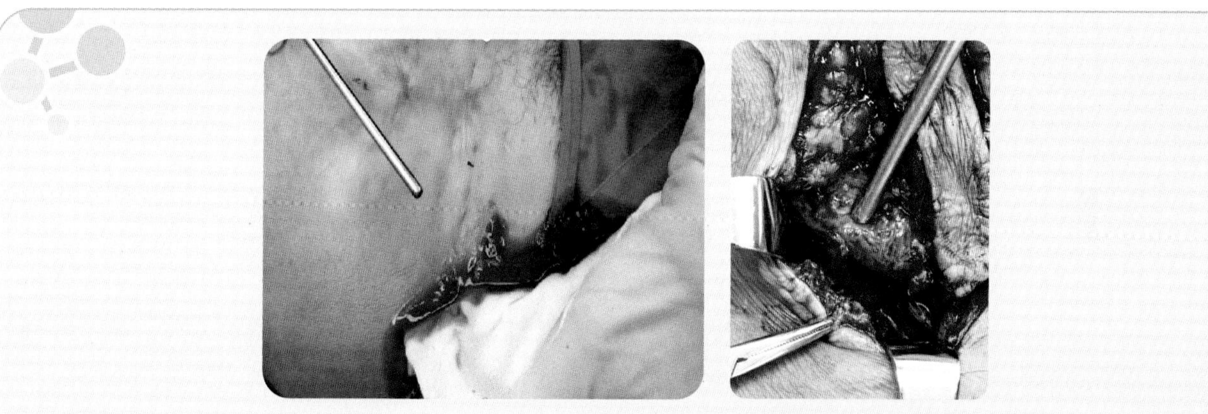

Figure 5.4.3 Intraoperative Observations

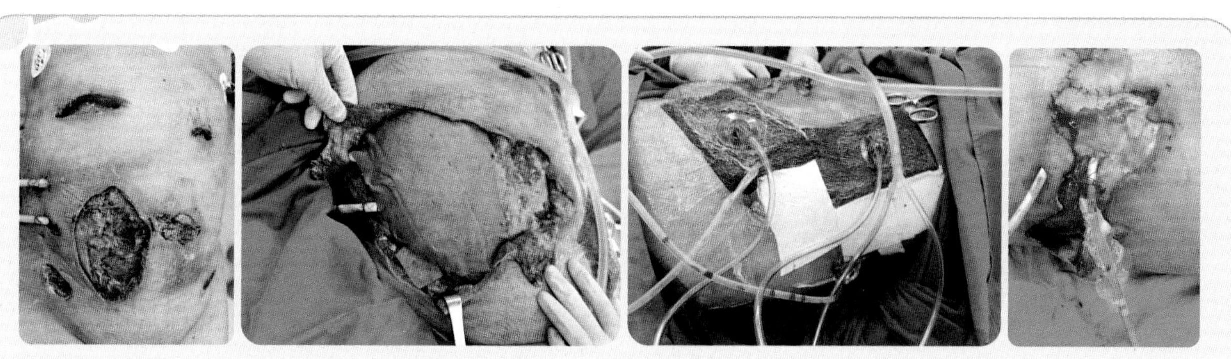

Figure 5.4.4 Multiple debridement, VSD+ growth factor, fresh wound surface

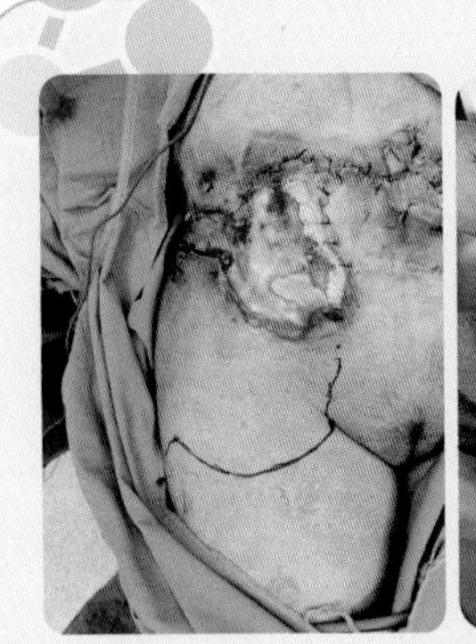
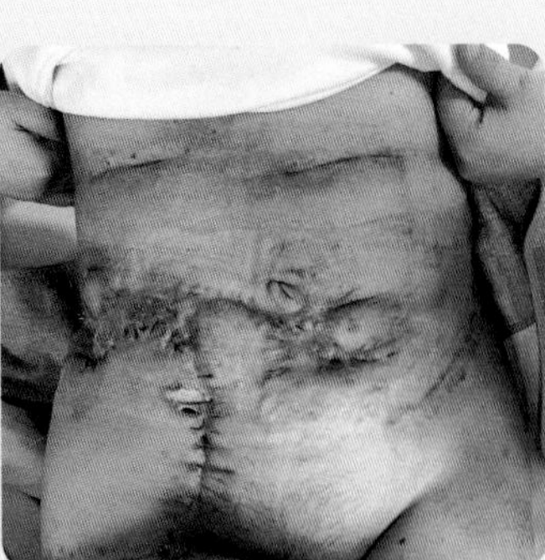
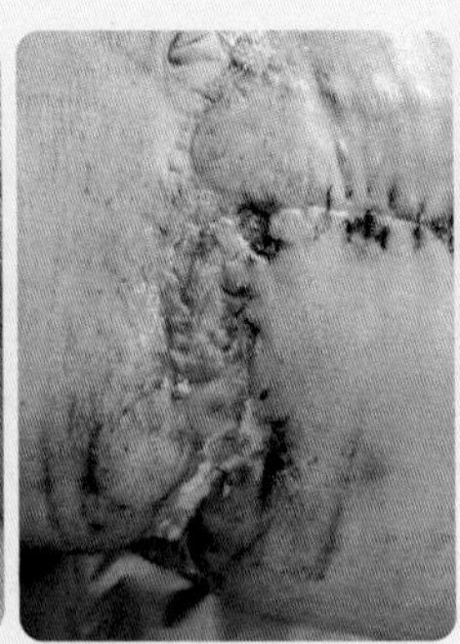
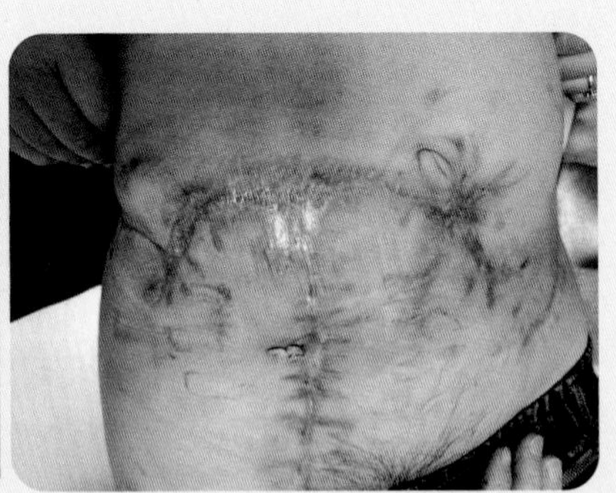

图 5.4.5 设计带蒂旋转皮瓣修复缺损腹壁，创面逐步愈合

（刘政军 赵 胜）

案例五 左大腿急性坏死性筋膜炎

◆ 致病原因

患者骑三轮车翻车跌入沟渠，压伤左大腿前侧，有 4 cm 伤口，伤口在当地医院缝合，现有急性坏死性筋膜炎。

◆ 症状与体征

左大腿伤后 3 天，左大腿出现胀痛难忍，并逐渐加重，寒战，乏力，心悸，气促，发热，体温 38.3 ℃，表情淡漠，反应迟钝，全身湿冷，面色苍白。左大腿广泛性肿胀，前侧皮肤皮革样变，散在花斑，坏死皮肤边界不清，局部皮肤有疱皮并破溃脱落，大腿前侧有 4 cm 缝合伤口，皮肤波动阳性，压之从伤口有洗肉水样黏稠液体溢出，局部温度轻度增高，压痛敏感（图 5.5.1 ~ 图 5.5.3）。左小腿内侧广泛性红肿，局部温度高，压痛敏感，局部波动阳性，局部皮肤皮革样变。足趾活动良好，足背动脉搏动减弱，足部感觉正常，足部血运良好，髂腹股沟淋巴结轻度肿大，压痛阳性。

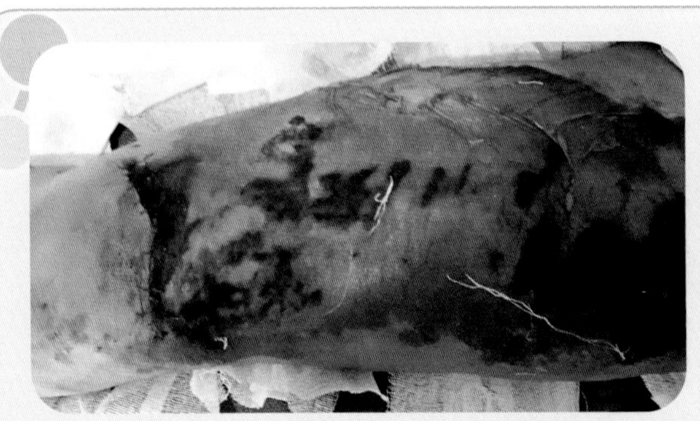

图 5.5.1 左大腿皮肤大面积坏死，皮肤皮革样变

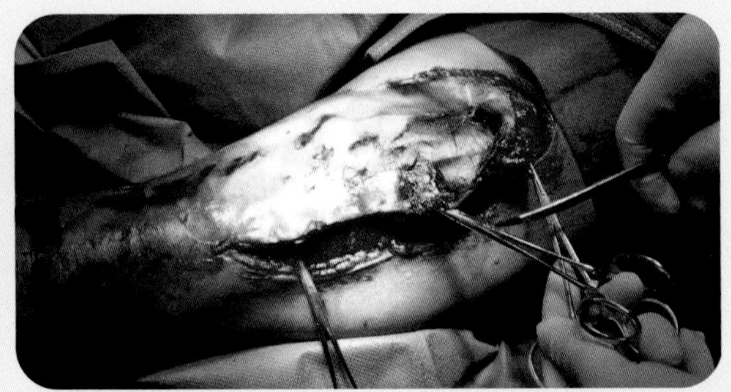

图 5.5.2 手术切开大腿皮肤，皮肤和皮下脂肪广泛游离

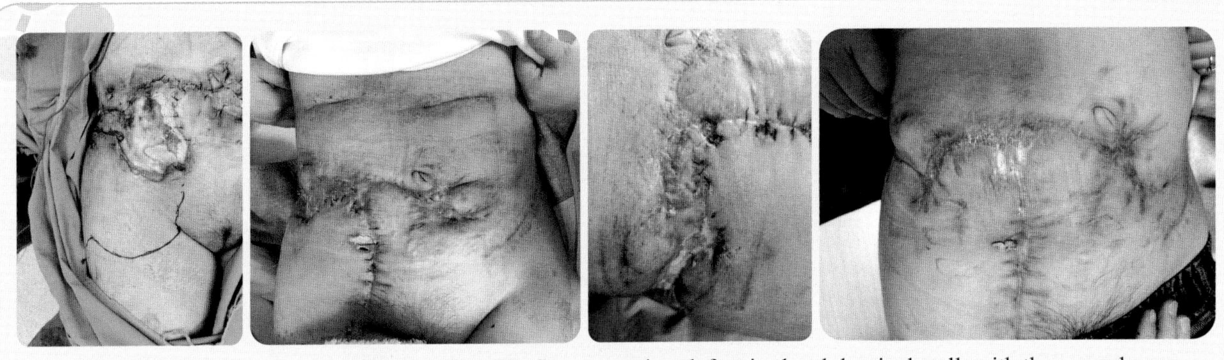

Figure 5.4.5 Design a pedicled rotating skin flap to repair a defect in the abdominal wall, with the wound gradually healing

(Liu Zhengjun, Zhao Sheng)

Case 5 Acute necrotizing fasciitis of left thigh

◆ Cause of illness

The patient overturned on a tricycle and fell into a ditch, injuring the front side of their left thigh with a 4 cm wound. The wound was sutured at a local hospital and currently has acute necrotizing fasciitis.

◆ Signs and symptoms

Three days after the left thigh injury, there was unbearable swelling and pain in the left thigh, which gradually worsened, accompanied by chills, fatigue, palpitations, shortness of breath, fever, a body temperature of 38.3 ℃, indifferent expression, slow response, damp and cold body, and pale complexion. Widespread swelling in the left thigh, leather like changes in the skin on the front side, scattered flower spots, unclear boundaries of necrotic skin, and local skin with blister skin that has ruptured and fallen off. There is a 4cm suture wound on the front side of the thigh, with positive skin fluctuations. When pressed, there is a sticky liquid resembling a washing meat sample overflowing from the wound, and the local temperature slightly increases, with sensitive tenderness (Figure 5.5.1-Figure 5.5.3). Widespread redness and swelling on the inner side of the left calf, high local temperature, sensitive tenderness, positive local fluctuations, and leather like changes in the local skin. Good toe movement, weakened dorsalis pedis artery pulsation, normal foot sensation, good foot blood supply, mild swelling of iliac and inguinal lymph nodes, positive tenderness.

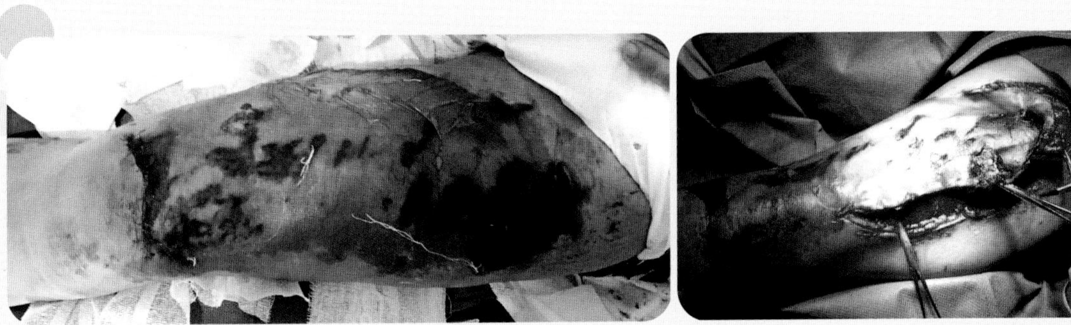

Figure 5.5.1 Large area necrosis of the left thigh skin and leather like transformation of the skin

Figure 5.5.2 Surgical incision of thigh skin, extensive free skin and subcutaneous fat

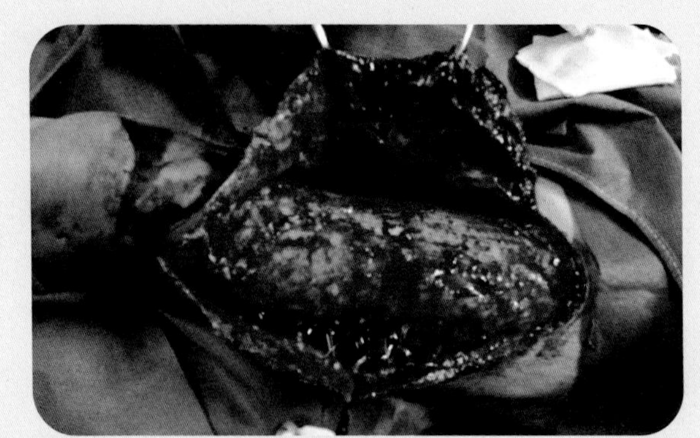

图 5.5.3　大腿皮肤广泛性游离，皮下有大量洗肉水样黏稠液体

◆ 治疗方案

1. 患者入院后立即进行细菌培养 + 药物敏感试验。

2. 患者入院后立即完善术前准备，在腰硬联合麻醉下行坏死皮肤、组织切除，脓液清除术。术中切除大腿和小腿大面积坏死皮肤皮下脂肪和坏死筋膜，并用双氧水、碘伏和生理盐水反复冲洗创腔，大腿创面有 33 cm × 18 cm 创面，几乎环绕整个大腿，大腿后侧皮肤广泛剥脱，右腿内侧 8 cm × 6 cm，创面深达肌筋膜层，术中吸引黏稠洗肉水样渗出液约 1200 mL。重组人碱性成纤维细胞生长因子喷洒创面，使用 VSD 治疗（图 5.5.4 ~ 图 5.5.7）。

3. 术后抬高患肢、局部冰敷减少渗出，持续 VSD+ 重组人碱性成纤维细胞生长因子滴注创面，细菌培养未出结果前，给予广谱抗菌药物覆盖治疗，局部红外线理疗促进改善血液循环。

4. 术后 3 天根据细菌培养给予敏感抗菌药物，预防深静脉血栓，给予气压泵治疗。

5. 术后 5 天拆除 VSD 装置，创面新鲜新鲜程度不够，故再次使用 VSD，促进创面新鲜，为植皮消灭创面缩短时间窗（图 5.5.8）。

6. 第二次 VSD+ 重组人碱性成纤维细胞生长因子滴注冲洗治疗 4 天，拆除 VSD 装置，大腿和小腿内侧创面新鲜，创面肉芽组织红润，渗血活跃，创面达到植皮条件（图 5.5.9）。

7. 选择腰硬联合麻醉，根据 2 个创面缺损面积，于右侧大腿切取中厚游离皮片，分别移植于大腿和小腿内侧，皮片边缘缝合，喷洒重组人碱性成纤维细胞生长因子，油纱覆盖创面，后棉垫加压包扎（图 5.5.10、图 5.5.11）。

8. 植皮术后 7 天，换药见植皮完全成活，并督促患者下地康复训练；术后 12 天，植皮完全成活，患者康复出院（图 5.5.12、图 5.5.13）。

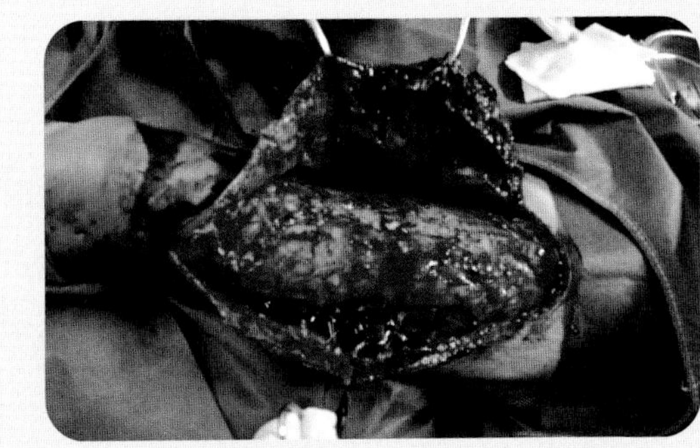

Figure 5.5.3 Widespread free thigh skin, with a large amount of flesh washing water like viscous liquid under the skin

◆ Treatment plan

1. The patient should undergo bacterial culture and drug sensitivity testing immediately after admission.

2. After admission, the patient immediately completed preoperative preparation, performed necrotic skin and tissue resection, and pus removal surgery under lumbar epidural anesthesia. During the surgery, large areas of necrotic skin, subcutaneous fat, and fascia in the thigh and calf were removed, and the wound cavity was repeatedly washed with hydrogen peroxide, iodine, and physiological saline. The thigh wound had a size of 33 cm × 18 cm, almost surrounding the entire thigh, and the skin on the back of the thigh was extensively peeled off. The inner side of the right leg was 8 cm × 6 cm, and the wound depth reached the myofascial layer. About 1200 mL of viscous, flesh washing exudate was aspirated during the surgery. Recombinant human basic fibroblast growth factor was sprayed onto the wound surface and treated with VSD (Figure 5.5.4- Figure 5.5.7).

3. After surgery, elevate the affected limb and apply local ice to reduce exudation. Continuously inject VSD+ recombinant human basic fibroblast growth factor into the wound. Before bacterial culture yields results, provide broad-spectrum antibacterial drug coverage treatment and local infrared therapy to promote improved blood circulation.

4. Three days after surgery, sensitive antibacterial drugs were administered based on bacterial culture to prevent deep vein thrombosis, and pneumatic pump treatment was given.

5. Five days after surgery, the VSD device was removed, but the freshness of the wound was not sufficient. Therefore, VSD was used again to promote wound freshness and shorten the time window for skin grafting to eliminate the wound (Figure 5.5.8).

6. The second VSD+ recombinant human basic fibroblast growth factor infusion and flushing treatment lasted for 4 days. The VSD device was removed, and the wounds on the inner side of the thigh and calf were fresh. The granulation tissue on the wounds was red and actively oozing blood, and the wounds met the conditions for skin grafting (Figure 5.5.9).

7. Choose spinal epidural anesthesia, cut medium thick free skin grafts from the right thigh based on the defect area of two wounds, transplant them onto the inner side of the thigh and calf, suture the edges of the skin grafts, spray recombinant human basic fibroblast growth factor, cover the wound with oil gauze, and then apply pressure with cotton pads for bandaging (Figure 5.5.10, Figure 5.5.11).

8. After 7 days of skin grafting, the dressing was changed and the skin graft was found to be completely alive, and the patient was urged to undergo rehabilitation training on the ground; After 12 days of surgery, the skin graft completely survived and the patient recovered and was discharged (Figure 5.5.12, Figure 5.5.13).

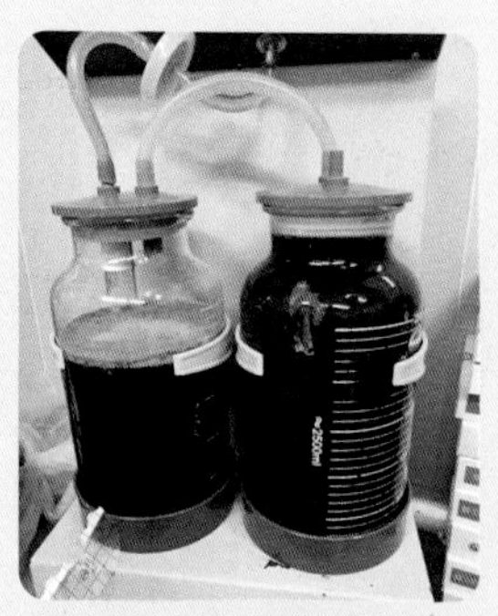
图 5.5.4 左大腿和小腿吸引 1200 mL 洗肉水液体，冲洗液体 1800 mL

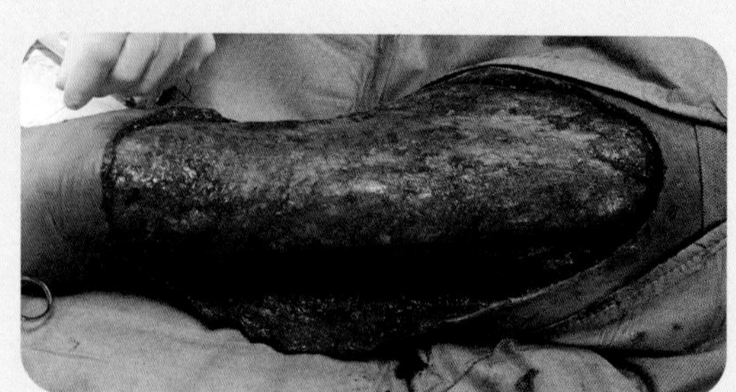
图 5.5.5 左大腿坏死和小腿坏死皮肤切除，裸露大面创面

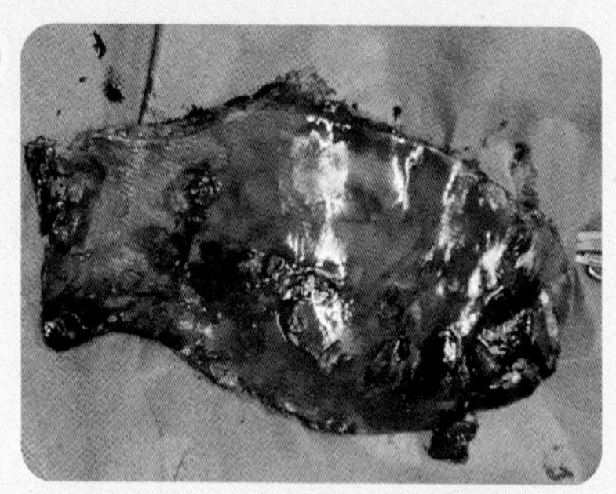
图 5.5.6 大腿坏死皮肤切除

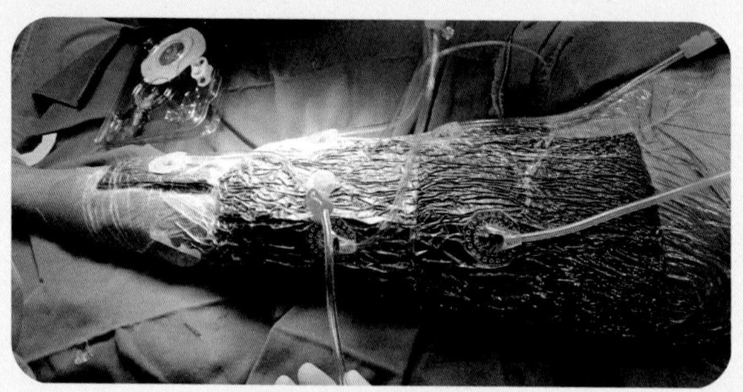
图 5.5.7 VSD+ 生长因子滴注冲洗治疗

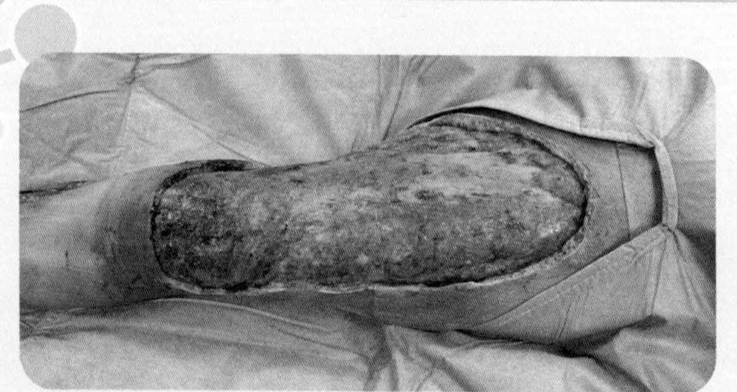
图 5.5.8 第一次负压治疗 5 天，创面不新鲜

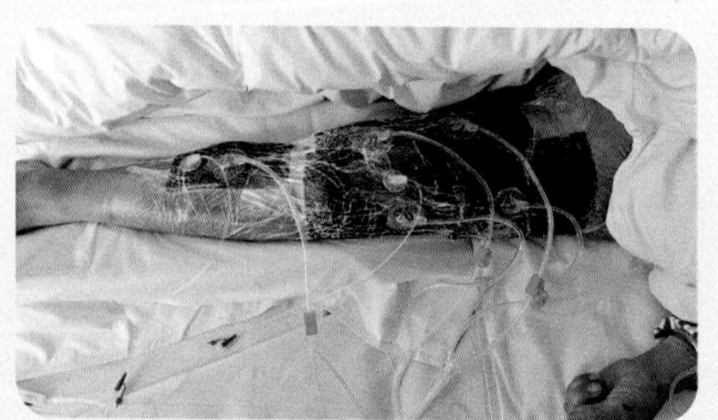
图 5.5.9 第二次 VSD+ 生长因子滴注冲洗治疗

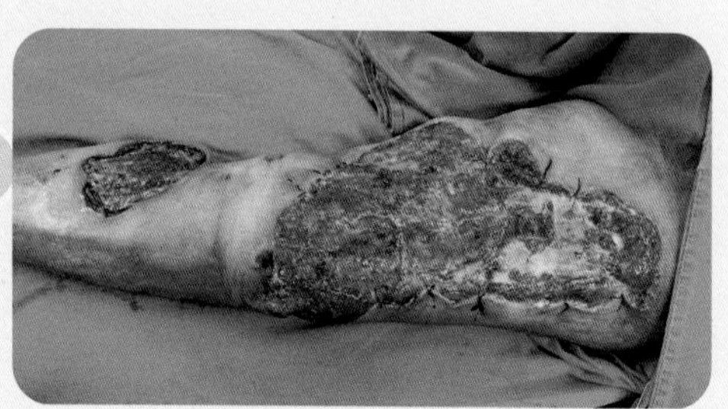
图 5.5.10 第二次负压治疗后，创面新鲜，为了缩小创面，减张缝合

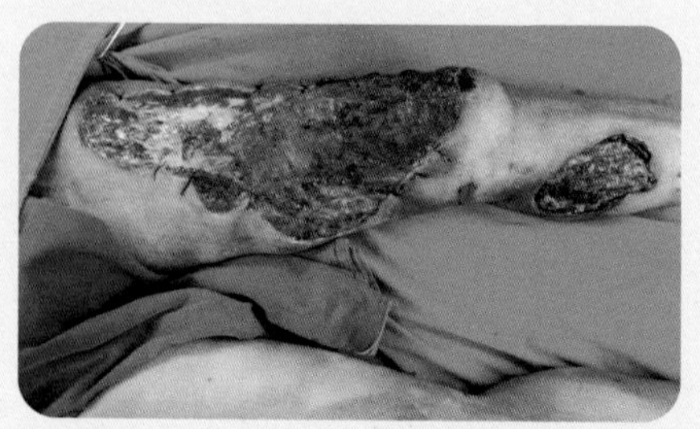
图 5.5.11 大腿和小腿创面新鲜，小腿创面边缘有部分创面坏死

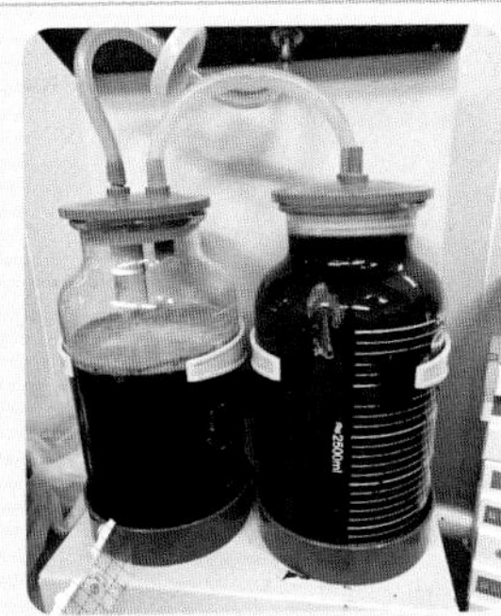
Figure 5.5.4 The left thigh and calf attract 1200 mL of meat wash solution, and 1800 mL of wash solution

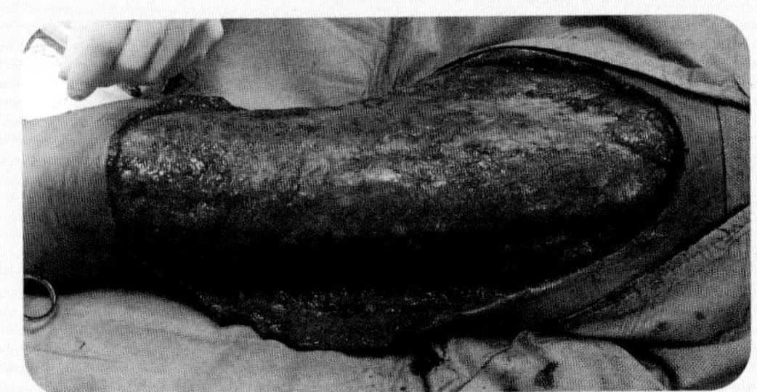
Figure 5.5.5 Removal of necrotic skin on the left thigh and calf, exposing a large surface wound

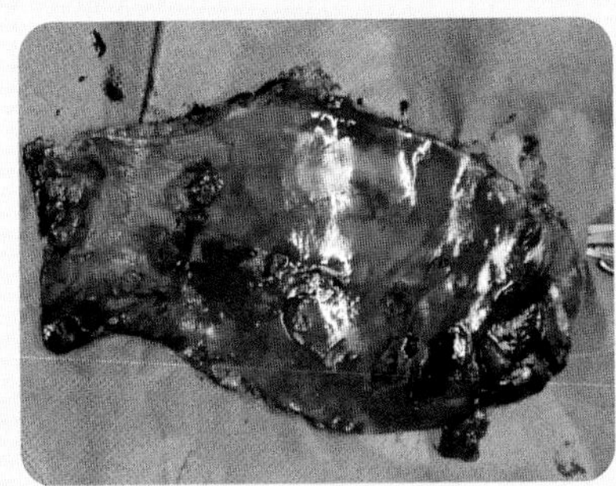
Figure 5.5.6 Removal of necrotic skin on the thigh

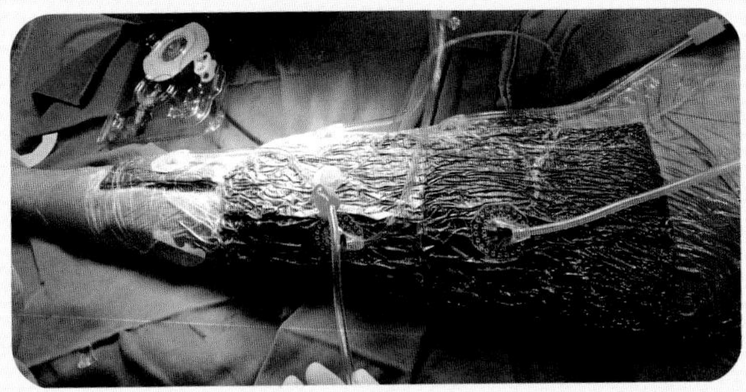
Figure 5.5.7 VSD+ growth factor drip irrigation treatment

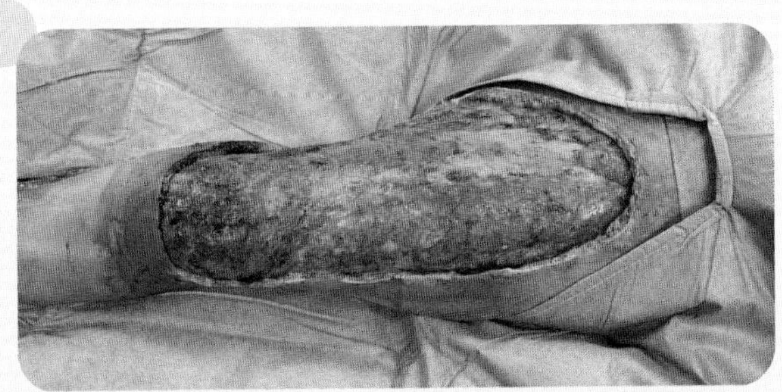
Figure 5.5.8 First negative pressure treatment for 5 days, wound not fresh

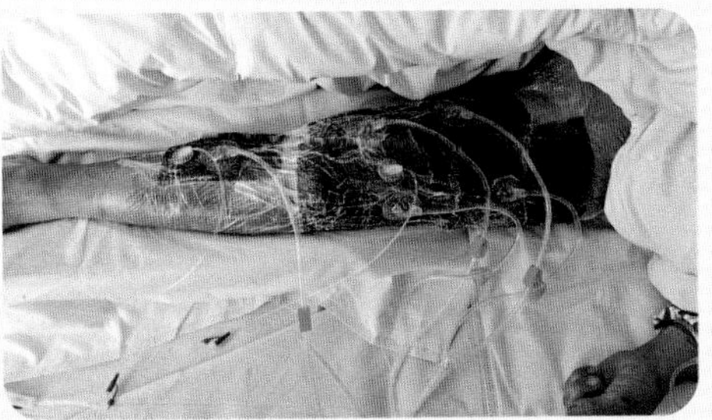
Figure 5.5.9 Second VSD+ growth factor drip irrigation treatment

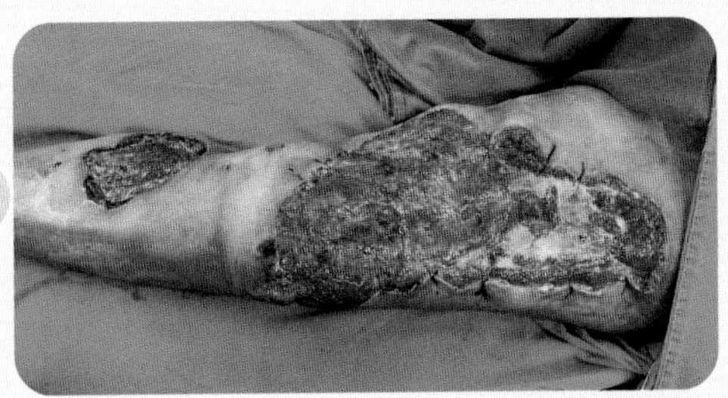
Figure 5.5.10 After the second negative pressure treatment in the wound was fresh. In order to reduce the wound size, tension reduction suturing was performed

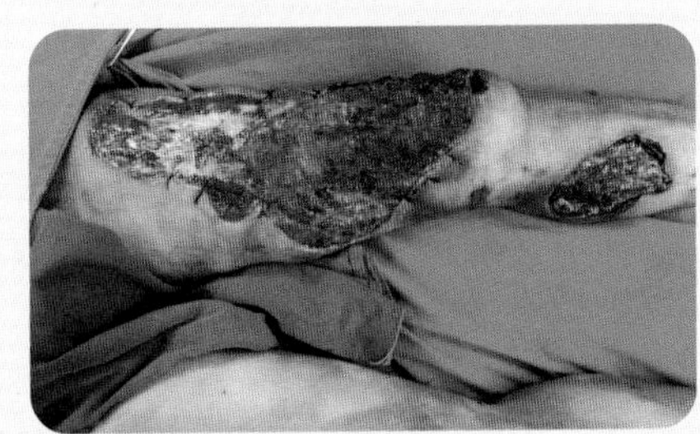
Figure 5.5.11 Fresh thigh and calf wounds, with partial necrosis at the edge of calf wounds

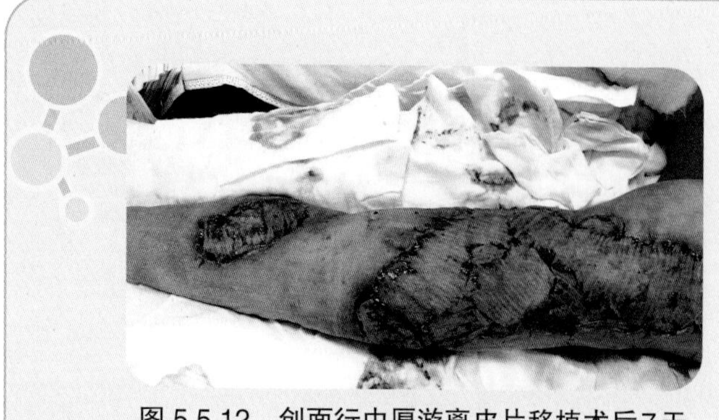

图 5.5.12　创面行中厚游离皮片移植术后 7 天，游离植皮成活

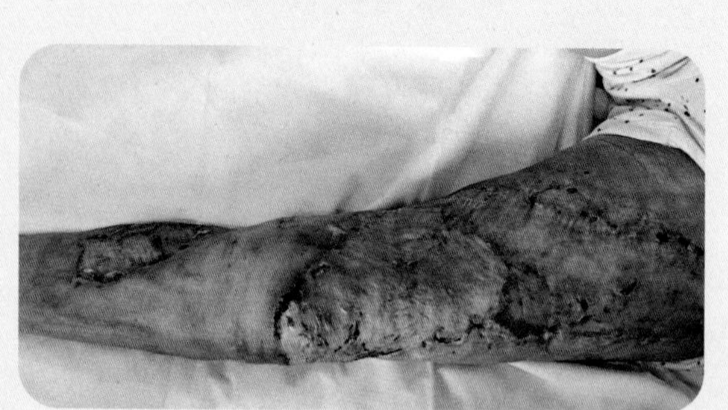

图 5.5.13　术后 12 天，植皮完全成活

（陈善亮　陈银炜）

案例六　小腿破溃经久不愈、钢板外露

◆ 致病原因

患者因车祸致左胫腓骨开放粉碎性骨折，术后出现皮肤坏死，钢板外露 38 年。

◆ 症状与体征

患者于 38 年前，因车祸致左小腿开放粉碎性骨折，在当地医院行胫骨骨折清创骨折复位钢板内固定术。术后出现胫前皮肤坏死，胫骨钢板外露，流脓水 38 年，在当地诊所行换药治疗至今。左小腿胫前有 8 cm × 4 cm 创面，局部皮缘内陷，可见钢板外露，创腔深部有黄白色脓性分泌物，味臭，局部肉芽组织老化，小腿胫前皮肤色素沉着，局部瘢痕较硬，局部皮温不高，无明显红肿，足背动脉波动消失，足底感觉正常，足趾屈曲良好，伸趾活动受限，踝关节僵硬（图 5.6.1、图 5.6.2）。下肢动脉超声，示小腿胫后动脉变细内膜增厚，胫前足背动脉闭塞，远端血流消失；股骨干和小腿 DR，示左侧胫骨和腓骨畸形愈合，胫骨中段可见虫蚀样变，有 3 枚螺钉松动脱落。

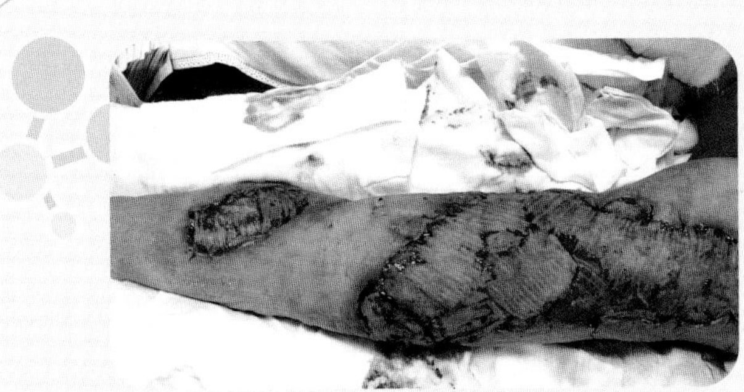

Figure 5.5.12 Seven days after performing medium thickness free skin graft transplantation on the wound, the free skin graft survived

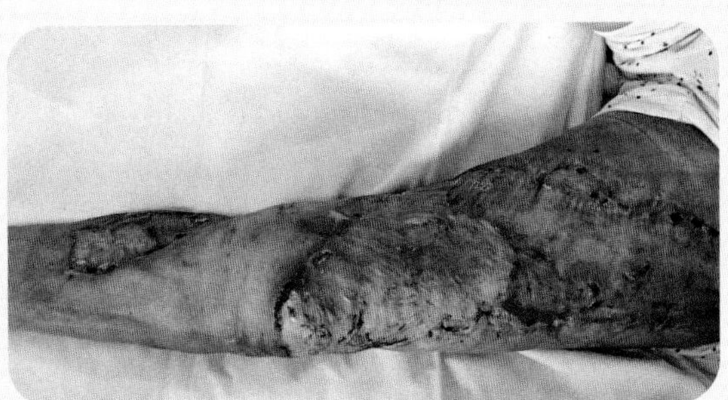

Figure 5.5.13 After 12 days of surgery, the skin graft completely survived

(Chen Shanliang, Chen Yinwei)

Case 6 Prolonged leg rupture and exposed steel plate

◆ Cause of illness

The patient suffered an open comminuted fracture of the left tibia and fibula due to a car accident. After surgery, skin necrosis occurred and the steel plate was exposed for 38 years.

◆ Signs and symptoms

The patient suffered an open comminuted fracture of the left lower leg due to a car accident 38 years ago, and underwent tibial fracture debridement, fracture reduction, and steel plate internal fixation surgery at a local hospital. After surgery, there was necrosis of the skin in front of the tibia, exposure of the tibial steel plate, and pus discharge for 38 years. The patient has been undergoing dressing change treatment at a local clinic until now. There is an 8 cm × 4 cm wound on the anterior tibia of the left lower leg, with a local inward retraction of the skin edge and visible steel plate exposure. There is yellow white purulent secretion in the deep part of the wound cavity, with a foul odor. The granulation tissue in the local area is aging, and the skin pigmentation in the anterior tibia of the lower leg is present. The local scar is relatively hard, and the skin temperature is not high, with no obvious redness or swelling. The fluctuation of the dorsalis pedis artery has disappeared, and the plantar sensation is normal. The toe flexion is good, but the toe extension is limited, and the ankle joint is stiff (Figure 5.6.1, Figure5.6.2). Lower limb arterial ultrasound shows thinning and thickening of the posterior tibial artery, occlusion of the anterior tibial dorsalis pedis artery, and disappearance of distal blood flow; DR of the femoral shaft and lower leg shows malunion of the left tibia and fibula, with insect like changes visible in the middle section of the tibia and three loose screws falling off.

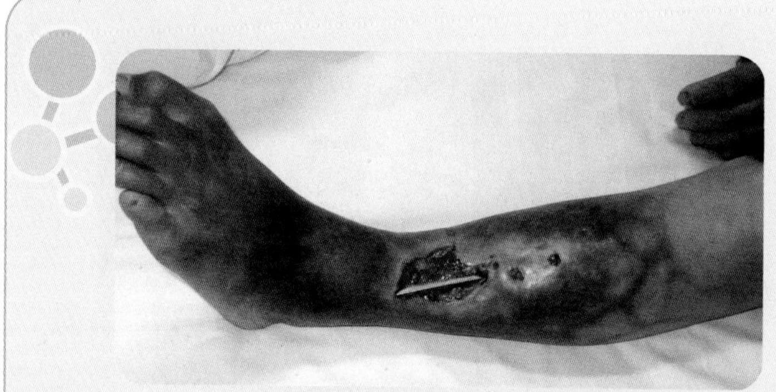

图 5.6.1 左侧胫前见 8 cm × 4 cm 创面，钢板外露，局部有脓性分泌物溢出

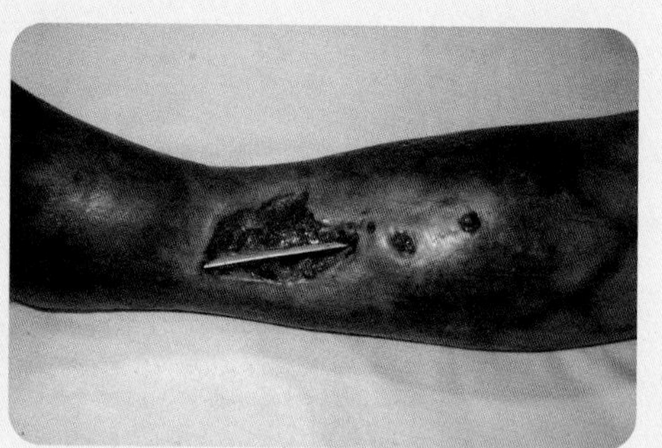

图 5.6.2 局部创面红肿明显

◆ 治疗方案

1. 患者入院后立即进行细菌培养 + 药物敏感试验。

2. 根据细菌培养选用敏感抗菌药物静脉滴注。

3. 腰硬联合麻醉下行创面清创感染增生肉芽组织水肿清除，钢板螺钉取出，扩大胫骨骨髓腔，死骨清除，双氧水、碘伏、生理盐水反复冲洗感染腔，之后采用 VSD，连续冲洗 7 天，然后局部细菌再次培养，经过综合治疗后未见细菌生长。

4. 腓肠神经营养血管皮瓣移植术

4.1 清创术：切除创腔内陷皮缘，刮出污秽无生机肉芽组织，胫骨骨髓腔内有肉芽组织增生，创面肉芽组织整体新鲜。胫前皮肤缺损 11 cm × 5 cm，骨外露 8 cm。

4.2 皮瓣设计：皮瓣轴线，外踝尖与跟腱中点连线，中点至腘窝中点连线。旋转点，外踝上 5 ~ 7 cm 为旋转点，解剖面为深筋膜层，面积 12 cm × 6 cm，筋膜蒂宽 3 cm。

4.3 皮瓣移植：按着皮瓣设计线，依次切开皮肤皮下脂肪，达肌筋膜，于蒂部解剖腓肠神经和小隐静脉并保留在皮瓣内，皮瓣边缘缝合固定，防止深浅筋膜分离滑脱。皮瓣游离结束后，皮瓣供区直接缝合，将皮瓣行受区供区缝合，皮瓣下放置三枚橡皮条引流，皮瓣外观和血供良好。包扎伤口。

5. 术后给予扩容、解痉镇痛、抗感染治疗，3 天拔引流条，12 天拆线，3 周下地负重行走功能训练。

6. 术后 6 个月复查，骨感染愈合，皮瓣愈合良好（图 5.6.3）。

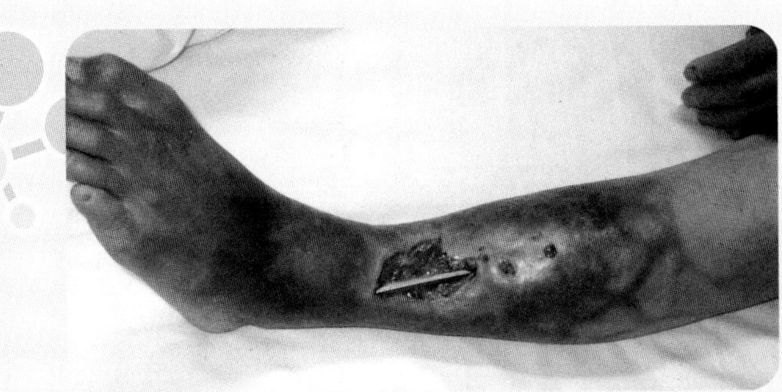
Figure 5.6.1 An 8 cm × 4 cm wound on the left anterior tibia, with exposed steel plate and localized purulent discharge

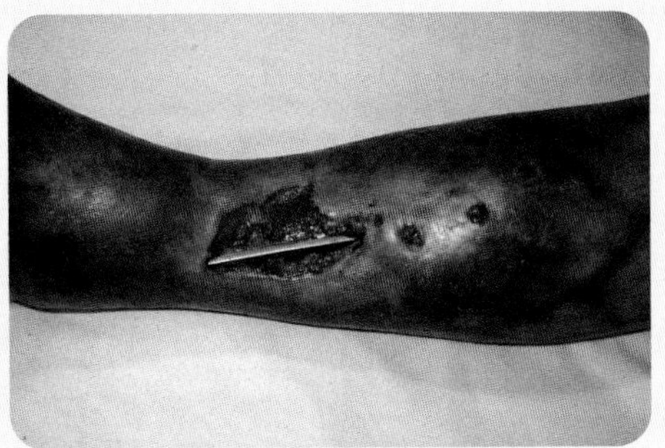
Figure 5.6.2 Local wound with obvious redness and swelling

◆ Treatment plan

1. The patient should undergo bacterial culture and drug sensitivity testing immediately after admission.

2. Select sensitive antibacterial drugs for intravenous infusion based on bacterial culture.

3. Under combined spinal and epidural anesthesia, wound debridement, infection, hyperplasia, granulation tissue edema, and removal were performed. Steel plate screws were removed, and the tibial bone marrow cavity was enlarged to remove dead bone. The infected cavity was repeatedly rinsed with hydrogen peroxide, iodine, and physiological saline, followed by VSD for 7 consecutive days. Local bacteria were then cultured again, and no bacterial growth was observed after comprehensive treatment.

4. Gastrocnemius nerve nutritional vascular flap transplantation

4.1 Debridement surgery: Remove the edge of the sunken skin in the wound cavity, scrape off the dirty and lifeless granulation tissue, and promote granulation tissue proliferation in the tibial bone marrow cavity. The granulation tissue on the wound surface is fresh as a whole. The skin defect in front of the tibia is 11 cm × 5 cm, and the bone is exposed by 8 cm.

4.2 Skin flap design: The axis of the skin flap is the line connecting the tip of the lateral malleolus and the midpoint of the Achilles tendon, and the line connecting the midpoint to the midpoint of the popliteal fossa. The rotation point is located 5-7 cm above the lateral ankle, and the anatomical plane is the deep fascia layer, with an area of 12 cm × 6 cm and a fascial pedicle width of 3 cm.

4.3 Skin flap transplantation: Following the design line of the skin flap, sequentially cut open the subcutaneous fat of the skin, reach the fascia, dissect the sural nerve and small saphenous vein at the pedicle and preserve them in the skin flap. Suture and fix the edge of the skin flap to prevent the separation and slippage of the deep and shallow fascia. After the free movement of the skin flap is completed, the donor area of the skin flap is directly sutured, and the donor area of the skin flap is sutured. Three rubber strips are placed under the skin flap for drainage, and the appearance and blood supply of the skin flap are good. Wrap the wound.

5. Postoperative treatment includes dilation, spasmolysis, analgesia, and anti-infection therapy. The drainage strip is removed after 3 days, the stitches are removed after 12 days, and the weight-bearing walking function training is performed for 3 weeks.

6. After 6 months of postoperative follow-up, the bone infection healed and the skin flap healed well (Figure 5.6.3).

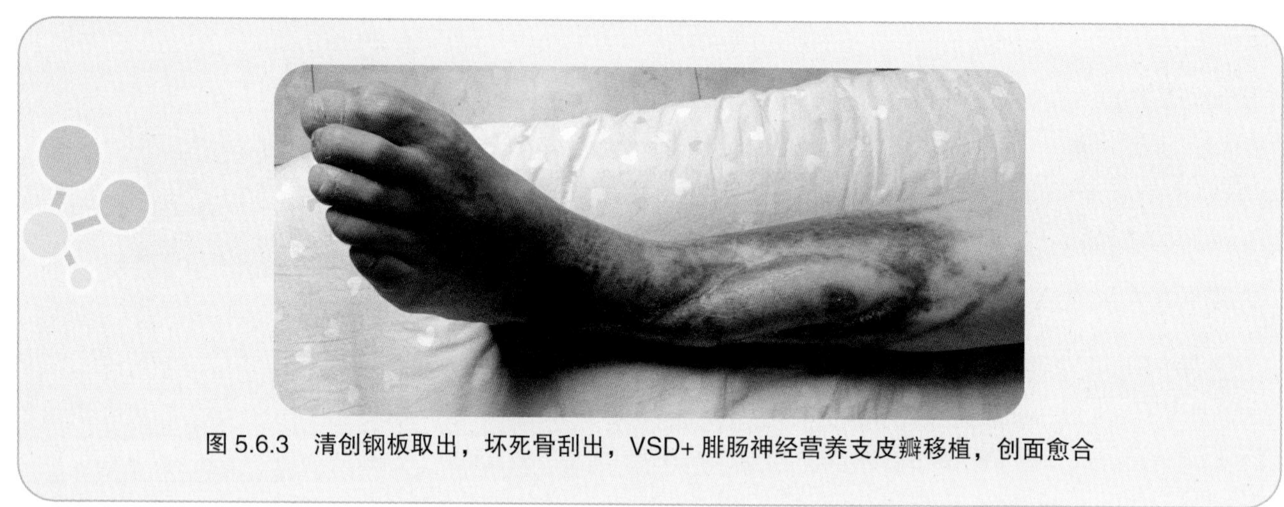

图 5.6.3　清创钢板取出，坏死骨刮出，VSD+ 腓肠神经营养支皮瓣移植，创面愈合

（陈善亮）

案例七　小腿坏死性筋膜炎

◆ 致病原因

患者糖尿病史 18 年，平时口服二甲双胍维持血糖，右小腿疖肿反复破溃流脓 4 月余，曾经在当地医院多次切开引流。

◆ 症状与体征

右小腿广泛性肿胀，膝关节至足部散在多发溃疡，溃疡有大量黄色脓液流出，可触及无数个皮下炎症结节，皮温增高，较大结节波动明显，触之顺着破溃处溢出大量脓液，小腿后侧波动明显，膝关节、足踝关节活动受限，足背动脉搏动微弱，足趾活动良好，足底感觉减退，腹股沟浅表淋巴结无明显增大（图 5.7.1）。

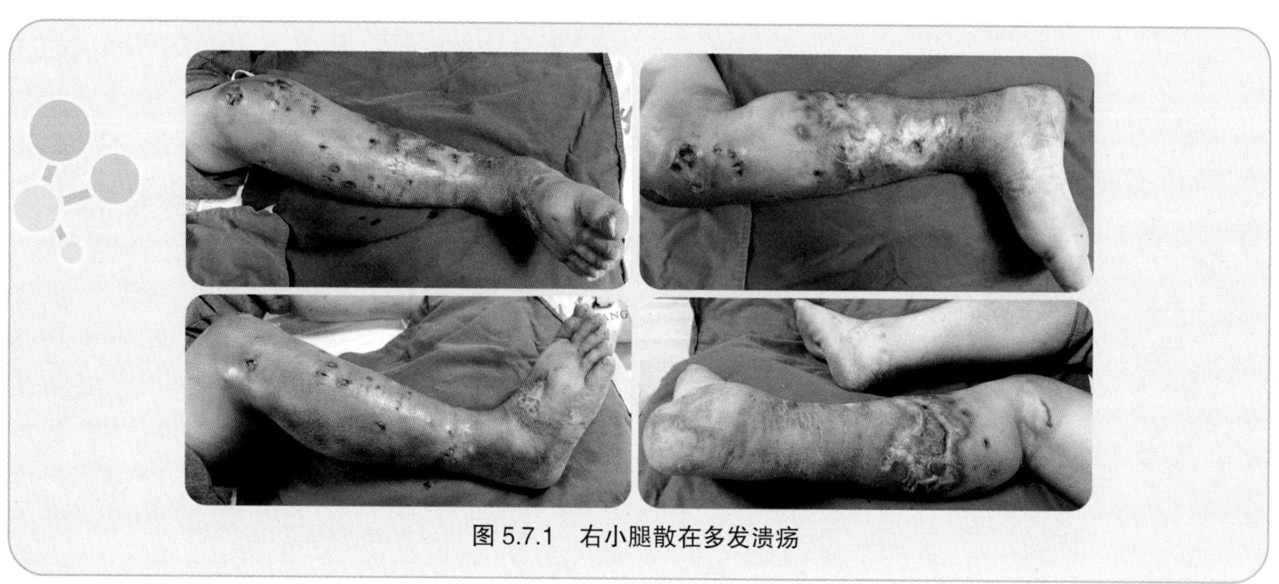

图 5.7.1　右小腿散在多发溃疡

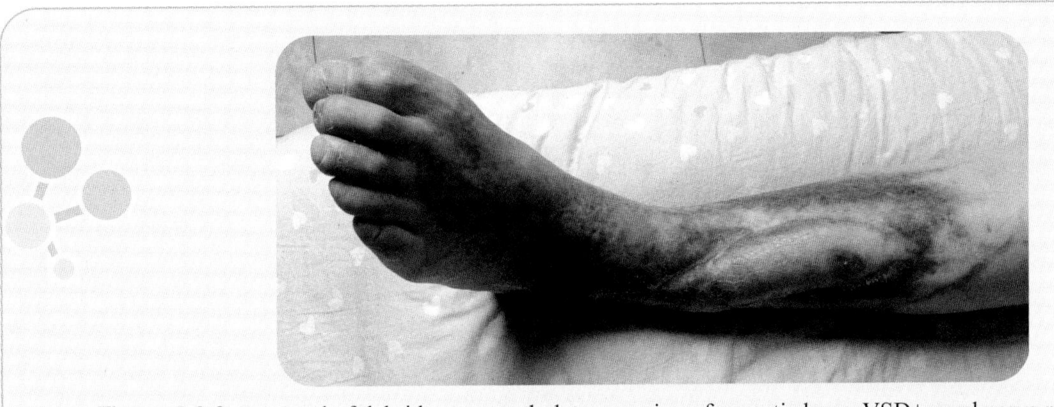

Figure 5.6.3 Removal of debridement steel plate, scraping of necrotic bone, VSD+ sural nerve nutritional branch skin flap transplantation, wound healing

(Chen Shanliang)

Case 7 Necrotizing fasciitis of the lower leg

◆ Cause of illness

The patient has a history of diabetes for 18 years. He usually takes metformin orally to maintain blood sugar. The right calf boil has repeatedly broken and festered for more than 4 months. He has been cut and drained many times in the local hospital.

◆ Signs and symptoms

Widespread swelling in the right lower leg, scattered multiple ulcers from the knee joint to the foot, with a large amount of yellow pus flowing out of the ulcers. Countless subcutaneous inflammatory nodules can be felt, and the skin temperature increases. The larger nodules fluctuate significantly, and a large amount of pus overflows along the rupture site. The posterior leg fluctuates significantly, and the knee and ankle joints are restricted in movement. The dorsalis pedis artery pulsation is weak, the toe movement is good, and the plantar sensation is reduced. There is no significant increase in the superficial inguinal lymph nodes (Figure 5.7.1).

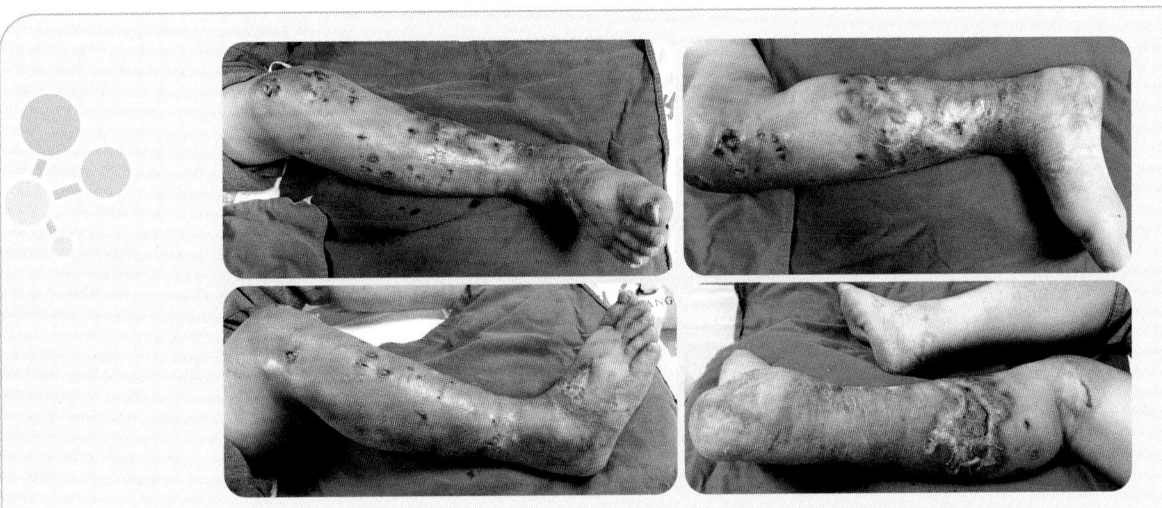

Figure 5.7.1 Scattered multiple ulcers in the right calf

◆ 治疗方案

1. 入院后筛查全身基础疾病，积极治疗原发病，纠正血糖，手术前空腹血糖控制在 8 mmol/L 左右，改善心肺功能，脓液细菌培养 + 药物敏感试验，根据细菌培养给予敏感抗菌药物。

2. 于全麻下行小腿广泛切开，扩创，感染病灶切除、脓肿切开，冲洗术，切开各个肌间隙感染灶，充分打开感染灶，扩创引流，双氧水、碘伏、生理盐水多次反复浸泡冲洗，直至肉眼看到新鲜创面为止，坏死组织彻底切除并电凝止血，于深部感染腔放置 VSD。持续负压冲洗（图 5.7.2 ～图 5.7.5）。

3. 经过 3 天 VSD 冲洗，创面引流液有臭味，引流液污秽不清，考虑 VSD 装置网孔堵塞引流不畅所致。于全麻下再次清创切除坏死皮肤和部分感染坏死组织，再次更换 VSD 装置，回病房持续 VSD+ 重组人碱性成纤维细胞生长因子滴管持续冲洗，7 天后拆掉 VSD 装置，创面肉芽组织逐渐新鲜，但植皮局部肉芽组织新鲜程度不够，改用人工双层真皮敷料覆盖创面，待肉芽组织饱满、新鲜为止，为植皮奠定基础（图 5.7.6）。

4. 经过 2 次扩创引流更换 VSD 装置，人工双层真皮敷料覆盖后 10 天。打开人工真皮硅胶膜，小腿创面新鲜，肉芽组织饱满，创面渗血活跃，创面已经达到植皮条件（图 5.7.7）。

5. 于全麻下行中厚游离皮肤移植，于对侧大腿前侧，电动取皮点取皮，切取大张中厚皮肤。游离移植于受区创面，皮片间用 5/0 细丝线拼接缝合，皮片切开无数个细小空洞，有利于创面渗出，防止渗出液将皮肤浮起，受区和供区应用凡士林油纱加压包扎（图 5.7.8）。

6. 术后 10 天拆开植皮区敷料，见植皮完全成活，边缘有少许未愈合创面，凡士林油纱再次覆盖（图 5.7.9）。植皮术后 20 天，植皮完全成活，创面完全覆盖（图 5.7.10）。膝关节及足踝关节循序康复训练。指导患者出院后注意事项，防止二次复发，积极控制糖尿病及其并发症。

◆ Treatment plan

1. After admission, screen for underlying systemic diseases, actively treat the primary disease, correct blood sugar, control fasting blood sugar at around 8 mmol/L before surgery, improve cardiopulmonary function, perform pus bacterial culture + drug sensitivity test, and administer sensitive antibiotics based on bacterial culture.

2. Under general anesthesia, the calf is extensively incised, expanded, infected lesions are removed, abscesses are incised, and flushing surgery is performed. Various intermuscular spaces infected lesions are incised, and the infected lesions are fully opened. Expansion and drainage are performed, and hydrogen peroxide, iodine, and physiological saline are repeatedly soaked and flushed until the fresh wound surface is visible to the naked eye. The necrotic tissue is completely removed and electrocoagulation is used to stop bleeding. A VSD is placed in the deep infection cavity. Continuous negative pressure flushing (Figure 5.7.2- Figure 5.7.5).

3. After 3 days of VSD flushing, the wound drainage fluid had a foul odor and was not clear. It is considered that the blockage of the VSD device mesh caused poor drainage. Under general anesthesia, the necrotic skin and partially infected necrotic tissue were removed again through debridement and excision. The VSD device was replaced again, and the patient returned to the ward for continuous VSD and rinsing with recombinant human basic fibroblast growth factor droppers. After 7 days, the VSD device was removed, and the granulation tissue of the wound gradually became fresh. However, the freshness of the granulation tissue in the transplanted area was not sufficient. An artificial double-layer dermal dressing was used to cover the wound until the granulation tissue was full and fresh, laying the foundation for skin grafting (Figure 5.7.6).

4. After 2 rounds of expansion and drainage, the VSD device was replaced and covered with artificial double-layer leather dressing for 10 days. Open the artificial leather silicone membrane, the calf wound is fresh, the granulation tissue is full, the wound has active bleeding, and the wound has reached the conditions for skin grafting (Figure 5.7.7).

5. Under general anesthesia, a medium thick free skin transplant was performed. On the anterior side of the contralateral thigh, an electric skin sampling point was used to remove the skin, and a large medium thick skin was cut. Free transplantation is performed on the wound surface of the recipient area, and the skin patches are sutured together with 5/0 fine silk thread. The skin patches are cut into numerous small cavities to facilitate wound leakage and prevent exudate from floating the skin. Vaseline gauze is used to apply pressure and wrap the recipient and donor areas (Figure 5.7.8).

6. Ten days after surgery, the dressing in the skin graft area was removed, and it was found that the skin graft was completely alive, with a few unhealed wounds at the edges. Vaseline gauze was used to cover it again (Figure 5.7.9). After 20 days of skin grafting, the skin graft completely survived and the wound was completely covered (Figure 5.7.10). Sequential rehabilitation training for knee and ankle joints. Instruct patients to pay attention after discharge, prevent secondary recurrence, and actively control diabetes and its complications.

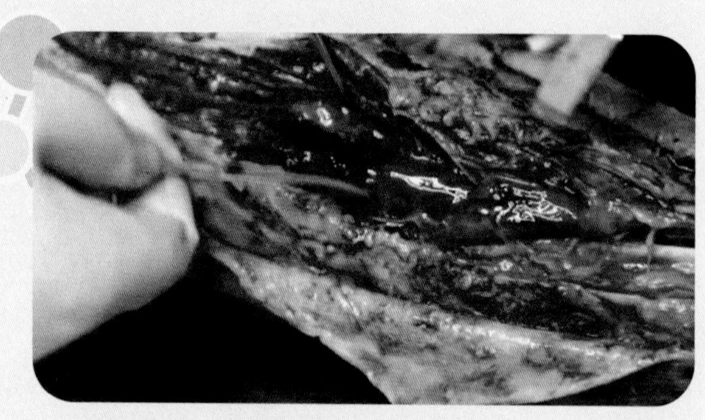

图 5.7.2　切开后见皮下和肌间隙中有大量稀薄脓液

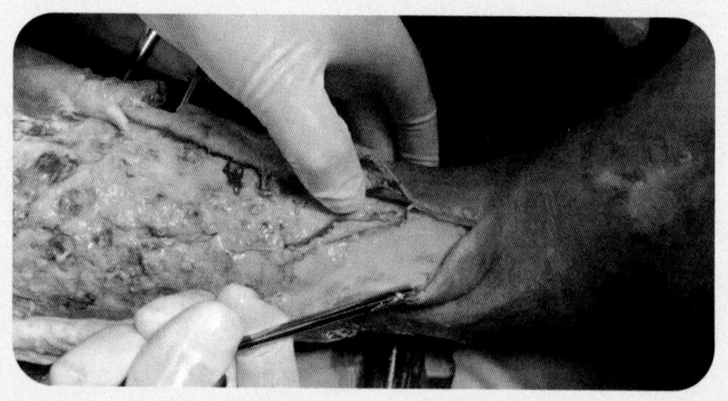

图 5.7.3　皮下脂肪层散在多发脓肿和炎性结节，足踝区有较大脓肿

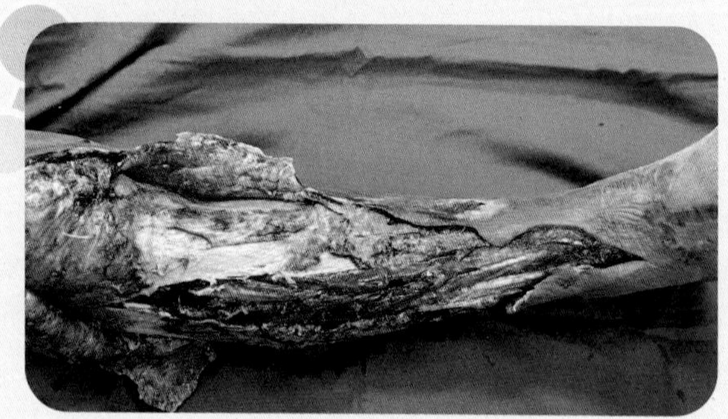

图 5.7.4　充分切开引流，清理脓腔和感染灶

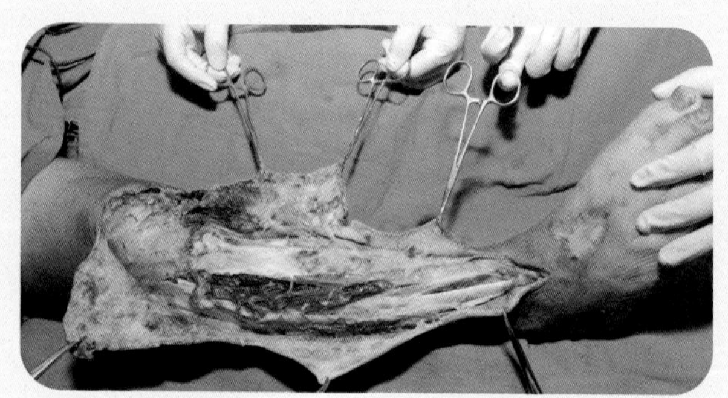

图 5.7.5　碘伏、双氧水、生理盐水反复冲洗，创面逐渐新鲜

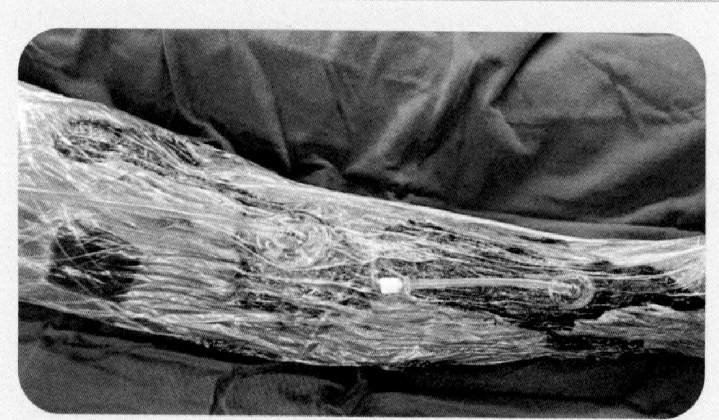

图 5.7.6　VSD 治疗 + 生长因子滴注持续冲洗

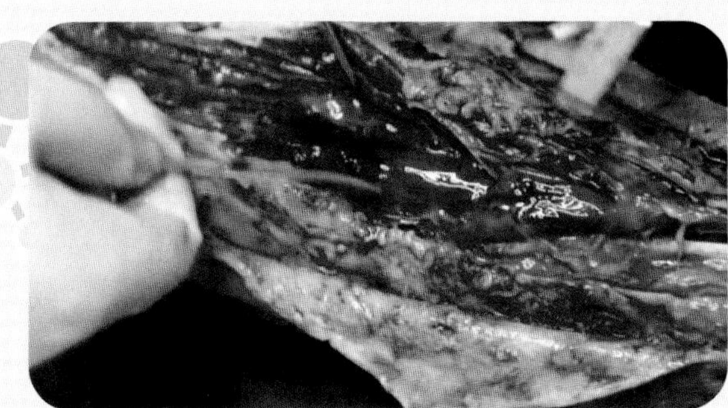

Figure 5.7.2 A large amount of thin pus in the subcutaneous and muscular spaces after incision

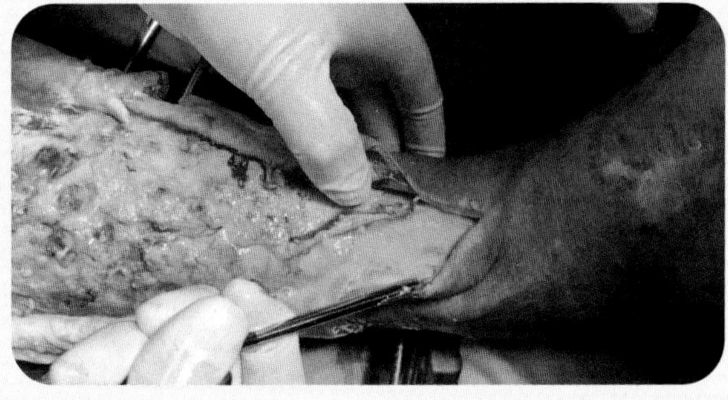

Figure 5.7.3 Scattered subcutaneous fat layer with multiple abscesses and inflammatory nodules, with larger abscesses in the ankle area

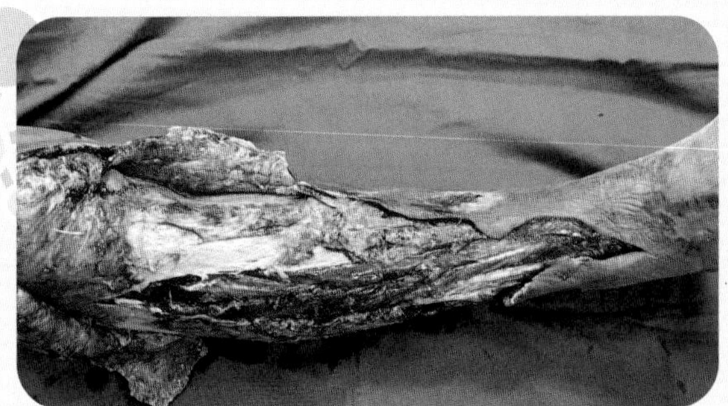

Figure 5.7.4 Fully incise and drain, clean the abscess cavity and infection site

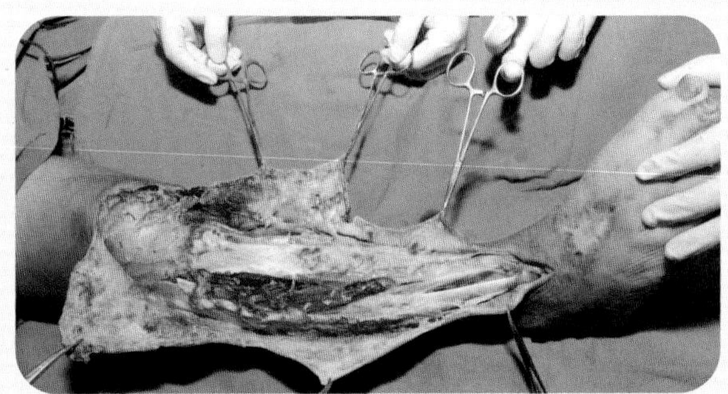

Figure 5.7.5 Repeated rinsing with iodine, hydrogen peroxide, and saline solution gradually freshens the wound surface

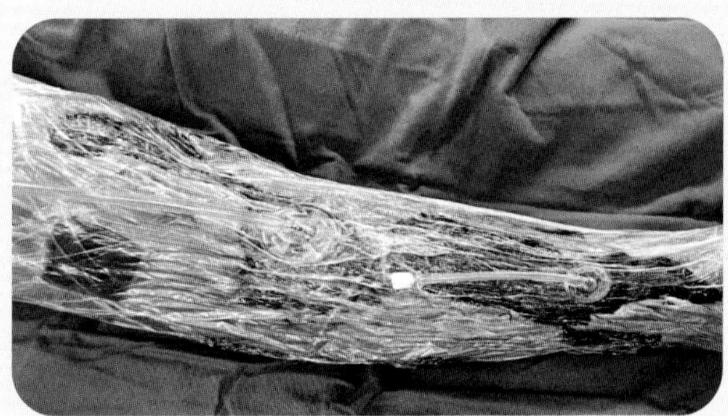

Figure 5.7.6 VSD treatment+continuous flushing with growth factor infusion

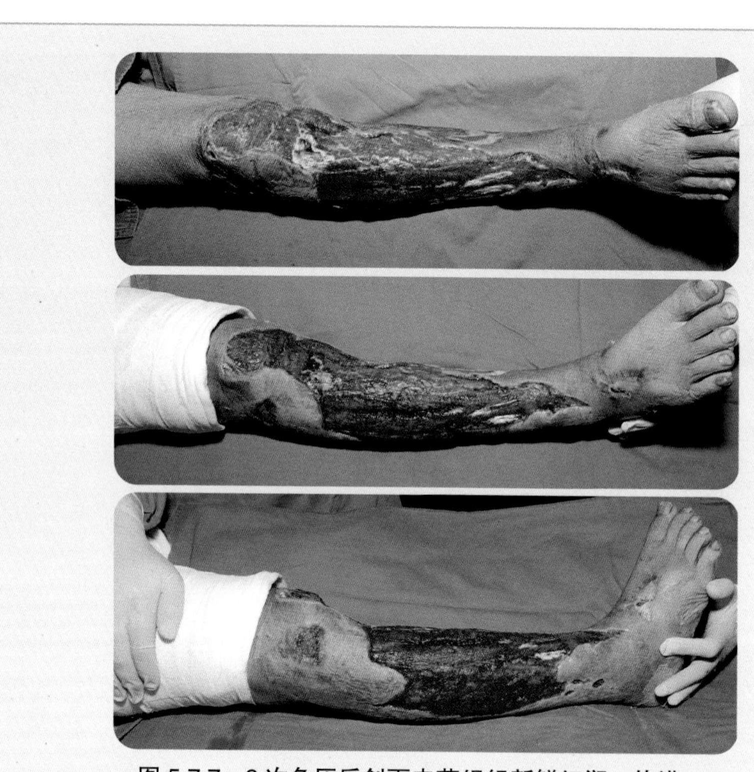

图 5.7.7　2 次负压后创面肉芽组织新鲜红润、饱满，远端部分肌腱外露

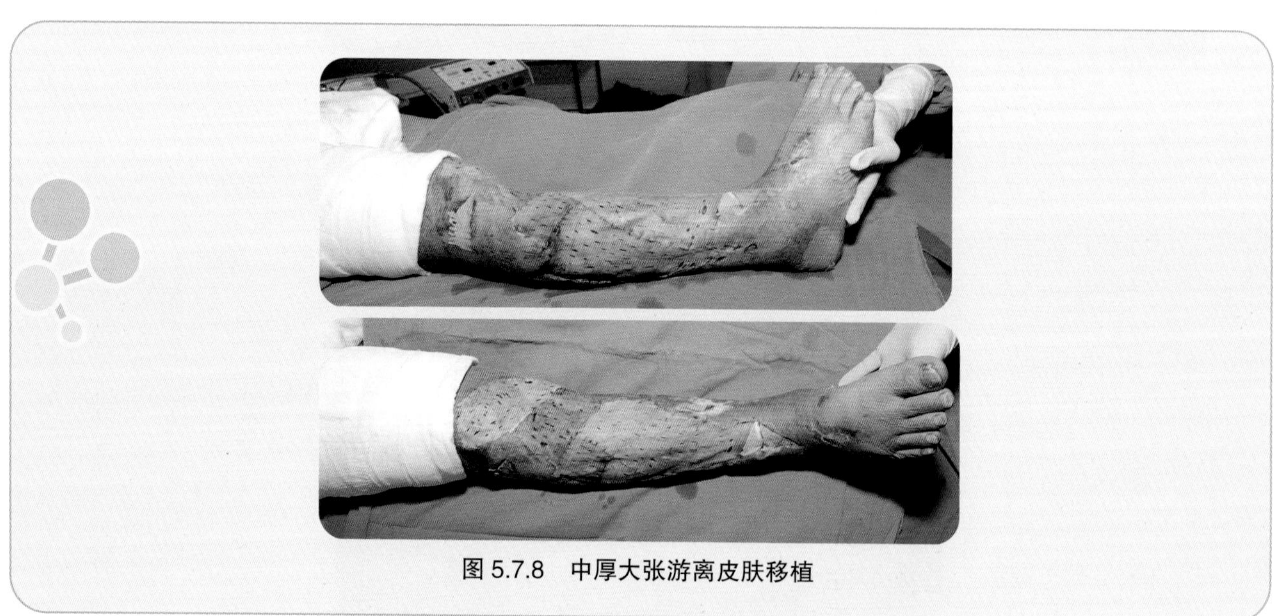

图 5.7.8　中厚大张游离皮肤移植

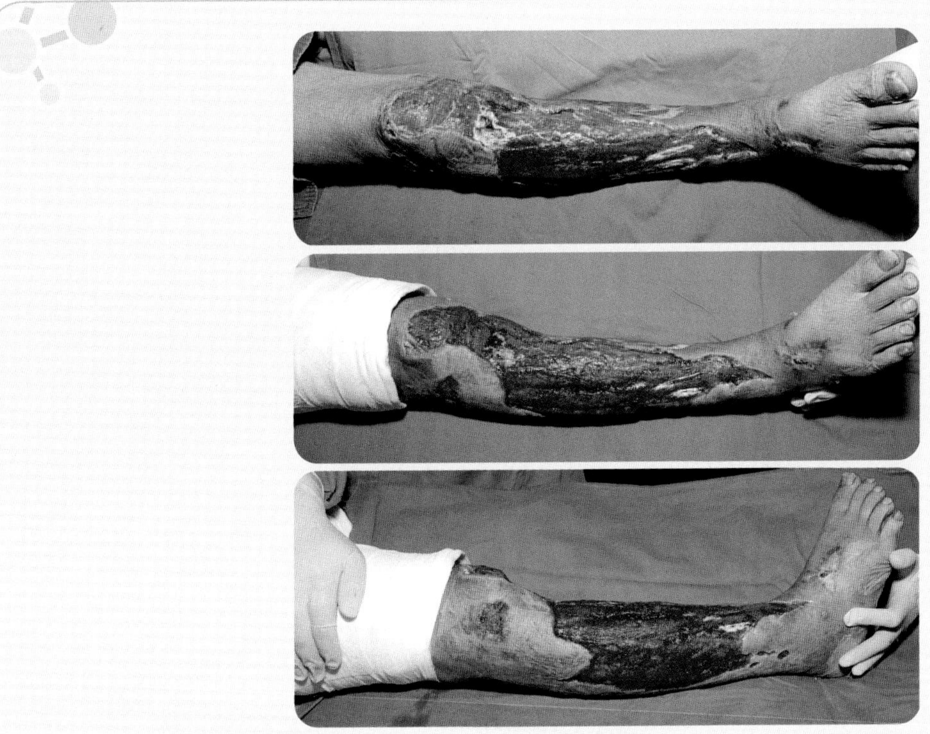

Figure 5.7.7 After 2 negative pressure cycles, the granulation tissue of the wound is fresh, rosy, and full, with the distal part of the tendon exposed

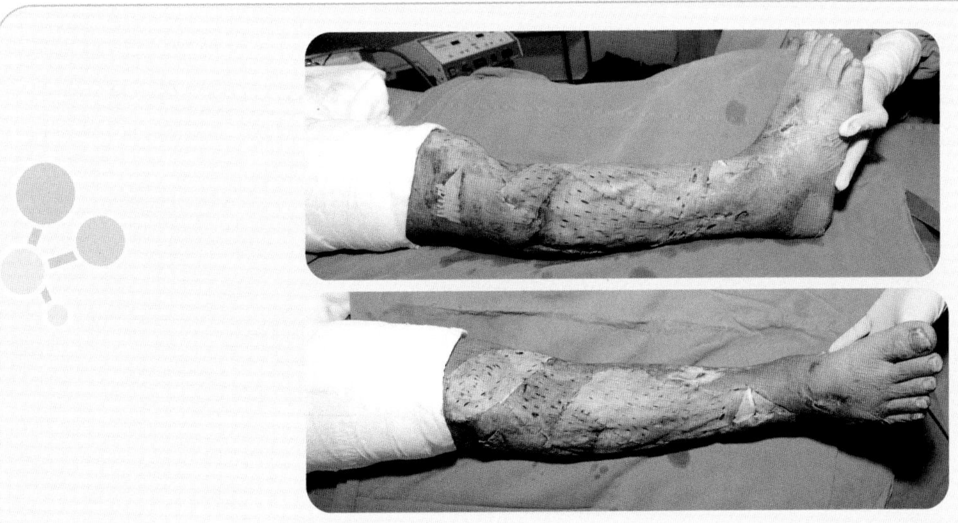

Figure 5.7.8 Medium thick and large open skin transplantation

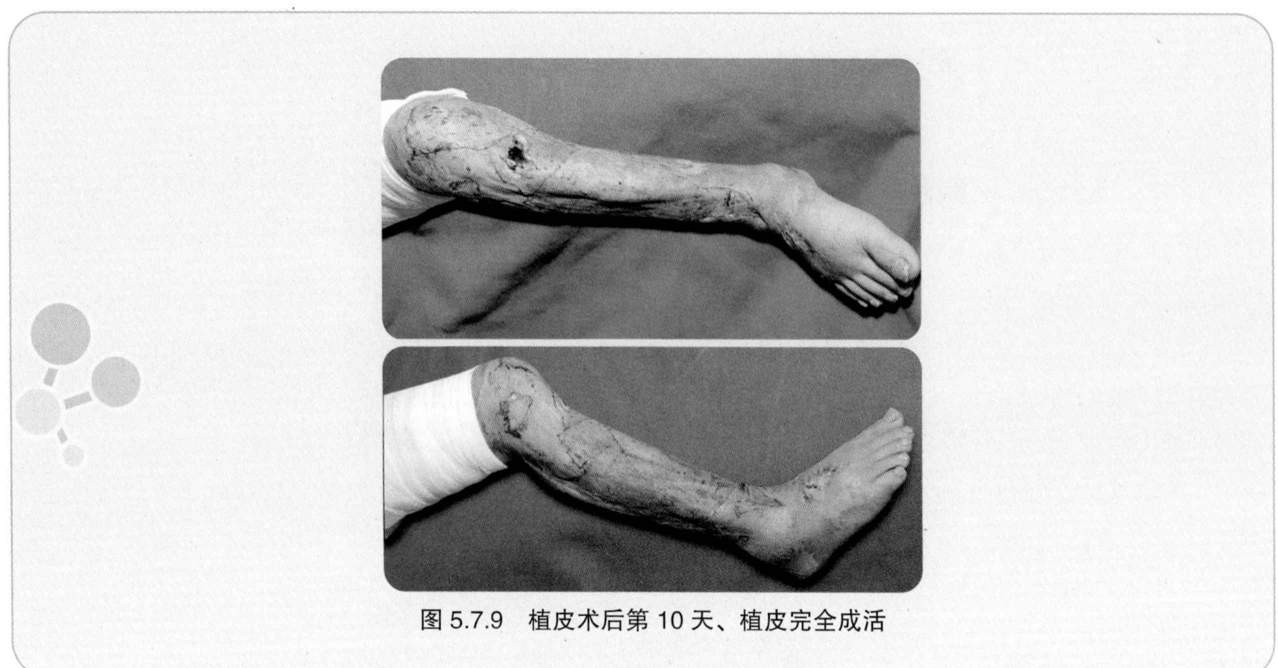

图 5.7.9 植皮术后第 10 天、植皮完全成活

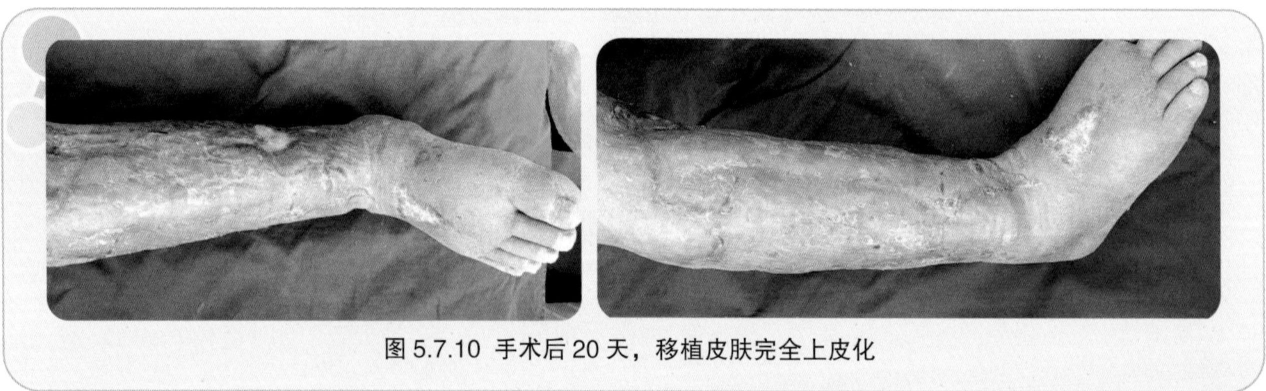

图 5.7.10 手术后 20 天，移植皮肤完全上皮化

（陈善亮）

案例八 坏死性脓皮病术后感染

◆ 致病原因

患者右足疱疹后溃疡不愈合 2 年，当地医院多次皮肤移植未愈合。

◆ 症状与体征

全身水肿，右足背创面大小约 13 cm × 9 cm，表面陈旧质脆肉芽组织，中央见坏死移植皮肤组织，少量脓性渗出，周边创面潜行腔隙，创面触痛明显，内踝周围皮肤血管炎表现（图 5.8.1）。

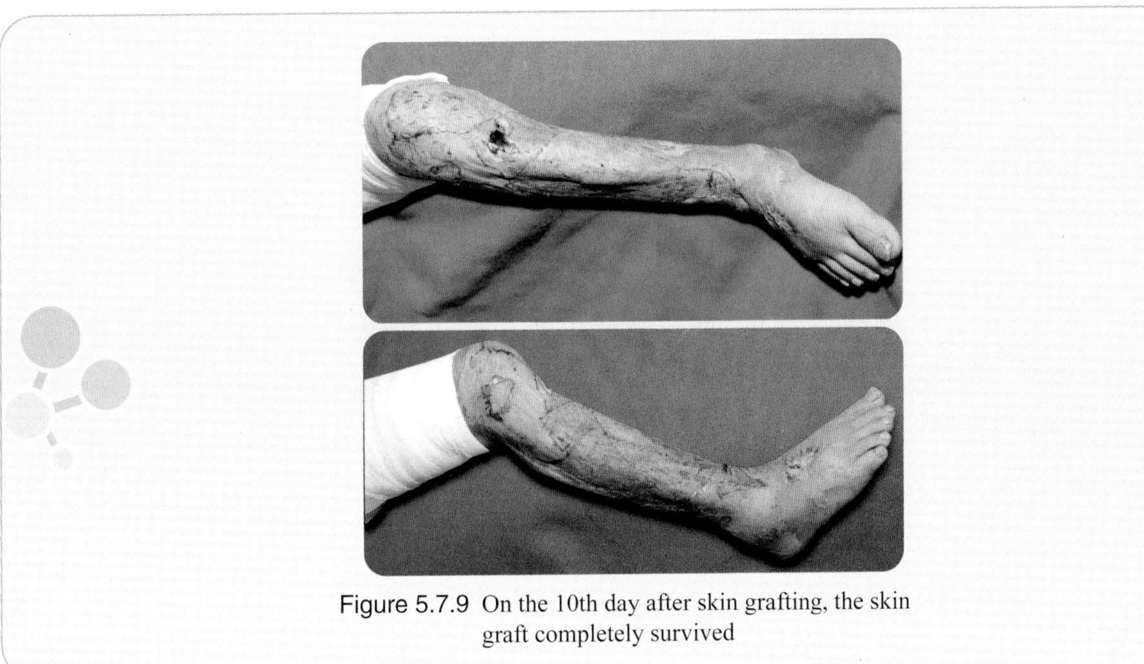

Figure 5.7.9 On the 10th day after skin grafting, the skin graft completely survived

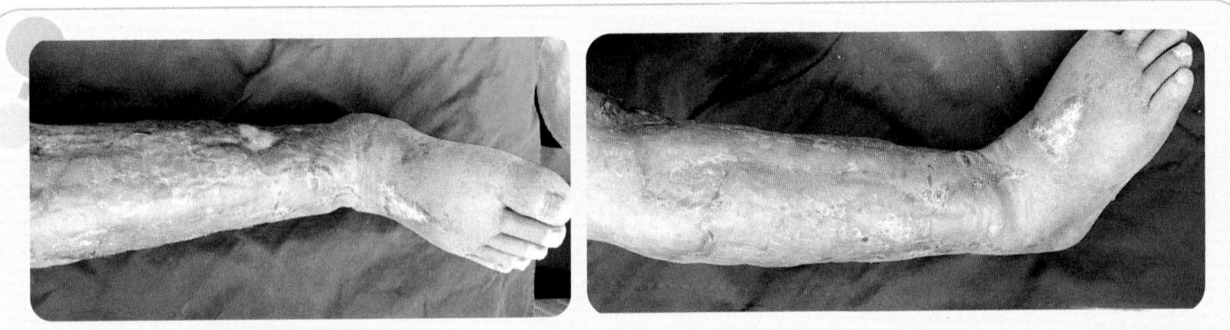

Figure 5.7.10 Complete epithelialization of transplanted skin 20 days after surgery

(Chen Shanliang)

Case 8 Postoperative infection in necrotizing pyoderma

◆ Cause of illness

The patient's right foot post herpetic ulcer did not heal for 2 years, and multiple skin transplants at the local hospital did not heal.

◆ Signs and symptoms

The whole body is swollen, and the size of the wound on the back of the right foot is about 13 cm × 9 cm. There is old and brittle granulation tissue on the surface, with necrotic transplanted skin tissue in the center and a small amount of purulent exudate. There are hidden cavities around the wound, and the wound is tender. The skin around the inner ankle shows vasculitis (Figure 5.8.1).

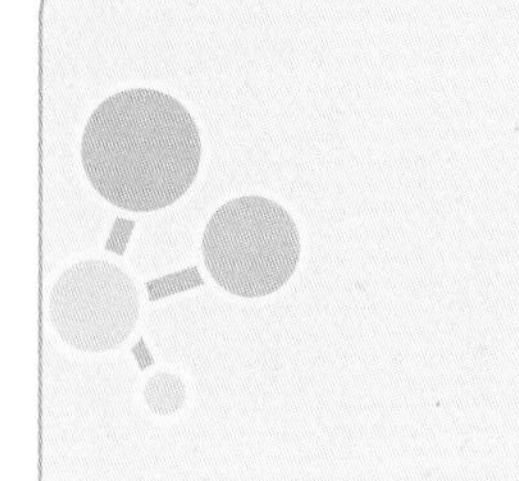

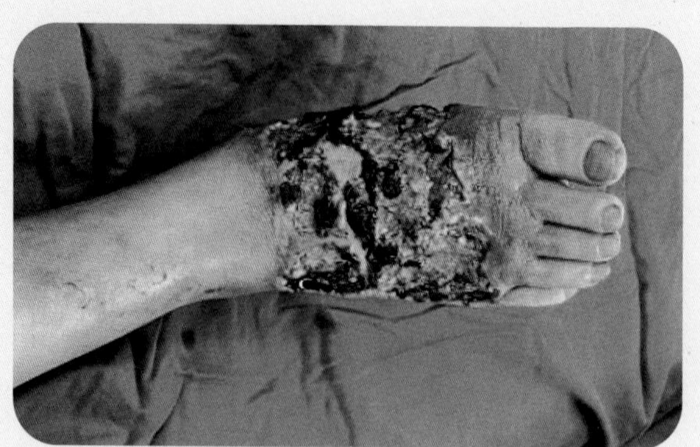

图 5.8.1　经历多次清创植皮创面未愈合

◆ 治疗方案

1. 二次清创 +VSD，创面肉芽组织健康干净，但创缘进展扩大伴脓性渗出，创面继续进展扩大，VSD 效果不理想（图 5.8.2）。

2. 清创换药，生长因子 + 新型碳敷料，创面浸渍扩大，创面控制仍不理想（图 5.8.3、图 5.8.4）。

3. MDT 讨论，明确病因为坏死性脓皮病，应用免疫抑制剂，甲泼尼龙、羟氯喹、沙利度胺等，中药清热利湿解毒滋阴养血；创面用生物纤维素敷料，创面周缘稳定，新鲜肉芽组织形成，经治疗创面愈合（图 5.8.5 ~ 图 5.8.7）。

此案例提示，临床面对慢性疑难创面的治疗时常需要多学科合作，明确病因。

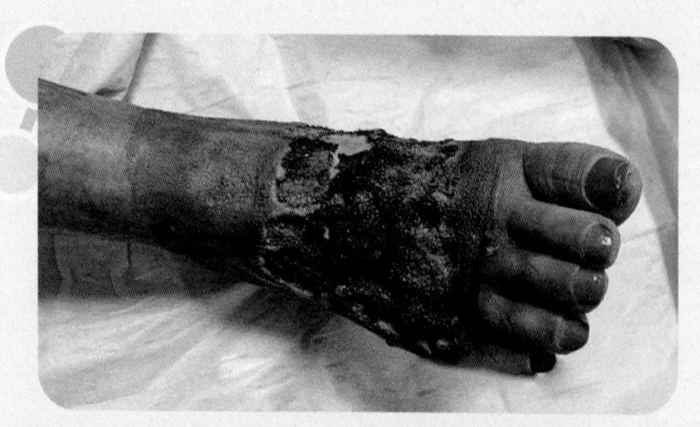

图 5.8.2　清创 +VSD 2 次，创面肉芽组织健康干净，但创缘进展扩大伴脓性渗出

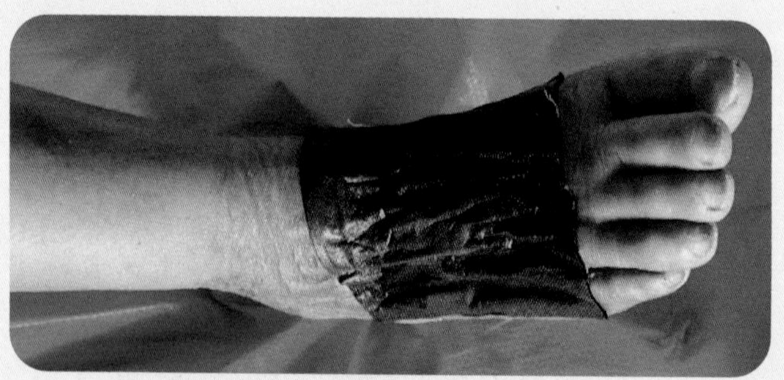

图 5.8.3　改用碳敷料 + 生长因子换药

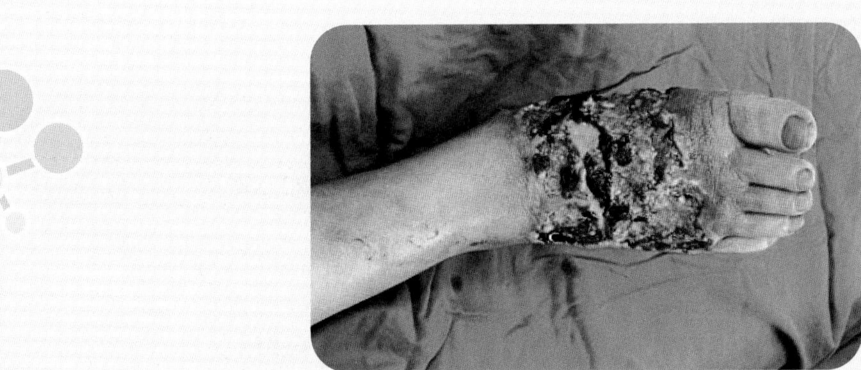

Figure 5.8.1 Failure to heal after multiple debridement and skin grafting wounds

◆ Treatment plan

1. After secondary debridement and VSD, the granulation tissue of the wound was healthy and clean, but the wound margin progressed and expanded with purulent exudation, and the wound continued to progress and expand, resulting in unsatisfactory VSD effect (Figure 5.8.2).

2. Debridement and dressing change, growth factor+ new carbon dressing, wound impregnation and expansion, but wound control is still not ideal (Figure 5.8.3, Figure 5.8.4).

3. MDT discussion, clarify the cause of necrotic pyoderma, apply immunosuppressive agents such as methylprednisolone, hydroxychloroquine, and thalidomide, and use traditional Chinese medicine to clear heat, remove dampness, detoxify, nourish yin, and nourish blood; The wound was treated with a biocellulose dressing, which stabilized the edge of the wound and formed fresh granulation tissue. After treatment, the wound healed (Figure 5.8.5- Figure 5.8.7).

This case suggests that clinical treatment of chronic difficult wounds often requires multidisciplinary collaboration to identify the underlying causes.

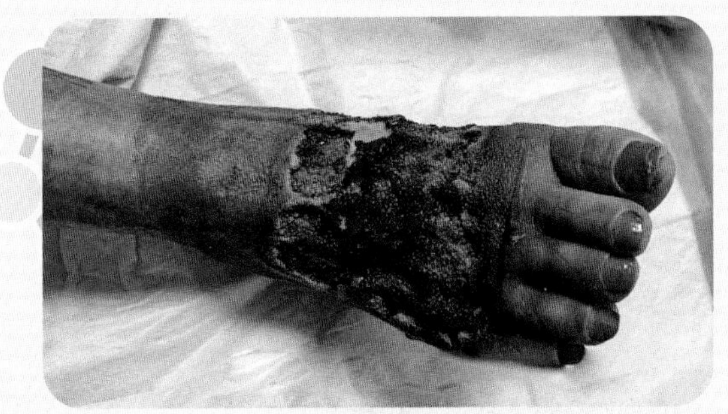

Figure 5.8.2 Clearing and VSD twice, the granulation tissue of the wound is healthy and clean, but the wound margin progresses and expands with purulent exudate

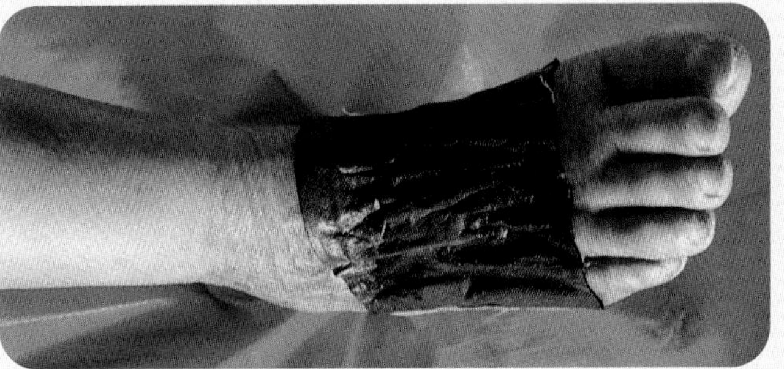

Figure 5.8.3 Switching to carbon dressing+growth factor dressing

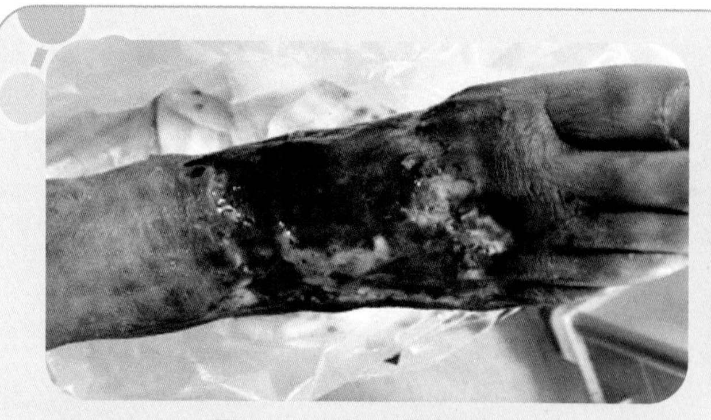

图 5.8.4　创面浸渍扩大

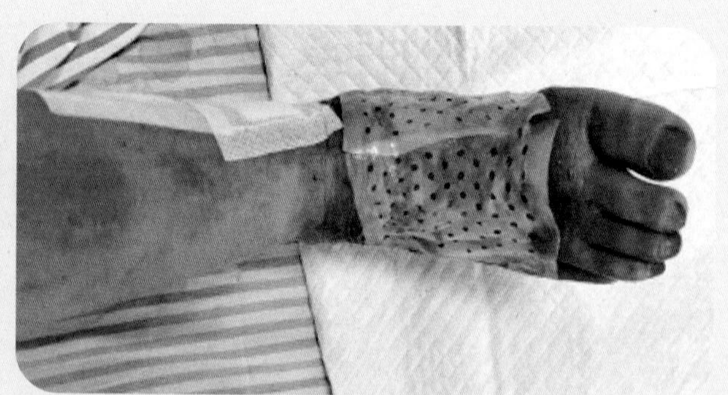

图 5.8.5　创面用生物纤维素敷料

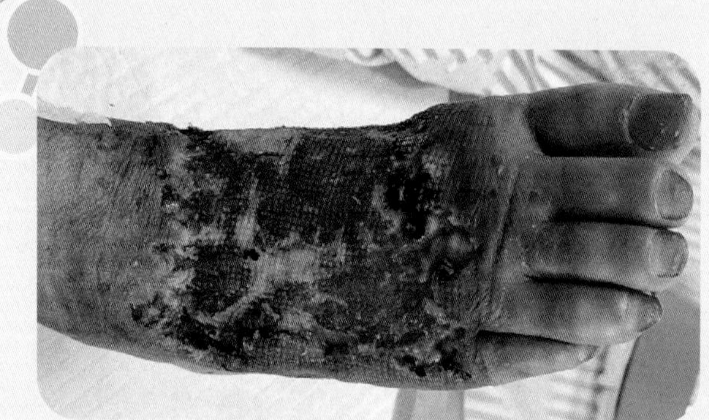

图 5.8.6　创面周缘稳定，新鲜肉芽组织形成

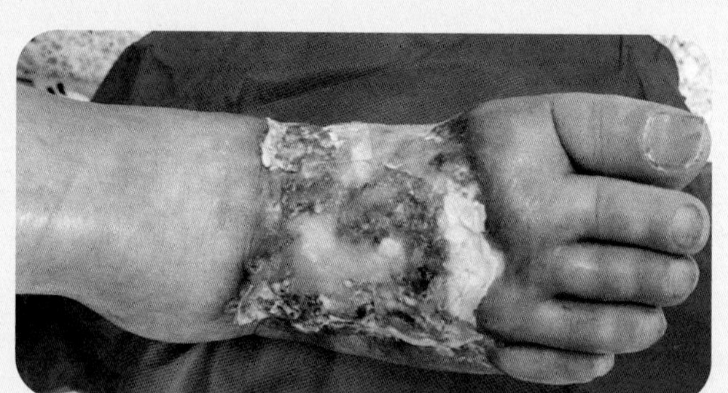

图 5.8.7　愈合创面

（王永高　王城磊）

案例九　造口旁疝术后切口感染

◆ 致病原因

患者行造口旁疝术，术后切口感染，合并糖尿病。

◆ 症状与体征

腹部创面 3 cm × 1 cm × 5.3 cm，75% 黄色，25% 红色，大量脓性渗出液，皮温略高。造口旁疝术后 13 天出现切口处持续性疼痛，发热（图 5.9.1）。B 超示炎症伴脓肿可能；脓肿培养金黄色葡萄球菌（+）；全腹 CT 示左下腹瘘口周围软组织肿胀伴多发渗出改变。

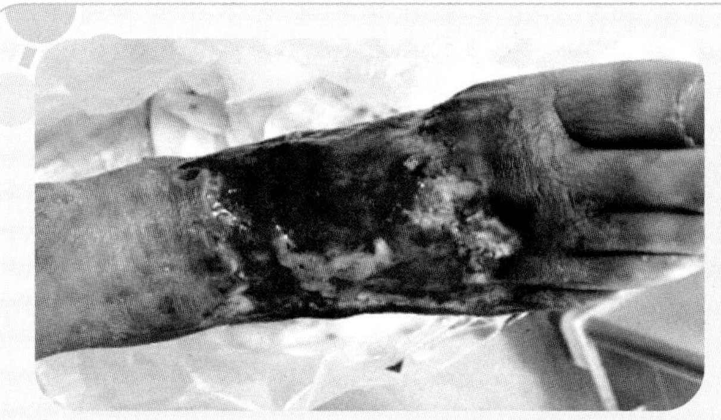
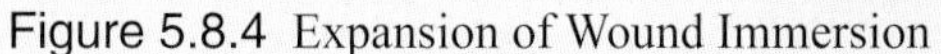

Figure 5.8.4 Expansion of Wound Immersion

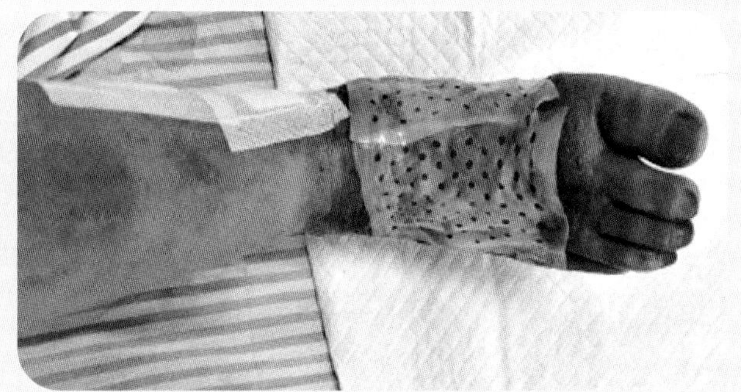

Figure 5.8.5 Biocellulose dressing for wounds

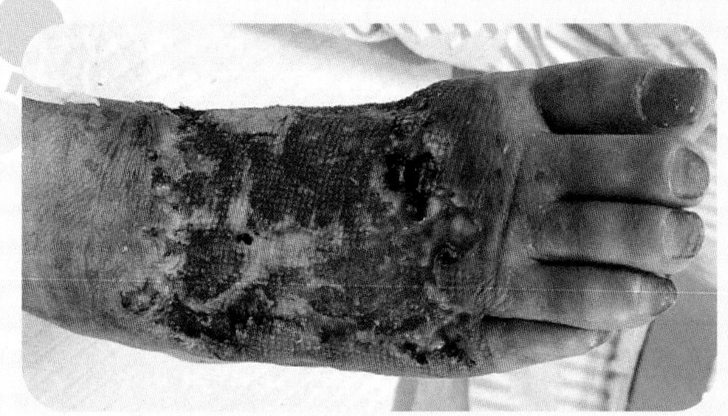

Figure 5.8.6 Stable wound perimeter and formation of fresh granulation tissue

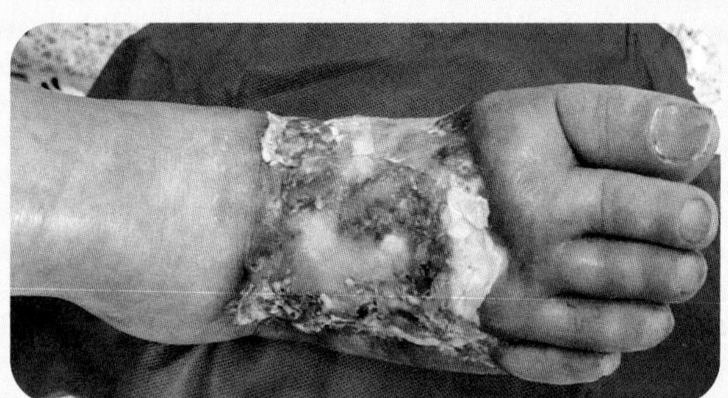

Figure 5.8.7 Healing wounds

(Wang Yonggao, Wang Chenglei)

Case 9 Postoperative incision infection in paraostomy hernia surgery

◆ Cause of illness

The patient underwent parastomy hernia, postoperative incision infection and diabetes.

◆ Signs and symptoms

Abdominal wound 3 cm × 1 cm × 5.3 cm, 75% yellow, 25% red, with a large amount of purulent exudate and slightly elevated skin temperature. Persistent pain and fever occurred at the incision site 13 days after the surgery for incisional hernia (Figure 5.9.1). B-ultrasound shows possible inflammation with abscess; Abscess culture of Staphylococcus aureus (+); Whole abdominal CT shows swelling of soft tissue around the left lower abdominal fistula with multiple exudative changes.

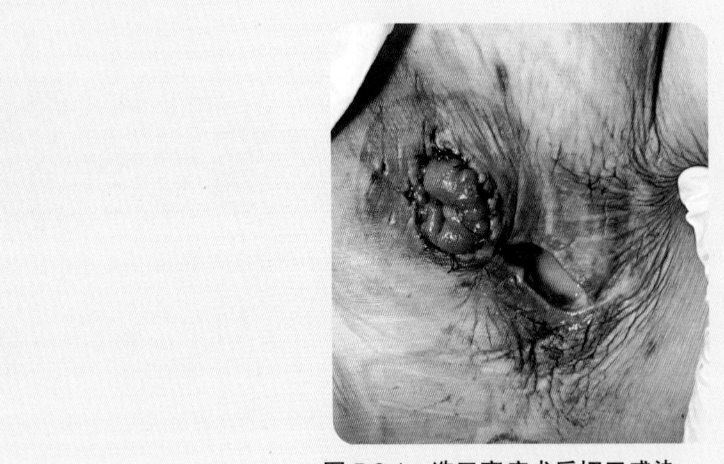

图 5.9.1　造口旁疝术后切口感染

◆ 治疗方案

1. 全身抗感染，控制血糖，做好饮食宣教。

2. 做好造口护理，避免粪便二次污染创面。

3. 积极清创，选择性使用新型伤口敷料局部抗感染，创面 3 cm × 1 cm × 5.3 cm，50% 黄色，50% 红色，清创 + 碘伏冲洗 + 生理盐水冲洗 + 亲水纤维银 + 水胶体 + 两件式凸面造口袋（图 5.9.2）。

4. 做好渗液管理，采用将伤口部分暴露于底盘外，充分引流，成纤维细胞生长因子促进创面肉芽组织生长。6 天后，创面 3 cm × 1 cm × 3.2 cm，100% 红色，中等渗液，加用成纤维细胞生长因子 + 硫酸银敷料（图 5.9.3）。12 天后，创面 2.8 cm × 1 cm × 2.1 cm，100% 红色，少量渗液（图 5.9.4）。

5. 及时床边缝合封闭创面，缩短创面愈合时间（图 5.9.5）。出院后 1 个月，伤口完全愈合（图 5.9.6）。

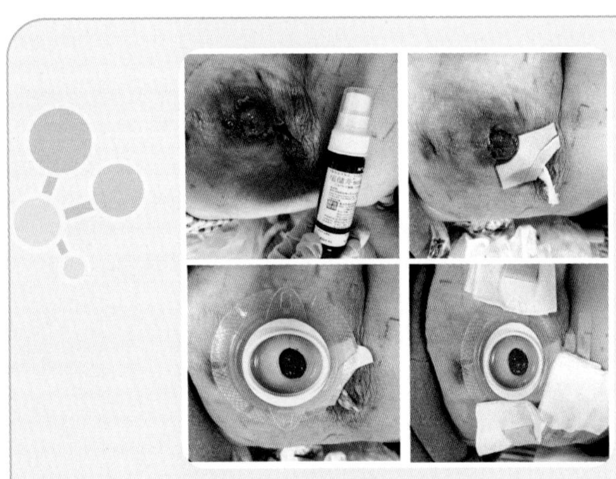

图 5.9.2　创面 3 cm × 1 cm × 5.3 cm，50% 黄色，50% 红色

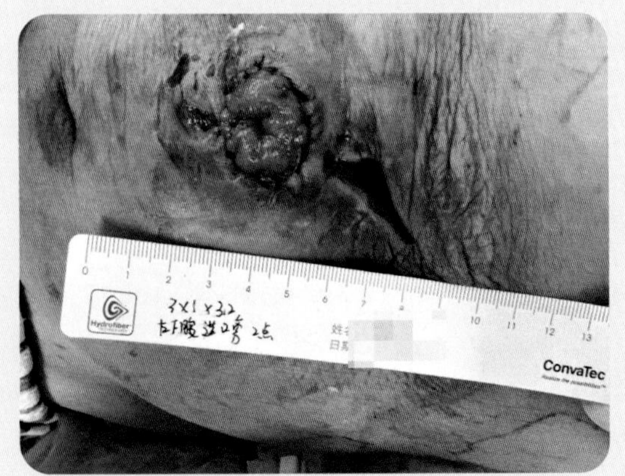

图 5.9.3　创面 3 cm × 1 cm × 3.2 cm，100% 红色，中等渗液

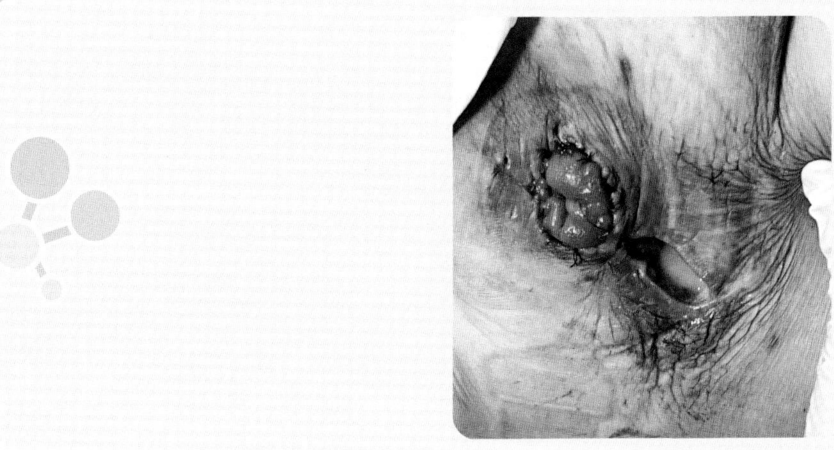

Figure 5.9.1 Postoperative incision infection in para stoma hernia surgery

◆ Treatment plan

1. Whole body anti infection, blood sugar control, and proper dietary education.

2. Take good care of the stoma to avoid secondary contamination of the wound with feces.

3. Actively clean the wound and selectively use a new type of wound dressing for local anti-infection. The wound is 3 cm × 1 cm × 5.3 cm, 50% yellow and 50% red. Clean the wound, rinse with iodine, saline, hydrophilic fiber silver, hydrogel, and two-piece convex surface ostomy bag (Figure 5.9.2).

4. Ensure proper management of exudate by exposing the wound area outside the chassis, ensuring adequate drainage, and promoting granulation tissue growth through fibroblast growth factor. After 6 days, the wound was 3 cm × 1 cm × 3.2 cm, 100% red, with moderate exudate, and fibroblast growth factor+ silver sulfate dressing was added (Figure 5.9.3). After 12 days, the wound was 2.8 cm × 1 cm × 2.1 cm, 100% red, and had a small amount of exudate (Figure 5.9.4).

5. Timely suture and seal the wound at the bedside to shorten the wound healing time (Figure 5.9.5). One month after discharge, the wound fully healed (Figure 5.9.6).

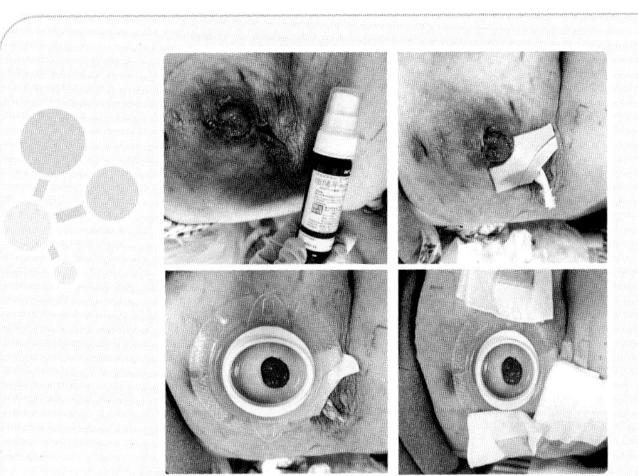

Figure 5.9.2 Wound size 3 cm × 1 cm × 5.3 cm, 50% yellow, 50% red

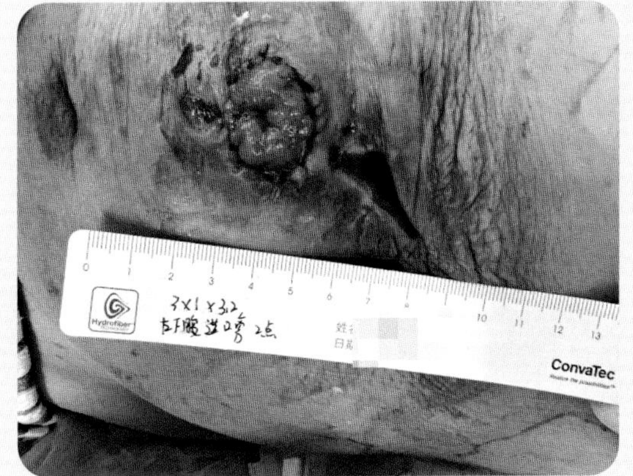

Figure 5.9.3 Wound size 3 cm × 1 cm × 3.2 cm, 100% red, moderate exudate

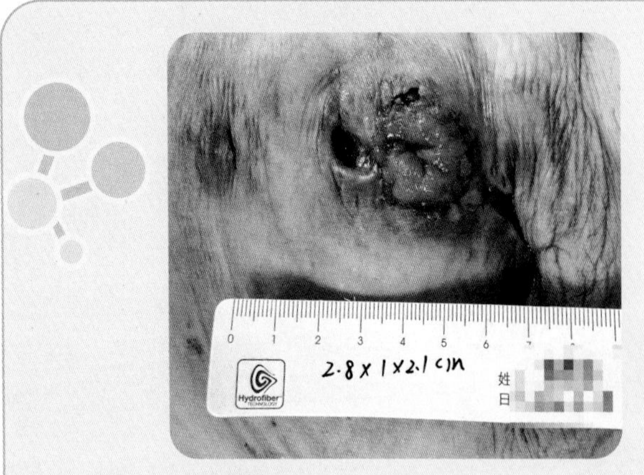

图 5.9.4　创面 2.8 cm × 1 cm × 2.1 cm，100% 红色，少量渗液

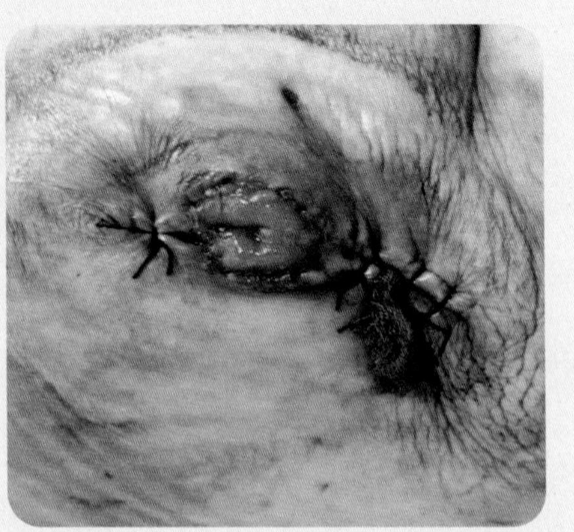

图 5.9.5　床边清创缝合，闭合伤口

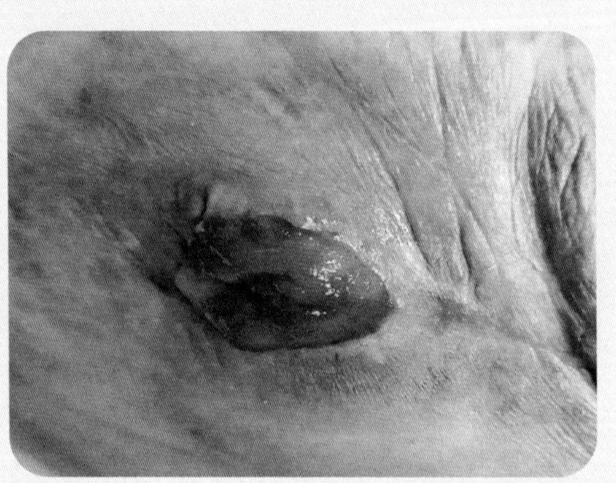

图 5.9.6　出院后 1 个月，伤口完全愈合

（邱巧如　王永高）

案例十　巨型五步蛇咬伤合并蛇伤性创面

◆ 致病原因

患者在竹林中被巨型五步蛇咬伤，创面坏死。

◆ 症状与体征

左上肢高度肿胀，进行性加重，并向肩部、胸部蔓延，上臂围右 35 cm、左 27 cm，皮肤大量水疱和血疱，左手指屈曲障碍，肌力减弱，左上肢感觉麻木，桡动脉搏动减弱（图 5.10.1）。实验室检查，血小板 11×10^9/L、纤维蛋白原 0.35 g/L。

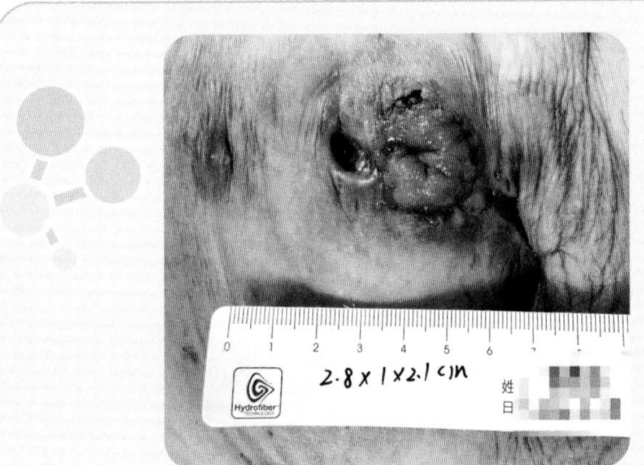

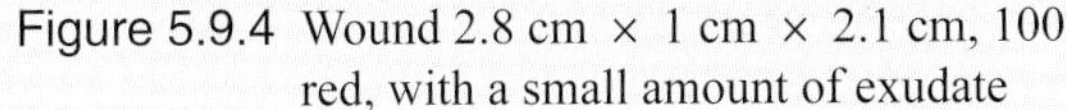

Figure 5.9.4 Wound 2.8 cm × 1 cm × 2.1 cm, 100% red, with a small amount of exudate

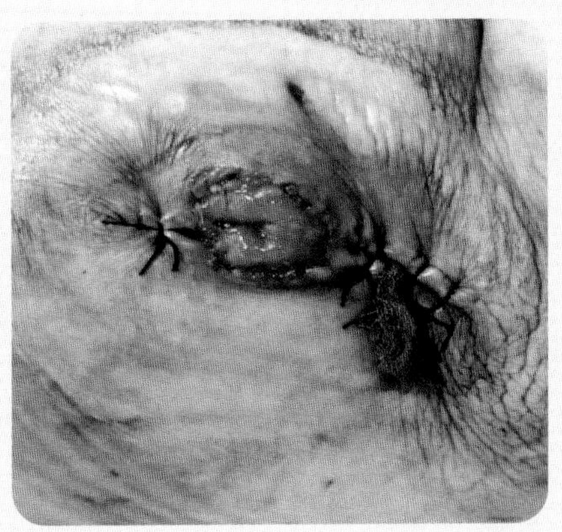

Figure 5.9.5 Bedside debridement and suturing, closing the wound

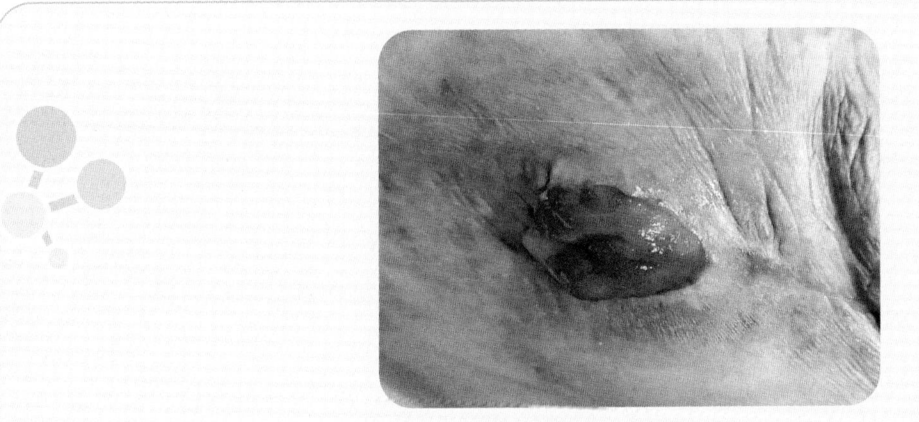

Figure 5.9.6 One month after discharge, the wound fully healed

(Qiu Qiaoru, Wang Yonggao)

Case 10 Giant five step snake bite combined with snake wound

◆ Cause of illness

The patient was bitten by a giant five step snake in the bamboo forest, and the wound died.

◆ Signs and symptoms

The left upper limb is highly swollen, progressively worsening, and spreading to the shoulder and chest. The circumference of the upper arm is 35 cm to the right and 27 cm to the left, with a large number of blisters and blood blisters on the skin. The left hand has difficulty bending the fingers, weakened muscle strength, numbness in the left upper limb, and decreased radial artery pulsation (Figure 5.10.1). Laboratory examination showed platelet count of 11×10^9/L and fibrinogen at 0.35 g/L.

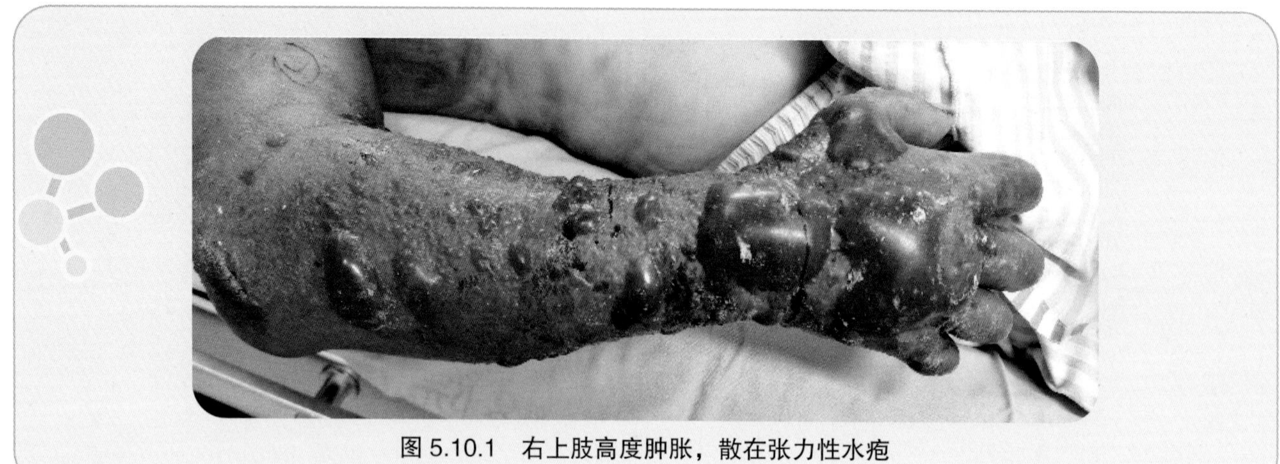

图 5.10.1　右上肢高度肿胀，散在张力性水疱

◆ 治疗方案

1. 分期治疗

1.1 急性出血期：左上肢皮下大片瘀斑，呈“蕲蛇斑”表现（图 5.10.2）。早期足量应用抗五步蛇毒血清，解毒利尿消肿治疗。

1.2 高危凝血期：凝血功能恢复后清创术、跳跃式小切口切开减压、抗感染等治疗（图 5.10.3）。

1.3 坏死期：细胞毒素可致细胞溶解，组织坏死，深达骨质层，并发感染。患者创面坏死深达肌层，侵及血管、神经等，清创切除坏死组织（图 5.10.4）。蛇毒导致组织坏死向近心端潜行性破坏，直达骨组织，再次彻底清创（图 5.10.5）。

2. 并发症处理：并发蛇毒诱导骨筋膜室综合征、蛇毒诱导的凝血病等，应早期足量应用抗蛇毒血清；创面累及皮下组织、肌腱、骨质等坏死，形成难愈性创面，应彻底清创 + 骨水泥填充 +VSD，继而皮瓣成形术（图 5.10.6）。

3. 中医中药辨证施治，中医可减少组织坏死、利于创面愈合，并减轻水肿和疼痛等。

4. 治疗 3 周后拆除骨水泥，邻近皮瓣移植，创面敷生长因子 + 银离子敷料，5 周后创面基本愈合（图 5.10.7、图 5.10.8）。

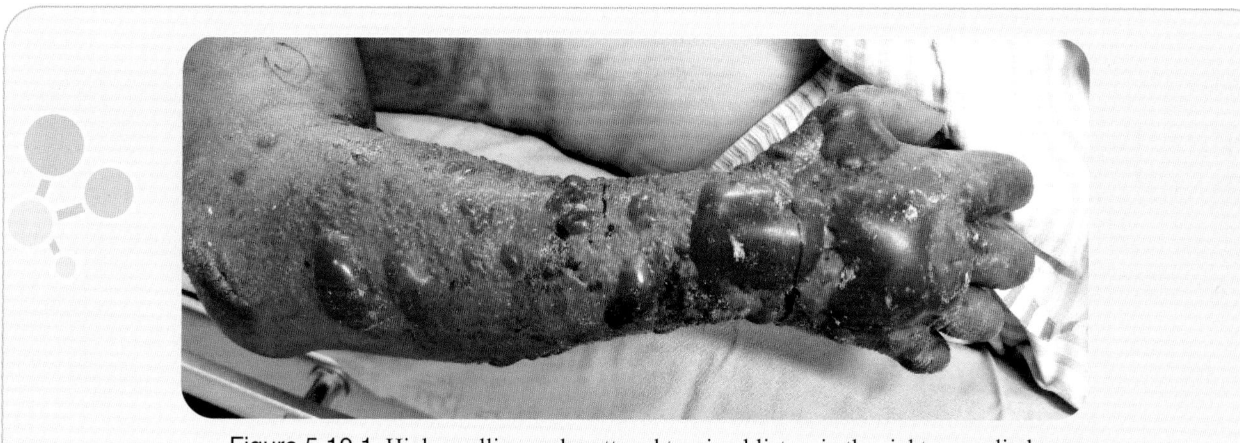

Figure 5.10.1 High swelling and scattered tension blisters in the right upper limb

◆ Treatment plan

1. Staged treatment

1.1 Acute bleeding phase: Large subcutaneous bruising on the left upper limb, presenting as "Qisnake spots" (Figure 5.10.2). Early and sufficient application of anti five step snake venom serum for detoxification, diuresis, and anti-inflammatory treatment.

1.2 High risk coagulation period: Treatment such as debridement, jumping small incision decompression, and anti infection after the recovery of coagulation function (Figure 5.10.3).

1.3 Necrosis stage: Cytotoxins can cause cell lysis, tissue necrosis, deep penetration into the bone layer, and concurrent infection. The patient's wound necrosis reached deep into the muscle layer, invading blood vessels, nerves, etc., and the necrotic tissue was removed by debridement (Figure 5.10.4). Snake venom causes tissue necrosis and stealthy destruction towards the proximal end, directly reaching bone tissue, and thorough debridement is performed again (Figure 5.10.5).

2. Complications management: If complications such as snake venom induced compartment syndrome and snake venom induced coagulation disease occur, early and sufficient use of anti snake venom serum should be applied; The wound involves necrosis of subcutaneous tissue, tendons, bone, etc., forming a difficult to heal wound. Thoroughly debridement, bone cement filling, and VSD should be performed, followed by skin flap reconstruction surgery (Figure 5.10.6).

3. Traditional Chinese Medicine (TCM) treatment based on syndrome differentiation can reduce tissue necrosis, promote wound healing, and alleviate edema and pain.

4. After 3 weeks of treatment, the bone cement was removed and adjacent skin flaps were transplanted. Growth factor and silver ion dressings were applied to the wound. After 5 weeks, the wound was basically healed (Figure 5.10.7, Figure 5.10.8).

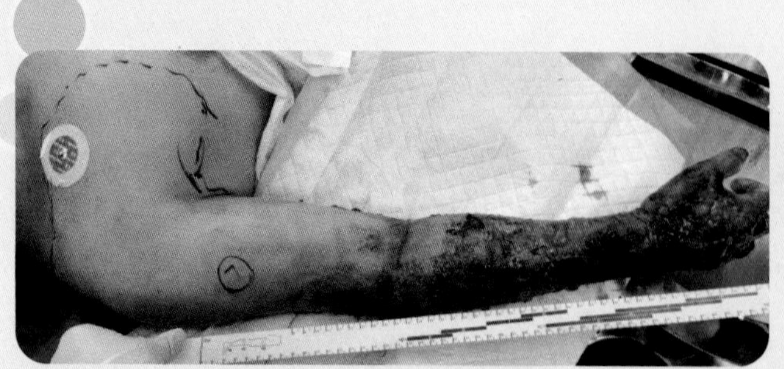
图 5.10.2　出血期，左上肢皮下大片瘀斑，呈“蕲蛇斑”表现

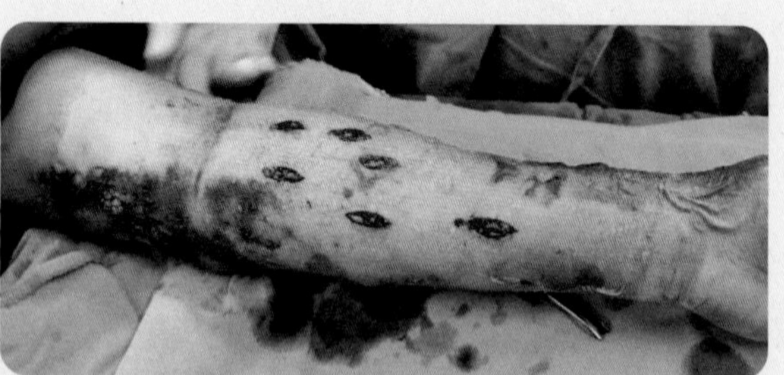
图 5.10.3　高危凝血期，清创 + 小切口跳跃式切开

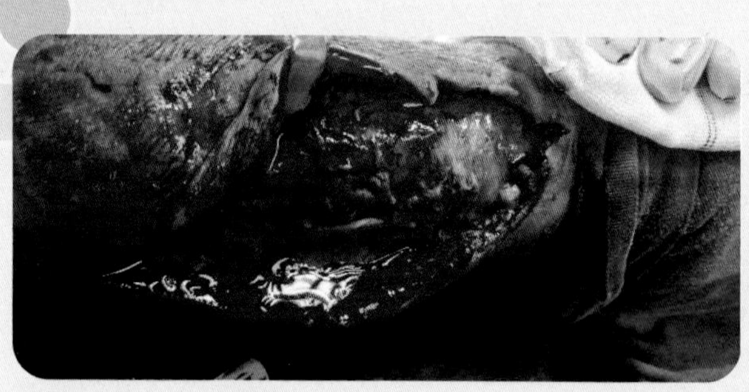
图 5.10.4　坏死期，创面坏死深达肌层，侵及血管、神经等

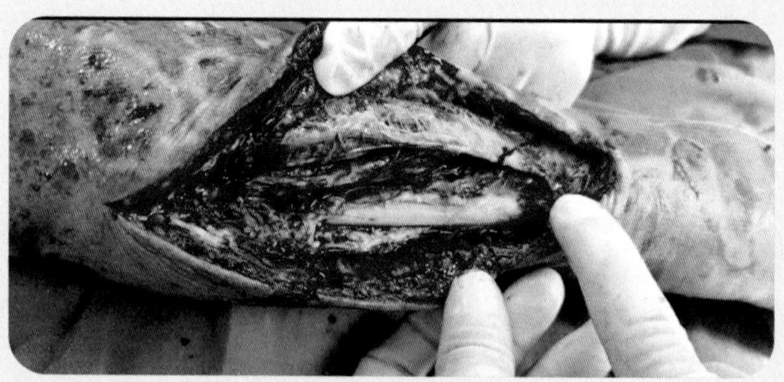
图 5.10.5　蛇毒导致组织坏死向近心端潜行性破坏，直达骨组织

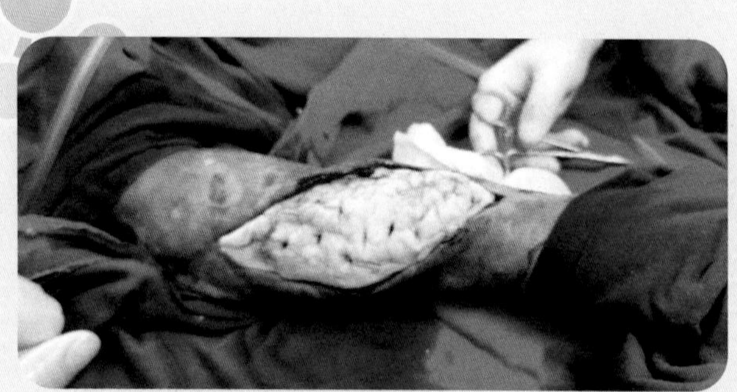
图 5.10.6　载药骨水泥 +VSD

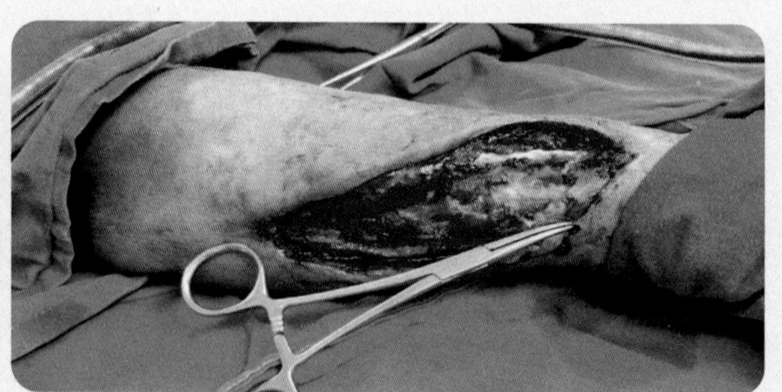
图 5.10.7　3 周后拆除骨水泥，邻近皮瓣移植

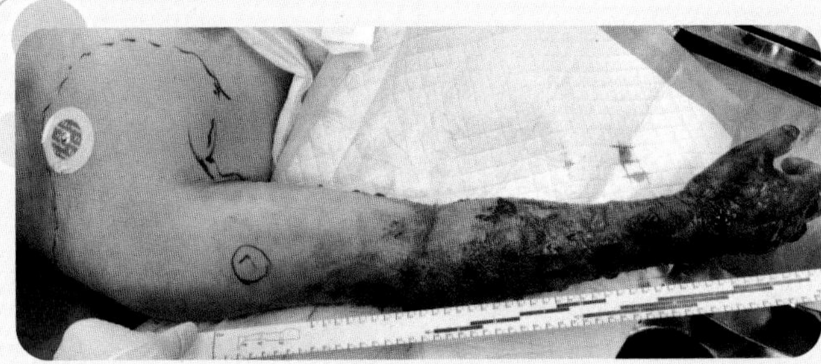

Figure 5.10.2 During the bleeding period, there is a large area of subcutaneous bruising on the left upper limb, which appears as a "snake spot"

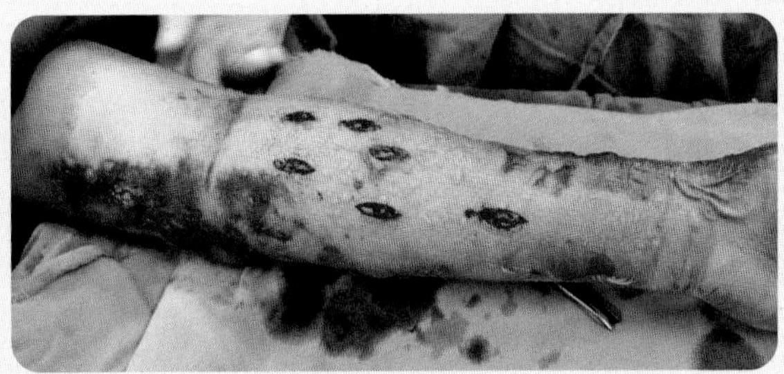

Figure 5.10.3 High risk coagulation period, debridement + small incision jumping incision

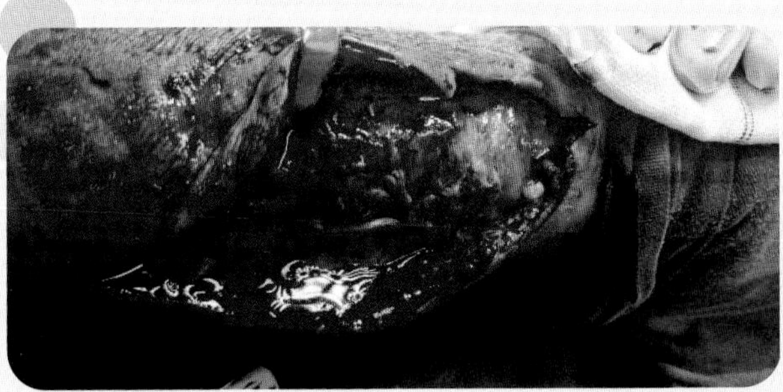

Figure 5.10.4 Necrosis stage, where the wound necrosis extends deep into the muscle layer and invades blood vessels, nerves, etc

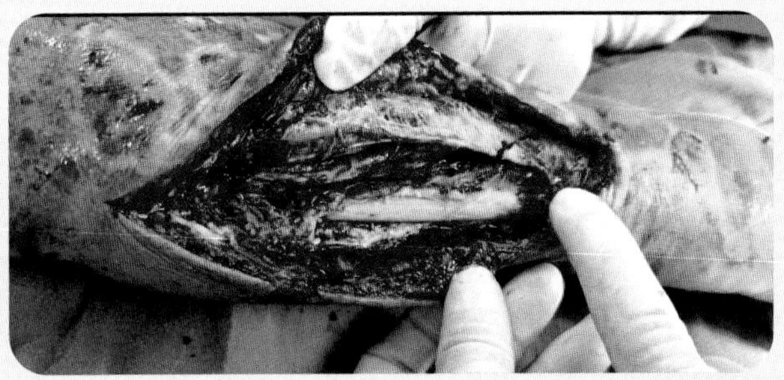

Figure 5.10.5 Snake venom causes tissue necrosis and stealthily destroys the proximal end, directly reaching the bone tissue

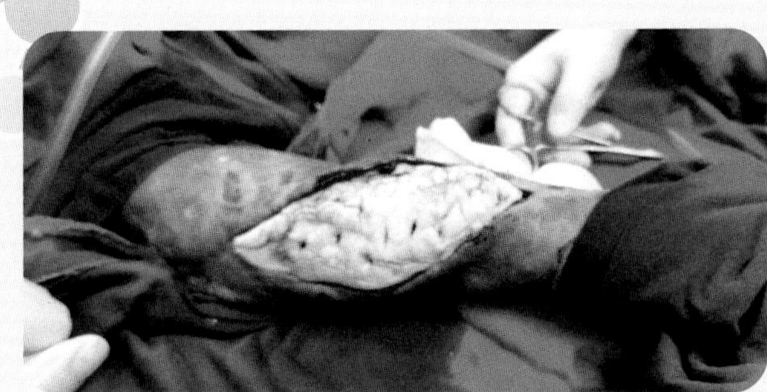

Figure 5.10.6 Drug loaded bone cement +VSD

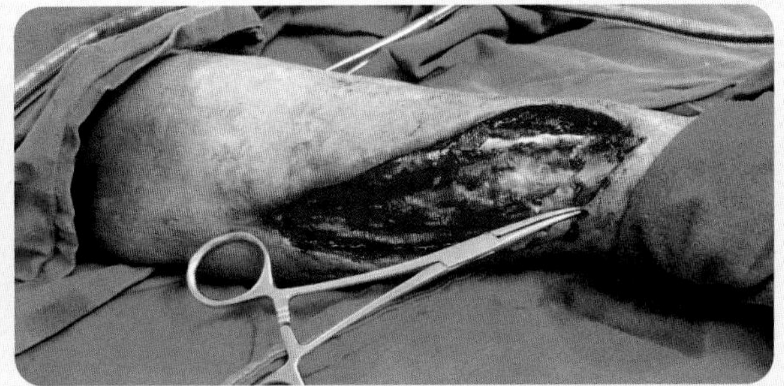

Figure 5.10.7 Removal of bone cement and adjacent skin flap transplantation after 3 weeks

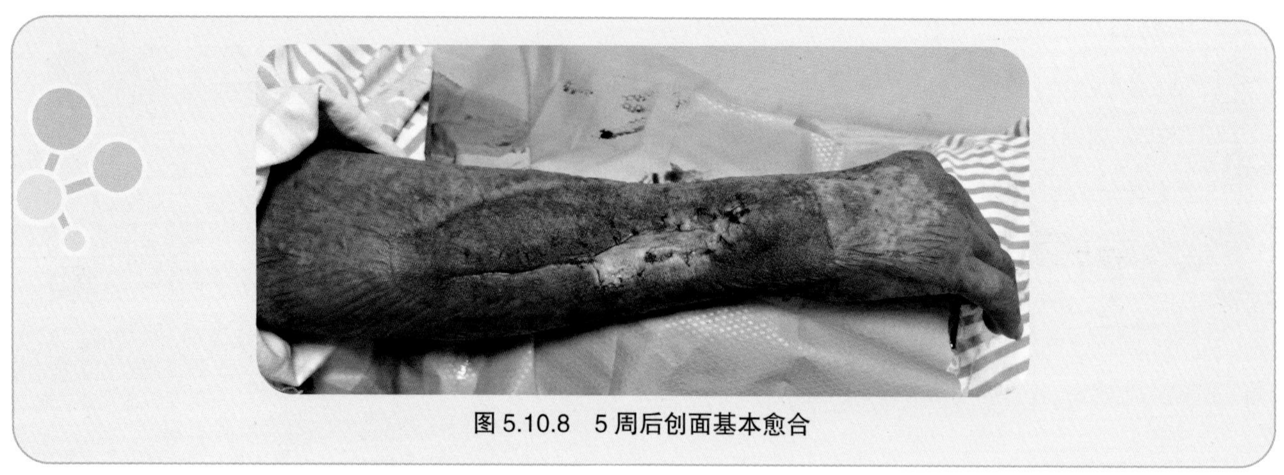

图 5.10.8　5 周后创面基本愈合

（王永高　谢　杰）

案例十一　蛇咬伤小腿坏死性筋膜炎

◆ 致病原因

患者被竹叶青毒蛇咬伤足踝区 7 天，伤后在当地医院注射抗蛇毒血清，并切开数个小切口引流。

◆ 症状与体征

右侧小腿剧痛难忍，精神萎靡，体温 38.6℃，四肢湿冷，心悸。右侧小腿至足踝部广泛性肿胀，足背动脉搏动消失，足底感觉减退，胫后动脉搏动微弱。足趾屈伸活动无力，小腿至足背部有多个切口，切口中有稀薄脓液和坏死肌肉组织溢出，小腿皮下波动明显，触痛明显，右下肢皮温增高，髂腹股沟淋巴结肿大，触痛明显（图 5.11.1）。

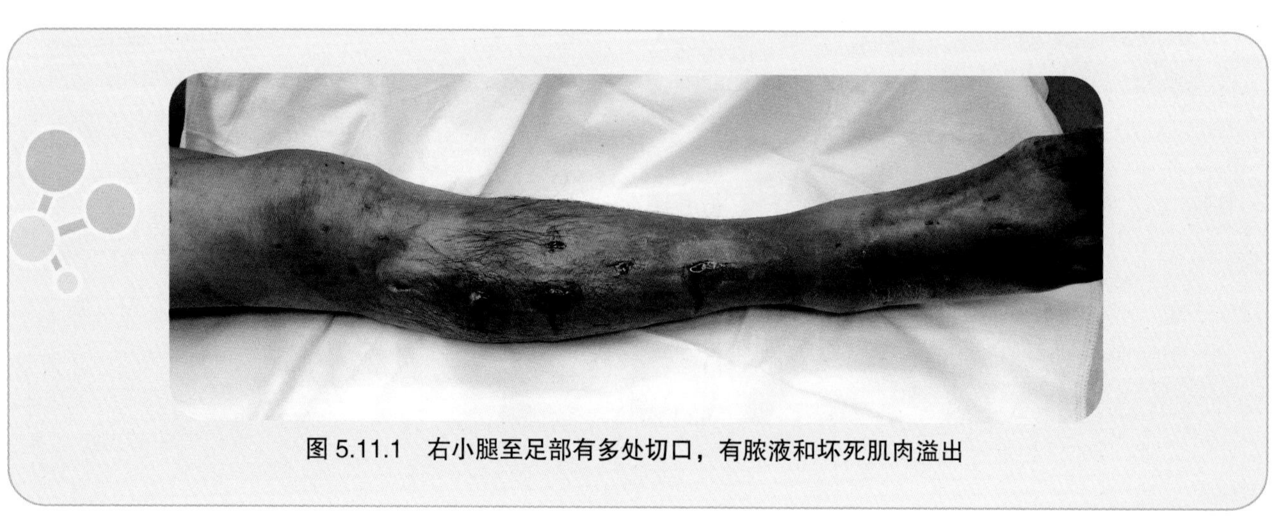

图 5.11.1　右小腿至足部有多处切口，有脓液和坏死肌肉溢出

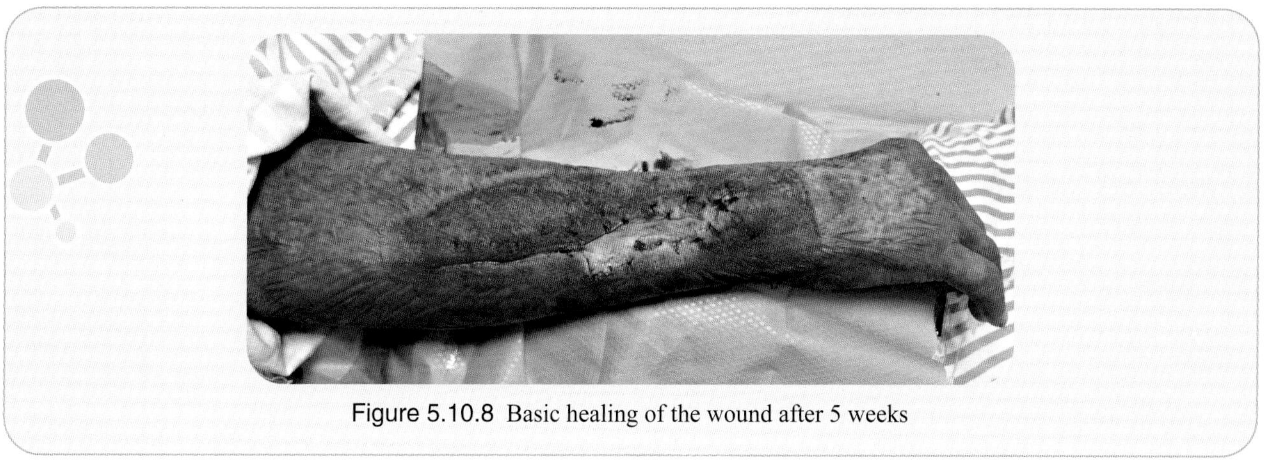

Figure 5.10.8 Basic healing of the wound after 5 weeks

(Wang Yonggao, Xie Jie)

Case 11 Necrotizing fasciitis of the calf caused by snake bite

◆ Cause of illness

The patient was bitten by a bamboo leaf green venomous snake in the ankle area for 7 days. After the injury, anti-snake venom was injected into the local hospital and several small incisions were made for drainage.

◆ Signs and symptoms

Severe pain in the right calf, mental exhaustion, body temperature of 38.6 ℃, wet and cold limbs, palpitations. Widespread swelling in the right calf to ankle, disappearance of dorsalis pedis artery pulsation, decreased plantar sensation, and weak posterior tibial artery pulsation. The toes have weak flexion and extension movements, and there are multiple incisions from the lower leg to the back of the foot. There is thin pus and necrotic muscle tissue overflowing from the incisions. The subcutaneous fluctuations of the lower leg are obvious, and the tenderness is significant. The skin temperature of the right lower limb is increased, and the iliac inguinal lymph nodes are enlarged, with obvious tenderness (Figure 5.11.1).

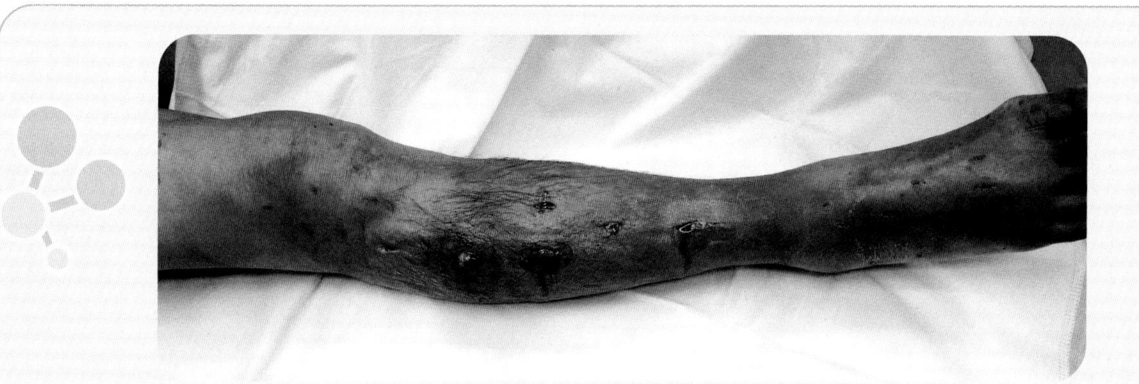

Figure 5.11.1 There are multiple incisions from the right calf to the foot, with pus and necrotic muscle overflowing

◆ 治疗方案

1. 患者入院时体温增高，精神萎靡，心悸气促，四肢湿冷，血压 80/40 mmHg。实验室检查，血常规检查见白细胞 21×10^9/L，中性粒细胞数 12.1×10^9/L、血红蛋白 82 g/L；B 型钠尿肽测定 39 000 pg/mL、肌酸激酶 236 IU/L，凝血功能正常；细菌培养，铜绿假单胞菌、药物敏感试验，对派拉西林 - 他唑巴坦和喹诺酮类药物敏感。

2. 根据症状和体征及辅助检查结果，结合小腿严重感染，考虑肌溶解引发感染中毒性休克，入院后立即积极抗休克并纠正失衡生命体征，导尿留置，吸氧，并给予广谱抗菌药物抗炎。

3. 休克纠正后，立即在全麻下行小腿切口扩创，坏死组织和感染病灶切除术，术中胫前肌群、小腿外侧肌群溶解液化坏死，胫前动脉静脉血栓并坏死，腓浅神经随肌肉坏死。胫前皮下脂肪液化坏死，胫前肌和小腿外侧肌间隙中有大量稀薄脓液。用吸引器吸出脓液渗出液，切除坏死肌肉皮下脂肪，胫腓骨裸露，部分骨膜坏死，直至肌肉组织新鲜渗血为止。活动出血点予以结扎，双氧水、碘伏和生理盐水反复浸泡冲洗消毒，安装 VSD 装置并封闭（图 5.11.2 ~ 图 5.11.5）。

4. 术后继续纠正全身状态，生命体征监护，肢体平放。VSD+ 重组人碱性成纤维细胞生长因子持续滴管冲洗，并观察渗出液颜色和创面气味。术后 3 天，再次清创并更换 VSD。创面较大的伤口，由于有大量液化坏死组织将 VSD 的网孔填塞，不利于充分引流，常规在术后 3 天再更换一次 VSD 装置，有利于起到负压吸引作用，术后检查贴膜漏液情况。

5. 二次 VSD 治疗 1 周，创面冲洗液逐渐干净，予以取下 VSD 装置，再次清创并直接闭合创面，伤口深部放置负压引流球两枚，包扎伤口，小腿石膏固定（图 5.11.6、图 5.11.7）。2 周后拆线，康复出院（图 5.11.8）。出院后定期随访，巩固治疗基础疾病，下肢康复训练。

◆ Treatment plan

1. When the patient was admitted, their body temperature increased, they were mentally lethargic, had palpitations and shortness of breath, their limbs were wet and cold, and their blood pressure was 80/40 mmHg. Laboratory examination, blood routine examination showed white blood cell count of 21 × 10^9/L, neutrophil count of 12.1 × 10^9/L, and hemoglobin level of 82 g/L; B-type natriuretic peptide was measured at 39 000 pg/mL, creatine kinase at 236 IU/L, and coagulation function was normal; Bacterial culture, Pseudomonas aeruginosa, drug sensitivity test, sensitivity to piperacillin tazobactam and quinolone drugs.

2. Based on symptoms, signs, and auxiliary examination results, combined with severe calf infection, it is considered that muscle dissolution may cause septic shock. Upon admission, active anti shock measures should be taken immediately, and imbalanced vital signs should be corrected. Urinary catheterization should be left in place, oxygen therapy should be administered, and broad-spectrum antibiotics should be given for anti-inflammatory purposes.

3. After shock correction, immediately under general anesthesia, the incision in the lower leg is expanded, necrotic tissue and infected lesions are removed, and during the operation, the anterior tibialis muscle group and lateral calf muscle group dissolve, liquefy and die, the anterior tibialis artery and vein thrombosis and necrosis occur, and the superficial peroneal nerve is necrotic along with the muscle. Subcutaneous fat liquefaction and necrosis in the anterior tibia, with a large amount of thin pus in the space between the anterior tibialis muscle and the lateral calf muscle. Use a suction device to aspirate the pus exudate, remove the necrotic subcutaneous fat of the muscle, expose the tibia and fibula, and partially necrotize the periosteum until fresh blood seeps from the muscle tissue. The bleeding points of the activity were ligated, and repeatedly soaked, rinsed, and disinfected with hydrogen peroxide, iodine, and saline solution. The VSD device was installed and sealed (Figure 5.11.2- Figure 5.11.5).

4. Continue to correct the overall body condition, monitor vital signs, and place limbs flat after surgery. VSD + recombinant human basic fibroblast growth factor continuous drip irrigation, and observation of exudate color and wound odor. Three days after surgery, the wound was cleared again and the VSD was replaced. For larger wounds, due to the large amount of liquefied necrotic tissue filling the VSD mesh, it is not conducive to sufficient drainage. It is customary to replace the VSD device again 3 days after surgery to facilitate negative pressure suction. After surgery, check the leakage of the film.

5. After one week of secondary VSD treatment, the wound flushing solution gradually cleared, and the VSD device was removed. The wound was cleared again and the wound was directly closed. Two negative pressure drainage balls were placed deep in the wound, and the wound was wrapped and fixed with calf plaster (Figure 5.11.6, Figure 5.11.7). Two weeks later, the stitches were removed and the patient recovered and was discharged (Figure 5.11.8). Regular follow-up after discharge to consolidate treatment of underlying diseases and lower limb rehabilitation training.

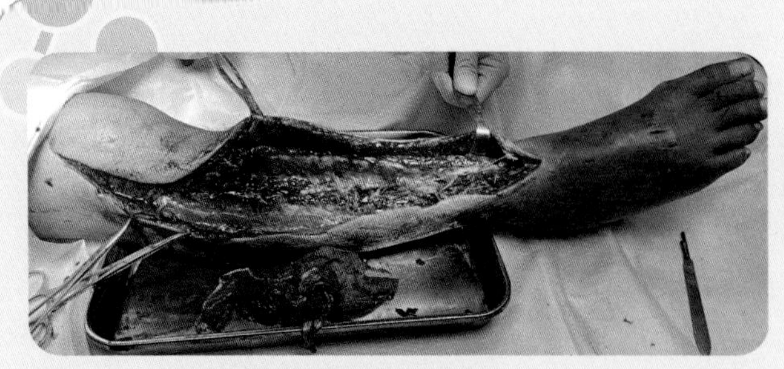

图 5.11.2　切开皮肤，皮下脂肪液化，胫前肌群，小腿外侧肌群大面积坏死

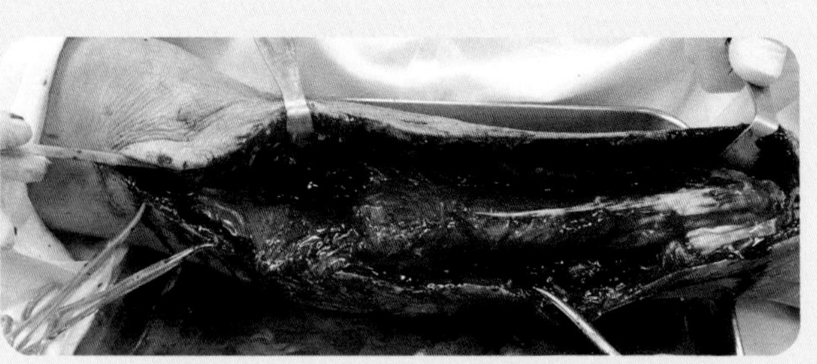

图 5.11.3　胫前肌群溶解液化坏死

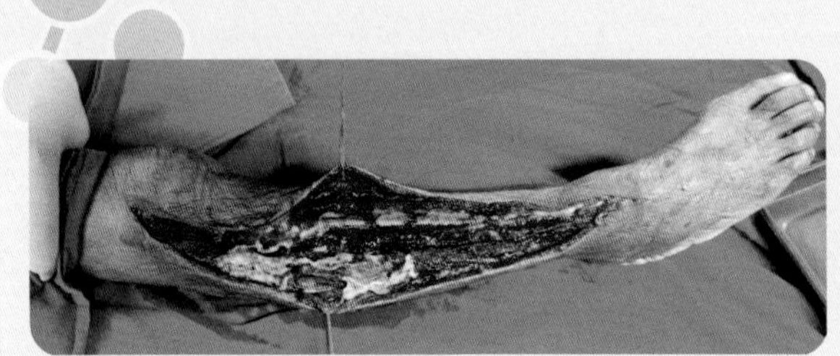

图 5.11.4　胫前肌群和小腿外侧肌群清除、胫前动静脉腓浅神经缺失，胫腓骨外露

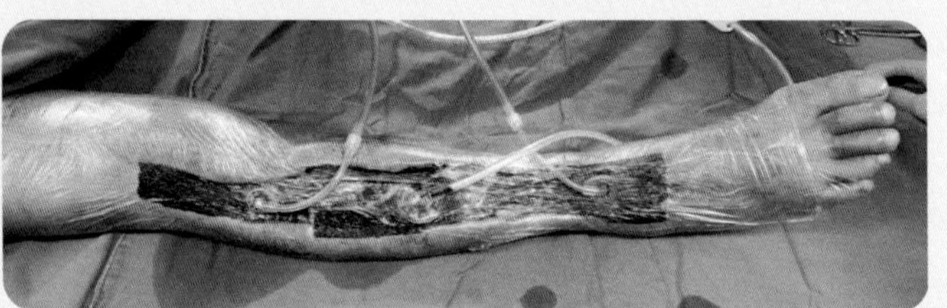

图 5.11.5　坏死肌群和感染灶切除后，应用 VSD

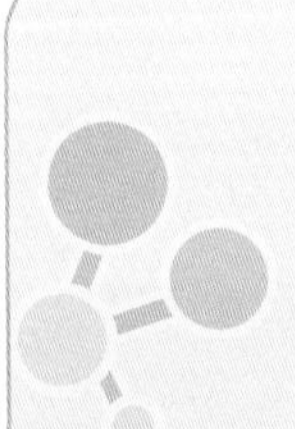

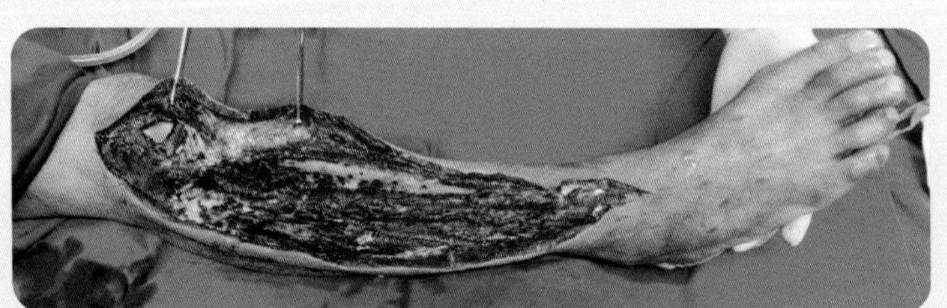

图 5.11.6　VSD+ 清创治疗后，创面较新鲜

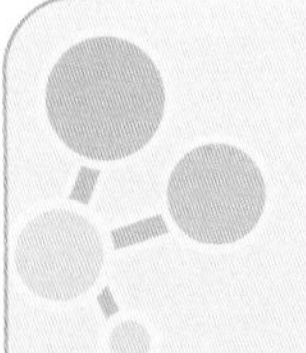

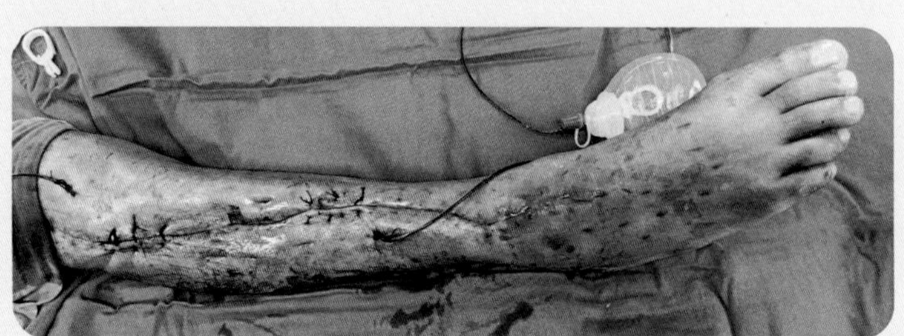

图 5.11.7　切口直接闭合，深部放置负压引流球

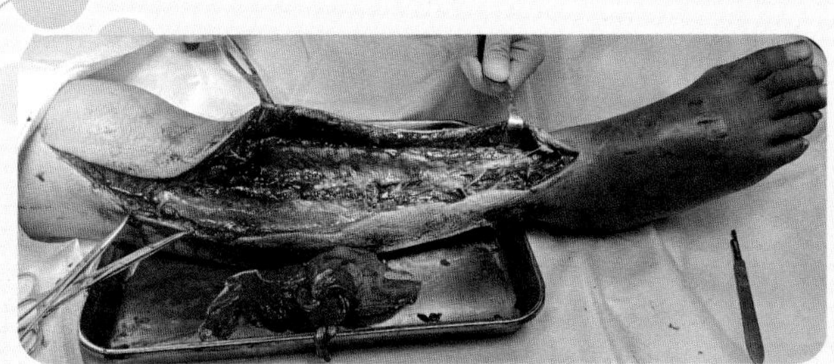

Figure 5.11.2 Skin incision, subcutaneous fat liquefaction, extensive necrosis of tibialis anterior muscle group and lateral calf muscle group

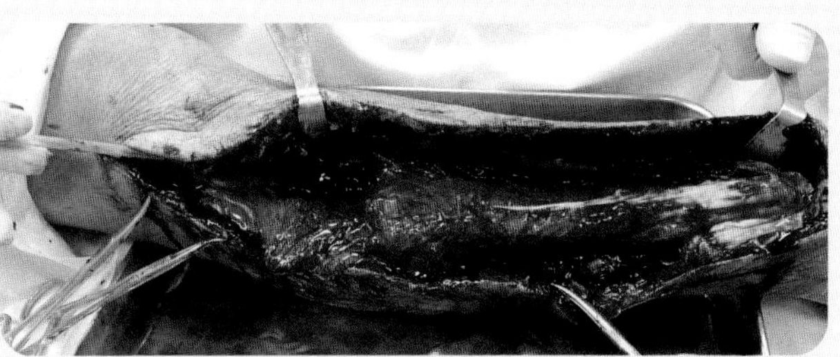

Figure 5.11.3 Dissolution, liquefaction and necrosis of anterior tibial muscle group

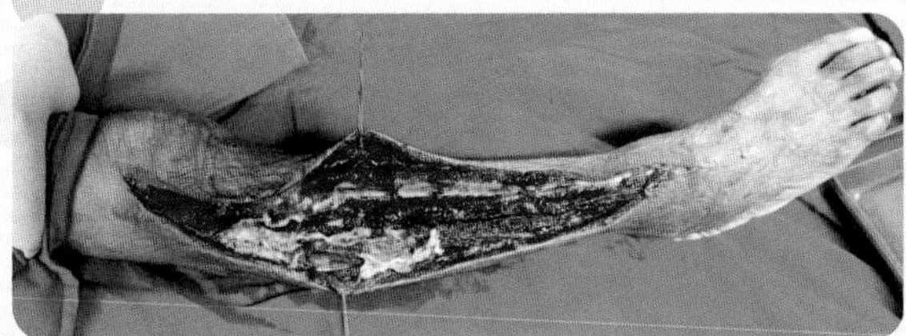

Figure 5.11.4 Clearance of tibialis anterior muscle group and lateral calf muscle group, loss of tibialis anterior arteriovenous peroneal nerve, and exposure of tibia and fibula

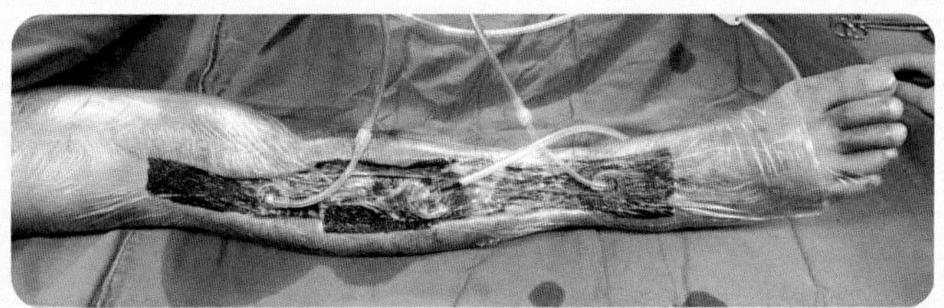

Figure 5.11.5 Application of VSD after resection of necrotic muscle group and infected lesion

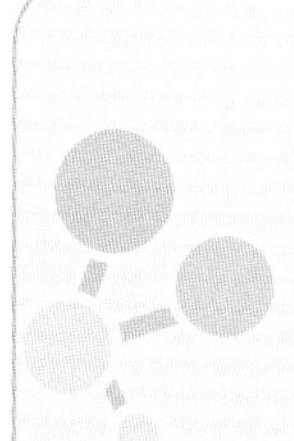

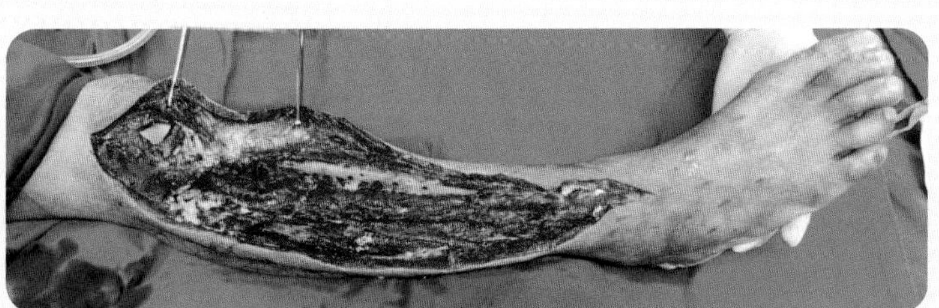

Figure 5.11.6 After VSD + debridement treatment, the wound appears fresher

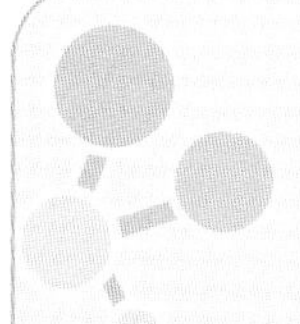

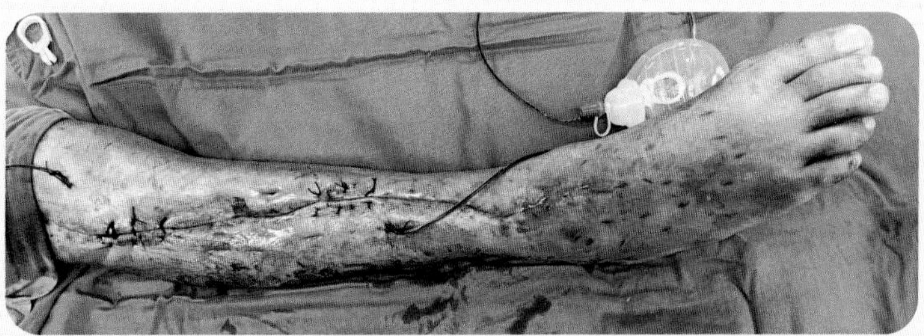

Figure 5.11.7 Close the incision directly and place a negative pressure drainage ball in the deep part

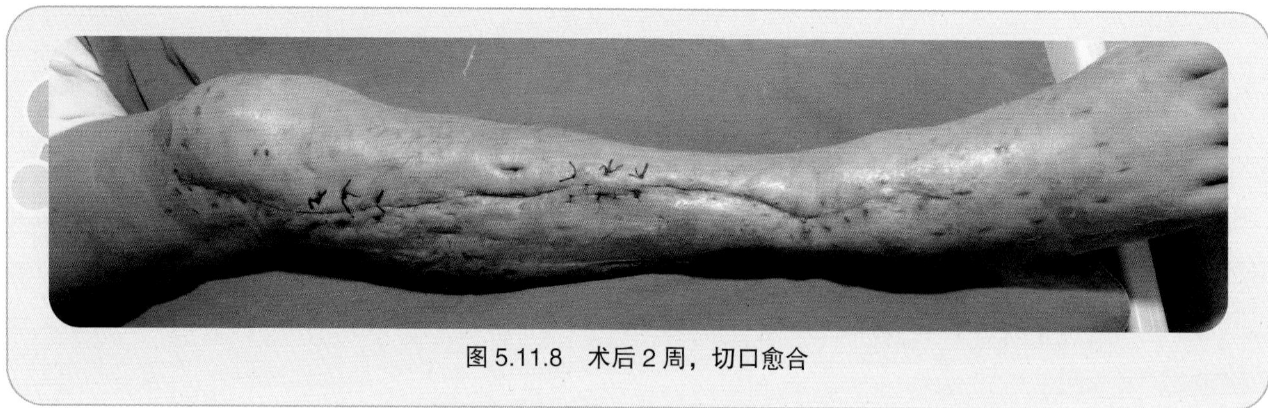
图 5.11.8　术后 2 周，切口愈合

（陈善亮）

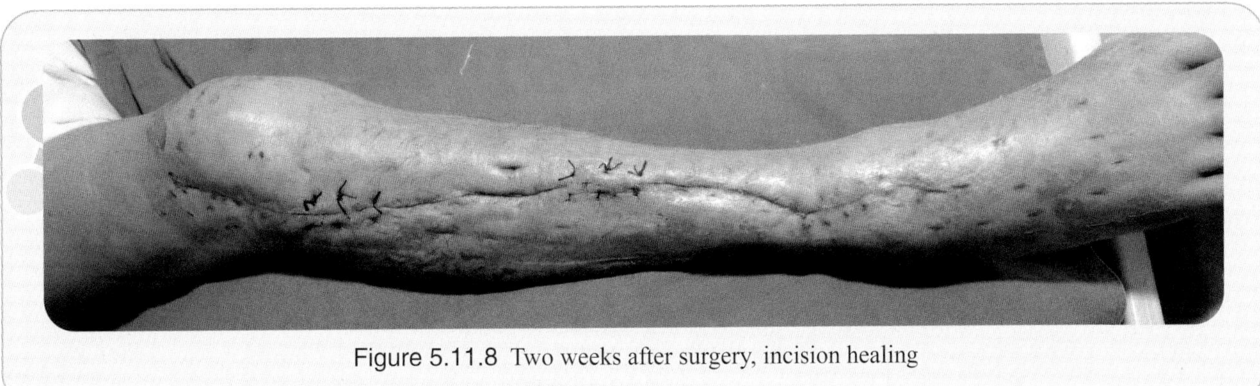

Figure 5.11.8 Two weeks after surgery, incision healing

(Chen Shanliang)

第 6 章

Chapter 6

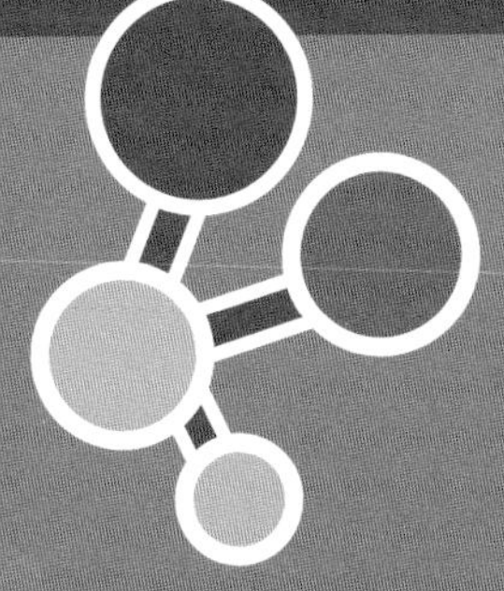

静脉性溃疡创面修复

Repair of Venous Ulcer Wounds

案例一　左侧内外踝静脉性溃疡

◆ 致病原因

患者，男性，78 岁，双侧大隐静脉曲张 31 年，双侧大隐静脉高位结扎分段剥脱术 9 年，双侧小腿破溃流脓经久不愈 12 年，既往因车祸致左侧髋关节骨折、股骨干粉碎骨折，膝关节粉碎骨折术后 39 年。

◆ 症状与体征

扶拐行走，跛行。左侧外踝有 9 cm × 5 cm 不规则溃疡，深达腓骨小头骨膜，局部有数条蛆虫蠕动，溃疡皮缘内陷，中心区有大量坏死组织，污秽不清，味臭，表面有白色脓性分泌物；左侧内踝有 4 cm × 4 cm 圆形溃疡，皮缘内陷，表面散在白色脓苔，局部无红肿，有大量炎性渗出（图 6.1.1、图 6.1.2）。小腿至足部色素沉着，皮肤角化硬化增厚，局部无红肿，小腿肌肉萎缩足背动脉和胫后动脉波动微弱，足底皮肤血液反流迟缓，皮温低，足底感觉正常。趾甲明显增厚，髋关节膝关节踝关节僵硬强直。

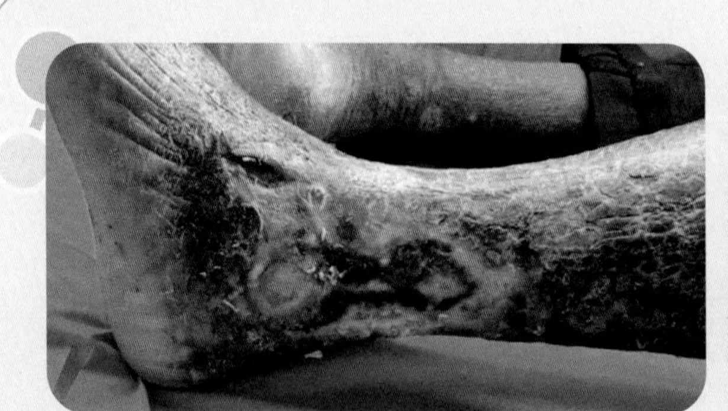

图 6.1.1　创面有大量蛆虫蠕动

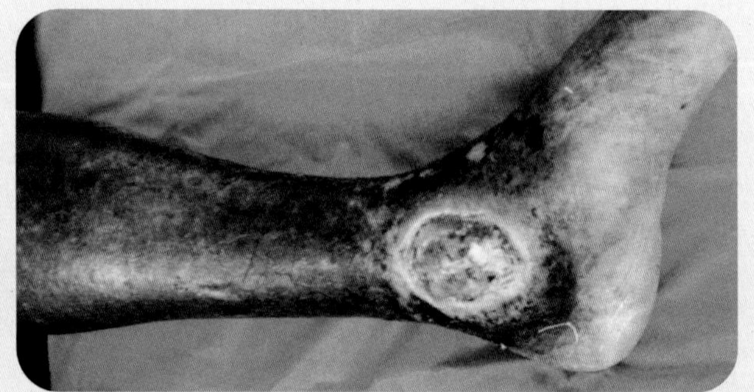

图 6.1.2　左侧可见圆形溃疡，表面有白色脓苔，局部污秽不清

◆ 治疗方案

1. 入院后积极治疗基础疾病，纠正心肺功能低下，控制血糖，纠正贫血和低蛋白血症，扩张外周血管，改善肢体血液循环，营养周围神经。

2. 根据细菌培养选用敏感抗菌药物。

3. 伤口每天清创，刮出溃疡面脓性分泌物和无生机肉芽组织，创面喷洒重组人碱性成纤维细胞生长因子，每天换药 2 次。

Case 1 Left medial and lateral ankle venous ulcer

◆ Cause of illness

The patient is a 78-year-old male with bilateral varicose veins of the great saphenous vein for 31 years. He underwent high-level ligation and segmental stripping of the great saphenous vein for 9 years. The patient also had persistent pus discharge from both calves for 12 years. He had a history of left hip fracture and comminuted fracture of the femoral shaft due to a car accident, and had a comminuted fracture of the knee joint 39 years after surgery.

◆ Signs and symptoms

Walking with crutches, limping. There is an irregular ulcer measuring 9 cm × 5 cm on the left lateral malleolus, which extends deep to the periosteum of the fibular head. Several maggots are wriggling locally, and the ulcer skin margin is invaginated. There is a large amount of necrotic tissue in the central area, which is dirty, smelly, and has white purulent discharge on the surface; There is a 4 cm × 4 cm circular ulcer on the left medial malleolus, with a sunken skin margin and scattered white pus coating on the surface. There is no local redness or swelling, and there is a large amount of inflammatory exudate (Figure 6.1.1, Figure 6.1.2). Pigmentation is present from the calf to the foot, with keratinized, hardened, and thickened skin. There is no local redness or swelling. The calf muscles are atrophied, and there is weak fluctuation in the dorsal and posterior tibial arteries. The blood reflux of the plantar skin is slow, the skin temperature is low, and the plantar sensation is normal. The toenails are significantly thickened, and the hip, knee, and ankle joints are stiff and rigid.

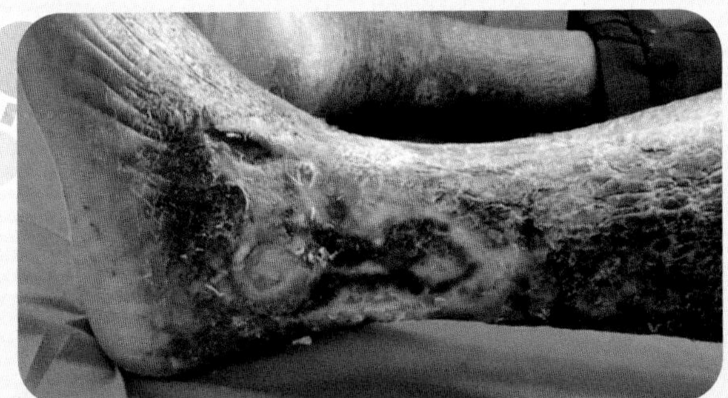

Figure 6.1.1 There are a large number of maggots wriggling on the wound surface

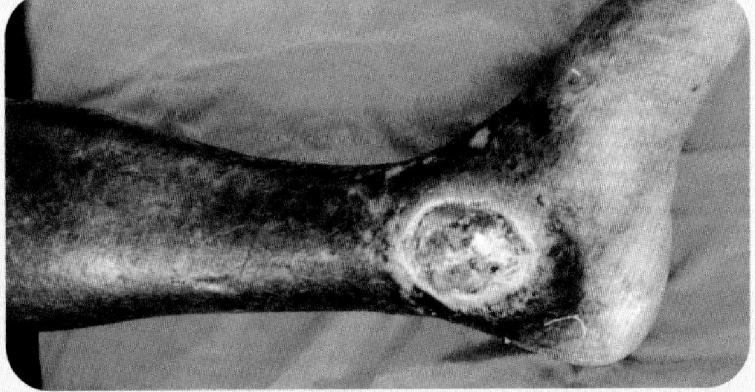

Figure 6.1.2 On the left side, a circular ulcer can be seen with white pus coating on the surface and unclear local contamination

◆ Treatment plan

1. Actively treat underlying diseases after admission, correct heart and lung dysfunction, control blood sugar, correct anemia and hypoalbuminemia, dilate peripheral blood vessels, improve limb blood circulation, and nourish peripheral nerves.

2. Select sensitive antibiotics based on bacterial culture.

3. Clean the wound daily, scrape off purulent secretions and lifeless granulation tissue from the ulcer surface, spray recombinant human basic fibroblast growth factor on the wound, and change dressing twice a day.

4. 中药熏洗下肢增厚角化皮肤，去除死削，蜂蜜凡士林软膏软化皮肤。

5. 红外线、微波局部理疗。

6. 基础疾病纠正后，采用 VSD+ 重组人碱性成纤维细胞生长因子局部滴注治疗，持续负压治疗 5 天，促进肉芽组织新鲜，饱满，改善局部血液循环，为创面植皮争取时间窗（图 6.1.3）。

7. VSD 治疗 5 天，拆除负压装置，创面新鲜，肉芽组织填满创面、出血活跃，植皮时机成熟，与全麻下行中厚游离皮片移植于外踝和内踝创面，创面喷洒重组人碱性成纤维细胞生长因子，油纱贴敷植皮区创面加压包扎（图 6.1.4、图 6.1.5）。

8. 术后 10 天，打开包扎敷料，植皮完全成活，创面完全愈合（图 6.1.6、图 6.1.7）。局部继续应用油纱敷料包扎，保护植皮区，宣教保护创面知识，防止创面二次破溃，康复出院。

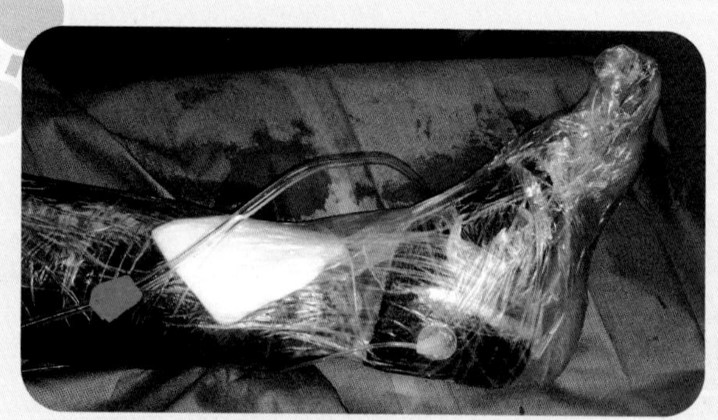

图 6.1.3　生长因子创面滴注 +VSD 治疗

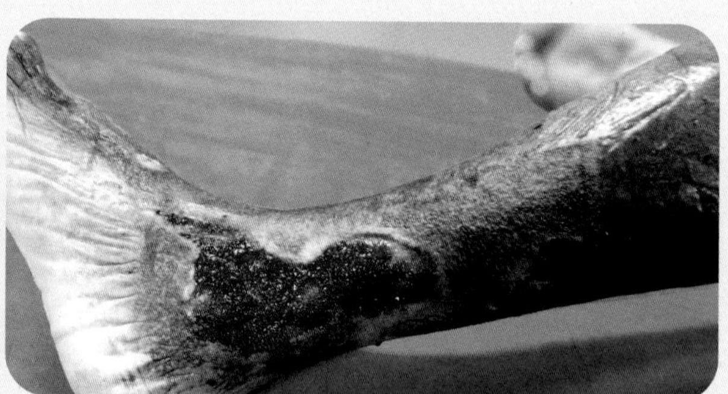

图 6.1.4　负压治疗 5 天，外踝创面饱满新鲜

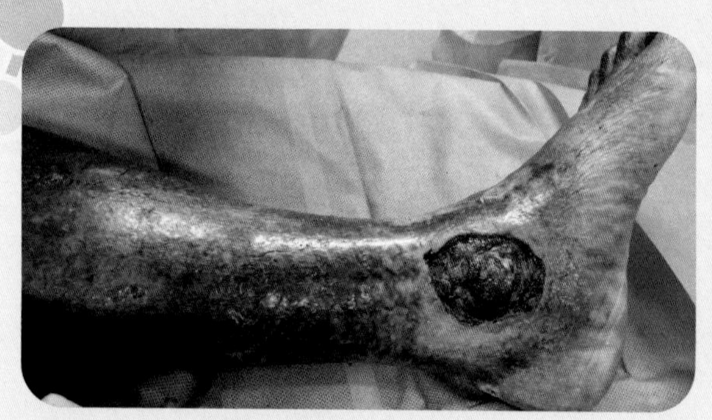

图 6.1.5　内踝创面新鲜，小腿皮肤广泛性色沉着

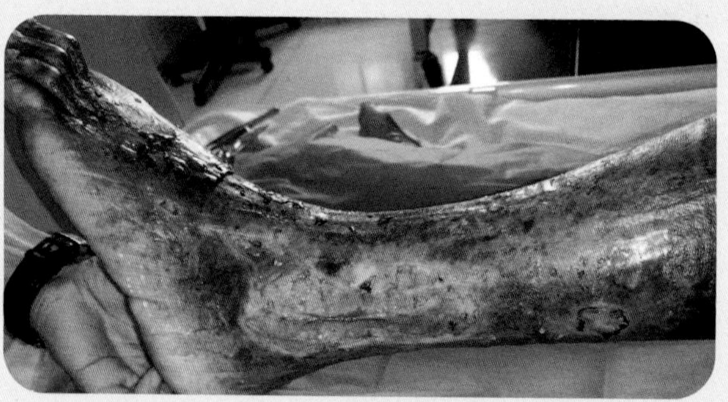

图 6.1.6　外踝中厚游离皮肤移植并成活

4. Use traditional Chinese medicine to fumigate and wash the thickened and keratinized skin of the lower limbs, remove dead skin, and soften the skin with honey Vaseline ointment.

5. Infrared and microwave local therapy.

6. After correcting the underlying disease, VSD + recombinant human basic fibroblast growth factor local infusion therapy was used, and negative pressure therapy was continued for 5 days to promote fresh and plump granulation tissue, improve local blood circulation, and create a time window for wound skin grafting (Figure 6.1.3).

7. VSD treatment lasted for 5 days. The negative pressure device was removed, the wound was fresh, granulation tissue filled the wound, bleeding was active, and the timing for skin grafting was ripe. Under general anesthesia, medium thick free skin grafts were transplanted onto the outer and inner ankle wounds. Recombinant human alkaline fibroblast growth factor was sprayed onto the wound, and oil gauze was applied to the skin grafting area for pressure bandaging (Figure 6.1.4, Figure 6.1.5).

8. Ten days after surgery, the dressing was opened and the skin graft survived completely, and the wound healed completely (Figure 6.1.6, Figure 6.1.7). Continue to apply oil gauze dressing locally, protect the skin graft area, educate on wound protection knowledge, prevent secondary rupture of the wound, and recover and discharge.

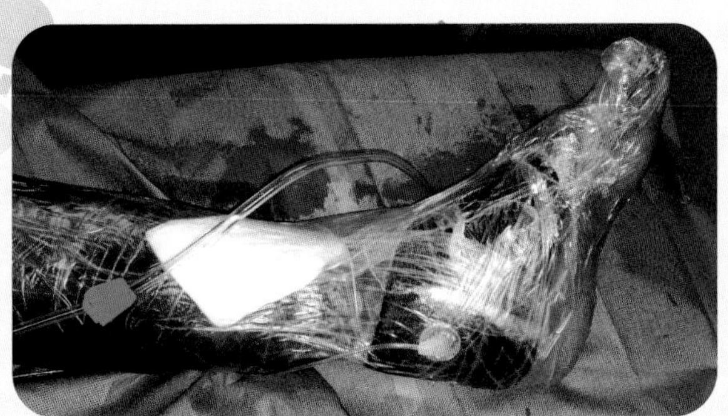

Figure 6.1.3 Growth factor wound infusion + VSD treatment

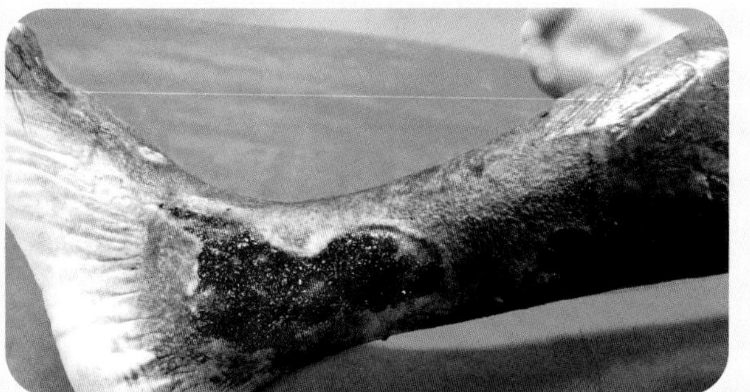

Figure 6.1.4 Negative pressure treatment for 5 days, the outer ankle wound is full and fresh

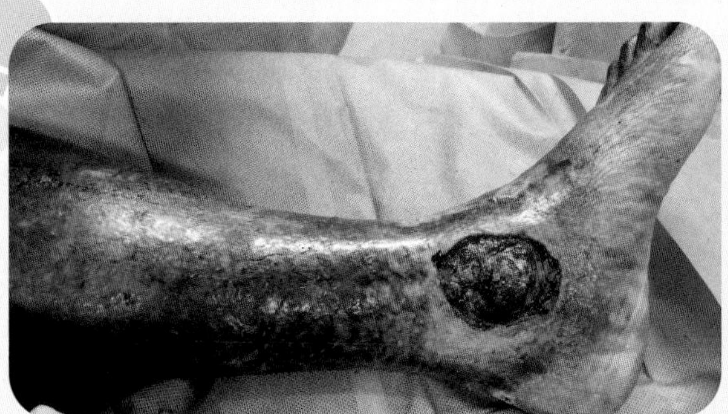

Figure 6.1.5 Fresh inner ankle wound and extensive pigmentation of calf skin

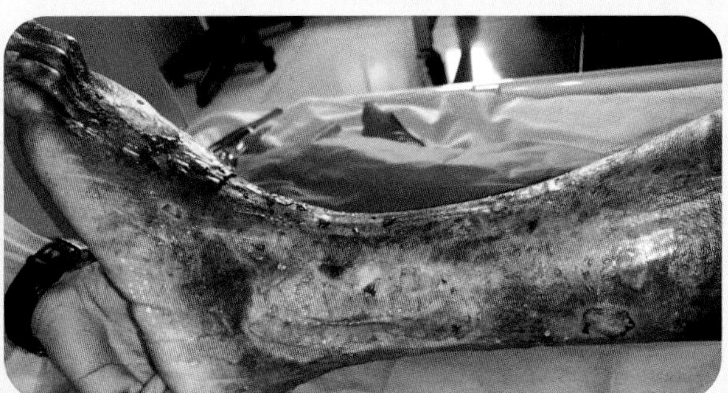

Figure 6.1.6 Transplantation and survival of thick free skin on the outer ankle

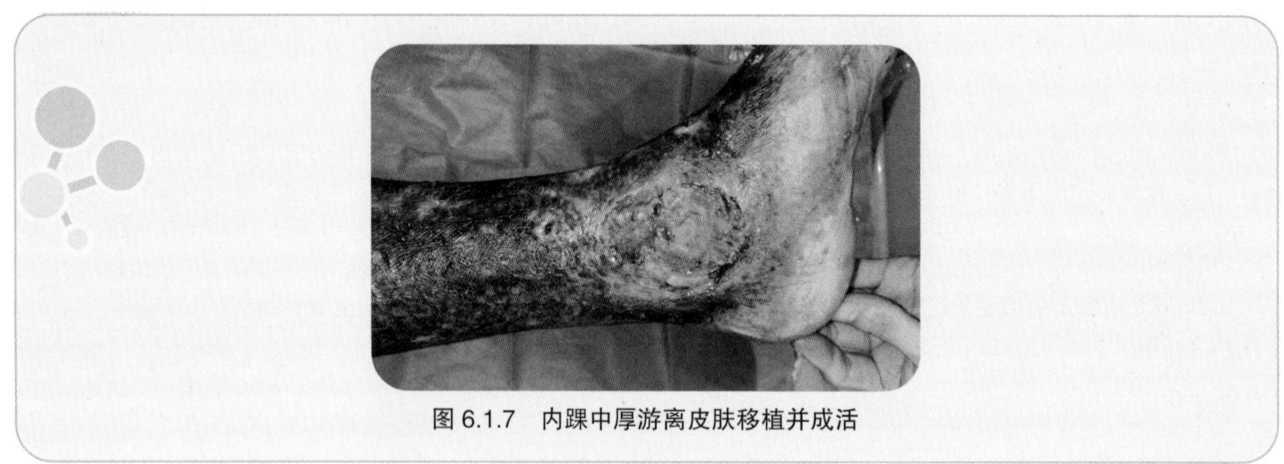

图 6.1.7　内踝中厚游离皮肤移植并成活

（陈善亮）

案例二　双下肢巨大静脉性溃疡

◆ 致病原因

患者双下肢长期皮肤瘀积性皮炎、瘙痒致下肢慢性溃疡。双下肢复杂性溃疡伴感染，双下肢静脉瓣膜功能不全伴浅静脉曲张

◆ 症状与体征

双小腿三处巨大溃疡，脓苔附着，右胫前创面 11.8 cm × 11 cm × 1 cm，深达肌层；左小腿内侧创面深达内踝 14 cm × 8 cm × 1 cm，左小腿外侧创面深达外踝 7.7 cm × 5.2 cm × 1 cm（图 6.2.1）。B 超示双下肢深静脉瓣膜功能不全。

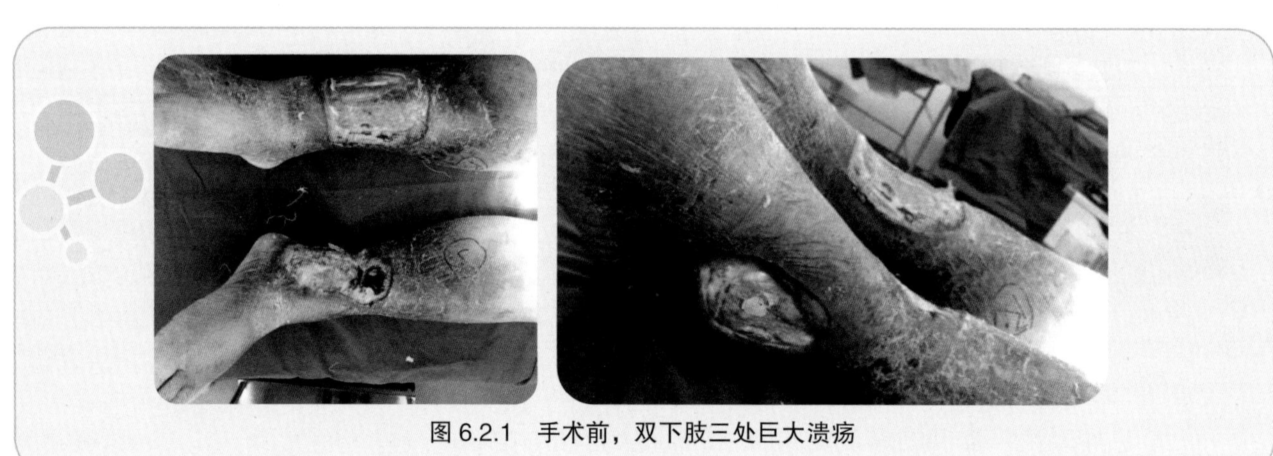

图 6.2.1　手术前，双下肢三处巨大溃疡

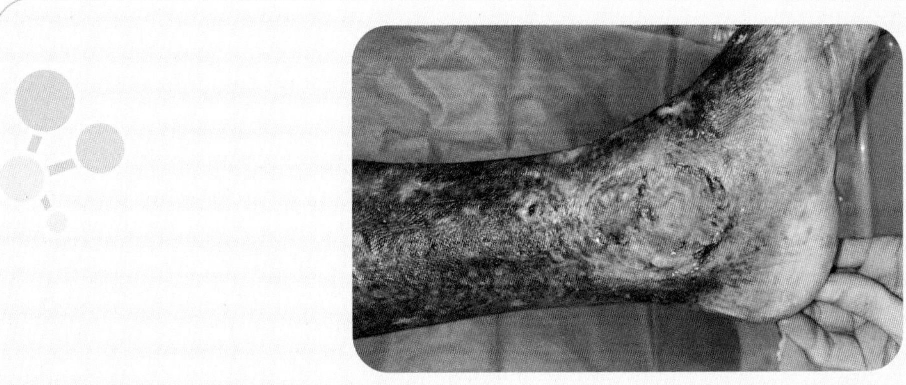

Figure 6.1.7 Transplantation and survival of middle thickness free skin on the inner ankle

(Chen Shanliang)

Case 2 Giant venous ulcers in both lower limbs

◆ Cause of illness

The patient has chronic ulcers in the lower limbs due to long-term skin stasis dermatitis and itching in both lower limbs. Complex ulcers with infection in both lower limbs, venous valve dysfunction with superficial varicose veins in both lower limbs

◆ Signs and symptoms

There are three huge ulcers on both lower legs, with pus coating attached. The wound on the right anterior tibia is 11.8 cm × 11 cm × 1 cm deep, reaching the muscle layer; The depth of the wound on the inner side of the left calf reaches 14 cm × 8 cm × 1 cm of the medial malleolus, and the depth of the wound on the outer side of the left calf reaches 7.7 cm × 5.2 cm × 1 cm of the lateral malleolus (Figure 6.2.1). Ultrasound shows deep vein valve dysfunction in both lower limbs.

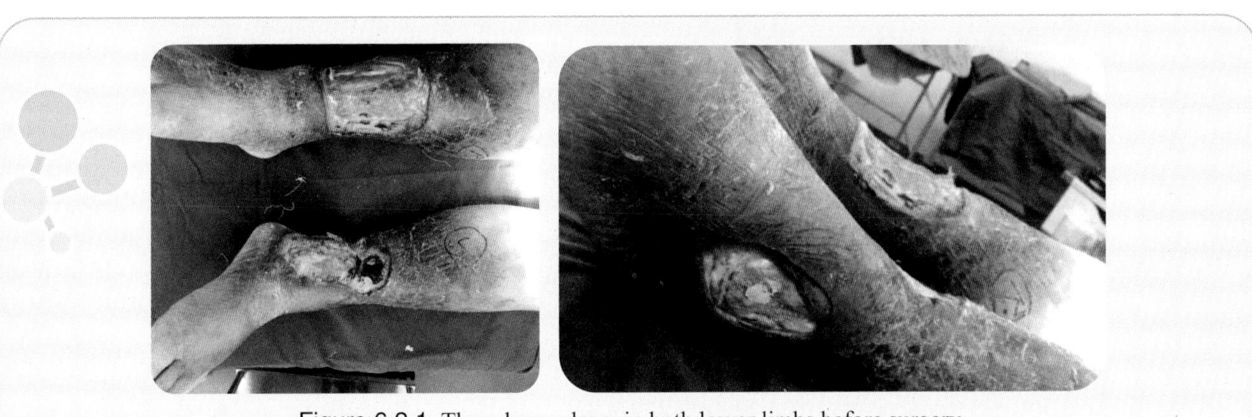

Figure 6.2.1 Three huge ulcers in both lower limbs before surgery

◆ 治疗方案

下肢复杂性溃疡，创面大而深，深达骨质，合并多重细菌感染，下肢静脉瓣膜功能不全，大隐静脉曲张伴穿通支反流。

1. 基础治疗，抬高患肢、压力治疗、中医治疗、抗生素应用。

2. 分期手术

2.1 一期：创面清创+VSD。测量坏死创面，双侧足靴区大创面深达右侧胫骨、左内踝和左外踝，彻底清创，切除坏死组织，VSD 治疗（图 6.2.2 ～图 6.2.4）。

2.2 二期：双下肢静脉造影 + 大隐静脉微波消融术 + 弹力绷带压力治疗。VSD 术后 2 周，肉芽组织生长，创面水肿，用银离子敷料 + 生长因子喷涂，加压包扎（图 6.2.5）。

2.3 三期：创面修复。创面床准备，创面深大，加强营养。3 次 VSD 后，创面肉芽组织新鲜，行邮票状皮肤移植术，外敷生长因子软纱，加压包扎（图 6.2.6）。

3. 创面移植皮成活，生长因子 + 银离子敷料换药，创面愈合（图 6.2.7、图 6.2.8）。

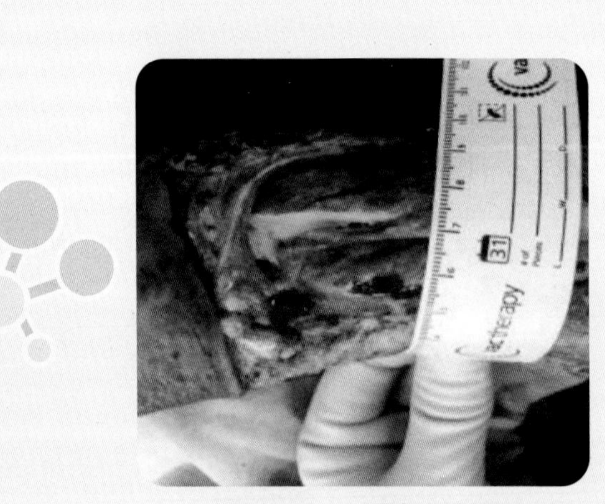

图 6.2.2　测量坏死创面

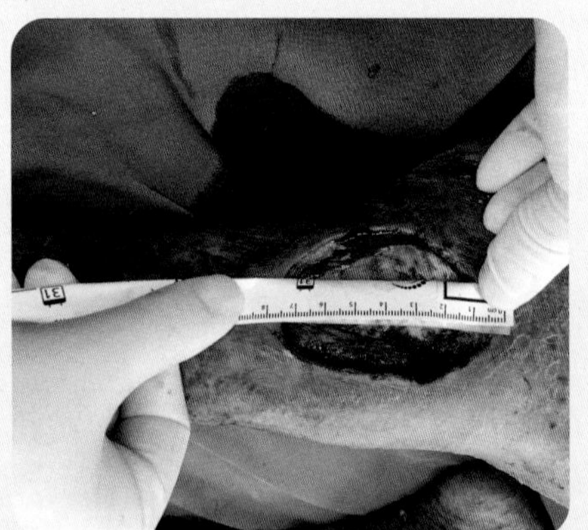

图 6.2.3　清创中，双侧足靴区大创面深达右侧胫骨、左内踝和左外踝，彻底清创，切除坏死组织

◆ Treatment plan

Complex ulcers in the lower limbs, with large and deep wounds reaching deep into the bone, combined with multiple bacterial infections, lower limb venous valve dysfunction, and large saphenous vein varicose veins with perforating branch reflux.

1. Basic treatment includes raising the affected limb, pressure therapy, traditional Chinese medicine treatment, and the use of antibiotics.

2. Staged surgery

2.1 Phase 1: Wound debridement + VSD. Measure necrotic wounds, with large wounds in the bilateral boot area reaching deep into the right tibia, left medial malleolus, and left lateral malleolus. Thoroughly clean the wound, remove necrotic tissue, and treat with VSD (Figure 6.2.2-Figure 6.2.4).

2.2 Phase II: Venography of both lower limbs + microwave ablation of the great saphenous vein + pressure therapy with elastic bandages. Two weeks after VSD surgery, granulation tissue grew and the wound became edematous. Silver ion dressings and growth factors were sprayed and pressure bandaged (Figure 6.2.5).

2.3 Phase III: Wound Repair. Preparation of wound bed, deep wound, and enhanced nutrition. After 3 VSDs, fresh granulation tissue was obtained from the wound, and a stamp like skin transplant was performed with external application of growth factor soft gauze and pressure bandaging (Figure 6.2.6).

3. The wound graft skin survived, growth factor + silver ion dressing was changed, and the wound healed (Figure 6.2.7, Figure 6.2.8).

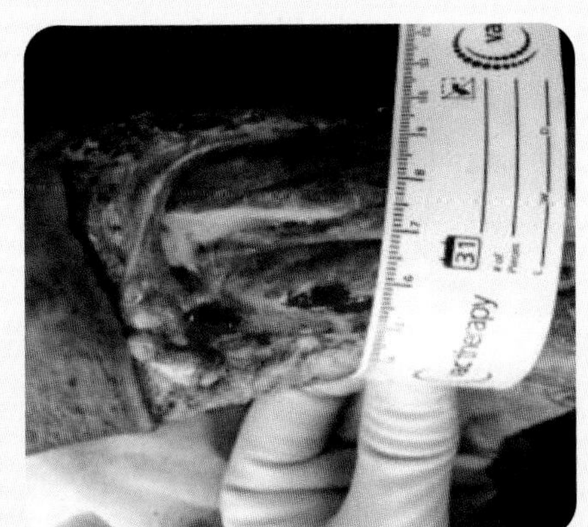

Figure 6.2.2 Measurement of necrotic wounds

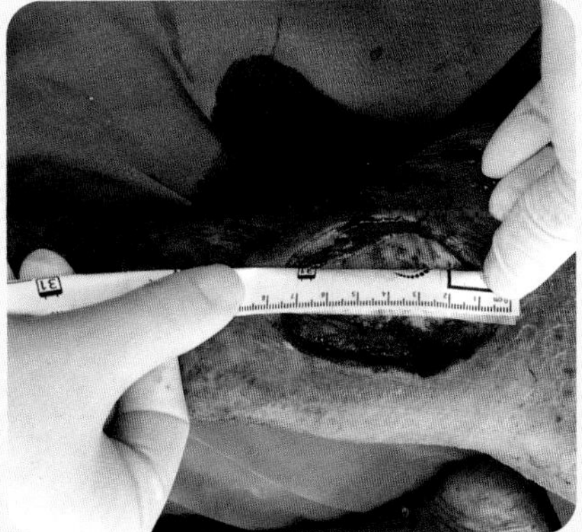

Figure 6.2.3 During debridement, the large wounds in the bilateral boot area extend deep to the right tibia, left medial malleolus, and left lateral malleolus. Thoroughly debridement is performed, and necrotic tissue is removed

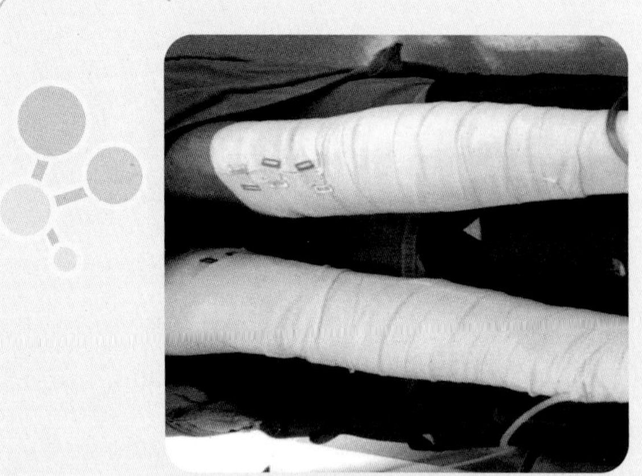
图 6.2.4　VSD

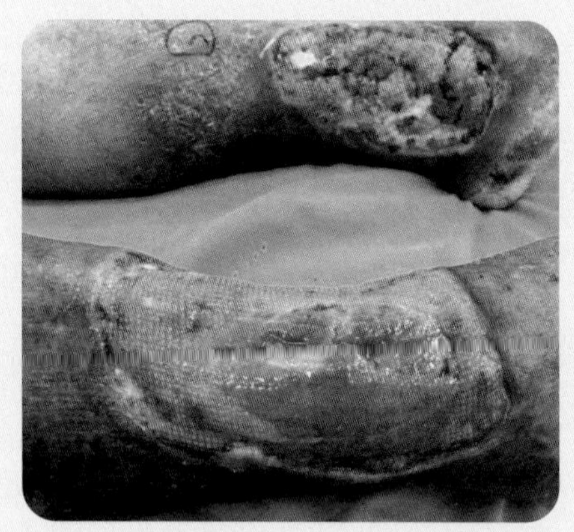
图 6.2.5　VSD 后 2 周，肉芽组织生长，创面水肿

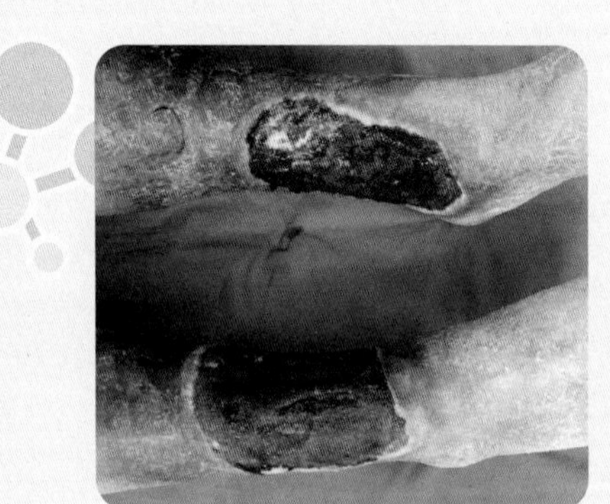
图 6.2.6　3 次 VSD 后，创面肉芽组织新鲜

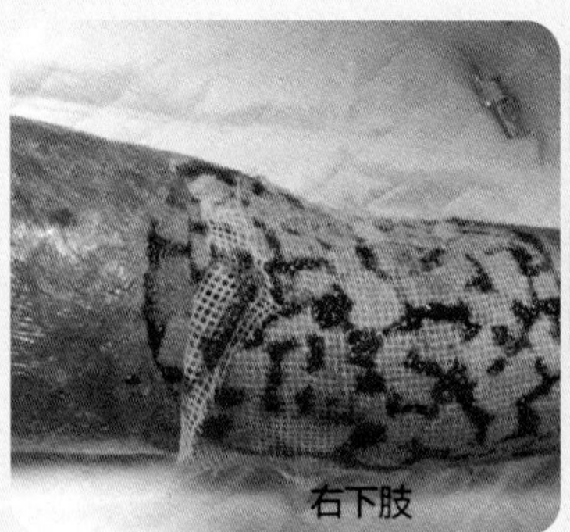

左下肢

图 6.2.7　移植皮成活，生长因子 + 银离子敷料换药

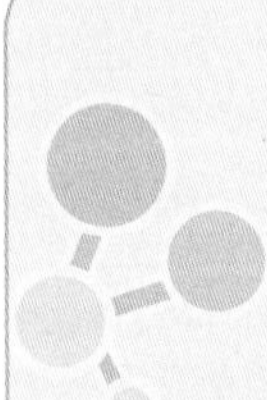

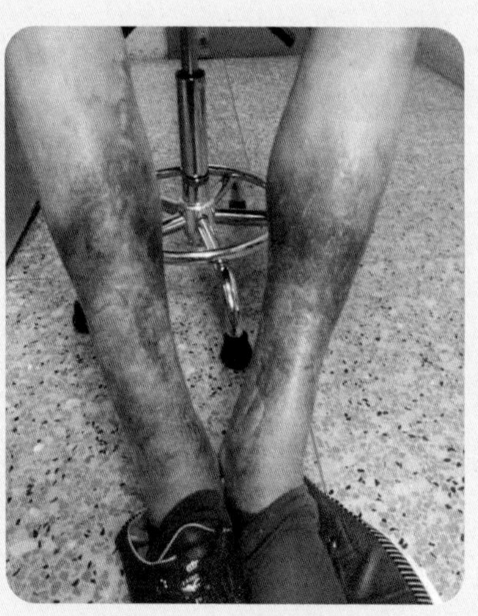
图 6.2.8　创面愈合

（王永高）

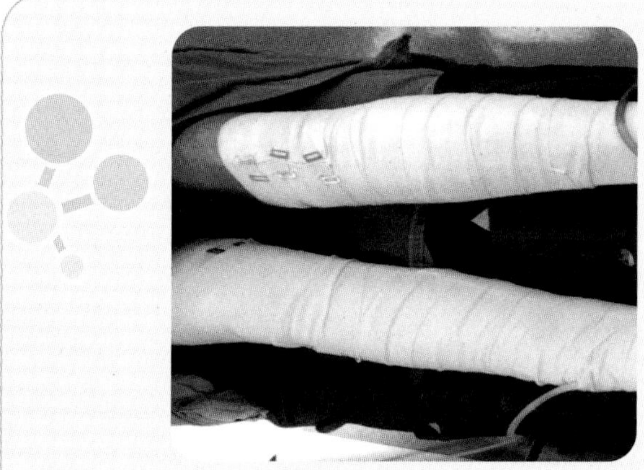

Figure 6.2.4 VSD

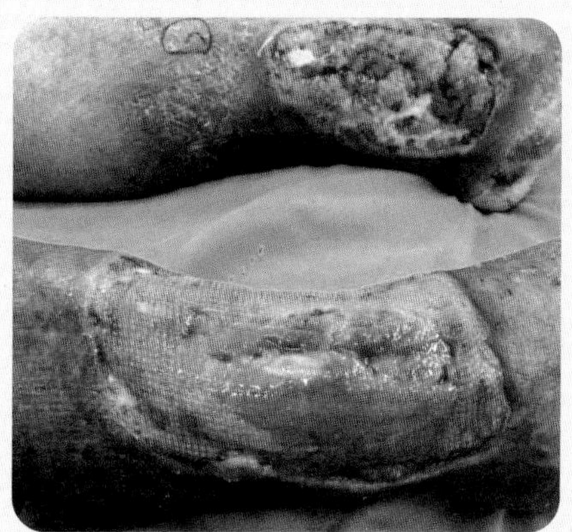

Figure 6.2.5 Two weeks after VSD, granulation tissue grows and the wound becomes edematous

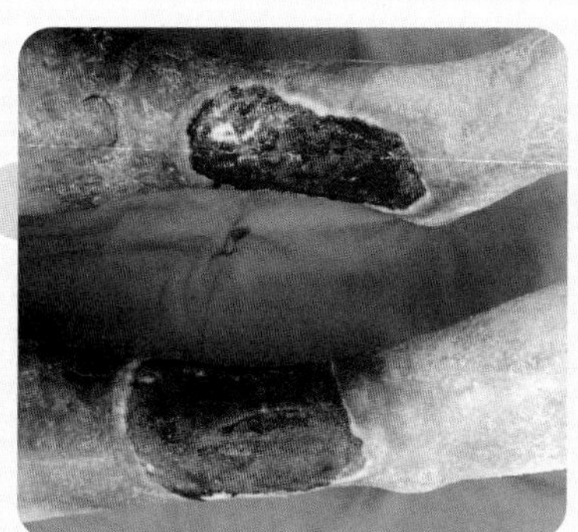

Figure 6.2.6 Fresh granulation tissue from the wound after 3 VSDs

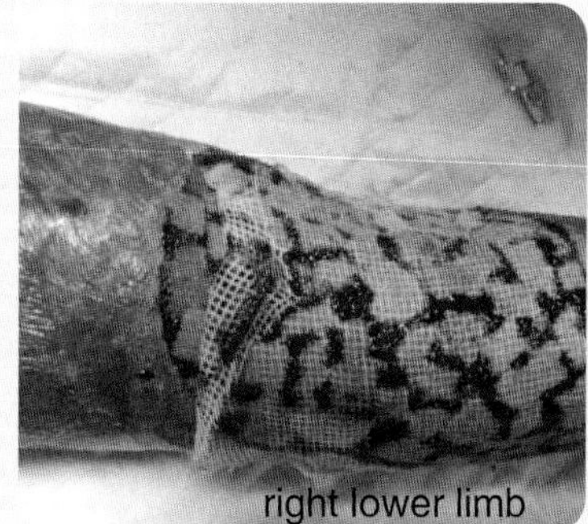

Figure 6.2.7 Survival of transplanted skin, growth factor + silver ion dressing change

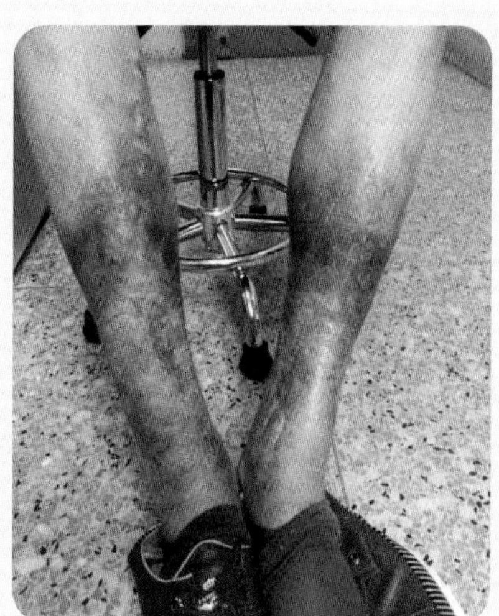

Figure 6.2.8 Wound healing

(Wang Yonggao)

案例三　双下肢多发溃疡、左髂静脉压迫综合征

◆ 致病原因

患者，88 岁，双下肢瘙痒、溃烂不愈 50 余年，诊断为双下肢多发溃疡、左髂静脉压迫综合征。

◆ 症状与体征

双小腿巨大创面，左小腿创面 20 cm × 15 cm × 1 cm，左足背创面 5 cm × 5 cm × 1 cm，右小腿创面 15 cm × 10 cm × 1 cm，创面大量脓苔，渗液多，周围皮肤色素沉着，覆盖中草药残渣，左下肢外侧创面见骨异常增生（图 6.3.1）。

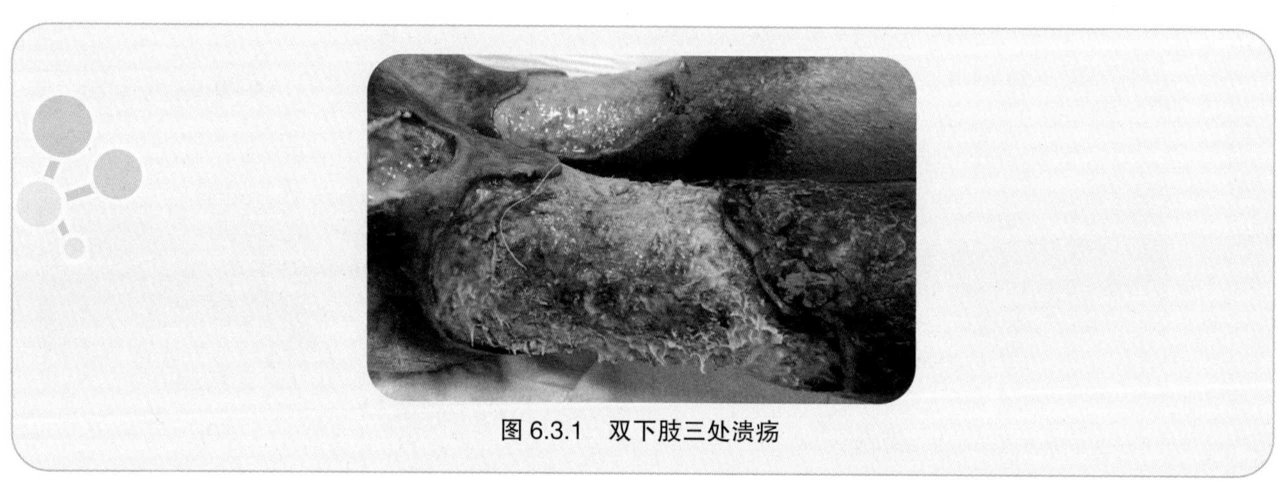

图 6.3.1　双下肢三处溃疡

◆ 治疗方案

1. 患者 88 岁，合并有高血压、陈旧性脑梗死、双下肢深静脉瓣膜功能不全及左髂静脉狭窄。

2. 清除坏死组织、增生骨组织，脓液细菌培养，坏死组织送病理。经过锐性清创、换药，湿性感染创面已逐渐收敛，达到干湿平衡，并施行 VSD、左小腿骨水泥覆盖、抗感染（图 6.3.2、图 6.3.3）。

3. 中西医 MDT 讨论，中医治拟清热解毒、活血通络。

4. 针对病因，行左下肢静脉造影 + 球囊扩张术，改善静脉回流。

5. 创面床准备，创面清创 + 载药骨水泥填充术 +VSD，术后创面定期换药（图 6.3.4）。

6. 术后 3 周，拆除骨水泥，创面基底新鲜肉芽组织生长，邮票状皮肤移植，敷生长因子的纱布垫，绷带加压包扎（图 6.3.5）。

7. 植皮后 10 天，双下肢创面基本成活（图 6.3.6）。

Case 3 Multiple ulcers in both lower limbs and left iliac vein compression syndrome

◆ Cause of illness

The patient is 88 years old, with itching and ulcers in both lower limbs that have not healed for more than 50 years. The diagnosis is multiple ulcers in both lower limbs and left iliac vein compression syndrome.

◆ Signs and symptoms

There are huge wounds on both lower legs, with wounds on the left leg measuring 20 cm × 15 cm × 1 cm, on the left foot back measuring 5 cm × 5 cm × 1 cm, and on the right leg measuring 15 cm × 10 cm × 1 cm. The wounds are covered with a large amount of pus and exudate, and the surrounding skin is pigmented and covered with residues of Chinese herbal medicine. Abnormal bone hyperplasia is observed on the outer side of the left lower limb (Figure 6.3.1).

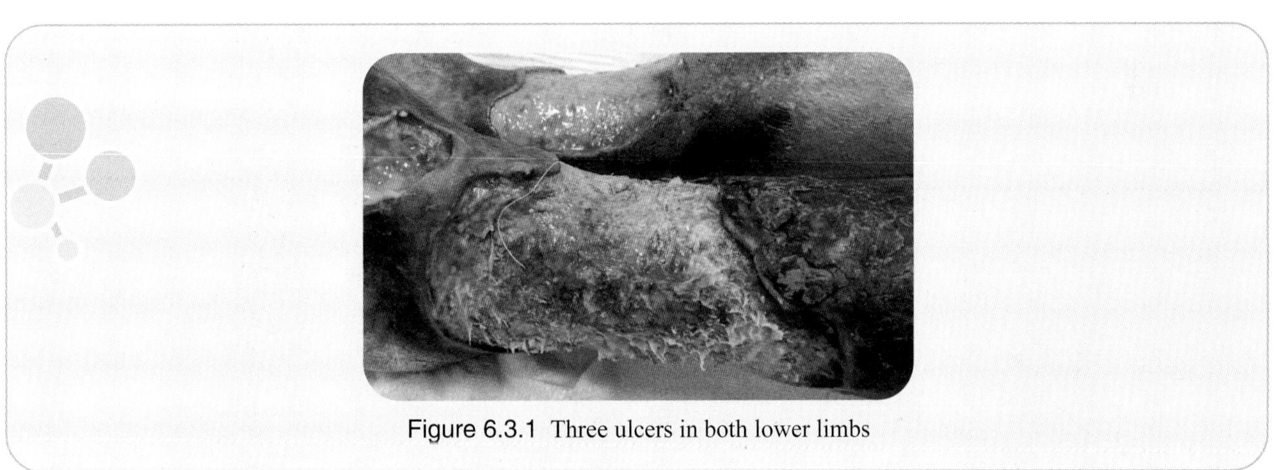

Figure 6.3.1 Three ulcers in both lower limbs

◆ Treatment plan

1. The patient is 88 years old and has comorbidities such as hypertension, old cerebral infarction, deep vein valve insufficiency in both lower limbs, and left iliac vein stenosis.

2. Remove necrotic tissue and hypertrophic bone tissue, culture pus bacteria, and send necrotic tissue for pathology. After sharp debridement and dressing change, the wet infected wound has gradually converged and reached dry wet balance, and VSD, left calf bone cement coverage, and anti-infection measures have been implemented (Figure 6.3.2, Figure 6.3.3).

3. MDT discussion on traditional Chinese and Western medicine, with the aim of clearing heat and detoxifying, promoting blood circulation, and unblocking meridians.

4. Based on the cause, perform left lower limb venography and balloon dilation to improve venous return.

5. Preparation of wound bed, wound debridement + drug loaded bone cement filling + VSD, and regular wound dressing changes after surgery (Figure 6.3.4).

6. Three weeks after surgery, the bone cement was removed, fresh granulation tissue was grown at the base of the wound, stamp shaped skin was transplanted, a gauze pad with growth factors was applied, and the bandage was compressed and wrapped (Figure 6.3.5).

7. 10 days after skin grafting, the wounds on both lower limbs were basically alive (Figure 6.3.6).

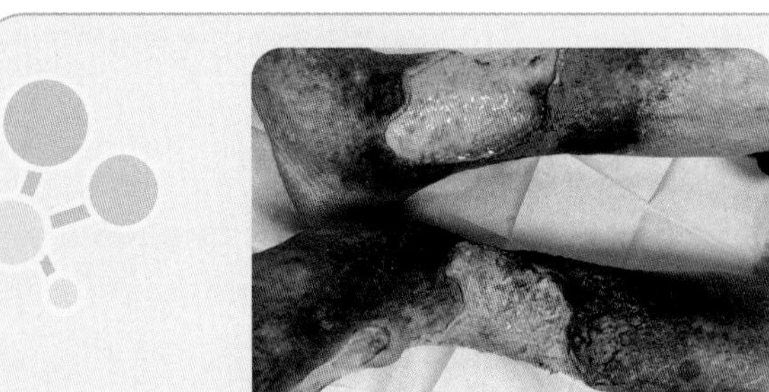

图 6.3.2　清除坏死组织、增生骨组织

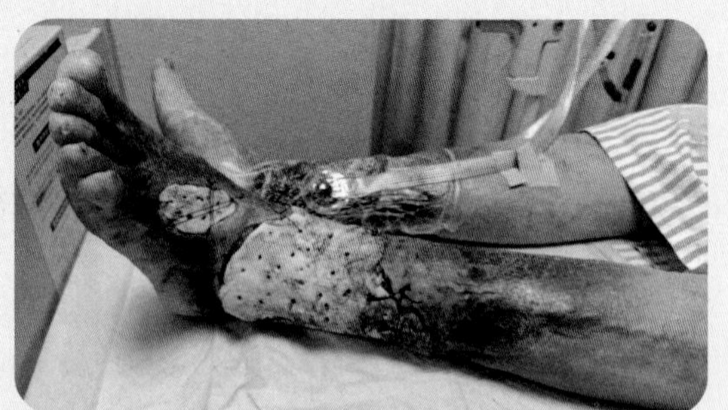

图 6.3.3　清创后右小腿 VSD、左小腿骨水泥覆盖

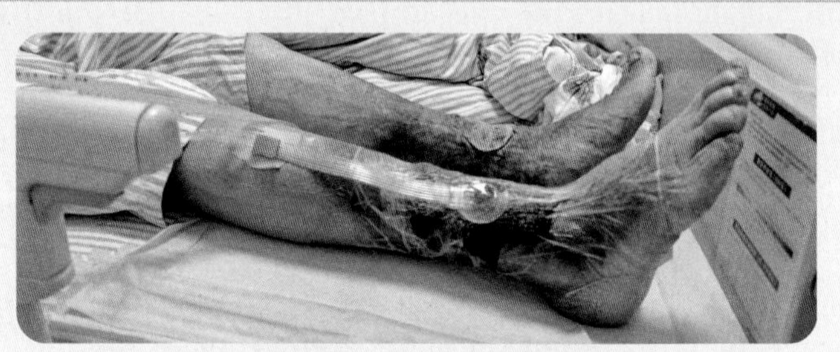

图 6.3.4　创面清创 + 载药骨水泥填充术 +VSD

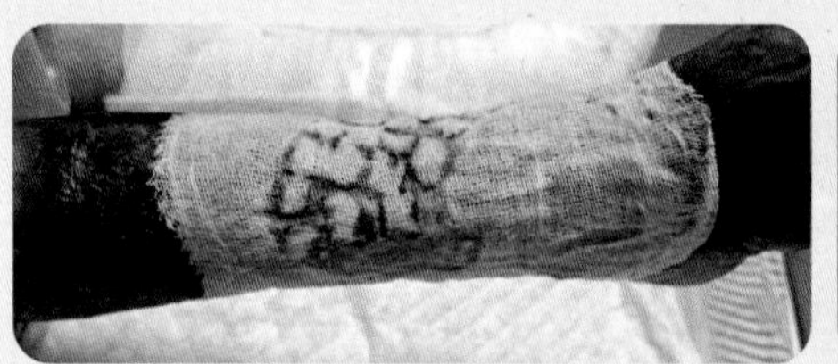

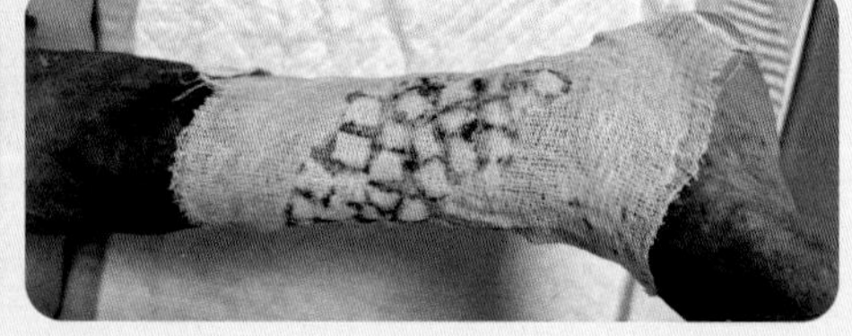

图 6.3.5　邮票状植皮

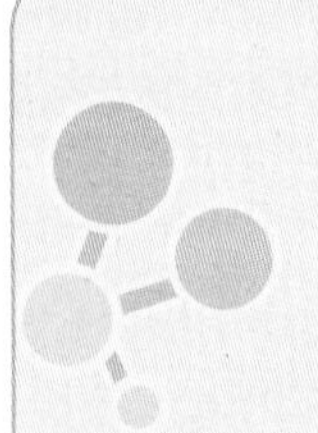

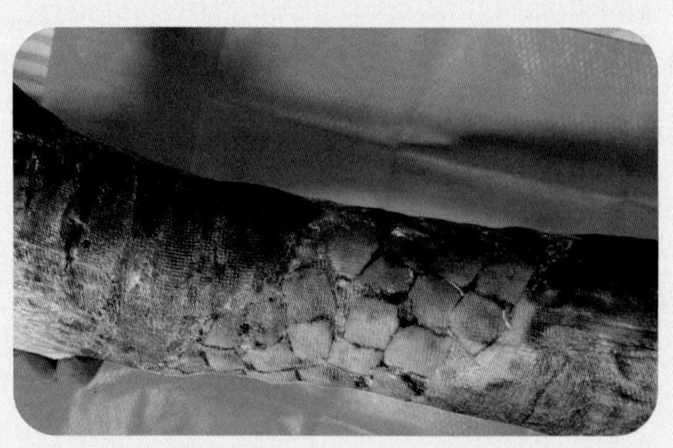

图 6.3.6　植皮后 10 天，双下肢创面基本成活

（王永高　王城磊）

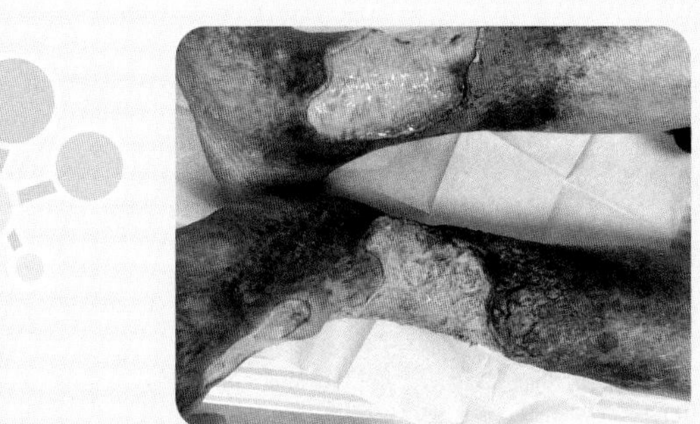

Figure 6.3.2 Removal of necrotic tissue and hypertrophic bone tissue

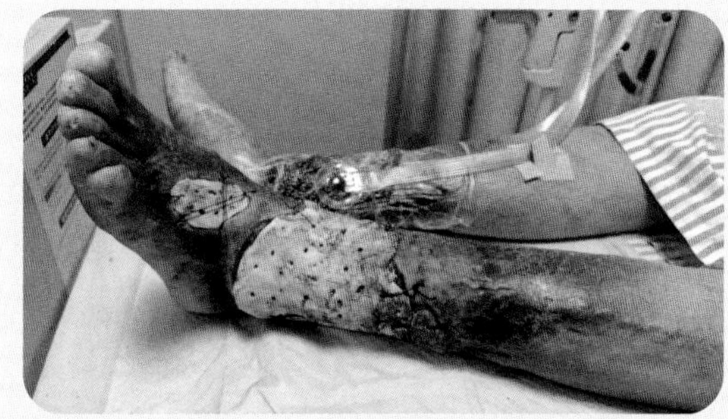

Figure 6.3.3 VSD in the right calf and cement coverage in the left calf after debridement

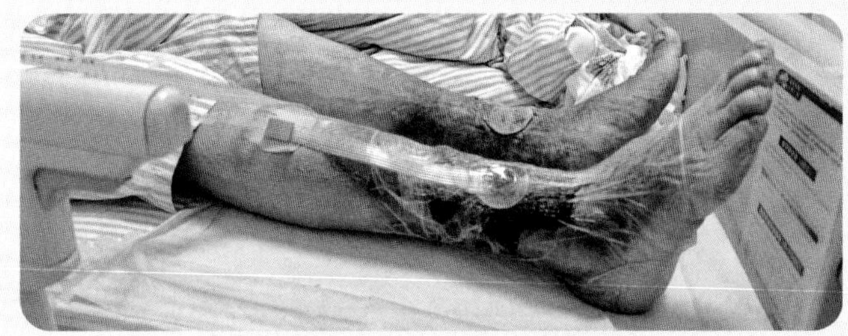

Figure 6.3.4 Wound debridement + drug loaded bone cement filling + VSD

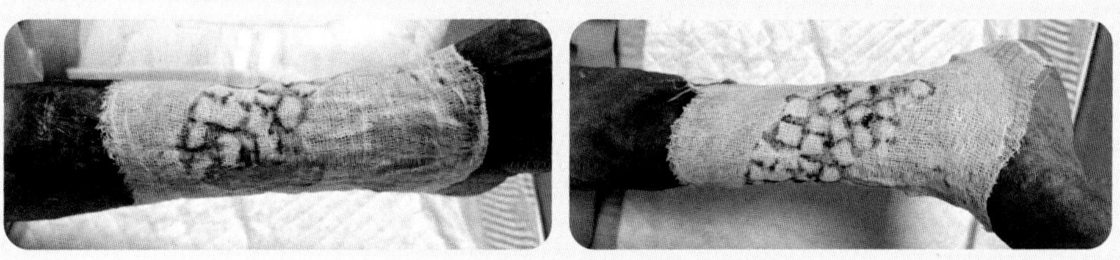

Figure 6.3.5 Stamp like skin graft

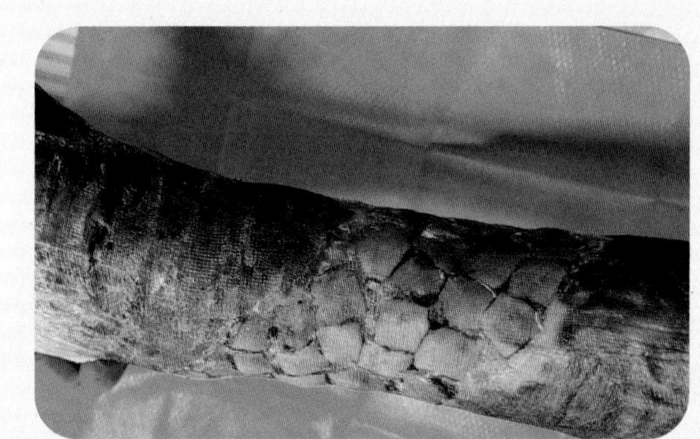

Figure 6.3.6 After 10 days of skin grafting, the wounds on both lower limbs have basically survived

(Wang Yonggao, Wang Chenglei)

案例四　左下肢内踝静脉性溃疡

◆ 致病原因

患者于 1 个月前出现下肢溃疡，自行使用溃疡散撒于创面，未到医院就诊。

◆ 症状与体征

左下肢内踝上方有一约 10.5 cm × 5.7 cm × 0.2 cm 溃疡，创面 75% 黄色组织，创面周围皮肤发黑，足背动脉搏动好，渗液大量，有异味，肢端温暖，数字疼痛量表评分，清创时疼痛评分 4 分（图 6.4.1）。

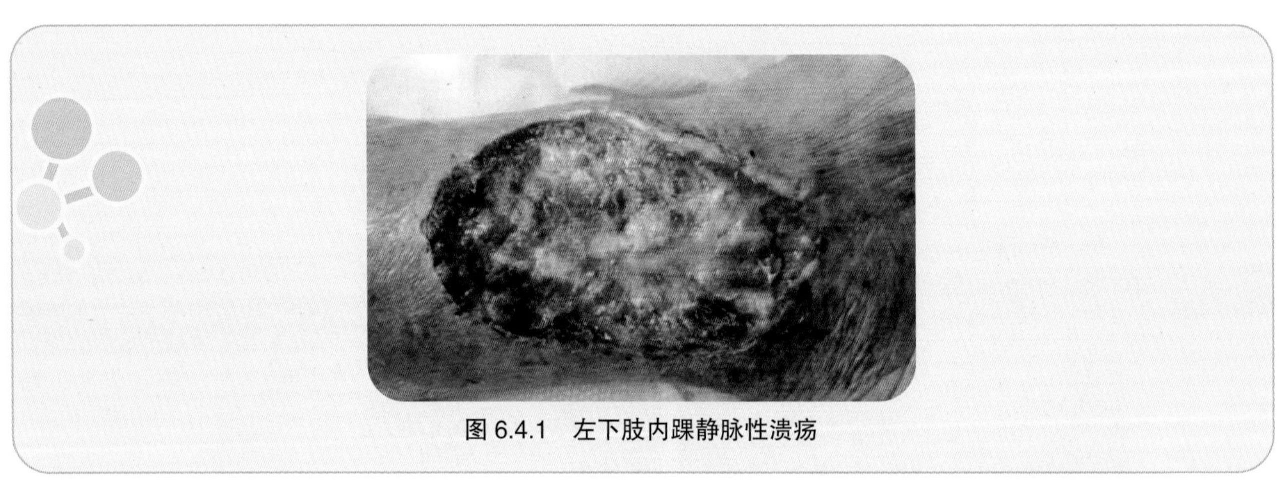

图 6.4.1　左下肢内踝静脉性溃疡

◆ 治疗方案

1. 伤口床准备（TIME 原则）、新型敷料选择、压力治疗、健康教育。

2. 压力治疗是治疗下肢静脉性溃疡最有效的方法。静脉溃疡所需的压力标准为 40 mmHg（5.3 kPa）。

3. 碘伏消毒创面及周围皮肤，0.9% 氯化钠注射液冲洗，用清创胶自溶清创，纤维银抗感染。自溶清创后伤口大小 7 cm × 4 cm × 0.2 cm，创面 50% 黄色组织，创面培养结果为大肠埃希菌。口服消炎药。创面予纤维银 + 纱布 + 弹力绷带包扎，隔日换药（图 6.4.2）。卧床休息时抬高左下肢，高于心脏水平，2 ~ 3 天换药一次。感染控制后，伤口大小 5 cm × 1.8 cm × 0.1 cm，创面 100% 红色组织，后使用生长因子促进上皮细胞爬行，泡沫敷料吸收渗液，弹力绷带包扎，创面基本愈合（图 6.4.3、图 6.4.4）。

4. 由于下肢静脉性溃疡伤口一般持续时间长，且易复发，易导致患者精神压力较大，应做好患者心理护理。

Case 4 Left lower limb internal ankle venous ulcer

◆ Cause of illness

The patient developed lower limb ulcers one month ago and self applied ulcer powder to the wound without seeking medical attention.

◆ Signs and symptoms

There is an ulcer measuring approximately 10.5 cm × 5.7 cm × 0.2 cm above the medial malleolus of the left lower limb. 75% of the wound is yellow tissue, and the skin around the wound is blackened. The dorsalis pedis artery has good pulsation, a large amount of exudate, and an unpleasant odor. The limb is warm and scored on the Digital Pain Scale, with a pain score of 4 points during debridement (Figure 6.4.1).

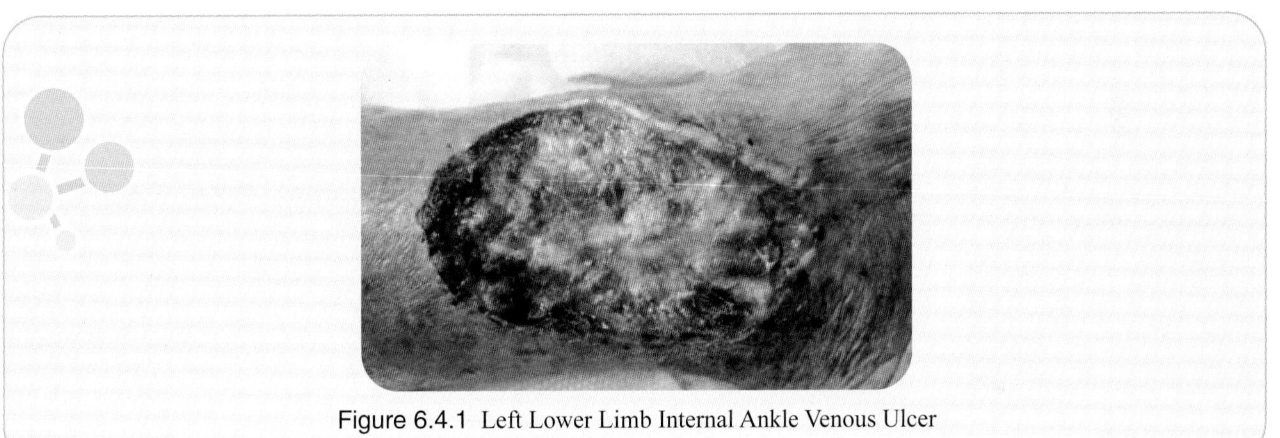

Figure 6.4.1 Left Lower Limb Internal Ankle Venous Ulcer

◆ Treatment plan

1. Wound bed preparation (TIME principle), selection of new dressings, pressure therapy, and health education.

2. Pressure therapy is the most effective method for treating lower limb venous ulcers. The pressure standard required for venous ulcers is 40 mmHg (5.3 kPa).

3. Disinfect the wound and surrounding skin with iodine, rinse with 0.9% sodium chloride injection, self dissolve with debridement gel, and use fiber silver to resist infection. After autolysis debridement, the wound size was 7 cm × 4 cm × 0.2 cm, with 50% yellow tissue on the wound. The wound culture result showed Escherichia coli. Oral anti-inflammatory drugs. The wound was wrapped with fibrous silver, gauze, and elastic bandage, and the dressing was changed every other day (Figure 6.4.2). Raise the left lower limb above the level of the heart during bed rest, and change dressing every 2-3 days. After the infection was controlled, the size of the wound was 5 cm × 1.8 cm × 0.1 cm, and the wound was 100% red tissue. After that, growth factors were used to promote the epithelial cells to crawl, foam dressings absorbed the exudate, and elastic bandages were used to bind the wound, and the wound was basically healed (Figure 6.4.3, Figure 6.4.4).

4. Due to the long duration and easy recurrence of lower limb venous ulcer wounds, patients are prone to significant mental stress and should receive proper psychological care.

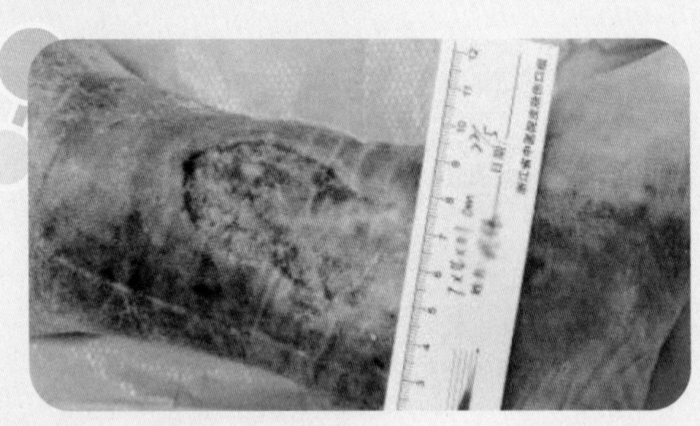

图 6.4.2　自溶清创后伤口大小 7 cm × 4 cm × 0.2 cm，创面 50% 黄色组织

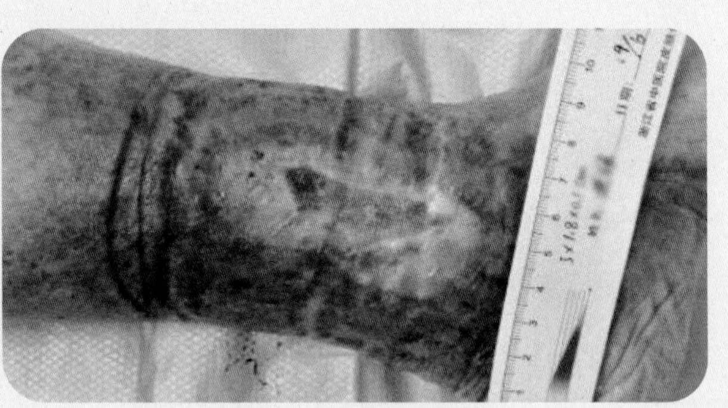

图 6.4.3　感染控制后，伤口大小 5 cm × 1.8 cm × 0.1 cm，创面 100% 红色组织

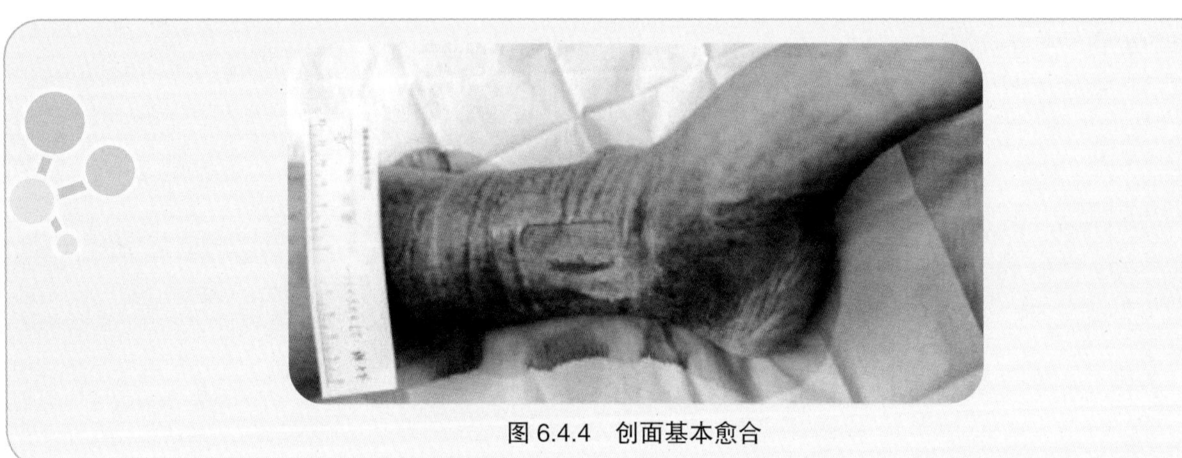

图 6.4.4　创面基本愈合

（沈晓娣　王永高）

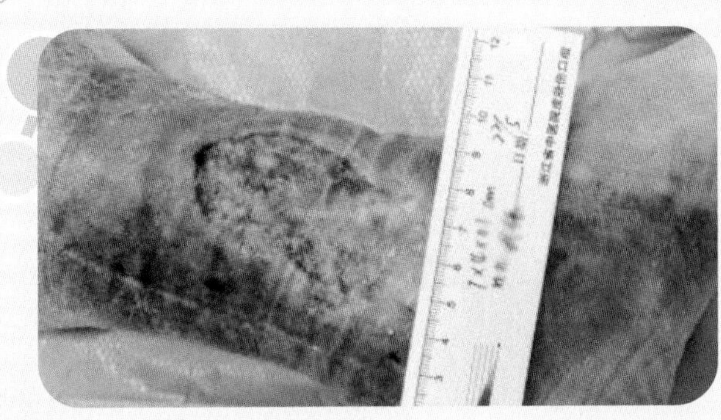

Figure 6.4.2 After autolysis debridement, the wound size is 7 cm × 4 cm × 0.2 cm, with 50% yellow tissue on the wound surface

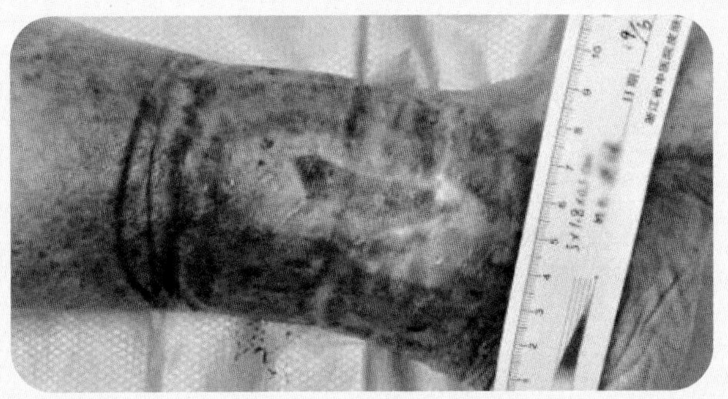

Figure 6.4.3 After infection control, the wound size is 5 cm × 1.8 cm × 0.1cm, with 100% red tissue on the wound surface

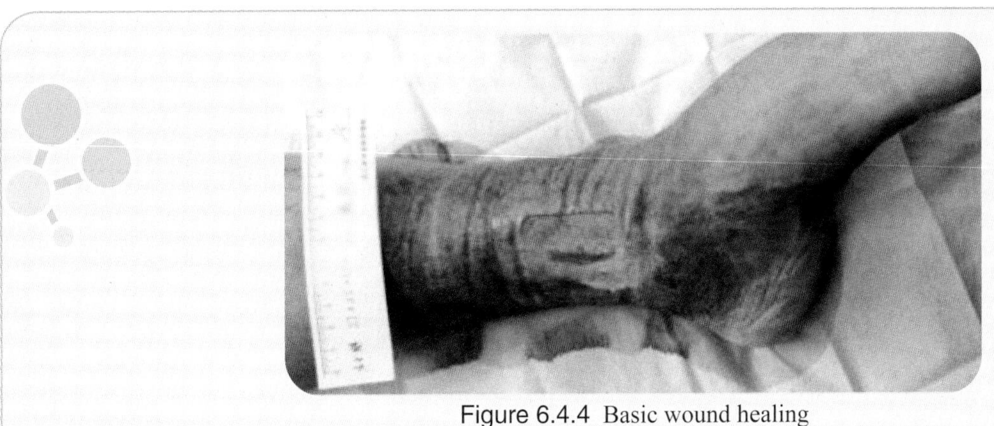

Figure 6.4.4 Basic wound healing

(Shen Xiaodi, Wang Yonggao)

第 7 章
Chapter 7

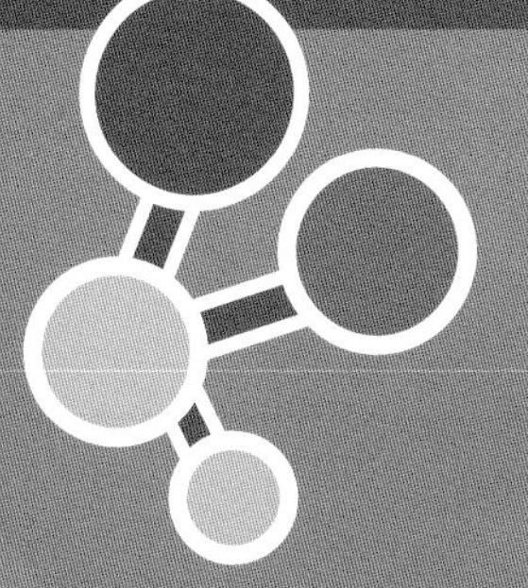

糖尿病性溃疡创面修复
Repair of Diabetes Ulcer Wounds

案例一　2 型糖尿病合并坏死性筋膜炎

◆ 致病原因

患者既往糖尿病病史 13 年，长期口服二甲双胍。3 天前买了一双新鞋，由于鞋子小而磨破了左足踇趾，压破了足背皮肤。

◆ 症状与体征

左足穿鞋小磨破后，左足胀痛 3 天，不能下地负重行走，肿胀疼痛并逐渐加重，寒战，乏力，心悸气短。左足广泛性肿胀，左足弥漫性红肿，局部温度高，广泛性压痛，足底和足背波动，以前足底部波动为主，前足底部可见白色脓性包块，局部波动明显（图 7.1.1、图 7.1.2）。足趾活动受限，左小腿凹陷性水肿，局部温度高，髂腹股沟淋巴结肿大，压痛明显。

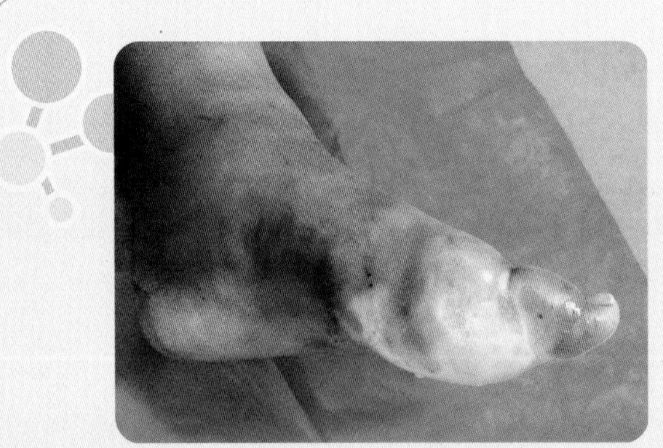
图 7.1.1　左足弥漫性肿胀

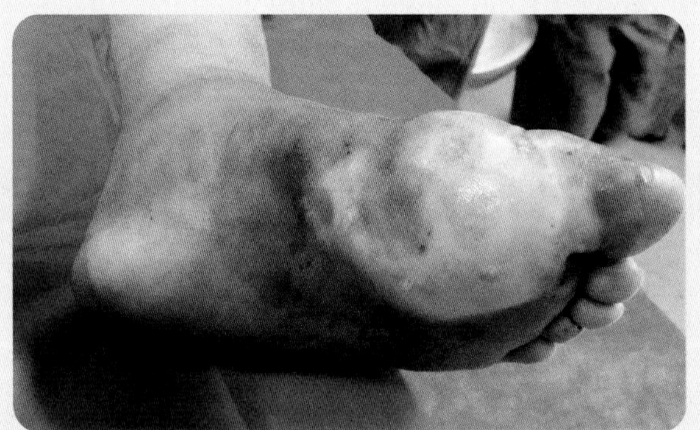
图 7.1.2　前足底可见白色脓性包块

◆ 治疗方案

1. 急诊入院后血液细菌培养，足部脓液细菌培养 + 药物敏感试验，根据细菌培养选用敏感抗菌药物，控制感染。

2. 积极治疗原发病，严格控制血糖，输新鲜红细胞悬液和冰冻血浆纠正贫血，输白蛋白纠正低蛋白血症。

3. 严格观察生命体征，预防因感染引发多器官功能衰竭，纠正低血容量休克和感染性休克。

4. 急诊行切开引流、扩大切开蜂窝组织感染病灶，切除坏死皮肤及坏死筋膜，充分扩大创腔开放引流，避免残留无效腔，创腔双氧水反复浸泡生理盐水冲洗，碘伏浸泡生理盐水冲洗，创腔填塞无菌纱布引流，

Case 1 Type 2 diabetes with necrotizing fasciitis

◆ Cause of illness

The patient had a history of diabetes for 13 years and took metformin orally for a long time. I bought a new pair of shoes 3 days ago, but due to their small size, I wore out my left toe and crushed the skin on the back of my foot.

◆ Signs and symptoms

After wearing shoes on the left foot, there was slight abrasion and pain, which lasted for 3 days. The left foot was unable to walk with heavy loads on the ground, and the swelling and pain gradually worsened. There were chills, fatigue, palpitations, and shortness of breath. Widespread swelling of the left foot, diffuse redness and swelling of the left foot, high local temperature, widespread tenderness, fluctuation of the sole and dorsum of the foot, mainly in the forefoot area, with white purulent masses visible at the bottom of the forefoot, and significant local fluctuations (Figure 7.1.1, Figure 7.1.2). Restricted toe movement, depressed edema in the left lower leg, high local temperature, swollen iliac and inguinal lymph nodes, and obvious tenderness.

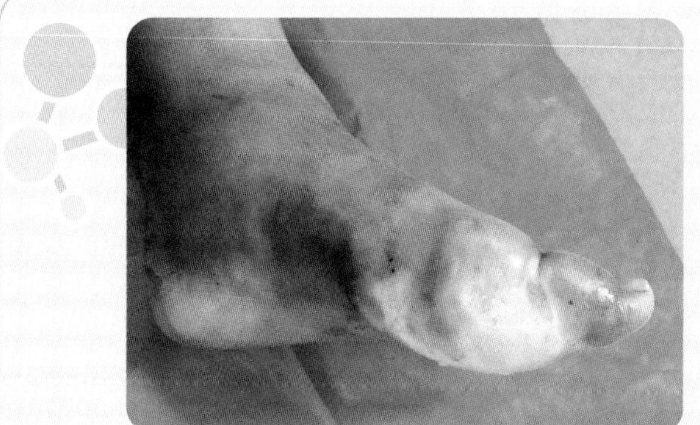

Figure 7.1.1 Diffuse swelling of left foot

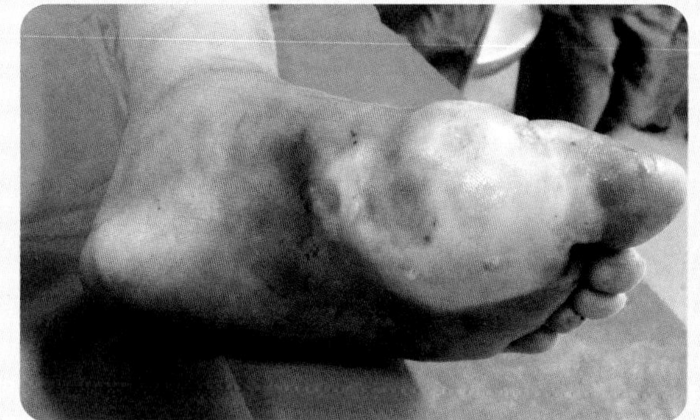

Figure 7.1.2 White purulent mass visible on the forefoot

◆ Treatment plan

1. After emergency admission, blood bacterial culture, foot pus bacterial culture+drug sensitivity test are conducted to select sensitive antibiotics based on bacterial culture and control infection.

2. Actively treat the primary disease, strictly control blood sugar, administer fresh red blood cell suspension and frozen plasma to correct anemia, and administer albumin to correct hypoalbuminemia.

3. Strictly observe vital signs, prevent multiple organ failure caused by infection, correct hypovolemic shock and septic shock.

4. In the emergency department, open and drain the wound, expand the incision of honeycomb tissue infection lesions, remove necrotic skin and fascia, fully expand the wound cavity for open drainage, avoid residual ineffective cavities, repeatedly soak the wound cavity in hydrogen peroxide and physiological saline for flushing, soak iodine in physiological saline for flushing, fill the wound cavity with sterile gauze for drainage, and wrap it with thick cotton pads. Due to the large amount of inflammatory exudate from the foot wound, reduce toxin reabsorption, and change the dressing three times a day (Figure 7.1.3-Figure 7.1.5).

厚棉垫包扎，由于足部创面有大量炎性渗出，减少毒素回吸收，每天 3 次更换敷料（图 7.1.3 ～图 7.1.5）。

5. 经过 5 天综合治疗，各项生化指标趋于恢复正常，足部创面渗出逐渐减少，每天换药时清创并剪除足部坏死皮肤，足部创面增大，几乎足背皮肤完全坏死，裸露大面积创面，创面肉芽组织水肿不新鲜，为了减少换药次数，促进创面新鲜和肉芽组织饱满，故采用 VSD+ 重组人碱性成纤维细胞生长因子滴注等综合治疗。负压治疗 7 天，拆除负压装置，足部创面新鲜，肉芽组织红润渗血活跃。于腰硬联合麻醉下行中厚游离皮肤移植，创面喷洒重组人碱性成纤维细胞生长因子，将游离皮肤移植于足部受区，皮肤边缘缝合，皮肤切开数个空洞，防止皮下渗出将皮肤浮起，油纱覆盖创面，加压包扎（图 7.1.6 ～图 7.1.10）。

6. 术后常规预防感染，积极预防全身并发症，治疗原发病。

7. 抬高患肢，局部理疗，预防深静脉血栓等综合治疗。

8. 术后 12 天拆线，皮肤完全成活，康复出院（图 7.1.11 ～图 7.1.13）。

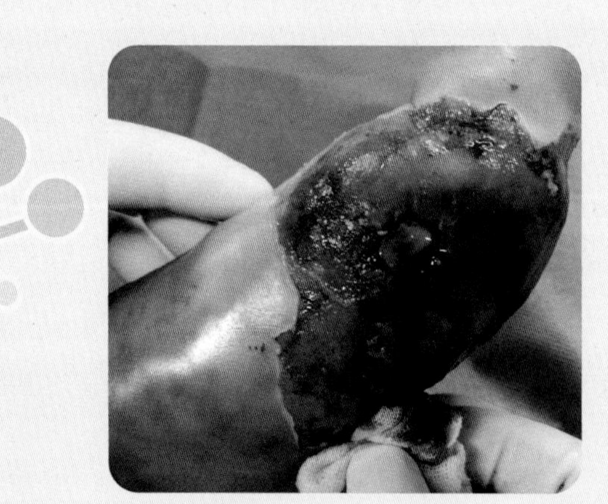

图 7.1.3　去除疱皮，可见皮肤破溃口，有稀薄白色脓液流出

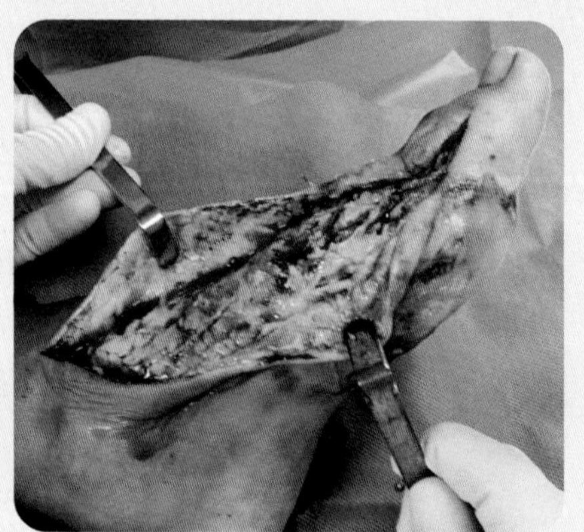

图 7.1.4　切开皮肤及皮下组织散在蜂窝样改变

5. After 5 days of comprehensive treatment, various biochemical indicators tended to return to normal, and the exudation of the foot wound gradually decreased. When changing dressing every day, the wound was cleared and the necrotic skin on the foot was removed. The foot wound increased in size, and almost the skin on the back of the foot was completely necrotic, exposing a large area of the wound. The granulation tissue of the wound was swollen and not fresh. In order to reduce the number of dressing changes, promote wound freshness and granulation tissue fullness, comprehensive treatment such as VSD+recombinant human alkaline fibroblast growth factor infusion was used. After 7 days of negative pressure treatment, the negative pressure device was removed, and the foot wound was fresh, with red granulation tissue and active bleeding. Under combined spinal and epidural anesthesia, medium thick free skin transplantation was performed. Recombinant human basic fibroblast growth factor was sprayed onto the wound surface, and the free skin was transplanted into the foot receiving area. The skin edges were sutured, and several holes were cut in the skin to prevent subcutaneous exudate from floating the skin. The wound was covered with oil gauze and pressure bandaged (Figure 7.1.6 - Figure 7.1.10).

6. Routine postoperative infection prevention, active prevention of systemic complications, and treatment of primary diseases.

7. Comprehensive treatment including raising the affected limb, local physical therapy, and prevention of deep vein thrombosis.

8. The stitches were removed 12 days after surgery, and the skin completely survived. The patient recovered and was discharged from the hospital (Figure 7.1.11 - Figure 7.1.13).

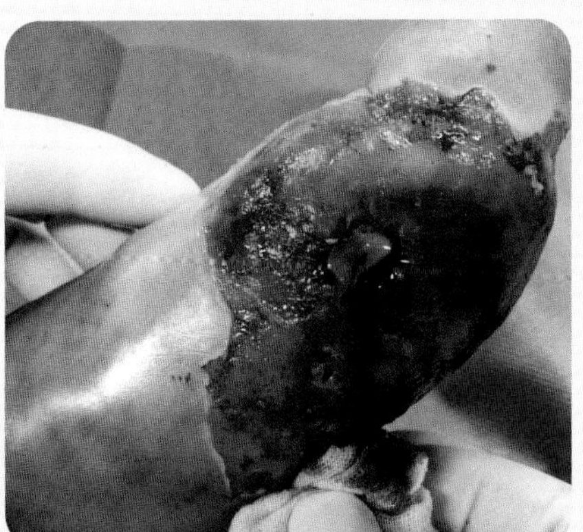

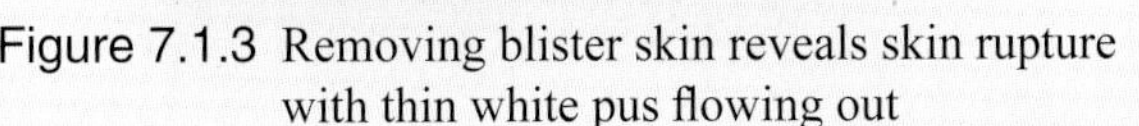

Figure 7.1.3 Removing blister skin reveals skin rupture with thin white pus flowing out

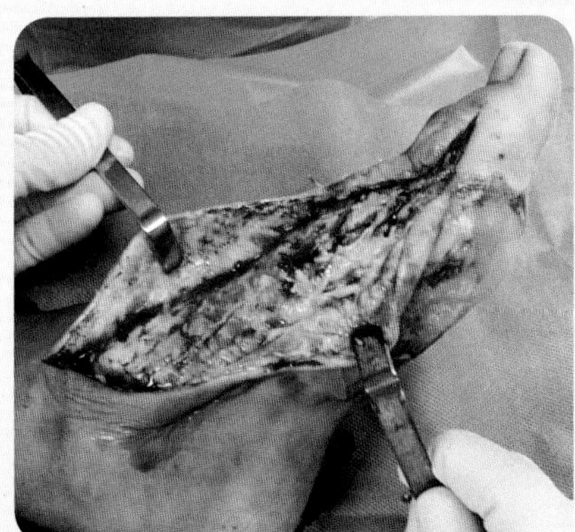

Figure 7.1.4 Scattered honeycomb like changes in skin and subcutaneous tissue after incision

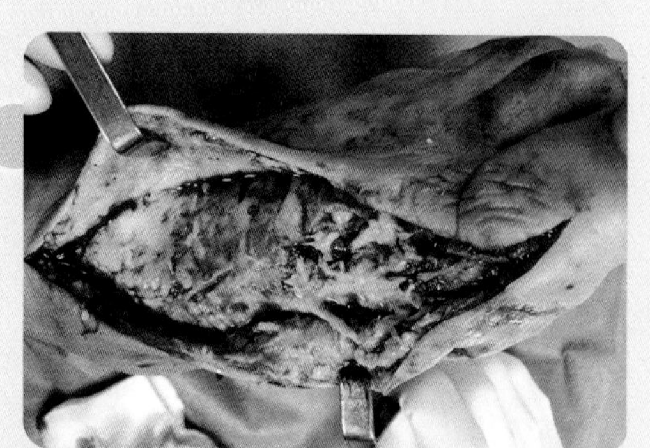

图 7.1.5　皮下广泛性水肿，蜂窝组织样改变，分隔中有大量脓液

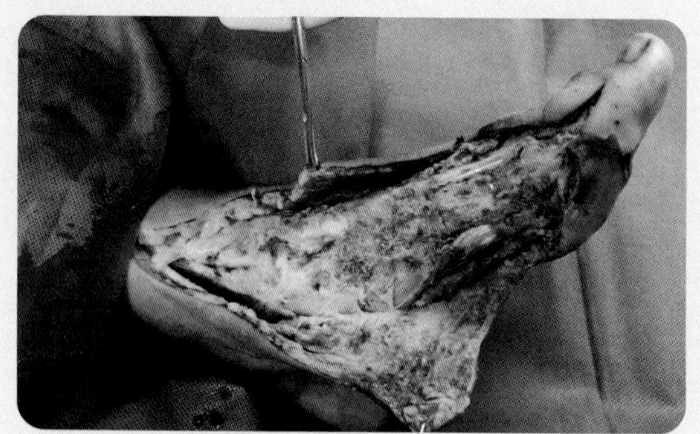

图 7.1.6　足部开放引流，坏死皮肤切除，并 VSD 治疗

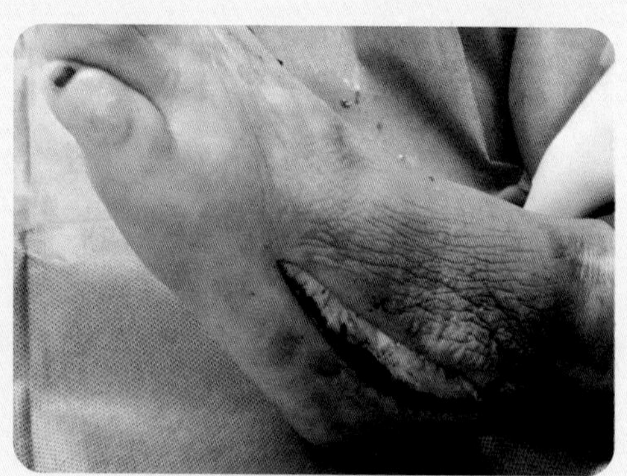

图 7.1.7　足外侧对口切开引流，皮肤起皱，肿胀逐渐消退

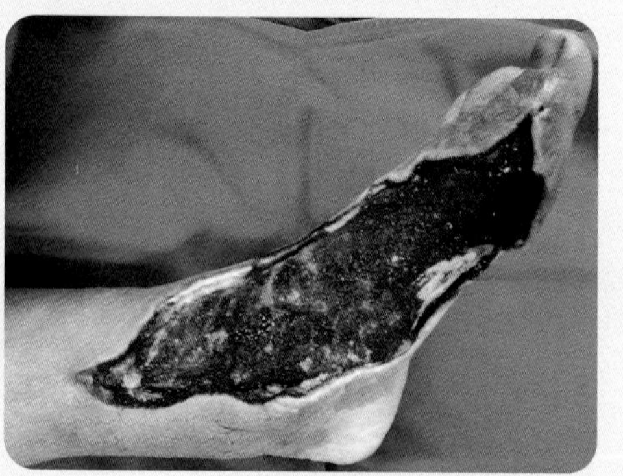

图 7.1.8　VSD+ 生长因子滴注 7 天，创面新鲜，肉芽组织红润

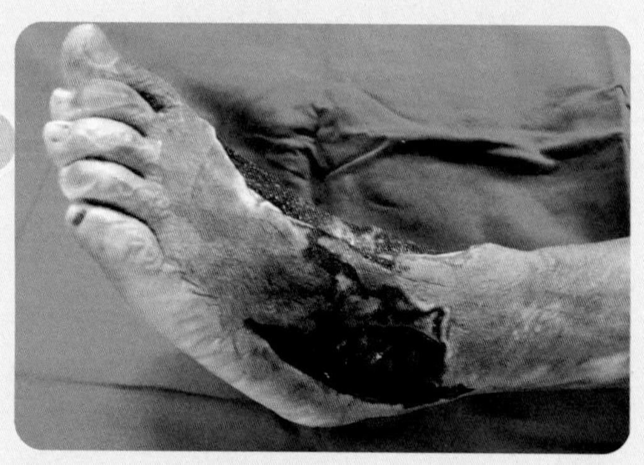

图 7.1.9　足外侧创面新鲜，足背有部分皮肤间桥相连

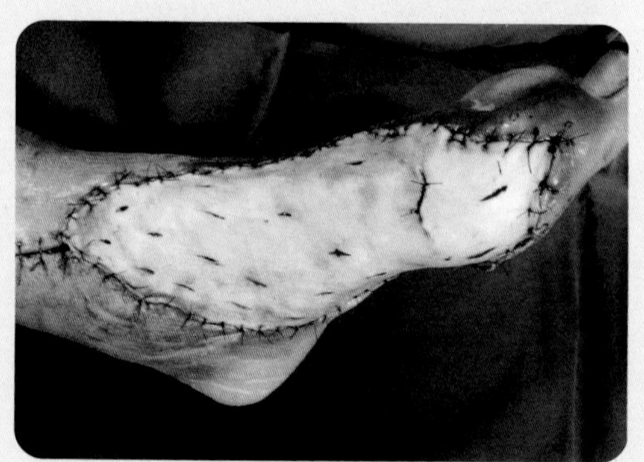

图 7.1.10　全厚皮肤游离移植

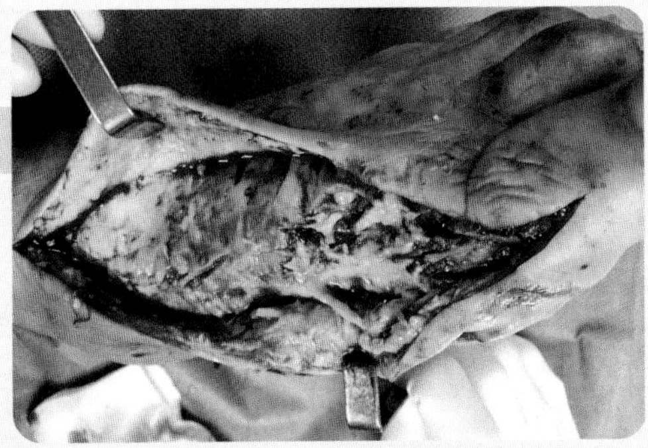

Figure 7.1.5 Widespread subcutaneous edema, honeycomb like changes, and large amounts of pus in the septa

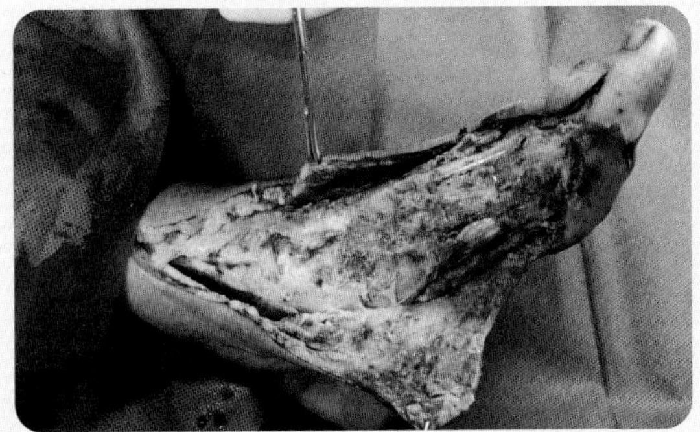

Figure 7.1.6 Foot open drainage, necrotic skin resection, and VSD treatment

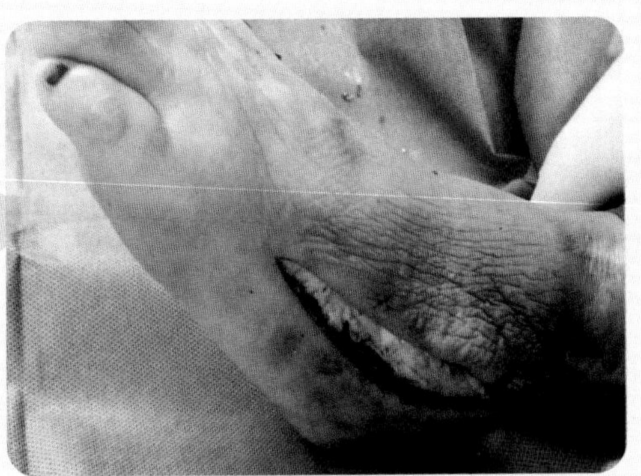

Figure 7.1.7 Opening and draining the lateral side of the foot, wrinkling of the skin, and gradual reduction of swelling

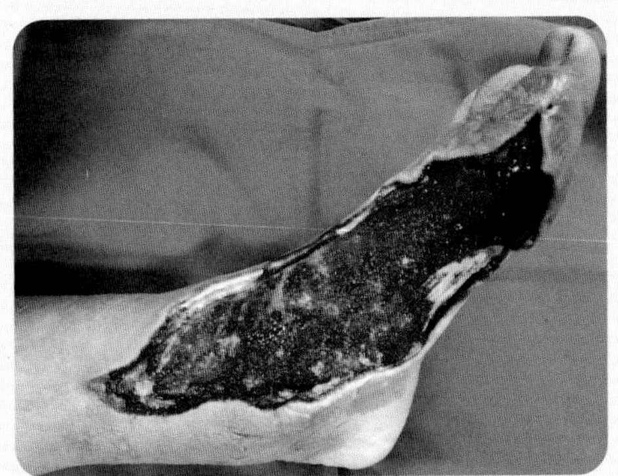

Figure 7.1.8 VSD+growth factor infusion for 7 days, fresh wound, and red granulation tissue

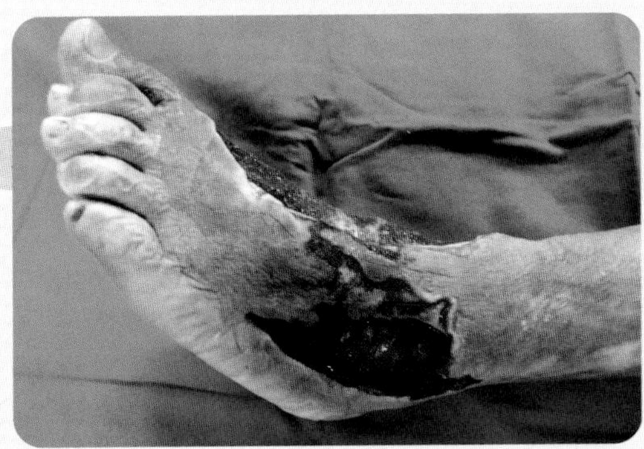

Figure 7.1.9 The wound on the lateral side of the foot is fresh, and there is a partial skin bridge connection on the dorsum of the foot

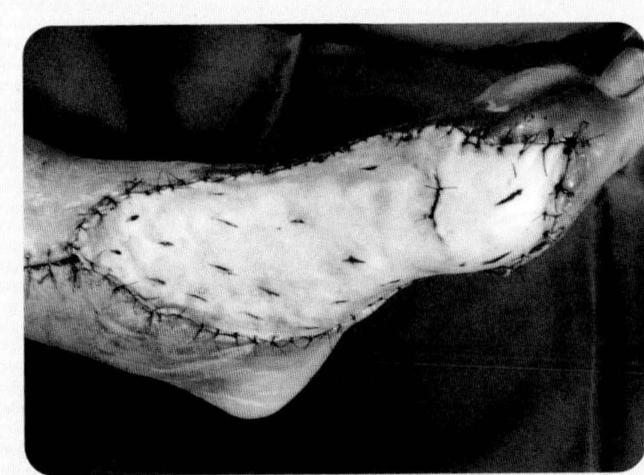

Figure 7.1.10 Full thickness skin free transplantation

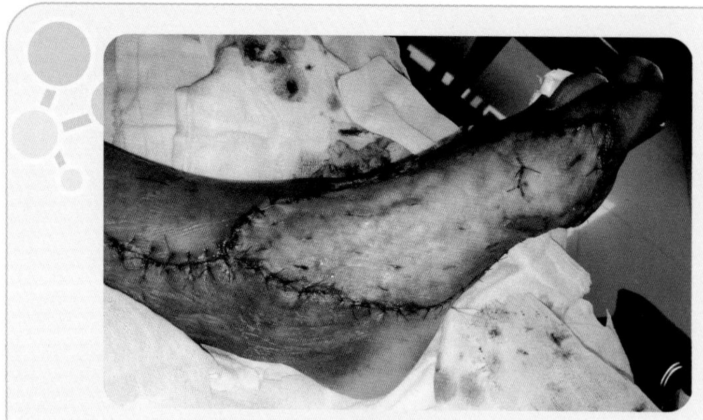

图 7.1.11　术后 12 天，植皮成活

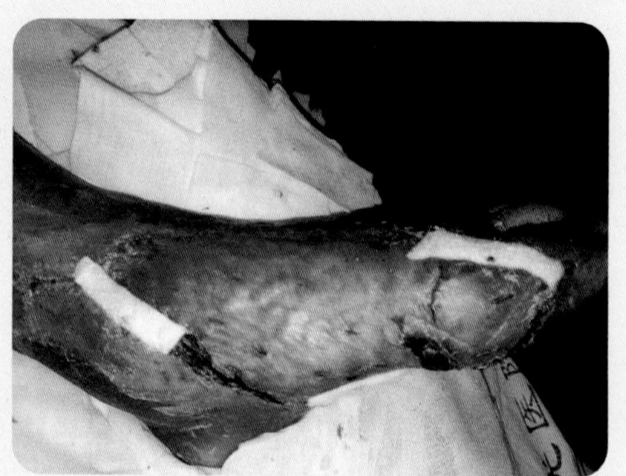

图 7.1.12　缝线已拆除

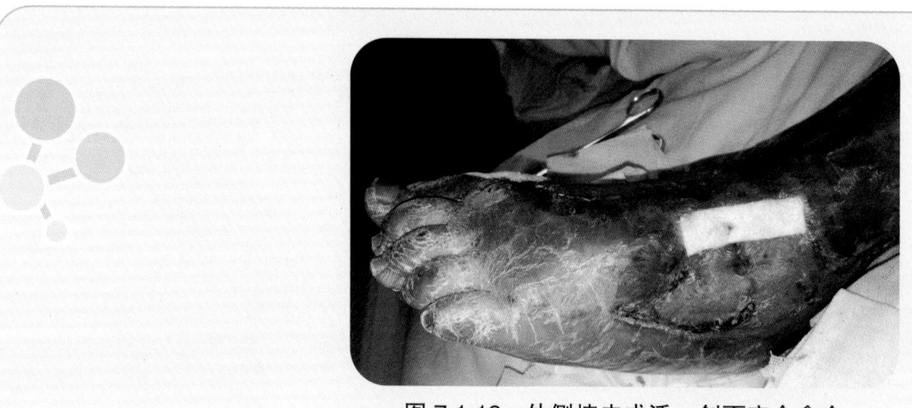

图 7.1.13　外侧植皮成活，创面完全愈合

（陈善亮）

案例二　左下肢动脉硬化闭塞、2 型糖尿病伴糖尿病足

◆ 致病原因

患者因左下肢动脉硬化闭塞、2 型糖尿病，引起左下肢动脉硬化闭塞症伴坏疽；2 型糖尿病足；慢性肾衰竭 5 期，长期维持血液透析状态；2 型糖尿病血糖控制不佳，伴有多个并发症；高血压。

◆ 症状与体征

左足**踇**趾变黑坏死，**踇**趾跖骨外露，有异味，少量渗液，左足底红肿破溃波及足底，患足皮温偏低，足背动脉搏动减弱（图 7.2.1）。脓液培养结果示奇异变形杆菌，给予敏感抗生素治疗。

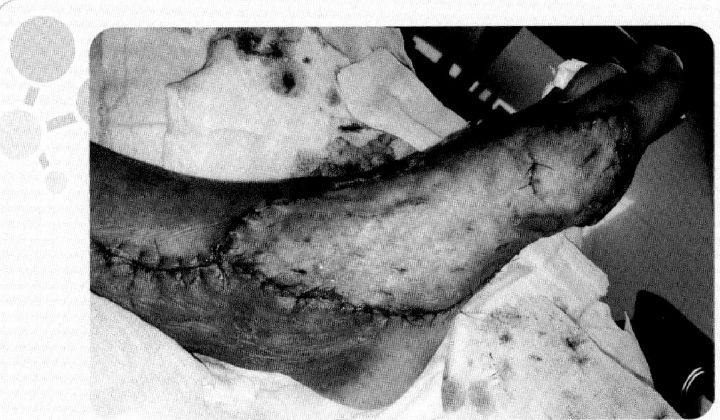

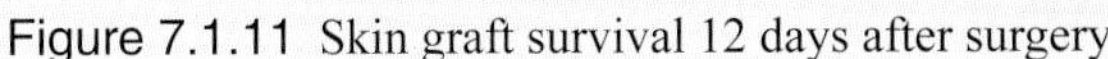

Figure 7.1.11 Skin graft survival 12 days after surgery

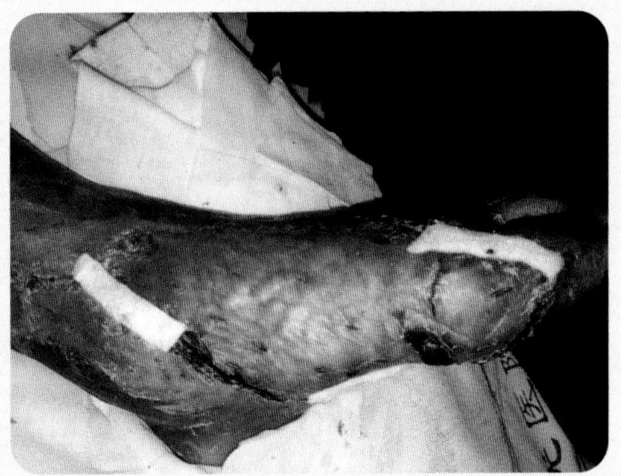

Figure 7.1.12 Suture removed

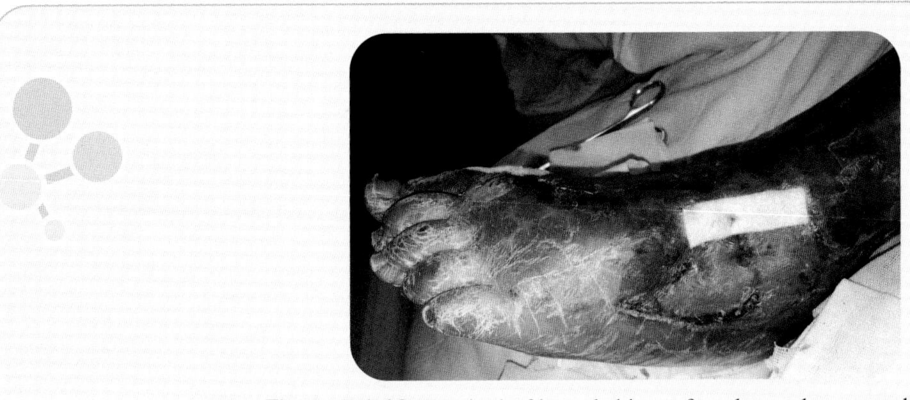

Figure 7.1.13 Survival of lateral skin graft and complete wound healing

(Chen Shanliang)

Case 2 Arteriosclerotic occlusion of left lower limb, type 2 diabetes with diabetes foot

◆ Cause of illness

The left lower extremity arteriosclerosis obliterans with gangrene were caused by the left lower extremity arteriosclerosis obliterans and type 2 diabetes; Type 2 diabetes foot; Chronic renal failure stage 5, long-term maintenance of hemodialysis status; Type 2 diabetes has poor blood sugar control and multiple complications; hypertension.

◆ Signs and symptoms

The left toe has turned black and necrotic, with exposed metatarsal bones and a strange odor. There is a small amount of exudate, and the left sole is red, swollen, and ulcerated, affecting the sole. The affected foot skin temperature is low, and the pulsation of the dorsal foot artery is weakened (Figure 7.2.1). The results of pus culture showed Proteus mirabilis, which was treated with sensitive antibiotics.

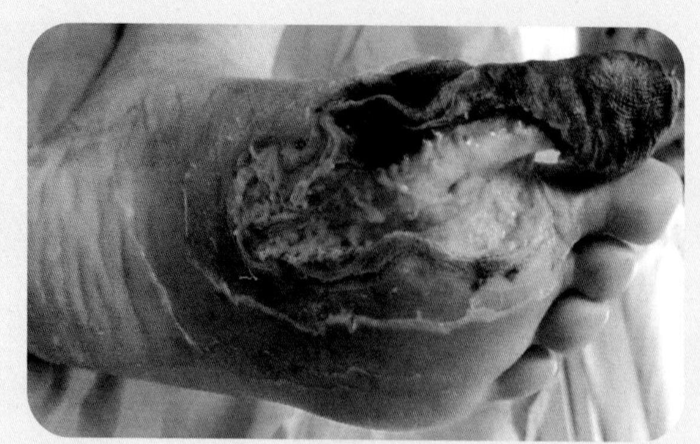

图 7.2.1　左足蹞趾变黑坏死、足底感染向近端蔓延

◆ 治疗方案

1. 基础疾病病因治疗（降糖、降压、营养支持、抗凝、纠正酸碱失衡、控制感染等），维持血液透析，中药内服。

2. 蚕食清创失活坏死组织，截除蹞趾，清洗创面，控制性损伤，改良型 VSD 治疗（图 7.2.2）。

3. 清创术后喷洒重组人碱性成纤维细胞生长因子加生理盐水 100 mL 冲洗创面 1 小时。

4. 创面肉芽组织新鲜，创面达到植皮条件，予以全厚皮封闭创面，再予 VSD（植皮术后不冲管）。创面全厚皮移植术后，皮片成活（图 7.2.3 ~ 图 7.2.5）。

5. 保足尽量维持"铁三角"（足跟、第 1 跖骨、第 5 跖骨）行走功能的稳定性。

6. 住院时间 3 个月以上，家属及患者有保足强烈愿望。

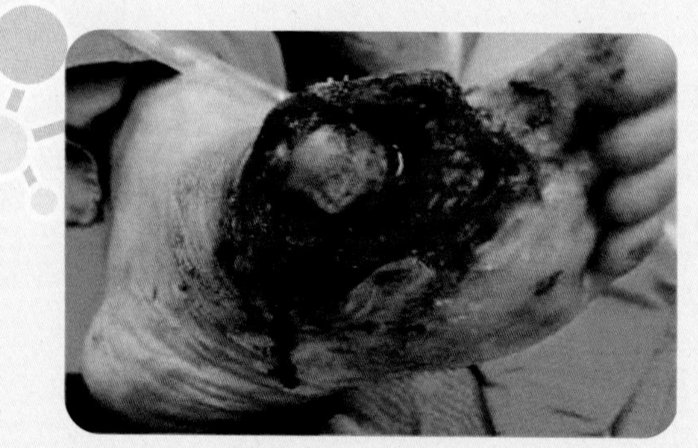

图 7.2.2　清创失活坏死组织，截除蹞趾，清洗创面

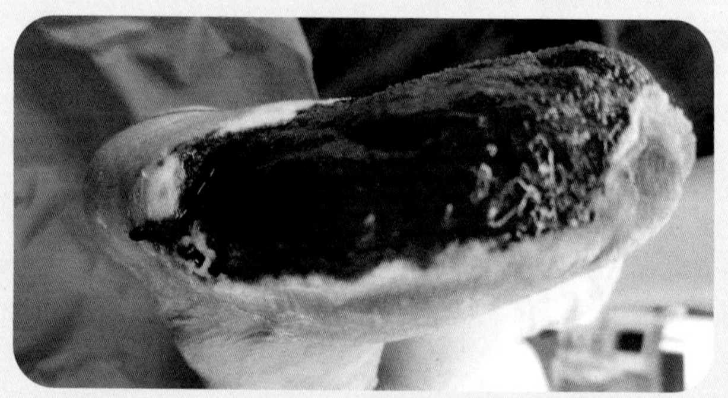

图 7.2.3　创面肉芽组织新鲜，达到植皮条件

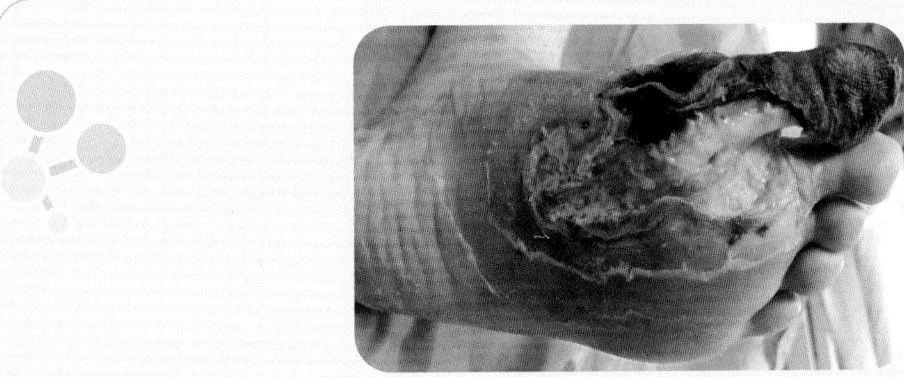

Figure 7.2.1 Blacking and necrosis of the left toe, with plantar infection spreading towards the proximal end

◆ Treatment plan

1. Treatment of underlying diseases (lowering blood sugar, lowering blood pressure, providing nutritional support, anticoagulation, correcting acid-base imbalances, controlling infections, etc.), maintenance of hemodialysis, and oral administration of traditional Chinese medicine.

2. Eat away the necrotic tissue from debridement, remove the toes, clean the wound, control the damage, and treat with modified VSD (Figure 7.2.2).

3. After debridement, spray recombinant human basic fibroblast growth factor and 100 mL of physiological saline to rinse the wound for 1 hour.

4. The granulation tissue on the wound is fresh, and the wound meets the conditions for skin grafting. Full thickness skin is applied to seal the wound, followed by VSD (no flushing after skin grafting). After full thickness skin transplantation on the wound, the skin graft survived (Figure 7.2.3-Figure7.2.5).

5. Keep the stability of the walking function of the "iron triangle" (heel, 1st metatarsal, 5th metatarsal) as much as possible.

6. Hospitalization for more than 3 months, with strong desire from family members and patients to ensure adequate care.

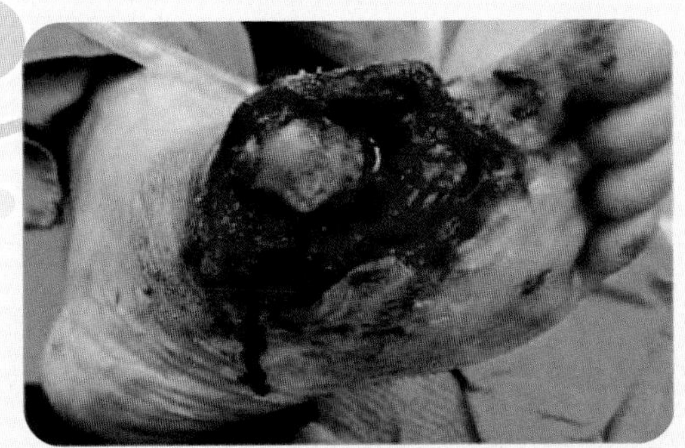

Figure 7.2.2 Debridement of necrotic tissue, toe amputation, and wound cleaning

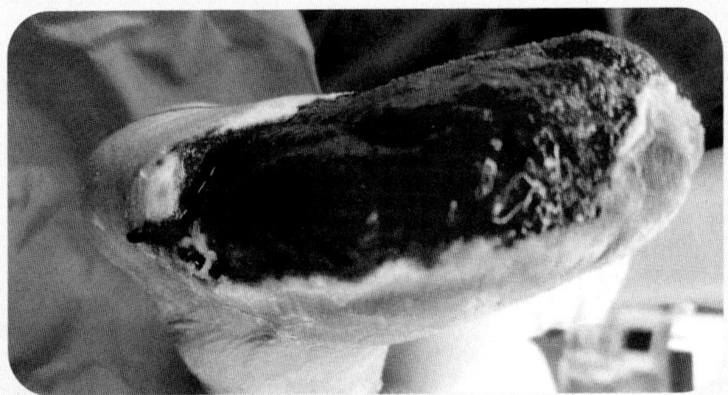

Figure 7.2.3 Fresh granulation tissue at the wound site, meeting the conditions for skin grafting

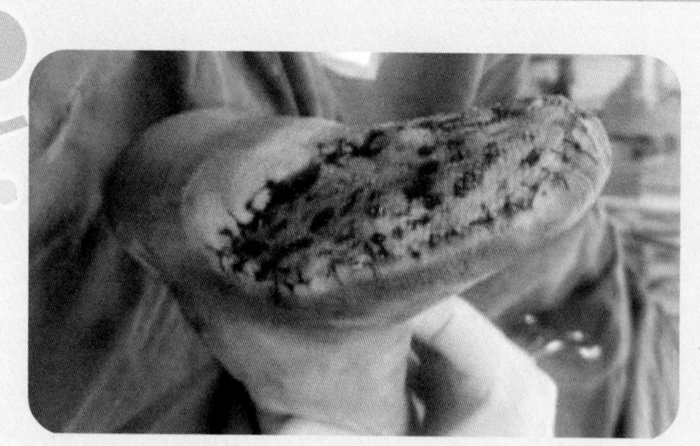

图 7.2.4　植皮术后 1 周创面

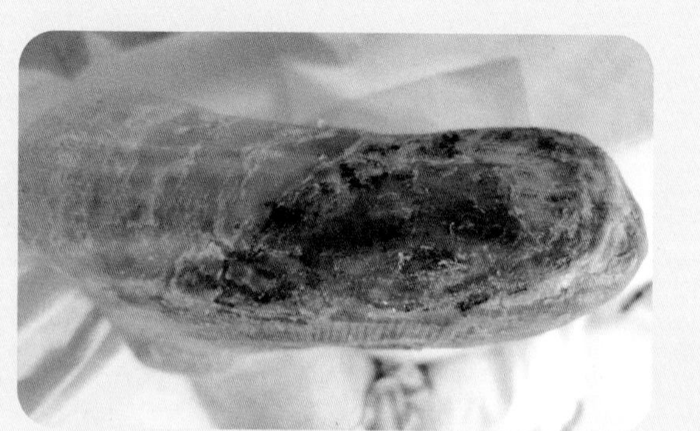

图 7.2.5　创面全厚皮移植术，皮片成活

（陈启鹏　乐世文）

案例三　2 型糖尿病伴糖尿病足

◆ 致病原因

患者因 2 型糖尿病，引起糖尿病足，伴坏死性筋膜炎、低蛋白血症、甲状腺功能减退、左心功能不全、高血压病 2 级（高危），有脑梗死病史。

◆ 症状与体征

神志淡漠，精神差，全身水肿，左足背破溃，少许坏死组织，伴脓性渗出物，左足第 2 趾可见破溃，大小约 1 cm × 2 cm 创面，左足外侧破溃，左足底可见约 5 cm × 3 cm 创面，可见脓性渗出物，左足肿胀明显，创面恶臭味（图 7.3.1）。左足背动脉可触及，足背皮温偏低。脓液培养结果，示咽峡炎链球菌（多耐），给予敏感抗生素治疗。

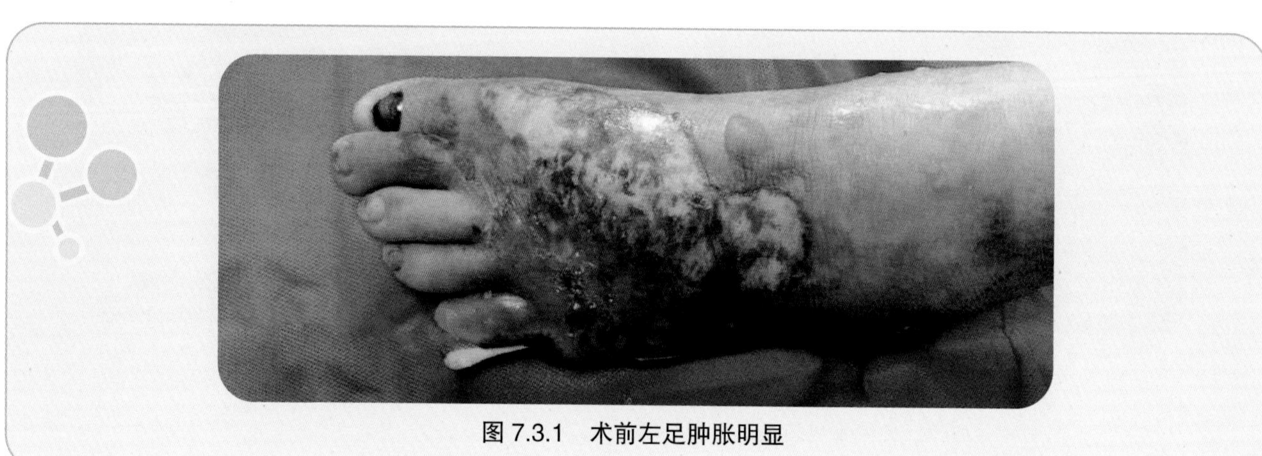

图 7.3.1　术前左足肿胀明显

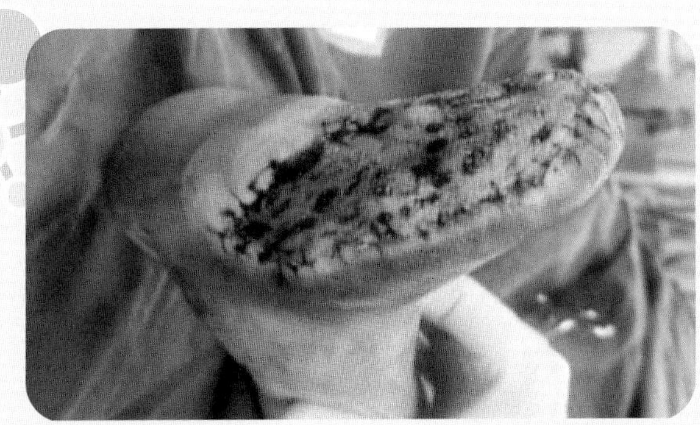
Figure 7.2.4 Wound one week after skin transplantation

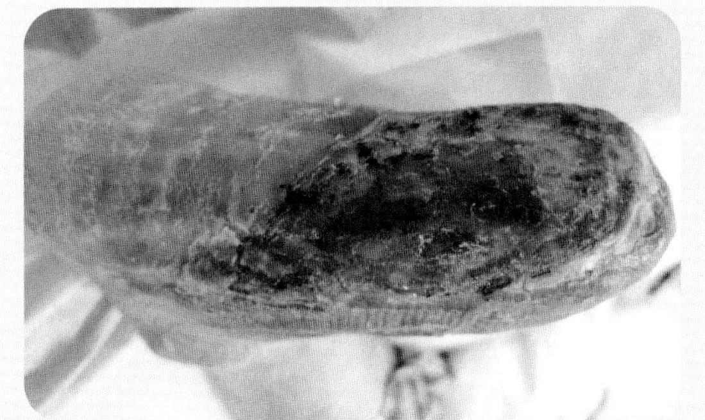
Figure 7.2.5 Full thickness skin transplantation on the wound, skin graft survival

(Chen Qipeng, Le Shiwen)

Case 3 Type 2 diabetes with diabetes foot

◆ Cause of illness

The patient had diabetes foot caused by type 2 diabetes, with necrotizing fasciitis, hypoproteinemia, hypothyroidism, left ventricular dysfunction, hypertension grade 2 (high-risk), and a history of cerebral infarction.

◆ Signs and symptoms

Faint mind, poor mental state, edema throughout the body, left foot dorsal rupture, slight necrotic tissue, accompanied by purulent exudate. A rupture can be seen on the second toe of the left foot, with a wound size of about 1 cm × 2 cm. The outer side of the left foot is ruptured, and a wound size of about 5 cm × 3 cm can be seen on the left sole, with purulent exudate visible. The left foot is swollen significantly, and the wound has a foul odor (Figure 7.3.1). The left dorsalis pedis artery is palpable, and the dorsalis pedis skin temperature is low. The result of pus culture showed Streptococcus pharyngitis (multidrug-resistant) and was treated with sensitive antibiotics.

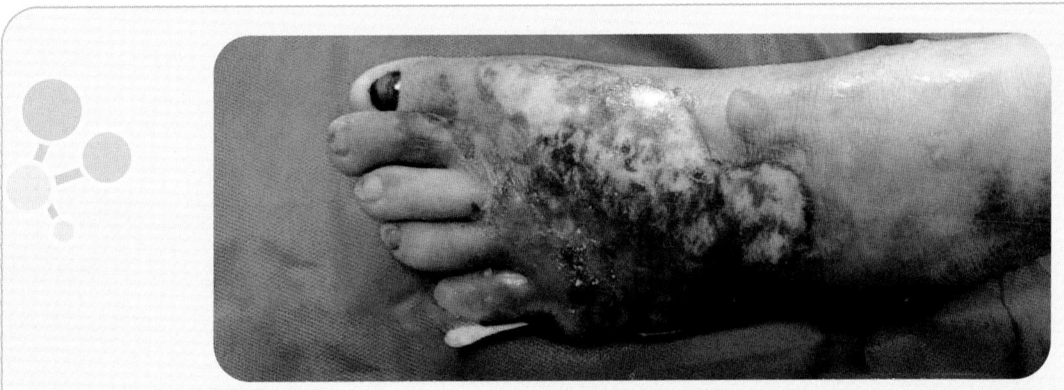
Figure 7.3.1 Significant swelling of the left foot before surgery

◆ 治疗方案

1. 基础疾病病因治疗（降糖、降压、营养支持、抗凝、纠正酸碱失衡、输血、纠正甲状腺功能减退、补充蛋白质、利尿、控制感染等），中药内服。

2. 蚕食清创，清除坏死组织，控制性损伤，改良型 VSD（图 7.3.2）。

3. 术后创面喷洒生长因子，每天重组人碱性成纤维细胞生长因子加生理盐水 100 mL 冲洗创面 1 小时。

4. 术后 1 周拆除 VSD，创面肉芽组织新鲜，创面达到植皮条件，予以全厚皮封闭创面，再予 VSD（植皮术后不冲管）。术后 1 周，皮片成活；术后 40 天，创面完全愈合（图 7.3.3 ～图 7.3.6）。

5. 住院时间 3 个月以上，家属及患者有保足强烈愿望。

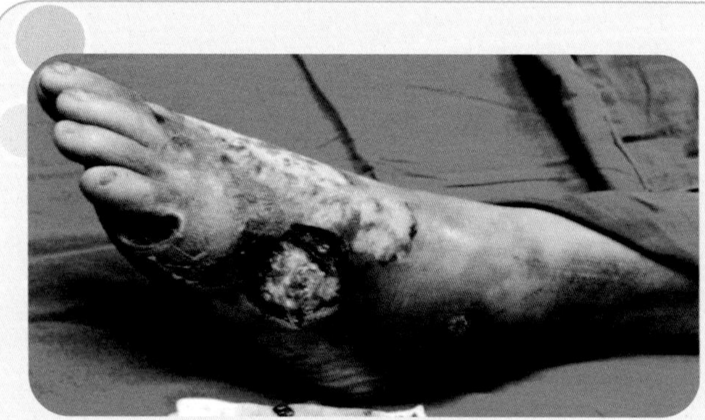

图 7.3.2　术中清除坏死组织

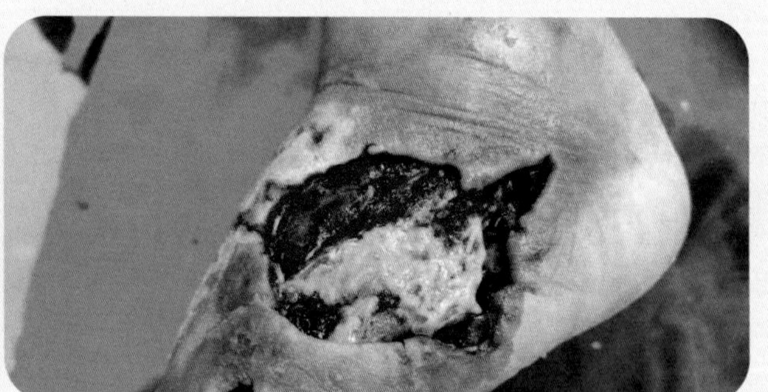

图 7.3.3　术后 1 周拆除 VSD

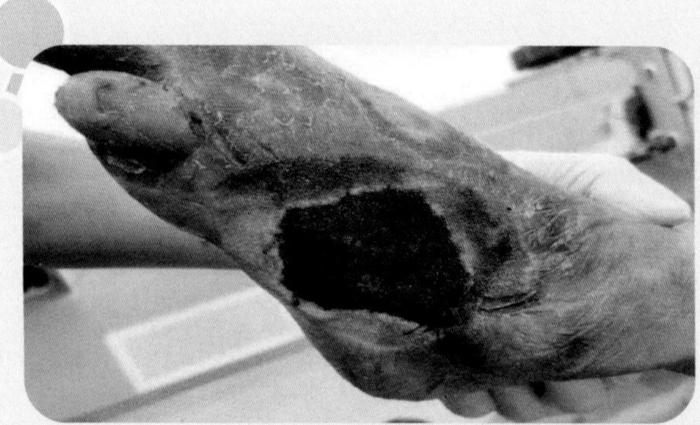

图 7.3.4　创面肉芽组织新鲜，植皮条件成熟

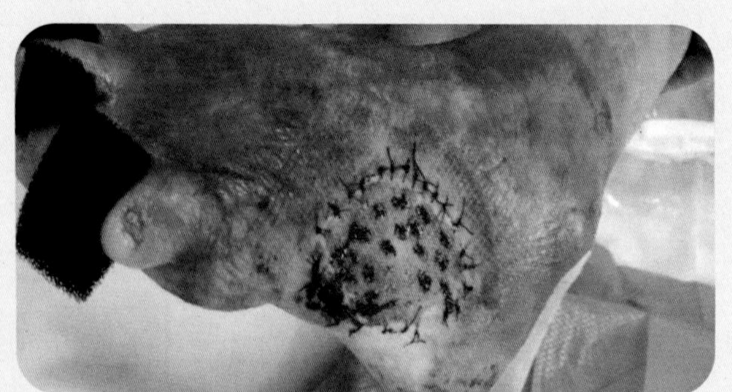

图 7.3.5　植皮术后 1 周，皮片成活

◆ Treatment plan

1. Treatment of underlying diseases (lowering blood sugar, lowering blood pressure, nutritional support, anticoagulation, correcting acid-base imbalance, blood transfusion, correcting hypothyroidism, supplementing protein, diuresis, controlling infections, etc.), taking traditional Chinese medicine orally.

2. Devouring debridement, removing necrotic tissue, controlling damage, modified VSD (Figure 7.3.2).

3. After surgery, spray growth factor onto the wound and rinse the wound with 100 mL of recombinant human basic fibroblast growth factor and physiological saline for 1 hour daily.

4. One week after surgery, the VSD was removed, the granulation tissue on the wound was fresh, and the wound met the conditions for skin grafting. Full thickness skin was applied to seal the wound, and then VSD was given (without flushing the tube after skin grafting). One week after surgery, the skin graft survived; 40 days after surgery, the wound completely healed (Figure 7.3.3- Figure 7.3.6).

5. Hospitalization for more than 3 months, with strong desire from family members and patients to ensure adequate care.

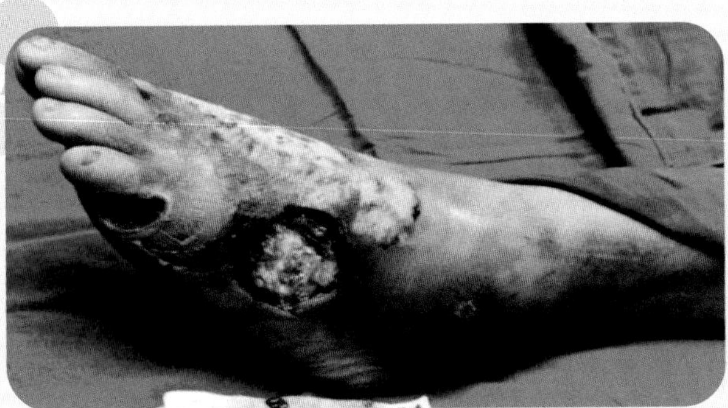

Figure 7.3.2 Intraoperative removal of necrotic tissue

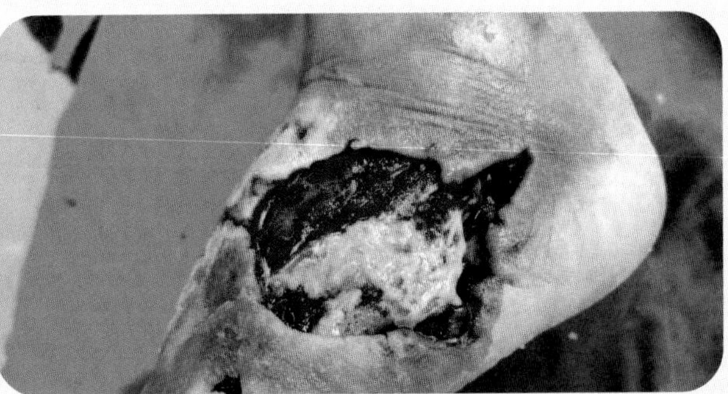

Figure 7.3.3 Removal of VSD 1 week after surgery

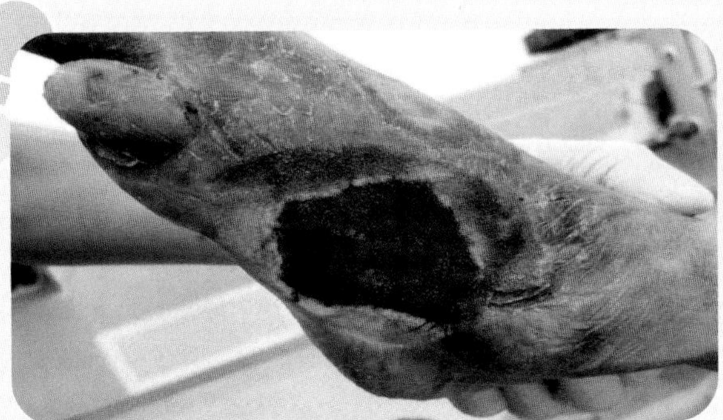

Figure 7.3.4 Fresh granulation tissue on the wound and mature skin grafting conditions

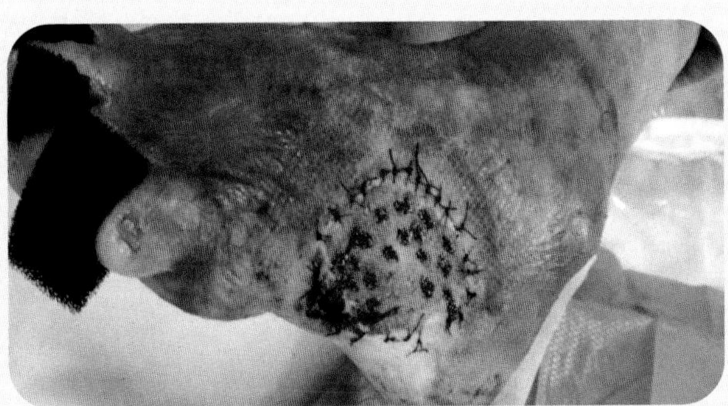

Figure 7.3.5 One week after skin grafting, skin graft survival

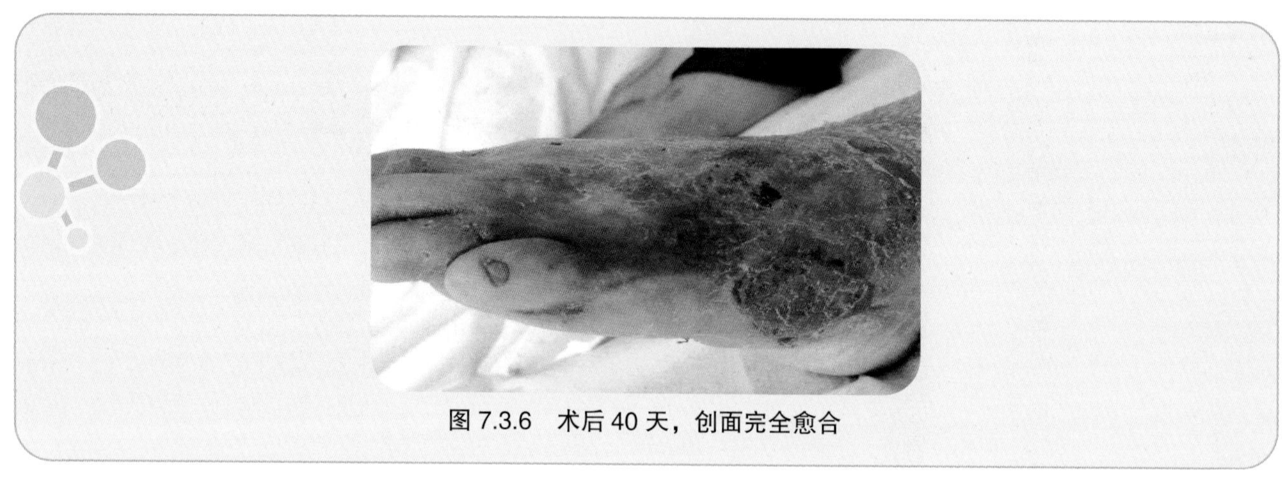
图 7.3.6　术后 40 天，创面完全愈合

（陈启鹏　乐世文）

案例四　2 型糖尿病合并右足跟坏死性筋膜炎

◆ 致病原因

患者因 2 型糖尿病，引起右足跟压疮坏死性筋膜炎，伴阿尔茨海默病（老年型）、左下肢动脉硬化症伴闭塞、血小板减少、多发性脑梗死。

◆ 症状与体征

右足跟可见约 2 cm × 3 cm × 0.5 cm 创面，创面中间可见黑痂，周围少许渗液，无明显。

◆ 治疗方案

1. 基础疾病病因治疗（营养支持、抗凝、纠正酸碱失衡、升高血小板、控制感染等），中药内服。

2. 蚕食清创，控制性损伤，改良型 VSD。术中可见足跟及足底筋膜坏死，大量脓性分泌物（图 7.4.1）。

3. 术后创面喷洒生长因子，每天重组人碱性成纤维细胞生长因子加生理盐水 100 mL 冲洗创面 1 小时。

4. 术后 1 月拆除 VSD，肉芽组织较新鲜；待创面肉芽组织新鲜，植皮条件成熟，予以全厚皮封闭创面，再予 VSD（植皮术后不冲管）；术后创面完全愈合（图 7.4.2 ~ 图 7.4.5）。

5. 住院时间 3 个月以上，家属及患者有保足强烈愿望。

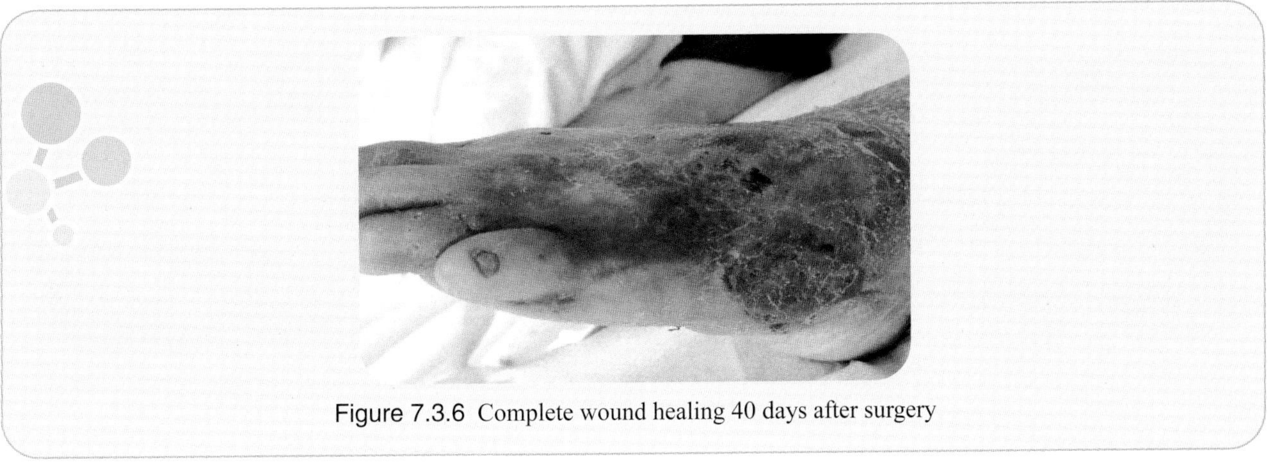

Figure 7.3.6 Complete wound healing 40 days after surgery

(Chen Qipeng, Le Shiwen)

Case 4 Type 2 diabetes with necrotizing fasciitis of right heel

◆ Cause of illness

The patient suffered from type 2 diabetes, which caused right heel pressure sore necrotizing fasciitis, accompanied by Alzheimer's disease (senile type), left lower extremity arteriosclerosis with occlusion, thrombocytopenia, and multiple cerebral infarction.

◆ Signs and symptoms

A wound of approximately 2 cm × 3 cm × 0.5 cm can be seen on the right heel, with a black scab visible in the middle of the wound and a small amount of exudate around it, but no obvious signs.

◆ Treatment plan

1. Treatment of underlying diseases (nutritional support, anticoagulation, correction of acid-base imbalance, elevation of platelets, control of infections, etc.), oral administration of traditional Chinese medicine.

2. Devouring debridement, controlling damage, and improving VSD. During the operation, necrosis of the heel and plantar fascia was observed, along with a large amount of purulent discharge (Figure 7.4.1).

3. After surgery, spray growth factor onto the wound and rinse the wound with 100 mL of recombinant human basic fibroblast growth factor and physiological saline for 1 hour daily.

4. One month after surgery, the VSD was removed and the granulation tissue was relatively fresh; When the granulation tissue of the wound is fresh and the conditions for skin grafting are mature, the wound should be sealed with full thickness skin, and then VSD (no flushing after skin grafting) should be given; The postoperative wound healed completely (Figure 7.4.2 - Figure 7.4.5).

5. Hospitalization for more than 3 months, with strong desire from family members and patients to ensure adequate care.

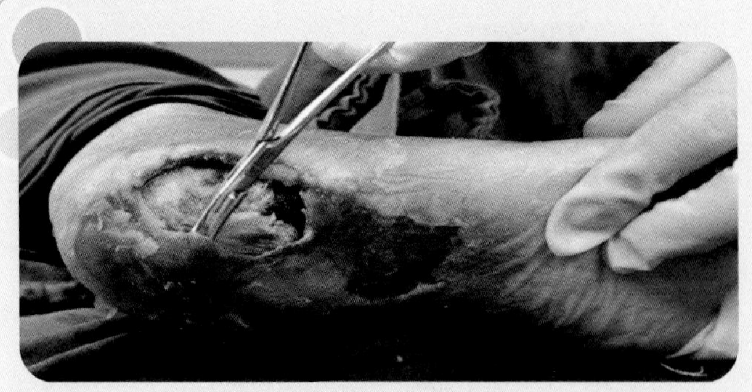

图 7.4.1　术中可见足跟及足底筋膜坏死，大量脓性分泌物

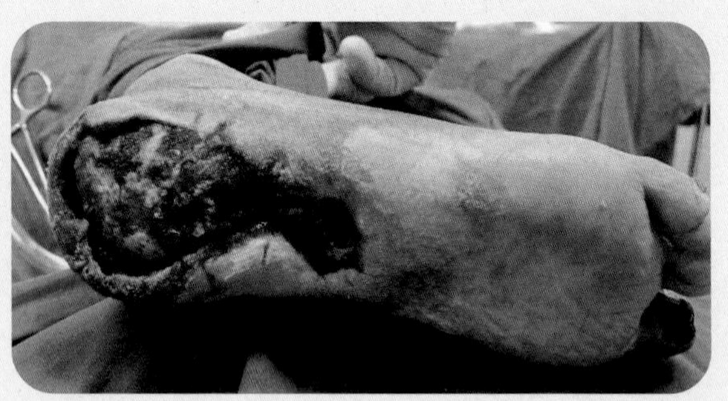

图 7.4.2　术后 1 个月拆除 VSD，肉芽组织较新鲜

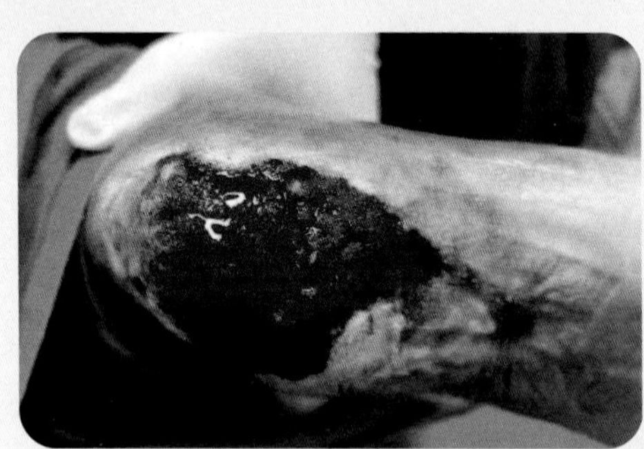

图 7.4.3　创面肉芽组织新鲜，植皮条件成熟

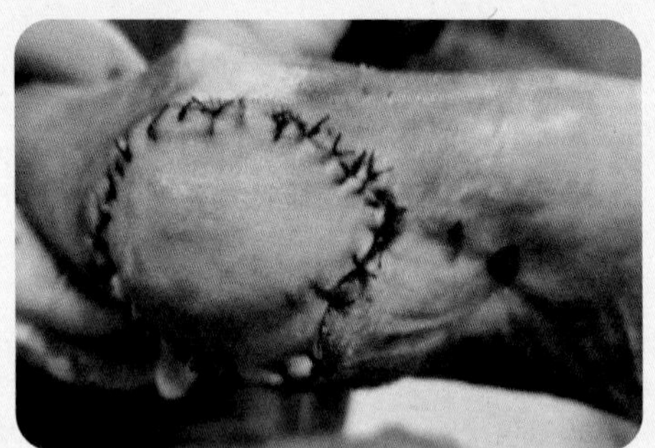

图 7.4.4　全厚皮植皮

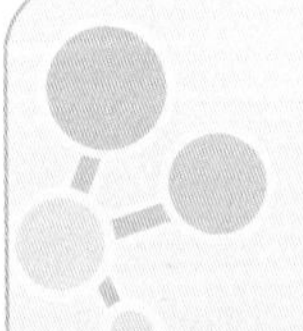

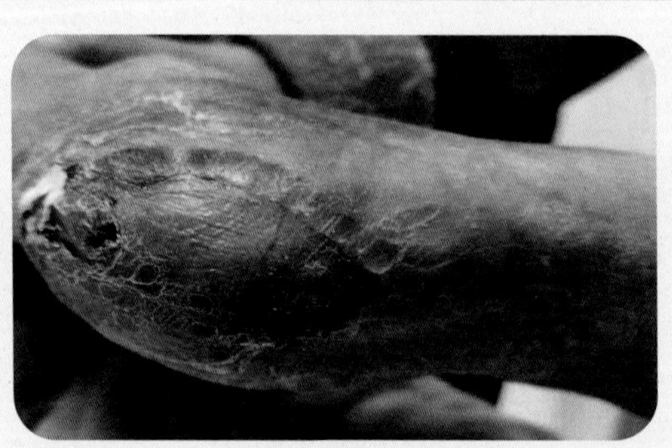

图 7.4.5　术后创面完全愈合

（陈启鹏　乐世文）

案例五　糖尿病足伴周围血管病变（Wagner 4 级）

◆ 致病原因

患者因有 2 型糖尿病，右足趾剪趾甲外伤出血，并发感染，第 4、第 5 趾坏死。

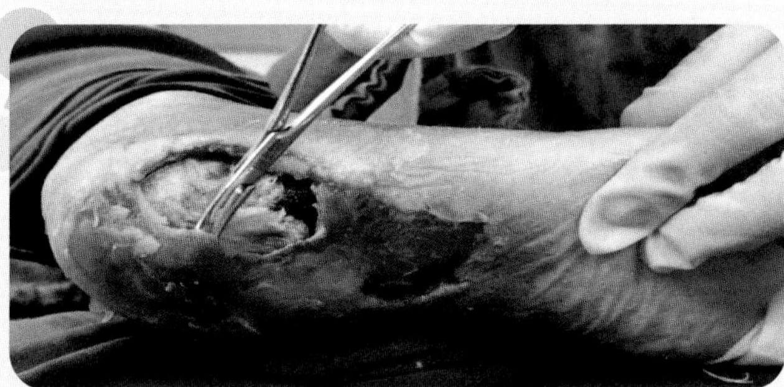

Figure 7.4.1 Necrosis of the heel and plantar fascia during surgery, with a large amount of purulent discharge

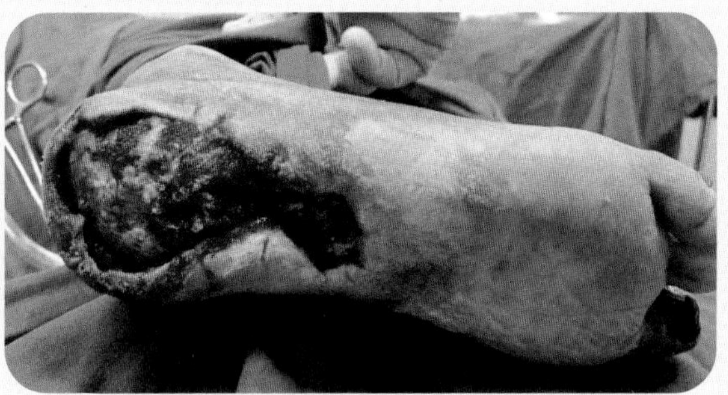

Figure 7.4.2 One month after surgery, VSD was removed and the granulation tissue was fresher

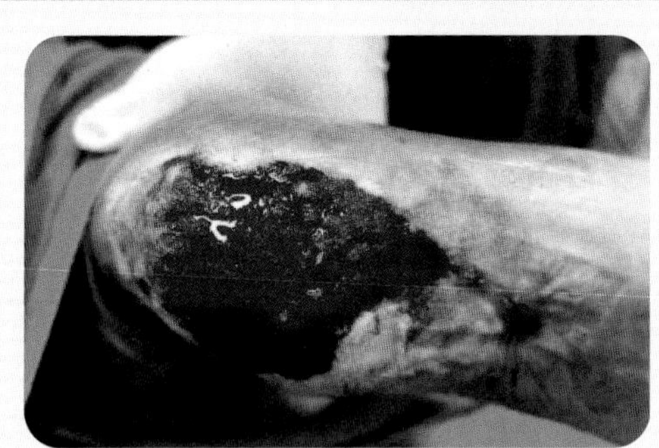

Figure 7.4.3 Fresh granulation tissue on the wound and mature skin grafting conditions

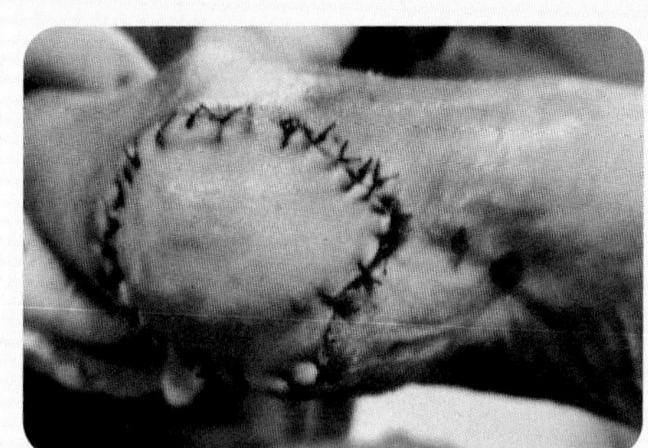

Figure 7.4.4 Full thickness skin graft

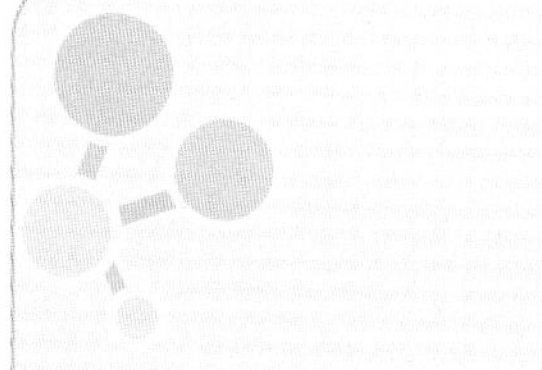

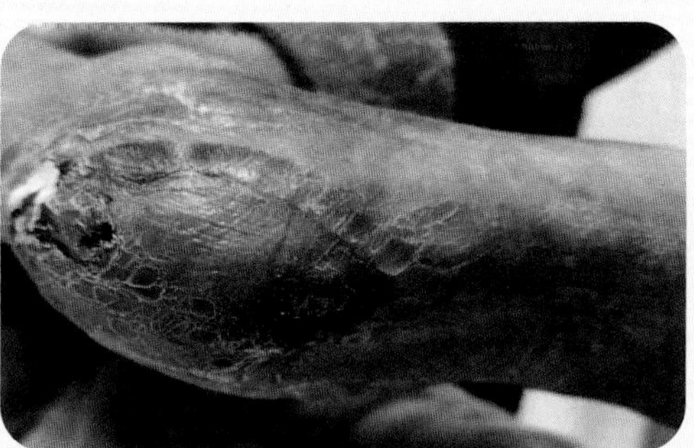

Figure 7.4.5 Complete wound healing after surgery

(Chen Qipeng, Le Shiwen)

Case 5 Diabetes foot with peripheral vascular disease (Wagner grade 4)

◆ Cause of illness

The patient suffered from type 2 diabetes, right toe nail cutting, trauma, bleeding, infection, and necrosis of the fourth and fifth toes.

◆ 症状与体征

既往右足第4趾已坏死截趾，第5趾干性坏死，跖趾关节处红肿、伴湿性坏死，足背动脉搏动未及，血糖控制欠佳（图7.5.1）。

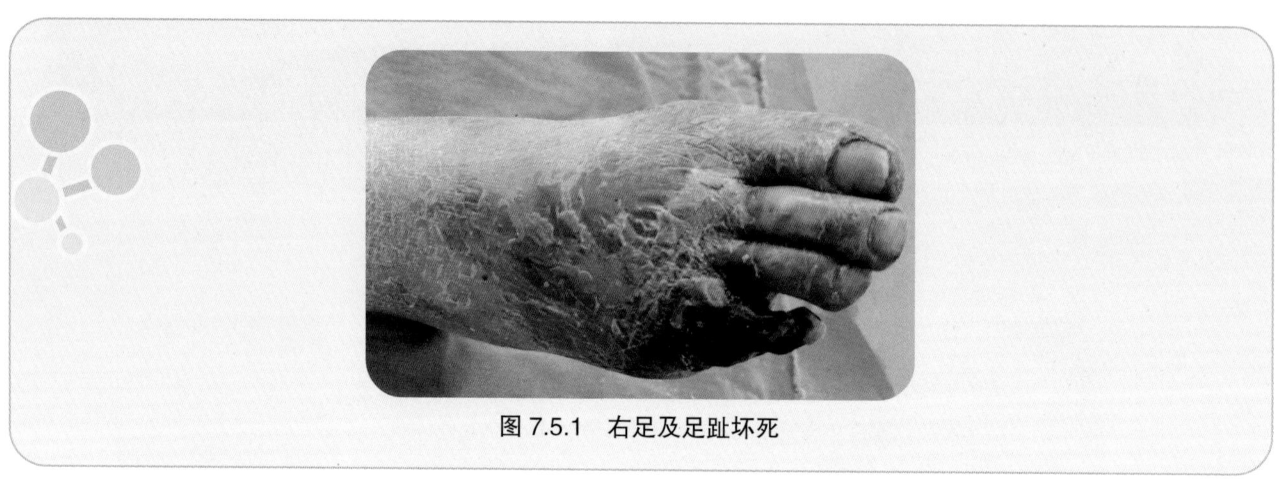

图7.5.1　右足及足趾坏死

◆ 治疗方案

1. 评估创面、血管、神经，评估糖尿病并发症及胰岛功能。

2. 处理急性并发症和评价重要脏器功能，经验性抗生素应用，中医辨证和中医外治，早期治则清热解毒、除湿化瘀。

3. 细菌培养，急诊手术行清创切开、引流，截趾、换药，目标是创面基本无臭味、坏死区缩小、脓腔及窦道开放或者引流（图7.5.2）。

4. 第二次手术，第5跖骨骨髓炎感染向近心端方向蔓延，彻底清创、跖骨部分切除（图7.5.3）。

5. 血管介入开通血管，改善血运，创面VSD引流，清热凉血等中药灌洗，促进创面肉芽组织生长；清创VSD 2次后，感染得到控制，载药骨水泥，并逐步降低抗生素强度。3周后拆除骨水泥，创面肉芽组织生长良好（图7.5.4～图7.5.6）。

6. 创面采用人工真皮移植修复，促进肉芽组织生长。

7. 家庭延展换药、康复指导，创面愈合（图7.5.7、图7.5.8）。

◆ Signs and symptoms

Previously, the fourth toe of the right foot had necrotic amputation, the fifth toe had dry necrosis, and the metatarsophalangeal joint was red and swollen with wet necrosis. The dorsal artery of the foot did not pulse, and blood glucose control was poor (Figure 7.5.1).

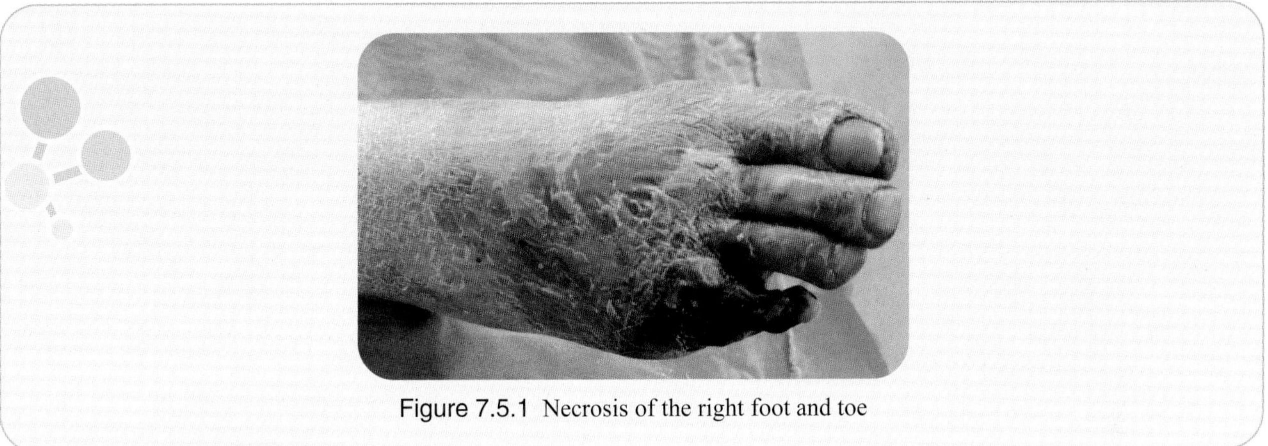

Figure 7.5.1 Necrosis of the right foot and toe

◆ Treatment plan

1. Evaluate the wound surface, blood vessels and nerves, and evaluate the complications of diabetes and pancreatic islet function.

2. To deal with acute complications and evaluate the function of important organs, empirical use of antibiotics, traditional Chinese medicine syndrome differentiation and external treatment, early treatment involves clearing heat and detoxifying, dehumidifying and removing blood stasis.

3. Bacterial culture, emergency surgery involves debridement, incision, drainage, toe amputation, and dressing change, with the goal of achieving a wound with minimal odor, reduced necrotic area, and opening or drainage of the purulent cavity and sinus tract (Figure 7.5.2).

4. In the second surgery, osteomyelitis infection of the 5th metatarsal bone spread towards the proximal end, and thorough debridement and partial resection of the metatarsal bone were performed (Figure 7.5.3).

5. Vascular intervention opens up blood vessels, improves blood flow, causes VSD drainage in wounds, and promotes granulation tissue growth through traditional Chinese medicine irrigation such as clearing heat and cooling blood; After two rounds of debridement of VSD, the infection was controlled, and drug loaded bone cement was used, gradually reducing the intensity of antibiotics. Three weeks later, the bone cement was removed and the granulation tissue on the wound grew well (Figure 7.5.4- Figure 7.5.6).

6. The wound is repaired using artificial dermal transplantation to promote granulation tissue growth.

7. Family extension dressing change, rehabilitation guidance, wound healing (Figure 7.5.7, Figure 7.5.8).

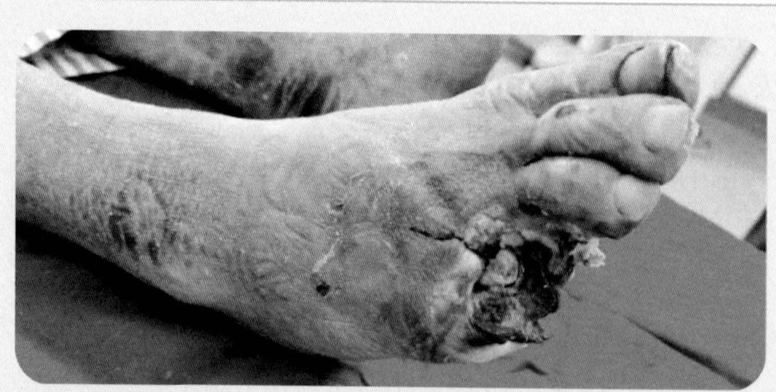

图 7.5.2　急诊手术，清创、截趾、换药

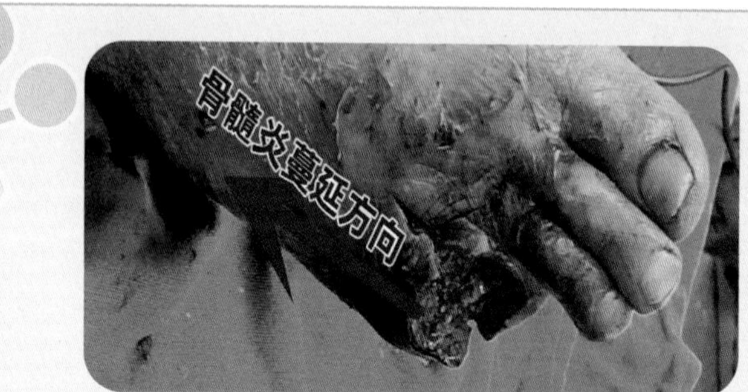

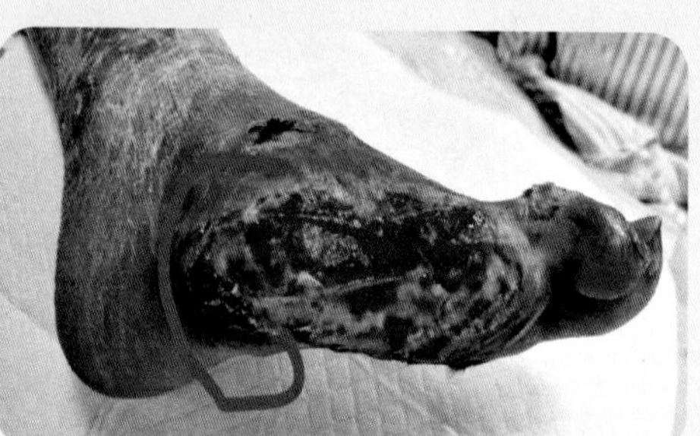

图 7.5.3　第二次手术，彻底清创、跖骨部分切除

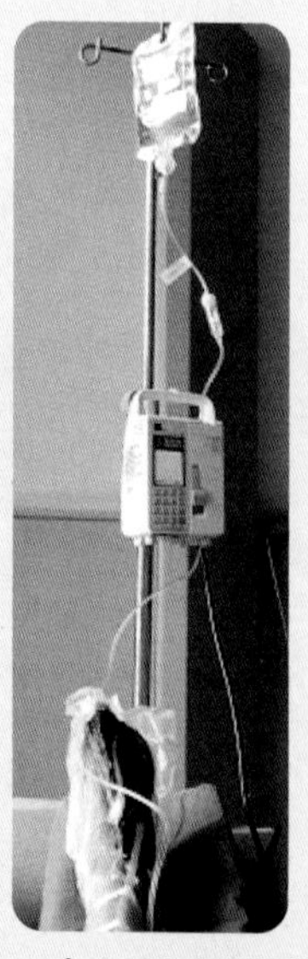

图 7.5.4　介入手术开通血管，创面 VSD 引流

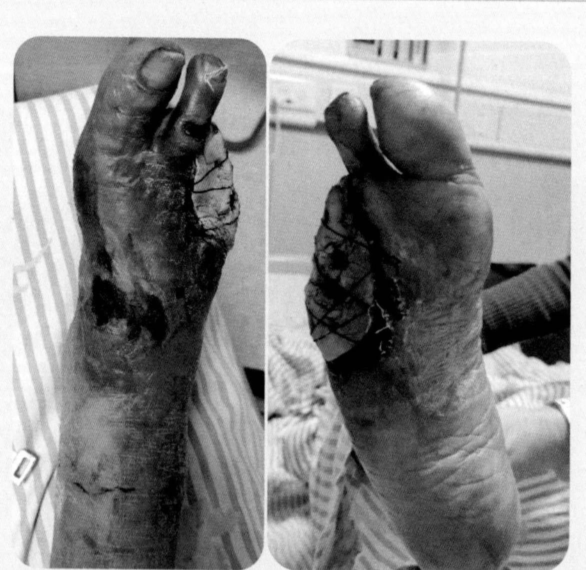

图 7.5.5　清创后载药骨水泥填充，换药

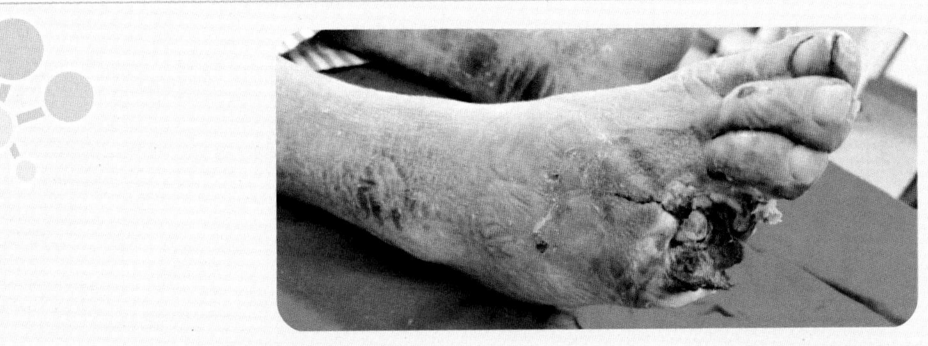

Figure 7.5.2 Emergency surgery, debridement, toe amputation, dressing change

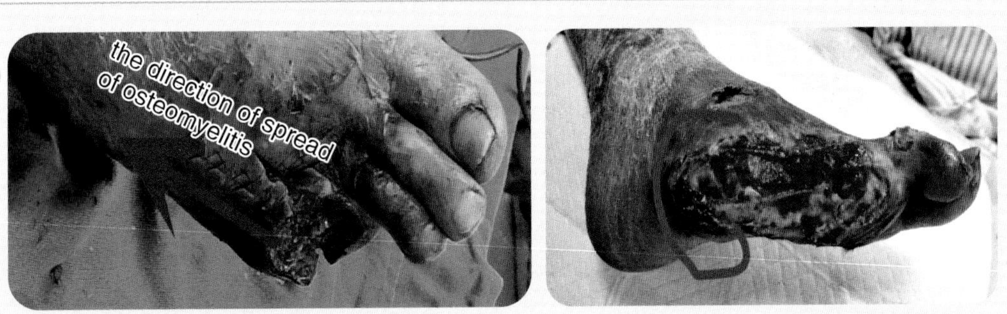

Figure 7.5.3 Second surgery, complete debridement and partial removal of metatarsal bone

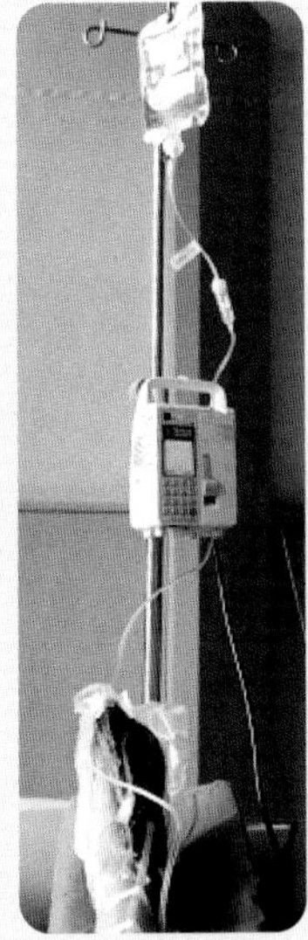

Figure 7.5.4 Interventional surgery to open blood vessels and drain VSD from the wound

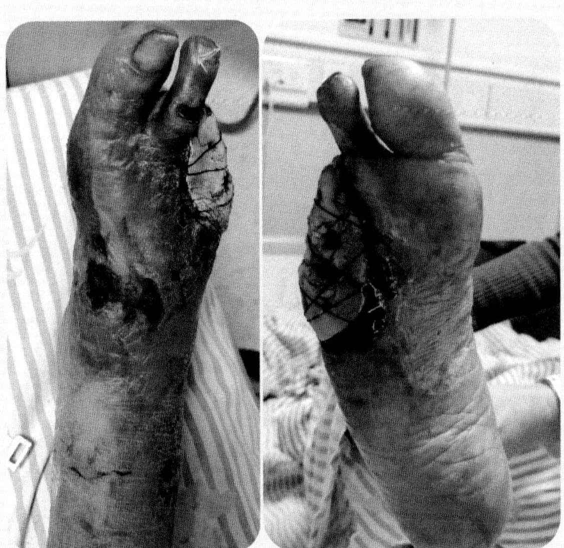

Figure 7.5.5 Filling with drug loaded bone cement after debridement and dressing change

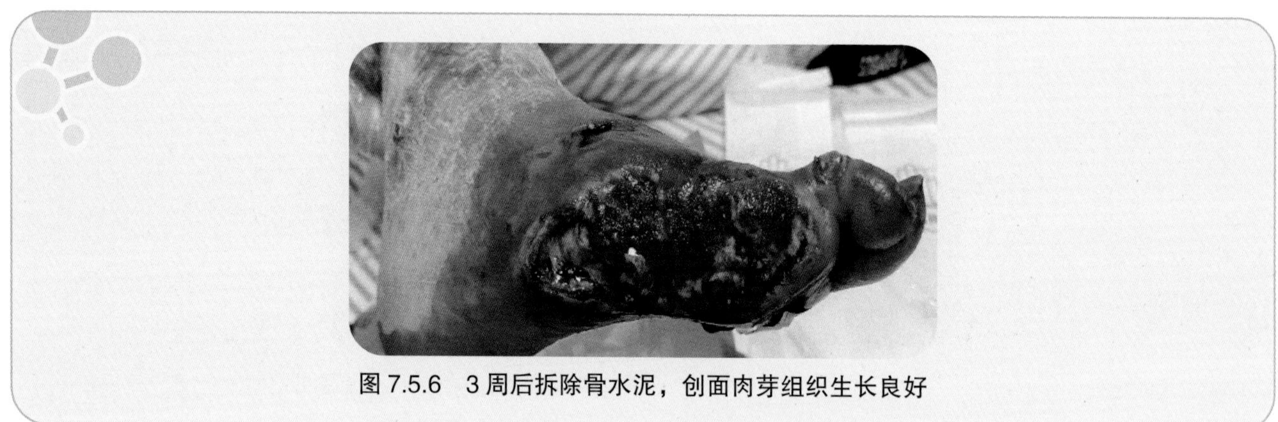
图 7.5.6　3 周后拆除骨水泥，创面肉芽组织生长良好

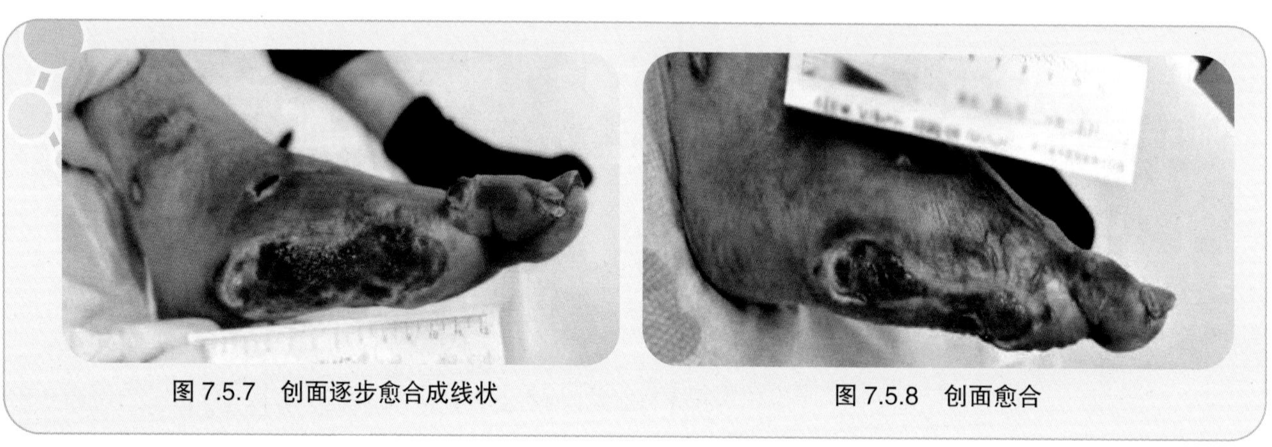
图 7.5.7　创面逐步愈合成线状

图 7.5.8　创面愈合

（王永高　倪斐琳）

案例六　2 型糖尿病伴糖尿病足、足跟慢性骨髓炎

◆ 致病原因

患者因左下肢动脉硬化闭塞、2 型糖尿病，引起左下肢动脉硬化闭塞症伴坏疽、高血压、特应性皮炎（中重度）、血小板功能异常、贫血、继发性甲状腺功能减退、糖尿病足、足跟慢性骨髓炎。

◆ 症状与体征

神清，精神软，消瘦，全身皮肤散发暗红色皮疹，伴有脱皮，未见水疱及渗液，可见抓痕，双手颤抖明显，握力尚可，双手上臂内侧可见 7 cm × 4 cm 的瘀斑，未见出血及渗液；左足第 3、第 5 趾发黑、溃烂，无出血及明显渗液，异味感明显，第 4 趾缺如，左足背皮温偏低，足背动脉搏动明显减弱，右足皮温尚可，足背动脉搏动正常（图 7.6.1）。

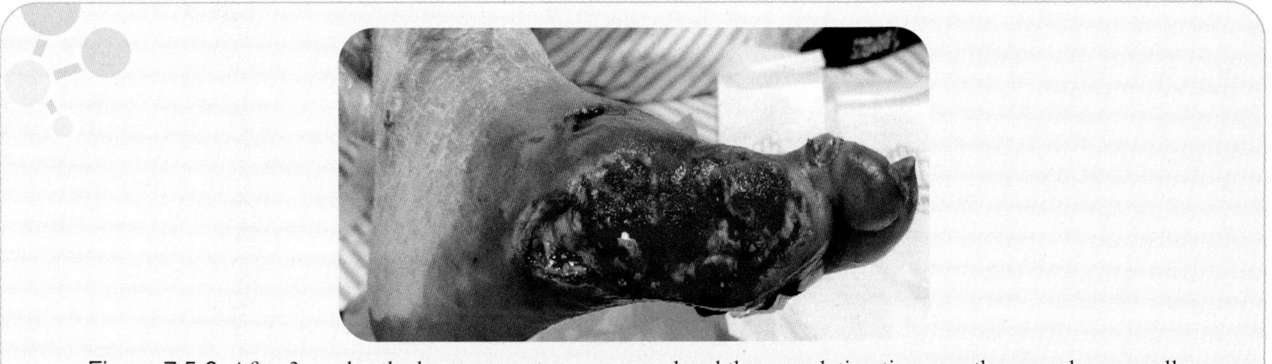

Figure 7.5.6 After 3 weeks, the bone cement was removed and the granulation tissue on the wound grew well

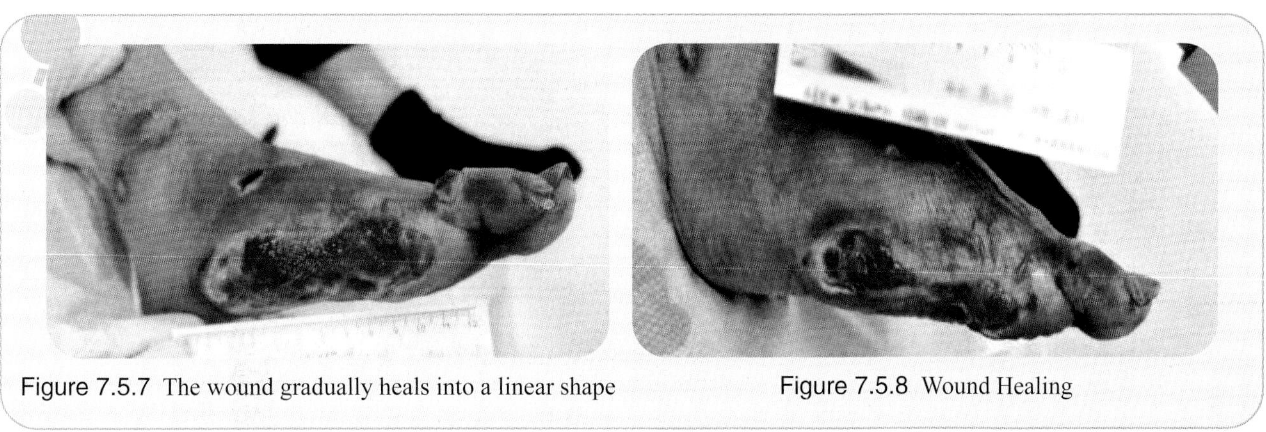

Figure 7.5.7 The wound gradually heals into a linear shape

Figure 7.5.8 Wound Healing

(Wang Yonggao , Ni Feilin)

Case 6 Type 2 diabetes with chronic osteomyelitis of foot and heel in diabetes

◆ Cause of illness

The patient had left lower extremity arteriosclerosis obliterans and type 2 diabetes, which caused left lower extremity arteriosclerosis obliterans with gangrene, hypertension, atopic dermatitis (moderate to severe), abnormal platelet function, anemia, secondary hypothyroidism, diabetes foot, heel chronic osteomyelitis.

◆ Signs and symptoms

Clear in mind, soft in spirit, thin, with a dark red rash on the skin all over the body, accompanied by peeling, no blisters or exudate, visible scratches, obvious tremors in both hands, decent grip strength, 7 cm × 4 cm bruising visible on the inner upper arm of both hands, no bleeding or exudate; The third and fifth toes of the left foot are blackened and ulcerated, with no bleeding or obvious exudation. There is a noticeable odor, and the fourth toe is absent. The temperature of the left foot dorsal skin is low, and the pulsation of the dorsal foot artery is significantly weakened. The temperature of the right foot skin is still acceptable, and the pulsation of the dorsal foot artery is normal (Figure 7.6.1).

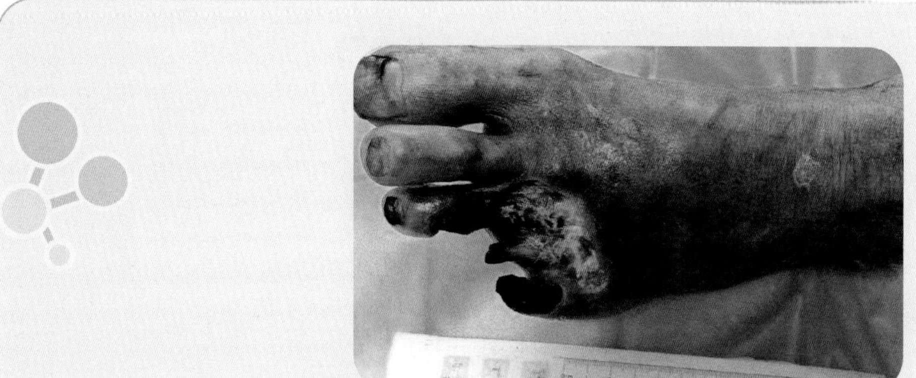

图 7.6.1　术前左足第 3、第 5 趾发黑、溃烂，第 4 趾缺如

◆ 治疗方案

1. 基础疾病病因治疗（降糖、降压、营养支持、抗凝、纠正贫血、纠正酸碱失衡、控制感染等），中药内服。

2. 蚕食清创，控制性损伤，改良型 VSD。术中清创坏死组织，截除左足第 2、第 3、第 5 趾及第 2 跖骨，截除左足第 1 趾骨（图 7.6.2、图 7.6.3）。

3. 术后每天使用重组人碱性成纤维细胞生长因子加生理盐水 100 mL 冲洗创面 1 小时。

4. 创面达到植皮条件后予以全厚皮封闭创面，再予封闭负压引流术（植皮术后不冲管）。术后创面逐渐愈合（图 7.6.4、图 7.6.5）。

5. 保足尽量维持“铁三角”（足跟、第 1 跖骨、第 5 跖骨）行走功能的稳定性。

6. 住院时间 3 个月以上，家属及患者有保足强烈愿望。

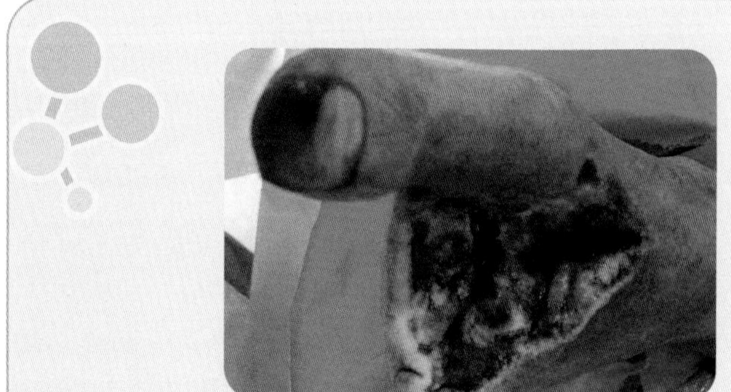

图 7.6.2　术中清创坏死组织，截除左足第 2、第 3、第 5 趾及第 2 跖骨

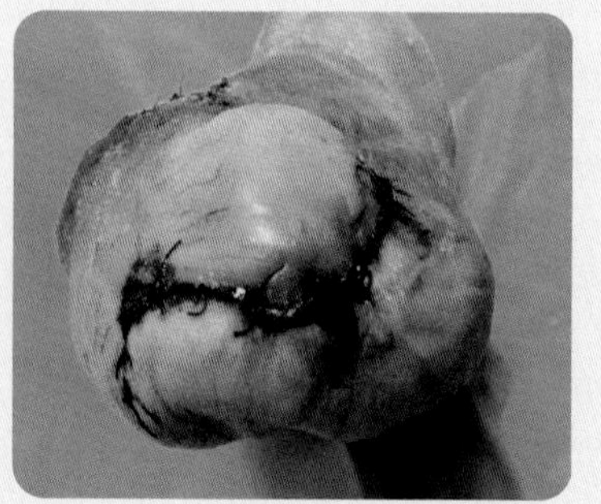

图 7.6.3　截除左足第 1 趾骨

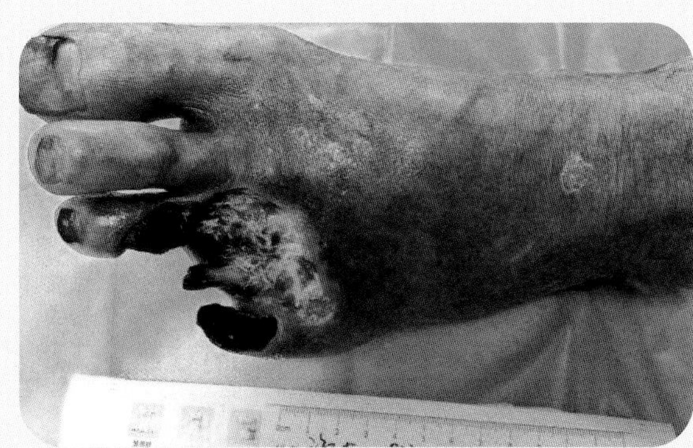

Figure 7.6.1 Preoperative blackening and ulceration of the third and fifth toes of the left foot, and absence of the fourth toe

◆ Treatment plan

1. Treatment of underlying diseases (lowering blood sugar, lowering blood pressure, nutritional support, anticoagulation, correcting anemia, correcting acid-base imbalance, controlling infections, etc.), taking traditional Chinese medicine orally.

2. Devouring debridement, controlling damage, and improving VSD. Intraoperative debridement of necrotic tissue, removal of the second, third, fifth toes, and second metatarsal bone of the left foot, and removal of the first toe bone of the left foot (Figure 7.6.2, Figure 7.6.3).

3. Rinse the wound with 100 mL of recombinant human basic fibroblast growth factor and physiological saline daily for 1 hour after surgery.

4. After the wound meets the conditions for skin grafting, full thickness skin will be used to seal the wound, followed by negative pressure drainage (without flushing the tube after skin grafting). The postoperative wound gradually healed (Figure 7.6.4, Figure 7.6.5).

5. Keep the stability of the walking function of the "iron triangle" (heel, 1st metatarsal, 5th metatarsal) as much as possible.

6. Hospitalization for more than 3 months, with strong desire from family members and patients to ensure adequate care.

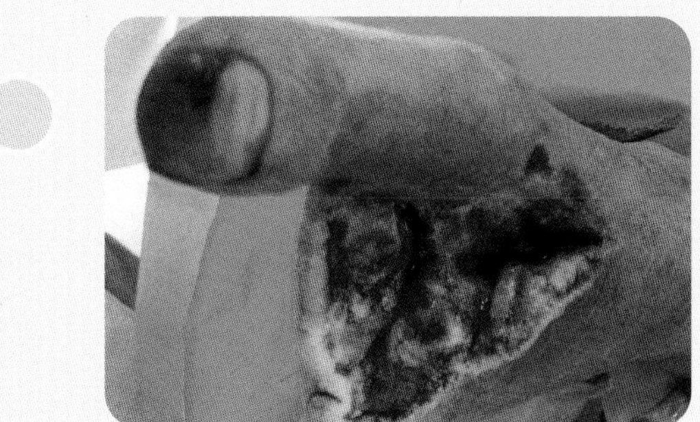

Figure 7.6.2 Intraoperative debridement of necrotic tissue, removal of left foot 2nd, 3rd, 5th toes and 2nd metatarsal bone

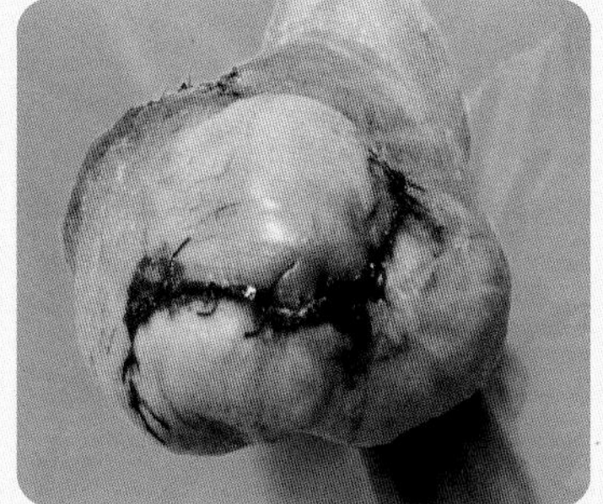

Figure 7.6.3 Removal of the first toe bone of the left foot

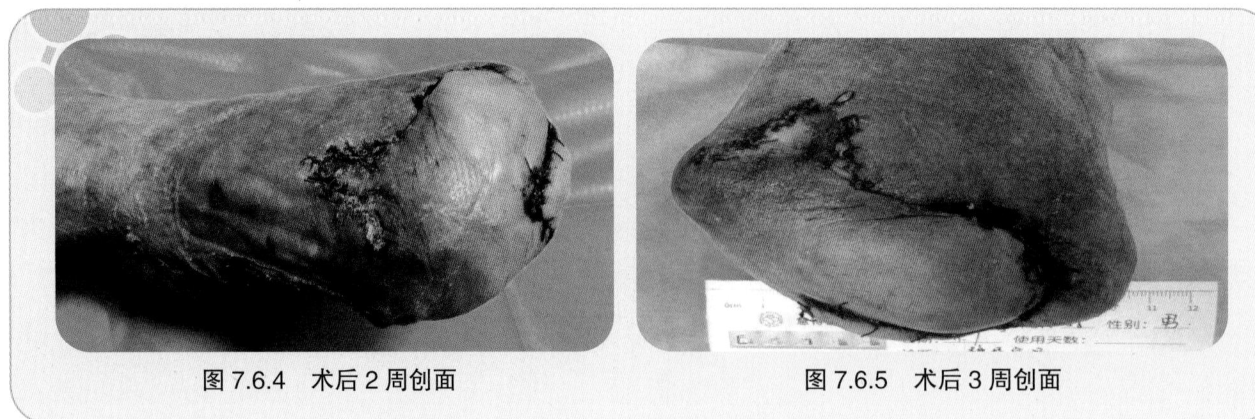

图 7.6.4　术后 2 周创面

图 7.6.5　术后 3 周创面

（陈启鹏　乐世文）

案例七　糖尿病足伴感染

◆ 致病原因

患者 2 型糖尿病病史 20 余年，右足外伤后红肿。

◆ 症状与体征

右足背大部红肿，面积约 14 cm × 9 cm，表面多发张力性水疱，破溃处见浑浊血性溢液，肤色紫暗，皮肤温度高，足背动脉触诊欠佳，末梢循环尚可，足背伸受限（图 7.7.1）。

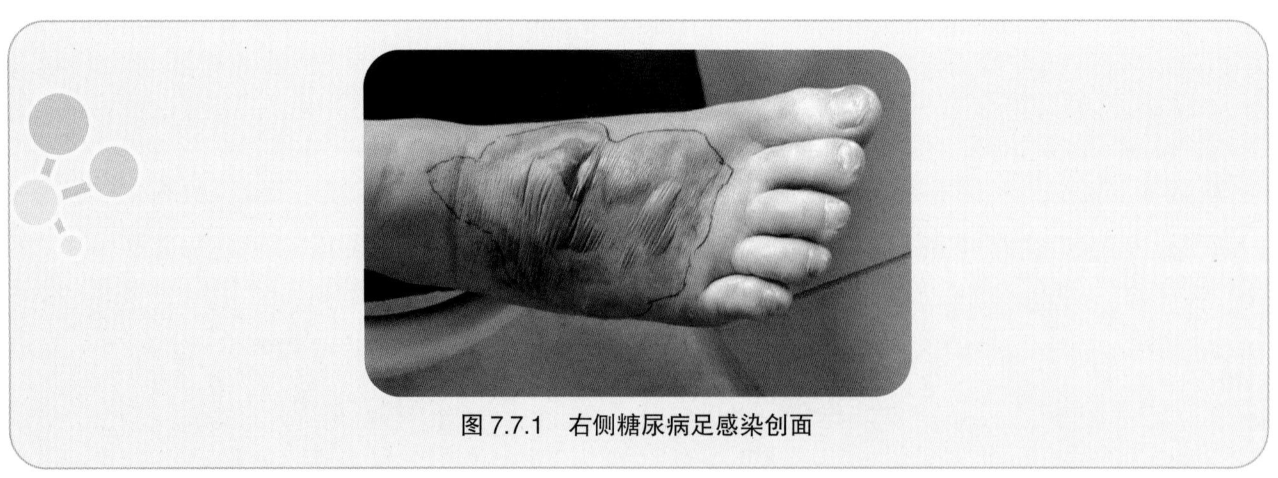

图 7.7.1　右侧糖尿病足感染创面

◆ 治疗方案

1. 评估创面、血管、神经，评估糖尿病并发症及胰岛功能。

2. 处理急性并发症和评价重要脏器功能，经验性抗生素应用；中医辨证，早期治则清热解毒、

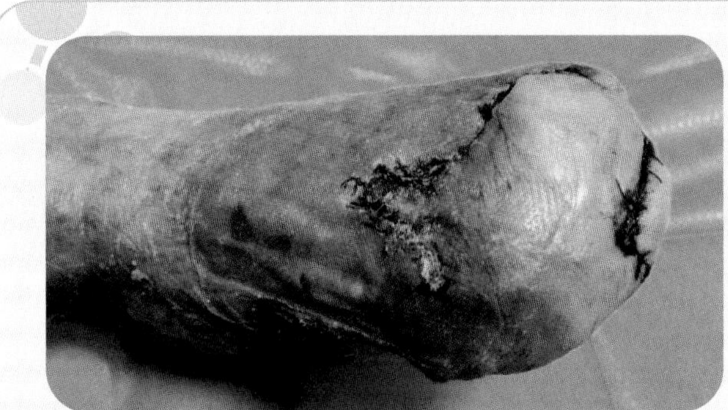

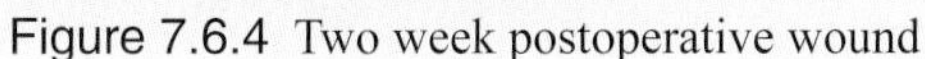

Figure 7.6.4 Two week postoperative wound

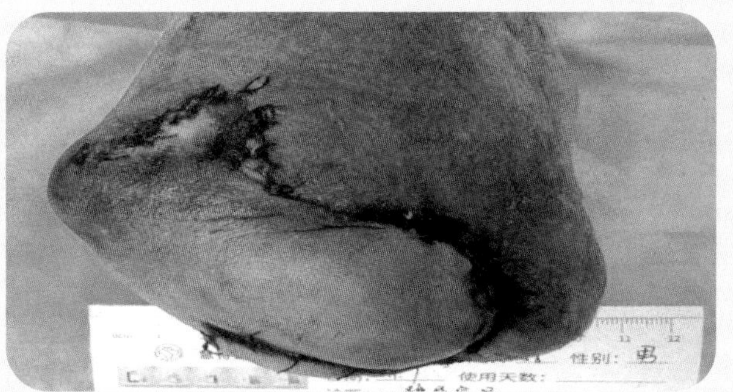

Figure 7.6.5 Three week postoperative wound

(Chen Qipeng, Le Shiwen)

Case 7 Diabetes foot with infection 

◆ Cause of illness

The patient had a history of type 2 diabetes for more than 20 years, and his right foot was red and swollen after trauma.

◆ Signs and symptoms

The right dorsum of the foot is mostly red and swollen, with an area of about 14 cm × 9 cm. There are multiple tension blisters on the surface, and turbid bloody discharge can be seen at the site of rupture. The skin color is dark purple, the skin temperature is high, and the palpation of the dorsalis pedis artery is poor. The peripheral circulation is still acceptable, but the dorsalis pedis extension is limited (Figure 7.7.1).

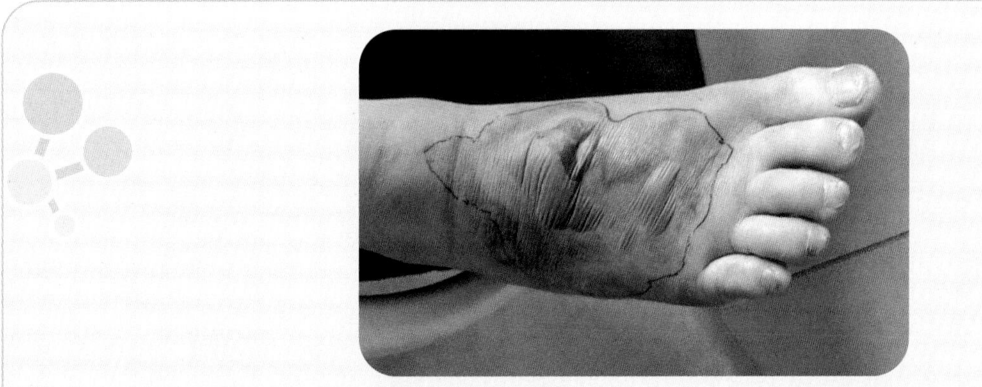

Figure 7.7.1 Infected wound of right diabetes foot

◆ Treatment plan

1. Evaluate the wound surface, blood vessels and nerves, and evaluate the complications of diabetes and pancreatic islet function.

2. Handling acute complications and evaluating important organ function, empirical use of antibiotics; In

除湿化瘀。

3. 早期清创切开、引流，细菌培养，目标是创面坏死区缩小、开放引流。

4. 蚕食清创 +VSD，感染控制后逐步降低抗生素强度。根据感染扩散方向，行卢氏切口清创、创面 VSD；清创后右足背创面 14 cm × 9 cm，趾背伸肌腱暴露（图 7.7.2、图 7.7.3）。

5. 腱周组织干枯变性，清创切除浅层坏死肌腱，人工真皮移植，采用人工真皮移植，生长因子 + 银离子敷料换药（图 7.7.4 ~ 图 7.7.6）。

6. 护理与康复：家庭延展换药、康复指导，2 个月创面愈合（图 7.7.7）。

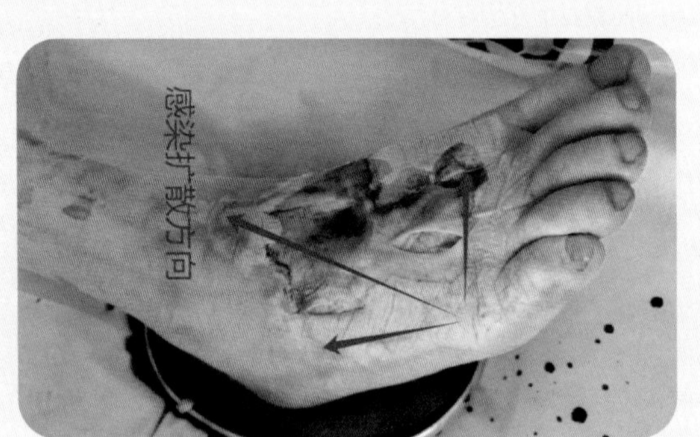

图 7.7.2 根据感染扩散方向，行卢氏切口清创、创面 VSD

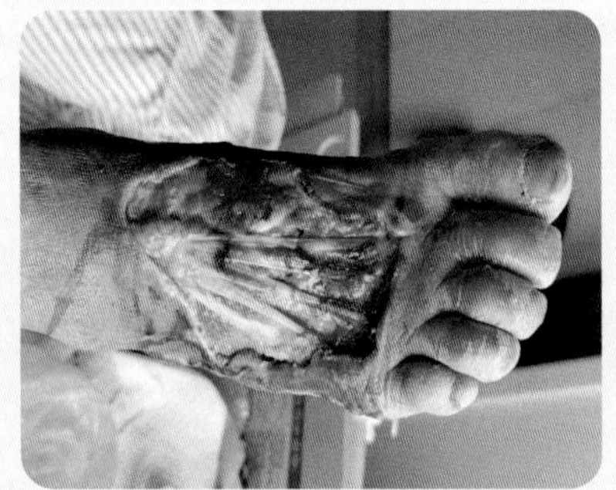
图 7.7.3 清创后右足背创面 14 cm × 9 cm，趾背伸肌腱暴露

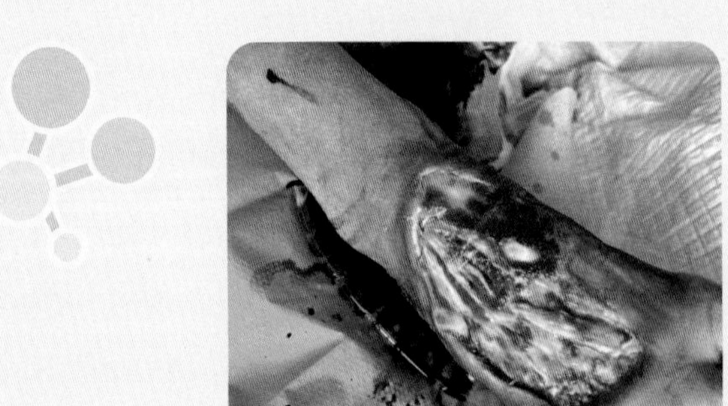
图 7.7.4 腱周组织干枯变性，清创切除浅层坏死肌腱，人工真皮移植

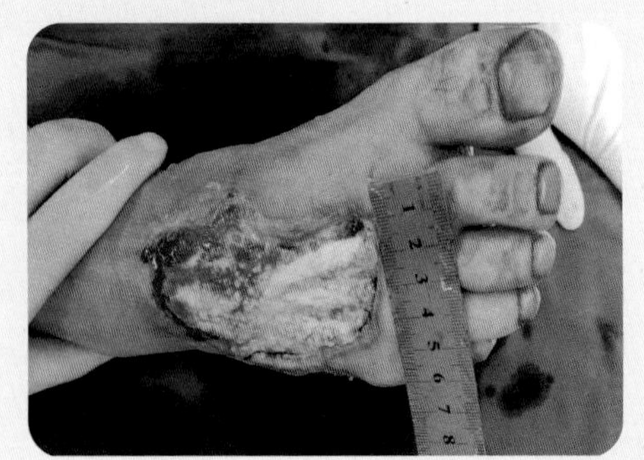
图 7.7.5 创面逐渐愈合

traditional Chinese medicine, early treatment involves clearing heat and detoxifying, removing dampness and removing blood stasis.

3. Early debridement, incision, drainage, bacterial culture, with the goal of reducing the necrotic area of the wound and opening drainage.

4. Consume debridement and VSD, gradually reduce antibiotic intensity after infection control. According to the direction of infection spread, perform Lu's incision debridement and VSD on the wound; After debridement, the wound on the back of the right foot was 14 cm × 9 cm, and the extensor tendon of the dorsal toe was exposed (Figure 7.7.2, Figure 7.7.3).

5. The peritendinous tissue became dry and degenerated, and superficial necrotic tendons were removed by debridement. Artificial dermis transplantation was performed, and growth factor+silver ion dressing was used for dressing change (Figure 7.7.4- Figure 7.7.6).

6. Nursing and Rehabilitation: Home extension dressing change, rehabilitation guidance, 2 months wound healing (Figure 7.7.7).

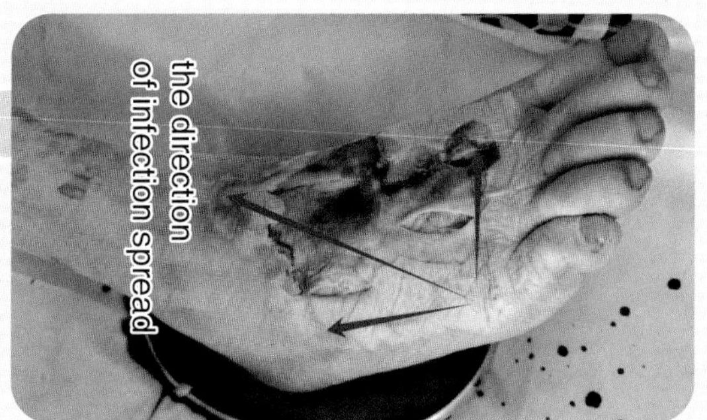

Figure 7.7.2 According to the direction of infection spread, perform wound debridement and VSD on the Lushi incision

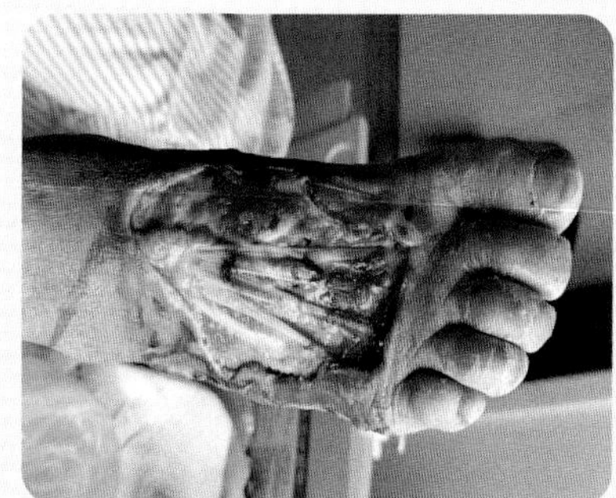

Figure 7.7.3 Right foot dorsal wound 14 cm × 9 cm after debridement, exposed extensor digitorum dorsi tendon

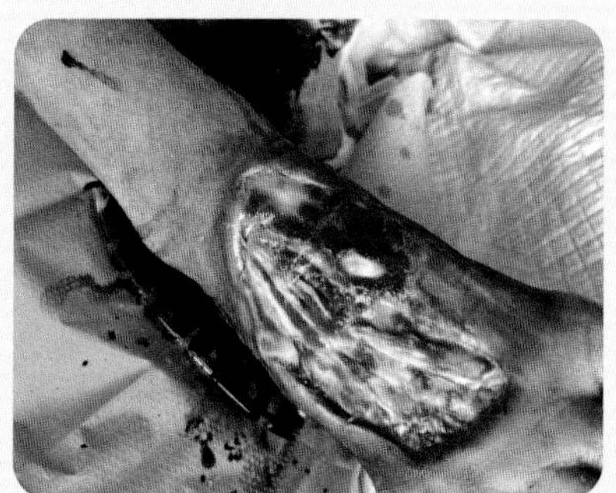

Figure 7.7.4 Dry and degenerated peritendinous tissue, debridement and resection of superficial necrotic tendons, and artificial dermal transplantation

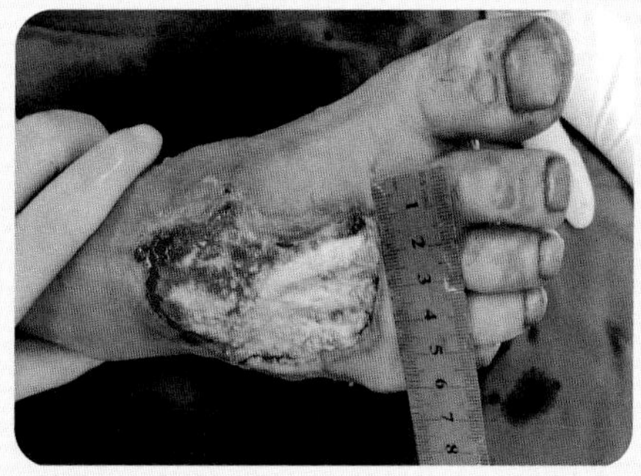

Figure 7.7.5 Gradual Healing of Wounds

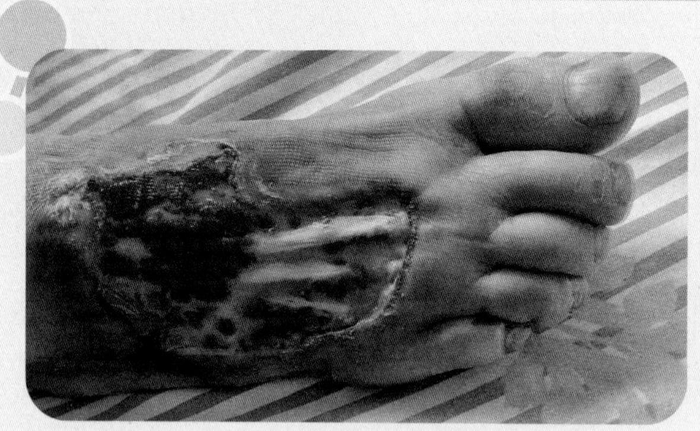
图 7.7.6　生长因子＋银离子敷料换药

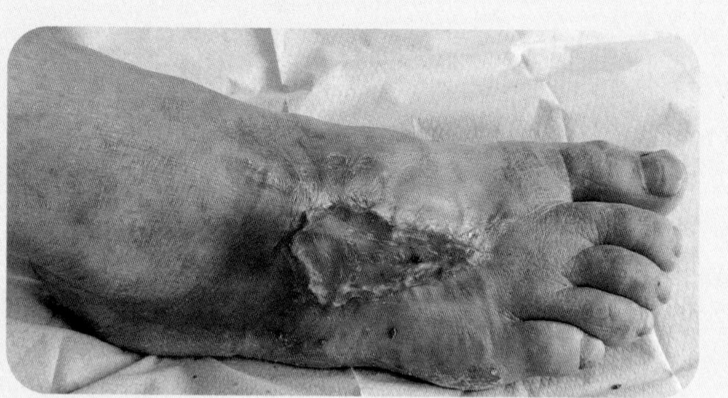
图 7.7.7　2 个月创面愈合

（王永高　王城磊）

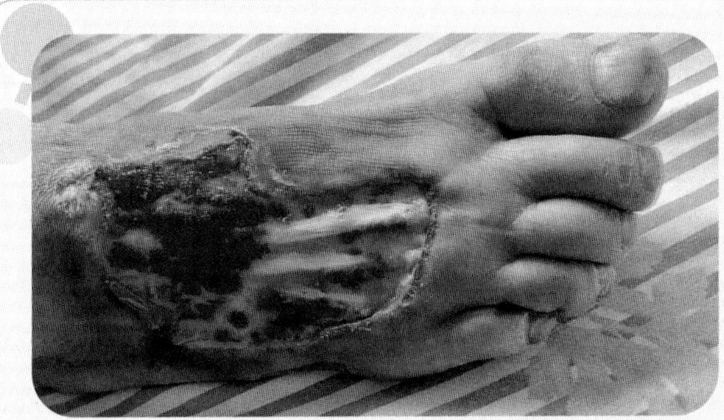

Figure 7.7.6 Growth factor + silver ion dressing dressing change

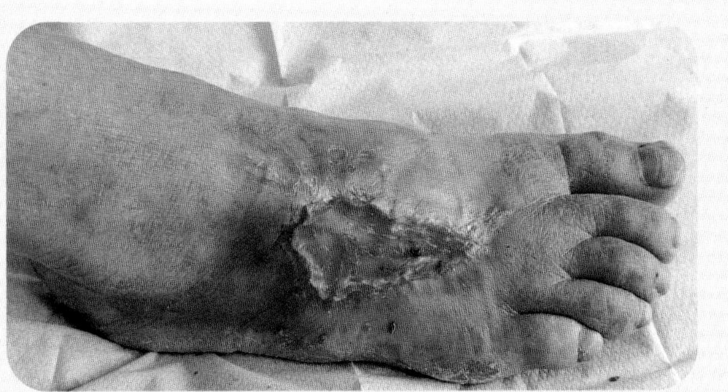

Figure 7.7.7 2 months wound healing

(Wang Yonggao, Wang Chenglei)

第 8 章
Chapter 8

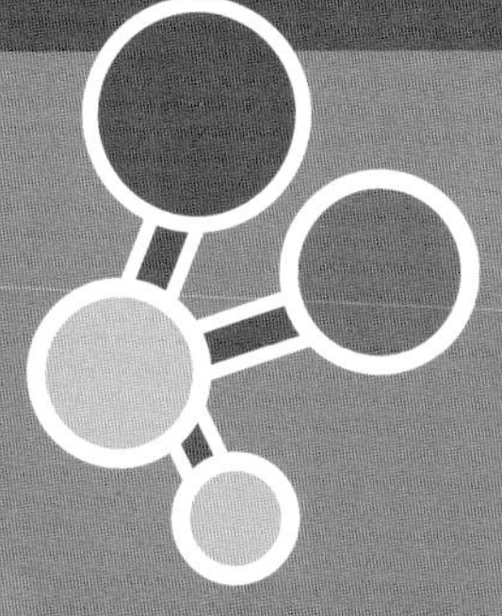

动脉性坏疽创面修复
Repair of Arterial Gangrene Wounds

案例一　双下肢动脉闭塞性脉管炎，双足坏死

◆ 致病原因

患者，男性，81 岁，长期吸烟饮酒，高血压病史 25 年，双下肢动脉闭塞性脉管炎，双足坏死。

◆ 症状与体征

双下肢间歇性疼痛跛行 5 年，夜间痛，肢体下垂疼痛缓解，疼痛时夜不能寐，口服曲马多片无缓解，双侧足趾发红，逐渐变黑坏死。左足从足踝远端变黑坏死，边界清楚，近端皮肤红肿明显，远端干瘪坏死，小腿中段以远端广泛性红肿，皮下有波动感，按压有大量稀薄发臭脓液顺着坏死边界流出，左侧膝关节以远端皮肤血液反流迟缓，皮温降低，腘动脉胫后动脉足背动脉波动消失，膝关节以下感觉减退，踝关节僵硬（图 8.1.1 ~ 图 8.1.3）。右足踝远端变黑坏死，远端有炎性渗出，皮下波动明显，坏死边界有脓性溢出，坏死边界不清晰，腘动脉、胫后动脉和足背动脉消失，小腿和足部皮肤发凉，血液反流迟缓，浅表静脉瘪陷（图 8.1.4）。

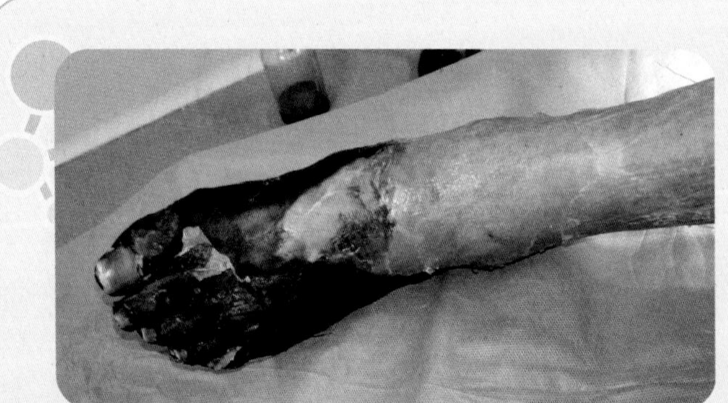
图 8.1.1　左足远端干瘪坏死，足踝远端红肿

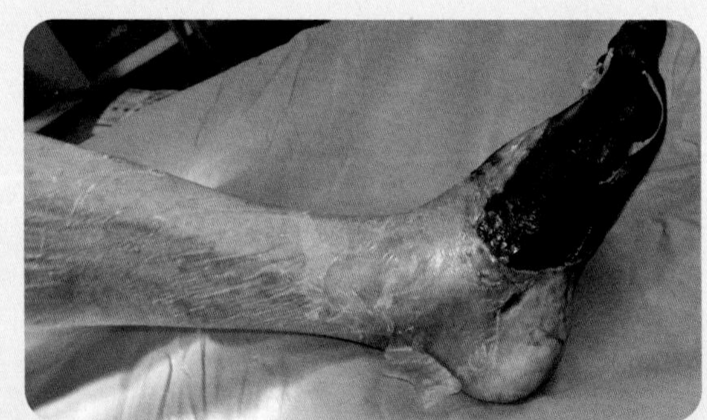
图 8.1.2　左小腿至足踝区皮下有波动，压之有稀薄脓液溢出

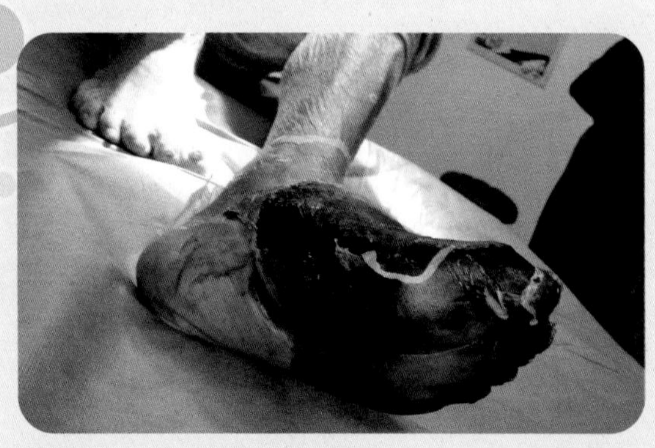
图 8.1.3　左足足底有脓液流出，中足远端坏死

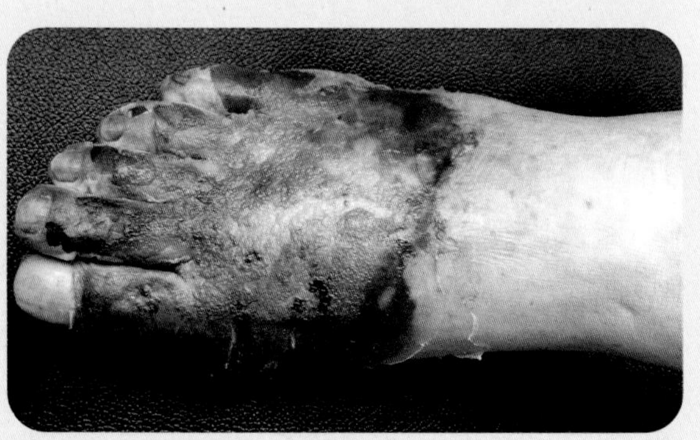
图 8.1.4　右足坏死，有湿性渗出

Case 1 Arterial occlusive vasculitis of both lower limbs, necrosis of both feet

◆ Cause of illness

The patient is an 81-year-old male who has been smoking and drinking for a long time. He has a history of hypertension for 25 years and has occlusive vasculitis in both lower limb arteries and necrosis in both feet.

◆ Signs and symptoms

Intermittent pain in both lower limbs, claudication for 5 years, nighttime pain, relief of limb sagging pain, insomnia during pain, no relief from oral tramadol tablets, redness of both toes, gradually turning black and necrotic. The left foot turns black and necrotic from the distal end of the ankle, with clear boundaries. The proximal skin is visibly red and swollen, while the distal end is dry and necrotic. The middle of the calf is extensively red and swollen from the distal end, with a wave like sensation under the skin. When pressed, a large amount of thin, foul smelling pus flows out along the necrotic boundary. The blood reflux of the skin at the distal end of the left knee joint is delayed, the skin temperature decreases, the fluctuation of the posterior tibial artery of the popliteal artery disappears, the sensation below the knee joint decreases, and the ankle joint becomes stiff (Figure 8.1.1-Figure 8.1.3). The distal end of the right ankle has turned black and necrotic, with inflammatory exudate and obvious subcutaneous fluctuations. There is purulent overflow at the necrotic boundary, and the necrotic boundary is unclear. The popliteal artery, posterior tibial artery, and dorsalis pedis artery have disappeared, and the skin of the calf and foot has become cold. Blood reflux is slow, and the superficial veins are sunken (Figure 8.1.4).

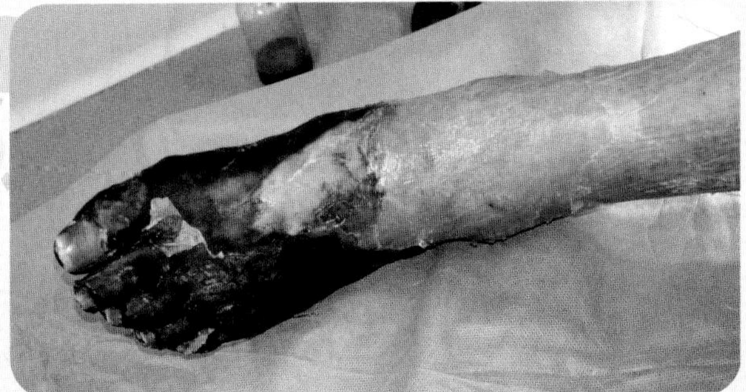

Figure 8.1.1 The distal end of the left foot is withered and necrotic, while the distal end of the ankle is red and swollen

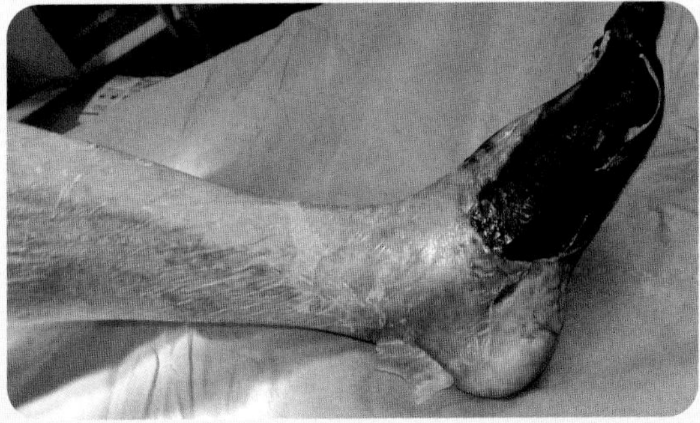

Figure 8.1.2 Subcutaneous fluctuations from the left calf to the ankle area, with thin pus overflowing under pressure

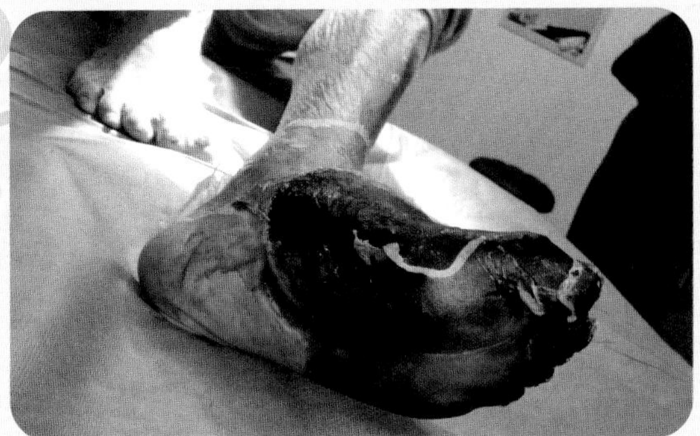

Figure 8.1.3 Purulent discharge from the sole of the left foot and necrosis of the distal midfoot

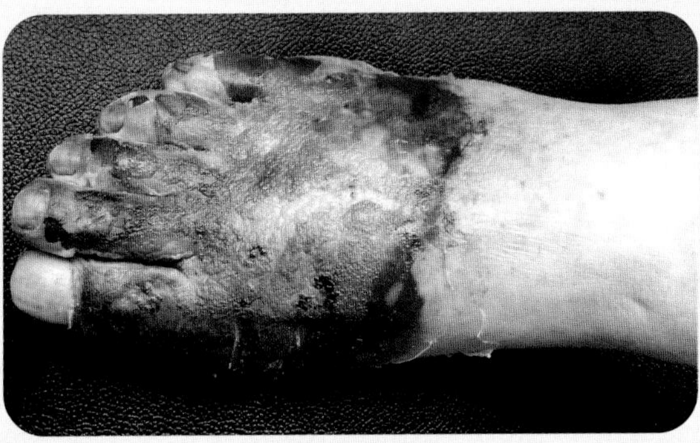

Figure 8.1.4 Right foot necrosis with wet exudation

◆ 治疗方案

1. 完善入院检查

1.1 下肢计算机体层血管成像（CTA）和超声检查，示髂外髂总动脉股动脉以远端广泛性完全闭塞并形成血栓，侧支循环建立不充分。肺部 CT、超声心电图检查，示心肺功能不全，伴有心包积液。

1.2 实验室检查：白细胞计数 9.3×10^9/L，血浆 D- 二聚体 1.3 μg/mL，尿酸 728 μmol/L，肌酐 263 μmol/L，总蛋白 56.8 g/L、白蛋白 35 g/L、β2 微球蛋白 3.9 mg/L，B 型钠尿肽 524.1 pg/mL，空腹血糖 6.61 mmol/L。

2. 入院后发起 MDT 会诊，纠正心肺功能不全，改善生命体征。

3. 调整全身状况后，于全麻下行高位截肢。伤口完全康复后，送回福利院康养（图 8.1.5、图 8.1.6）。

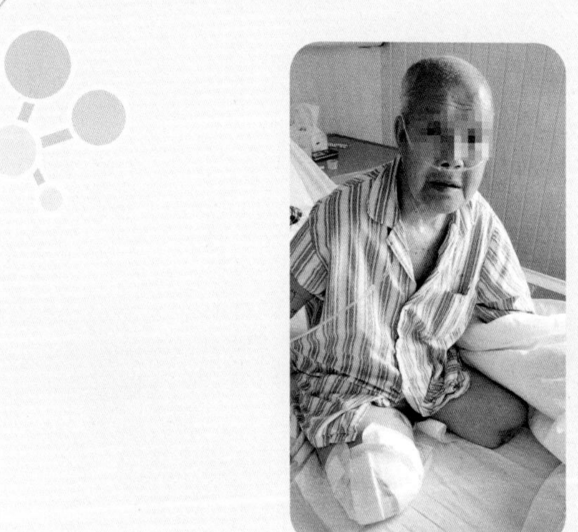

图 8.1.5　双大腿段高位截肢

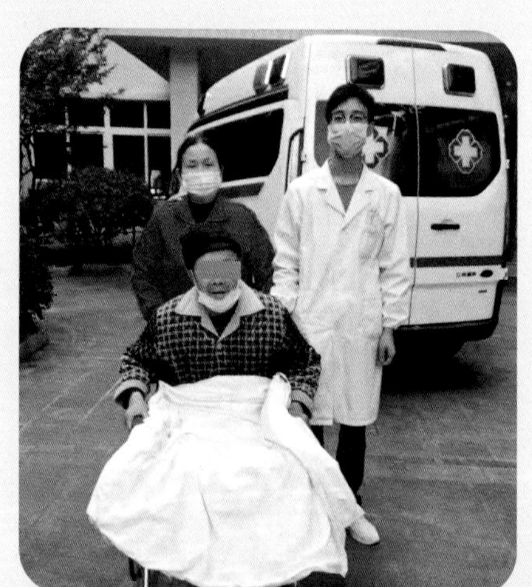

图 8.1.6　高位截肢后康复出院，送回养老院

（陈善亮）

案例二　左下肢大动脉闭塞合并长段骨外露

◆ 致病原因

患者，男性，78 岁，左下肢大动脉闭塞性脉管炎，合并长段骨外露。

◆ 症状和体征

患者为独居老人，左小腿、左足疼痛半年，抬高患肢疼痛加重、下垂后疼痛缓解。夜间疼痛加重，之后足趾逐渐变黑并向小腿蔓延坏死，足部和小腿皮肤肌肉组织开始腐烂脱落，自己用水果刀将坏死组织刮除，用旧衣布包扎伤口，未去医院治疗。端坐呼吸，呼吸急促，左足踝远端缺失，小腿中段远端皮肤缺损，

◆ Treatment plan

1. Improve admission examinations

1.1 Lower limb computed tomography angiography (CTA) and ultrasound examination showed extensive complete occlusion and thrombus formation in the distal end of the common iliac artery and femoral artery, with insufficient collateral circulation. Pulmonary CT and ultrasound electrocardiogram examination showed cardiopulmonary dysfunction, accompanied by pericardial effusion.

1.2 Laboratory examination: White blood cell count 9.3×10^9/L, plasma D-dimer 1.3 μg/mL, uric acid 728 μmol/L, creatinine 263 μmol/L, total protein 56.8 g/L, albumin 35 g/L, β2-microglobulin 3.9 mg/L, B-type natriuretic peptide 524.1 pg/mL, fasting blood glucose 6.61 mmol/L.

2. Initiate MDT consultation after admission to correct cardiopulmonary dysfunction and improve vital signs.

3. After adjusting the overall condition, perform high-level amputation under general anesthesia. After the wound fully recovers, it will be sent back to the welfare home for rehabilitation(Figure 8.1.5,Figure 8.1.6).

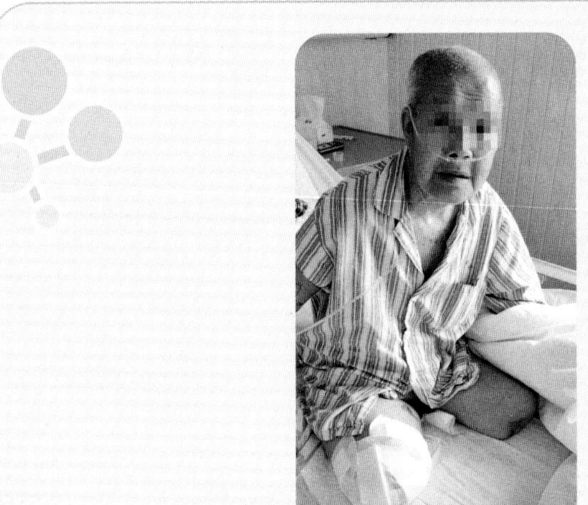

Figure 8.1.5 High amputation of both thigh segments

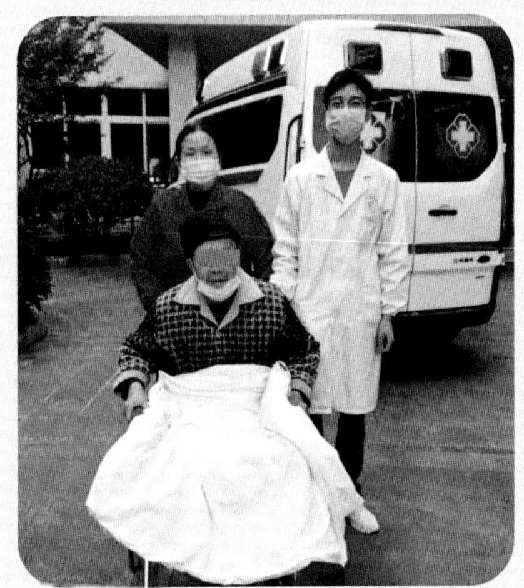

Figure 8.1.6 Rehabilitation and discharge after high amputation, sent back to welfare home

(Chen Shanliang)

Case 2 Left lower limb arterial occlusion with long segment bone exposure

◆ Cause of illness

Patient, male, 78 years old, with left lower limb arterial occlusive vasculitis and long segment bone exposure.

◆ Signs and symptoms

The patient is an elderly person living alone, with pain in the left calf and left foot for six months. The pain worsened when the affected limb was raised, and after sagging, the pain was relieved. The pain worsened at night, and then the toes gradually turned black and spread to the calves, causing necrosis. The skin and muscle tissues of the feet and calves began to rot and fall off. I used a fruit knife to scrape off the necrotic tissue and wrapped the wound with old clothing, but did not seek medical treatment. Sitting upright breathing, rapid breathing, missing

胫骨腓骨外露，皮肤软组织红肿，有大量脓性分泌物，创面布满蛆虫，味恶臭（图 8.2.1、图 8.2.2）。左膝关节屈曲僵硬。髂腹股沟区腘窝区动脉搏动消失。浅表腹股沟淋巴结肿大，压痛。右侧小腿至足踝部有大面积色沉，局部皮肤纤维化增厚，足背动脉搏动减弱，反流迟缓。足趾屈伸活动良好，感觉良好。

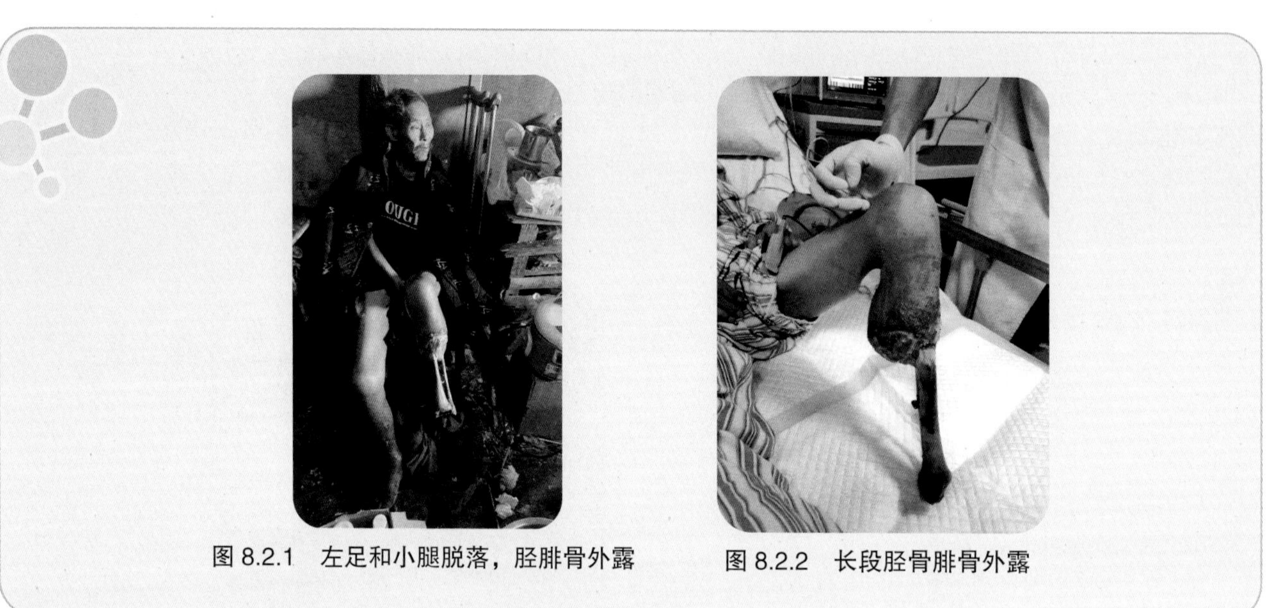

图 8.2.1　左足和小腿脱落，胫腓骨外露　　图 8.2.2　长段胫骨腓骨外露

◆ 治疗方案

由于有着严重心肺功能衰竭，积极治疗原发病，纠正心肺功能衰竭，加强基础护理，抗感染治疗，吸氧，雾化吸入纠正咳喘，促进排痰，导尿留置。

1. 完善入院检查

1.1 实验室检查: 血常规，白细胞计数 23.1×10^9/L、中性粒细胞计数 22.3×10^9/L、C- 反应蛋白 114.6 mg/L、超敏 C- 反应蛋白 5 mg/L、血红蛋白 106 g/L；血气分析，血糖 9.1 mmol/L，全血乳酸 2.04 mmol/L、碳酸氢根 31.1 mmol/L、二氧化碳分压 58.6 mmHg、D- 二聚体 1.5 μg/mL、白蛋白 26 g/L、乳酸脱氢酶 247 IU/L、肌酸激酶 968 IU/L、尿素氮 11.14 mmol/L、尿酸 449 μmol/L、B 型钠尿肽 35 000 pg/mL。

1.2 超声检查：左侧下肢髂总股动脉长段闭塞并由血栓形成，内膜增厚，无血流通过，全心增大，心包积液，三尖瓣中度反流，二尖瓣主动脉瓣反流，胸腔腹腔大量积液。

1.3 心电图：S-T 段改变、心肌缺血房室传导阻滞，心律失常改变。

1.4 肺部 CT：肺部大面积纤维钙化，两肺间质性肺炎，心影明显增大，烧杯样改变、心包积液。

2. 小腿脓性分泌物细菌培养 + 药物敏感试验，局部清创，驱除腐肉和蛆虫。伤口包扎换药为主，患者

distal left ankle, skin defect in the distal middle of the calf, exposed tibia and fibula, redness and swelling of skin and soft tissue, large amount of purulent secretion, wound covered with maggots, and foul odor (Figure 8.2.1, Figure 8.2.2). Left knee joint flexes and becomes stiff. The arterial pulsation in the iliac inguinal region and popliteal fossa area disappears. Swelling and tenderness of superficial inguinal lymph nodes. There is a large area of discoloration from the right calf to the ankle, local skin fibrosis and thickening, weakened dorsalis pedis artery pulsation, and delayed reflux. Good toe flexion and extension activity, feeling good.

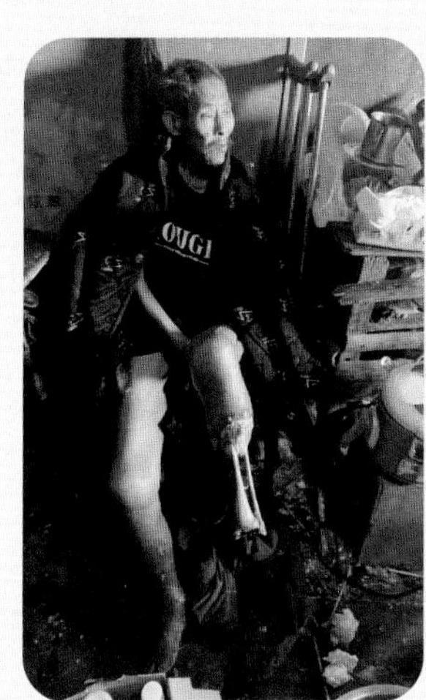

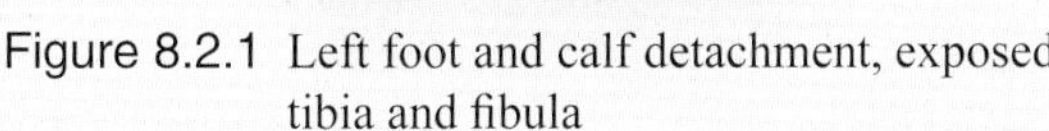

Figure 8.2.1 Left foot and calf detachment, exposed tibia and fibula

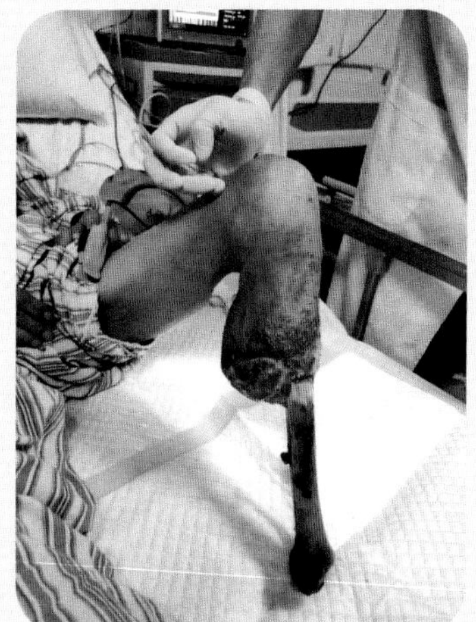

Figure 8.2.2 Long segment exposed tibia and fibula

◆ Treatment plan

Due to severe heart and lung failure, actively treating the primary disease, correcting heart and lung failure, strengthening basic nursing, anti infection treatment, oxygen therapy, nebulization inhalation to correct cough and asthma, promoting sputum discharge, and catheterization retention.

1. Improve admission examinations

1.1 Laboratory examination: blood routine, white blood cell count 23.1 × 10^9/L, neutrophil count 22.3 × 10^9/L, C-reactive protein 114.6 mg/L, high-sensitivity C-reactive protein 5 mg/L, hemoglobin 106 g/L; Blood gas analysis showed blood glucose at 9.1 mmol/L, whole blood lactate at 2.04 mmol/L, bicarbonate at 31.1 mmol/L, partial pressure of carbon dioxide at 58.6 mmHg, D-dimer at 1.5 μg/mL, albumin at 26 g/L, lactate dehydrogenase at 247 IU/L, creatine kinase at 968 IU/L, urea nitrogen at 11.14 mmol/L, uric acid at 449 μmol/L, and B-type natriuretic peptide at 35 000 pg/mL.

1.2 Ultrasound examination: Long segment occlusion of the common iliac and femoral artery in the left lower limb with thrombus formation, thickening of the endometrium, no blood flow passing through, enlargement of the entire heart, pericardial effusion, moderate tricuspid regurgitation, mitral and aortic regurgitation, and significant pleural and peritoneal effusion.

1.3 Electrocardiogram: S-T segment changes, myocardial ischemia atrioventricular block, arrhythmia changes.

1.4 Pulmonary CT: Large area fibrocalcifications in the lungs, interstitial pneumonia in both lungs, significant enlargement of the heart shadow, beaker like changes, pericardial effusion.

2. Bacterial culture and drug sensitivity test for purulent discharge from the calf, local debridement, and removal of carrion and maggots. The main focus is on wound dressing and dressing changes. For elderly people

为孤寡老人，对其发起医疗救助，每天精心护理，纠正多脏器衰竭为主（图 8.2.3 ～图 8.2.5）。

3. 小剂量输入白蛋白和红细胞悬液，纠正低蛋白血症和贫血，提高免疫力。

4. 心肺功能纠正后，各项化验指标明显改善。全麻下行清创，胫骨腓骨截除，局部转移皮瓣覆盖创面，伤口深部放置负压引流管。

5. 术后 48 小时拔出引流管，2 周拆线，康复出院。

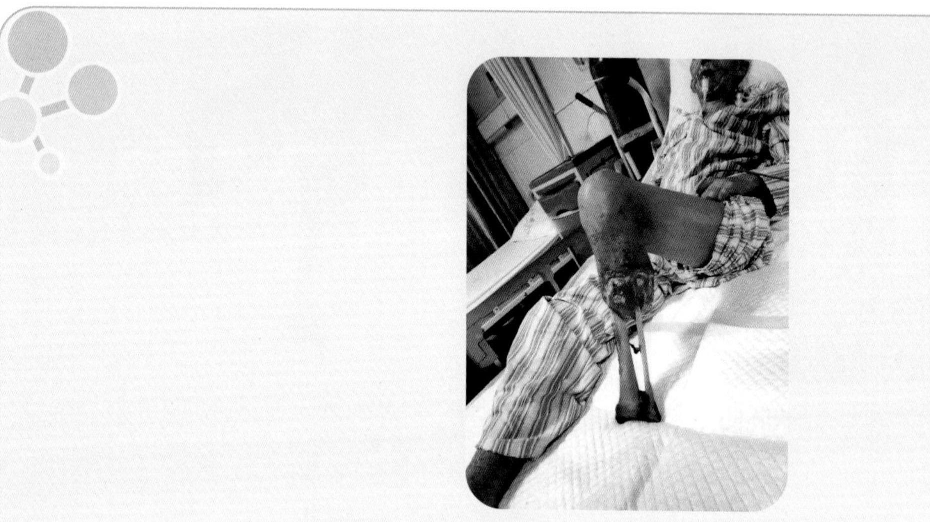

图 8.2.3　全身多脏器衰竭继发严重感染，创面每天换药为主

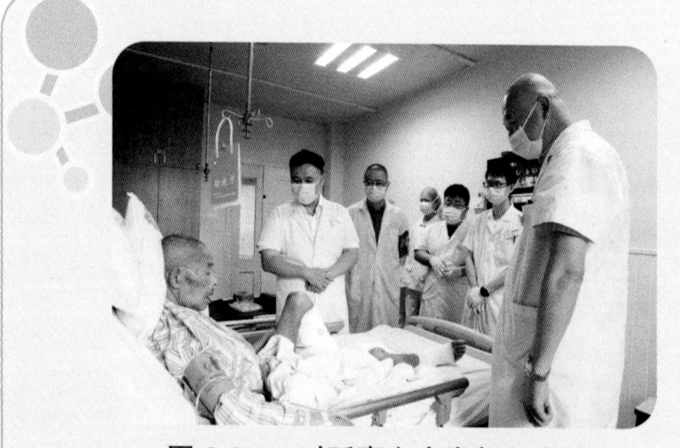

图 8.2.4　对孤寡老人发起医疗救助

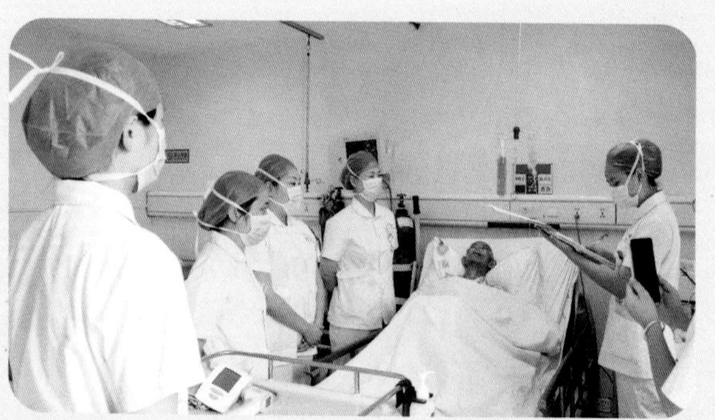

图 8.2.5　每天精心护理，纠正多脏器衰竭为主

（陈善亮）

living alone, medical assistance should be initiated, and meticulous care should be taken every day to correct multiple organ failure (Figure 8.2.3 - Figure 8.2.5).

3. Low dose administration of albumin and red blood cell suspension can correct hypoalbuminemia and anemia, and enhance immunity.

4. After the correction of cardiopulmonary function, various laboratory indicators improved significantly. Under general anesthesia, debridement was performed, the tibia and fibula were removed, and a local transfer skin flap was used to cover the wound. Negative pressure drainage was placed in the deep part of the wound.

5. Drainage was removed 48 hours after surgery, stitches were removed 2 weeks later, and the patient recovered and was discharged from the hospital.

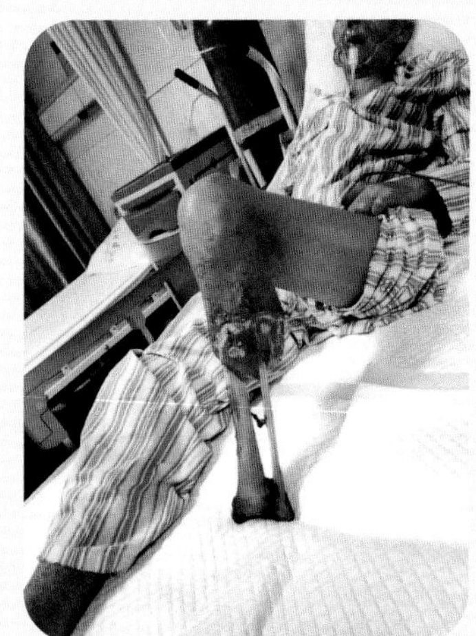

Figure 8.2.3 Severe infection triggered by systemic multiple organ failure, with daily dressing changes mainly on the wound surface

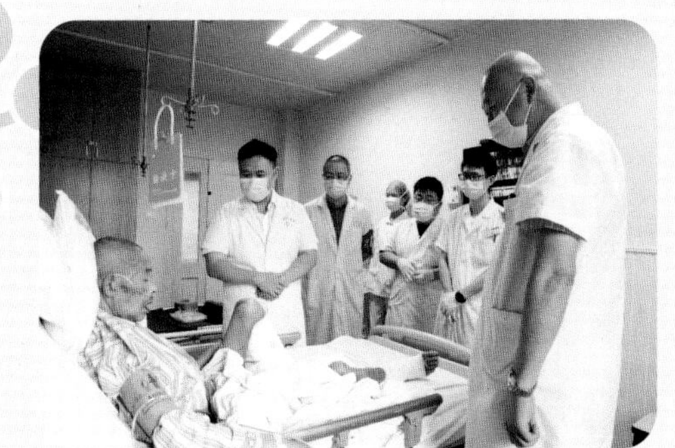

Figure 8.2.4 Initiate medical assistance for lonely and widowed elderly people

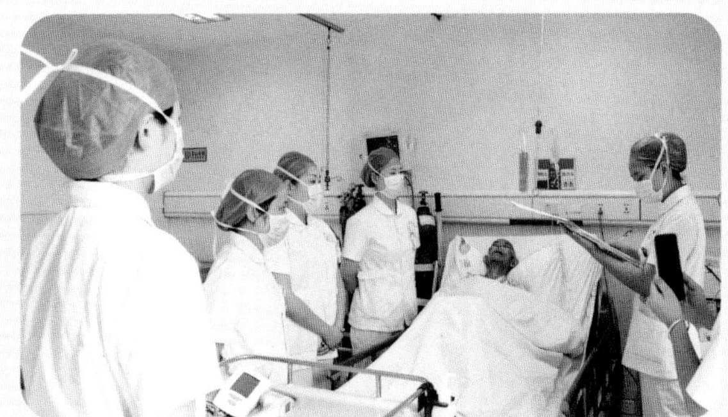

Figure 8.2.5 Daily meticulous care, focusing on correcting multiple organ failure

(Chen Shanliang)

案例三　急性下肢动脉栓塞序贯多器官功能衰竭合并下肢坏死性创面

◆ 致病原因

患者急性下肢动脉栓塞，血管介入开通后并发再灌注损伤、下肢骨筋膜室综合征、左小腿坏死性筋膜炎，导致双下肢坏死、感染，形成巨大创面，同时伴急性肺炎，2 型糖尿病伴肾性高血压、糖尿病性肾病；合并社区获得性肺炎伴胸腔积液、心功能Ⅳ级、呼吸性碱中毒、肝功能异常、低蛋白血症。

◆ 症状与体征

双膝以下皮温低、皮肤苍白花斑，双侧足背动脉搏动不可及，双侧小腿肿胀明显，双侧足趾多处发黑，触痛不明显。双侧足趾处皮肤发黑，双小腿可见水疱局部渗出。双下肢坏死，瘀斑，双下肢肿胀疼痛，下肢骨筋膜室综合征、感染加重、急性脑梗死，髂腰肌、腰大肌血肿，消化道出血，痂下感染（图 8.3.1 ~图 8.3.4）。

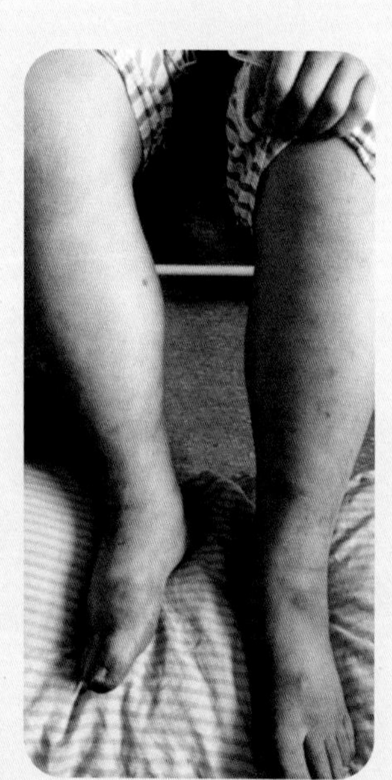

图 8.3.1　双下肢疼痛、肿胀，瘀斑

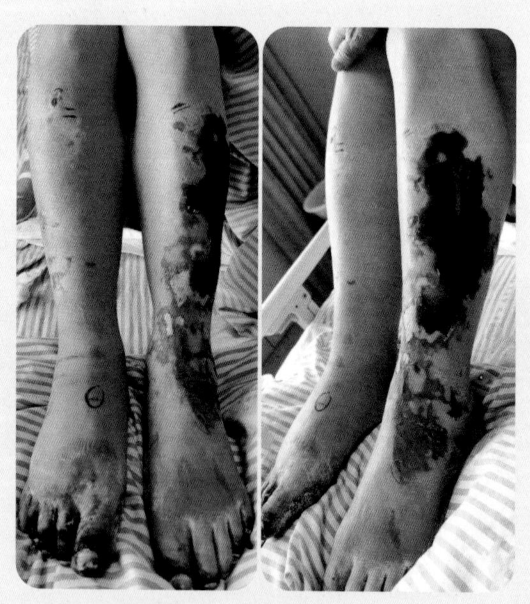

图 8.3.2　双下肢坏死

Case 3 Sequential multiple organ failure with lower limb necrotic wound caused by acute lower limb arterial embolism

◆ Cause of illness

The patient suffered from acute lower limb arterial embolism, followed by reperfusion injury, lower limb osteofascial compartment syndrome and left lower leg necrotizing fasciitis after vascular intervention was opened, resulting in necrosis and infection of both lower limbs, forming huge wounds, accompanied by acute pneumonia, type 2 diabetes with renal hypertension and diabetes nephropathy; Merge community-acquired pneumonia with pleural effusion, grade IV cardiac function, respiratory alkalosis, abnormal liver function, and hypoalbuminemia.

◆ Signs and symptoms

Low skin temperature below the knees, pale and spotted skin, unreachable pulsation of bilateral dorsalis pedis arteries, significant swelling of bilateral calves, multiple blackened areas of bilateral toes, and no obvious tenderness. The skin on both toes is blackened, and blisters can be seen locally oozing from both calves. Necrosis and bruising of both lower limbs, swelling and pain in both lower limbs, lower limb compartment syndrome, worsening of infection, acute cerebral infarction, iliopsoas and psoas muscle hematoma, gastrointestinal bleeding, and subcar infection (Figure 8.3.1 - Figure 8.3.4).

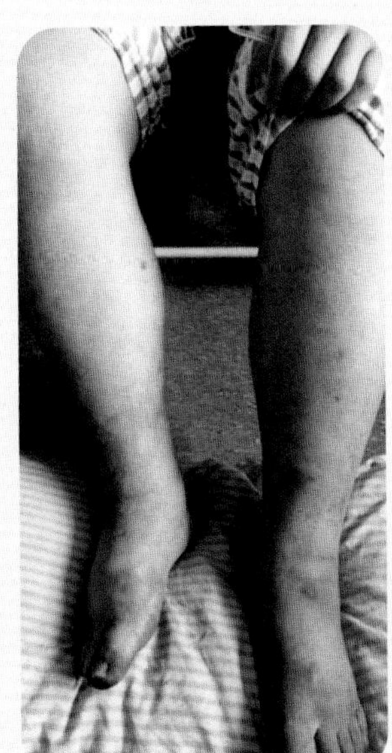

Figure 8.3.1 Pain, swelling, and bruising in both lower limbs

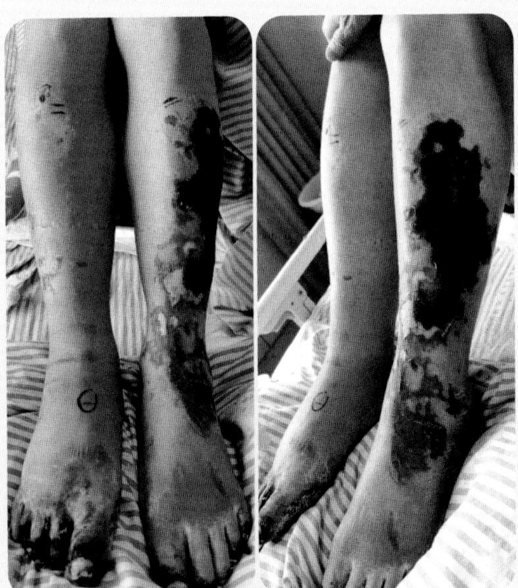

Figure 8.3.2 Necrosis of both lower limbs

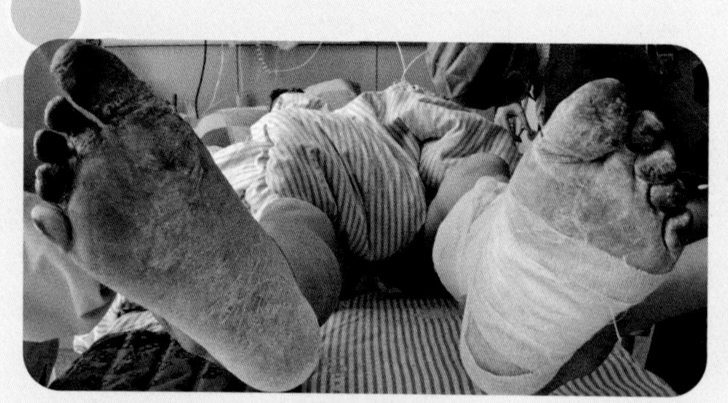
图 8.3.3 双下肢肿胀疼痛，合并多种疾病

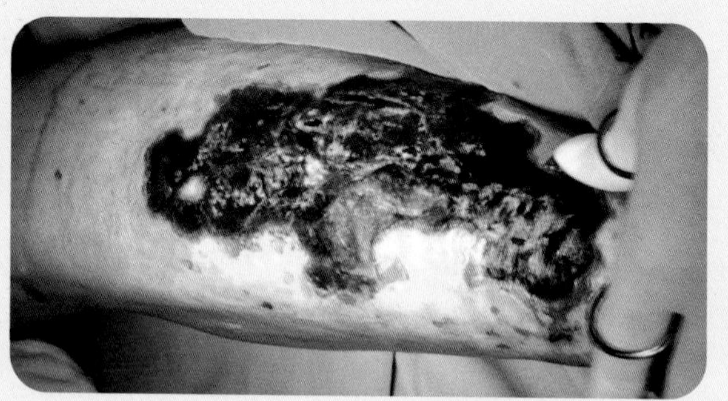
图 8.3.4 痂下感染

◆ 治疗方案

患者来自疫区，急性病容，病情复杂、危重、基础疾病多，患急性肺炎、糖尿病肾病，并发急性双下肢动脉栓塞入院，术后并发下肢骨筋膜室综合征、坏死性筋膜炎，多脏器功能衰竭，下肢大面积坏死。

1. 中西医 MDT 多次讨论，先排除新型冠状病毒性肺炎，急诊介入取栓术 + 抗凝治疗，同时治疗基础疾病。

2. 因并发脑出血、消化道出血、髂腰肌血肿，停用抗凝药，并输血、营养支持。

3. 左小腿坏死性筋膜炎、深筋膜室感染，左小腿胫骨前肌、腓骨长肌坏死，细菌培养为肺炎克雷伯菌，仅替加环素敏感。多次清创、换药、VSD，并抗感染治疗（图 8.3.5）。

4. 创面修复采取拉杆式闭合器辅助皮瓣转移术（图 8.3.6）。

5. 创面组织缺损大，病程漫长达 3 月余（图 8.3.7）。

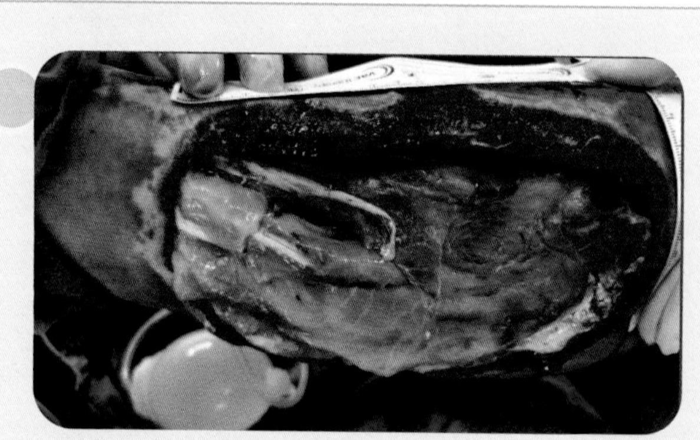
图 8.3.5 切痂清创术

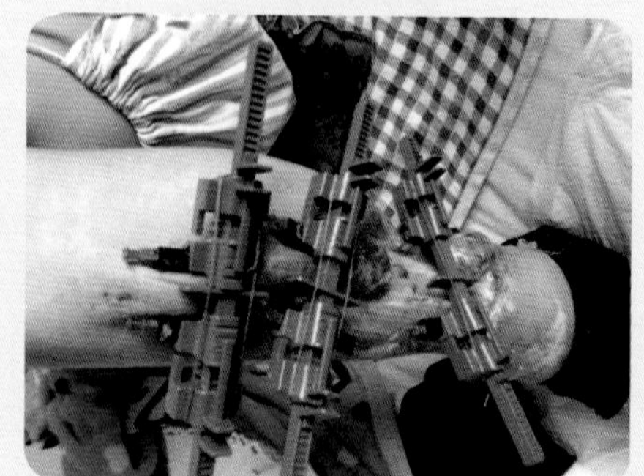
图 8.3.6 拉杆式闭合器及皮瓣转移术

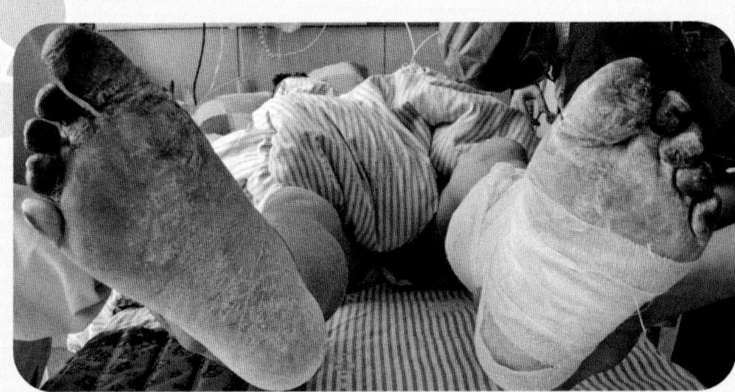

Figure 8.3.3 Swelling and pain in both lower limbs, combined with multiple diseases

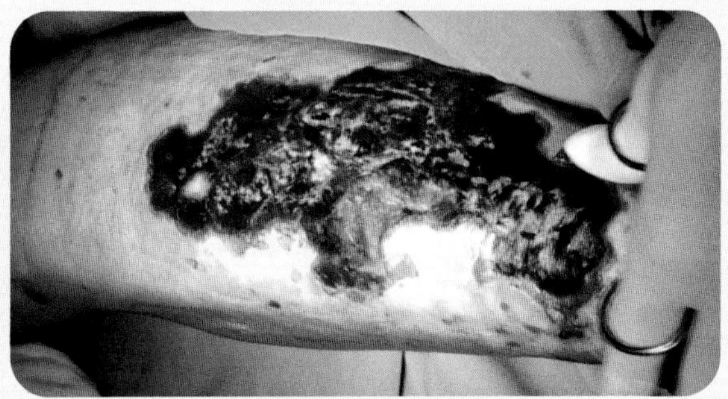

Figure 8.3.4 Subcrustal infection

◆ Treatment plan

The patient came from the epidemic area with acute appearance, complicated condition, critical condition, and many basic diseases. He suffered from acute pneumonia, diabetes nephropathy, and was admitted with acute arterial embolism of both lower extremities. After surgery, he was complicated with osteofascial compartment syndrome of lower extremities, necrotizing fasciitis, multiple organ failure, and massive necrosis of lower extremities.

1. MDT of traditional Chinese medicine and western medicine has been discussed for many times. First, novel coronavirus pneumonia was excluded, and emergency intervention embolectomy+anticoagulation treatment was performed, while basic diseases were treated.

2. Due to concurrent cerebral hemorrhage, gastrointestinal bleeding, and iliopsoas hematoma, anticoagulants were discontinued and blood transfusion and nutritional support were provided.

3. Necrotizing fasciitis and deep fascial compartment infection in the left calf, necrosis of the tibialis anterior muscle and peroneal longus muscle in the left calf, bacterial culture for Klebsiella pneumoniae, only sensitive to tetracycline. Multiple debridement, dressing changes, VSD, and anti infective treatment (Figure 8.3.5).

4. The wound repair adopts a pull rod closure device assisted flap transfer surgery (Figure 8.3.6).

5. The wound tissue defect is large, and the disease course is long for more than 3 months (Figure 8.3.7).

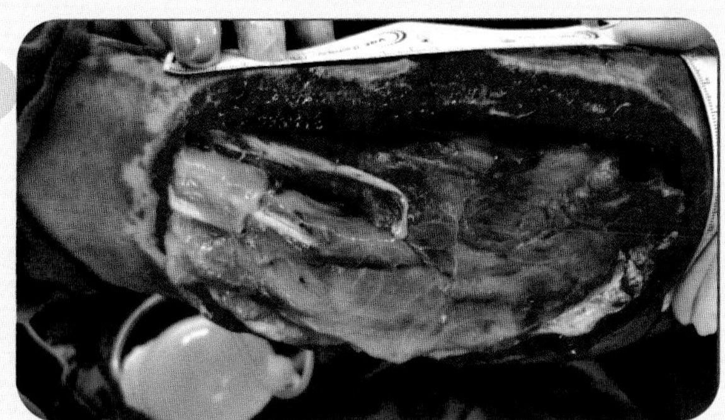

Figure 8.3.5 Keratotomy and debridement surgery

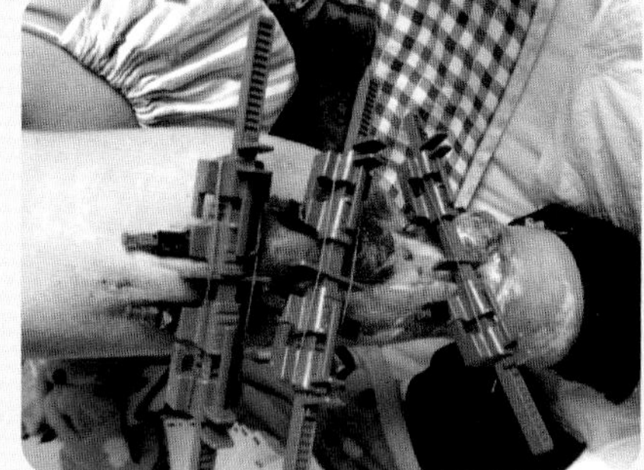

Figure 8.3.6 Pull rod closure device and flap transfer surgery

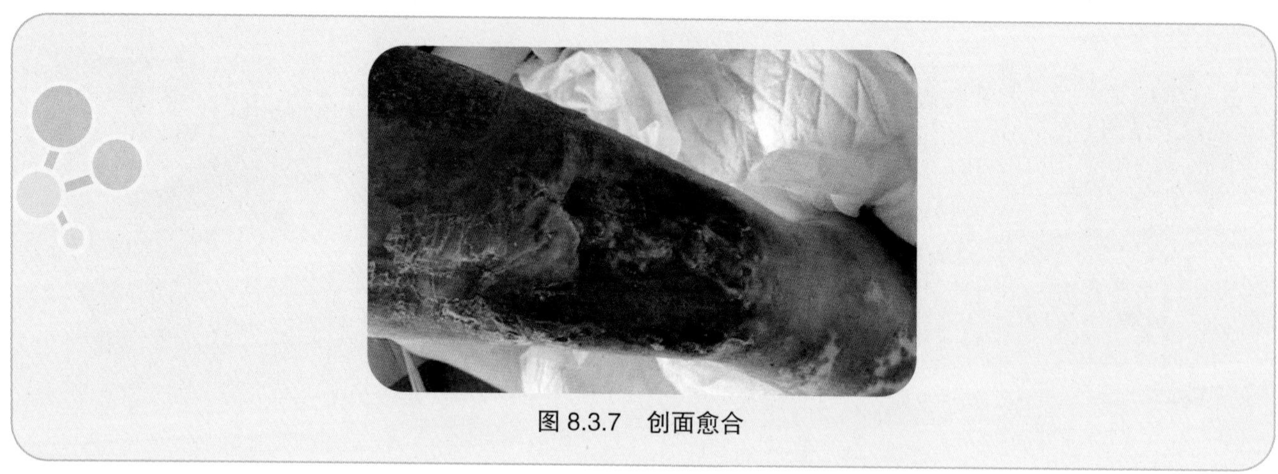

图 8.3.7　创面愈合

（王永高　黄　涛）

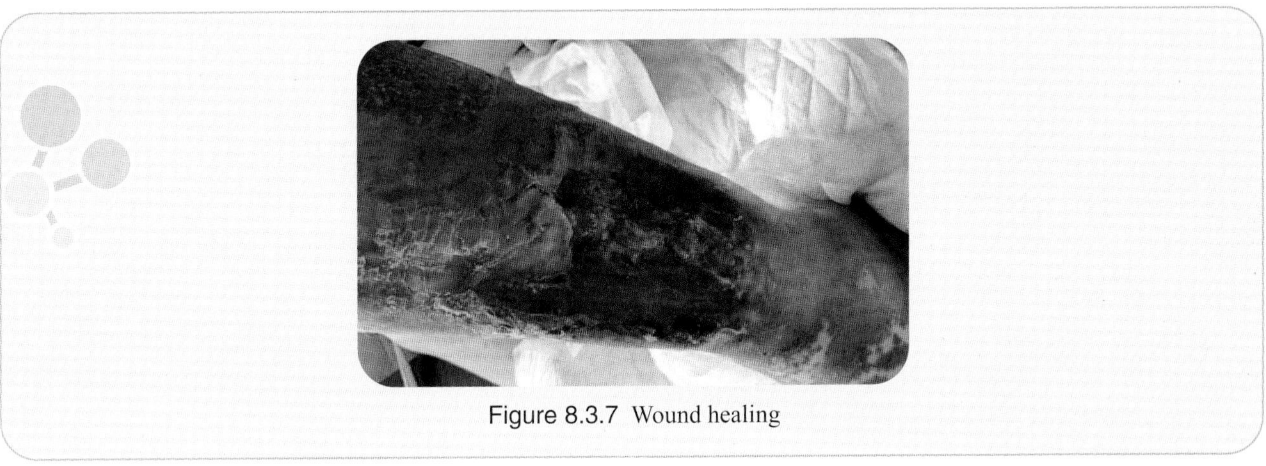

Figure 8.3.7 Wound healing

(Wang Yonggao, Huang Tao)

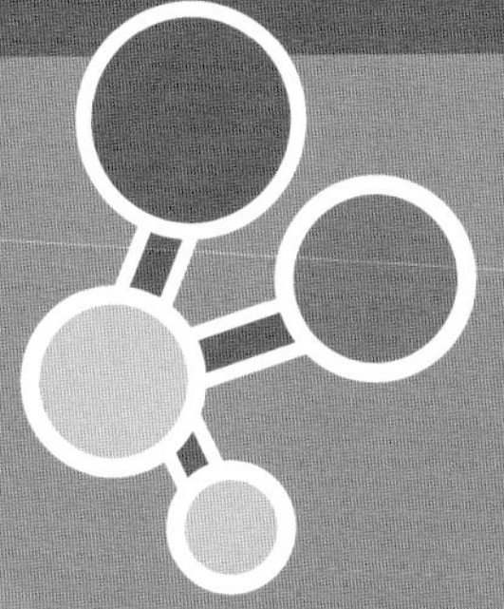

第 9 章
Chapter 9

恶性创面修复
Repair of Malignant Wounds

案例一　足跟部恶性黑色素瘤

◆ 致病原因

患者，男性，42 岁，出生时发现足跟部皮肤有玉米粒大小黑色斑点，随着年龄增长逐渐增大，遍布整个足跟，近 5 年来，中心区磨破，不愈合，疼痛，不敢负重，有黏液样渗出。时有愈合，走路再次磨破流血。

◆ 症状与体征

左侧足跟部有 6 cm × 7 cm 方形黑色肿物，略突起，表面凹凸不平，中心区有 1 cm 圆形溃疡，溃疡凹陷、有脓性分泌物、局部无红肿、轻度触痛、皮温不高、质地较硬，边界清楚（图 9.1.1）。全身浅表淋巴结无肿大。

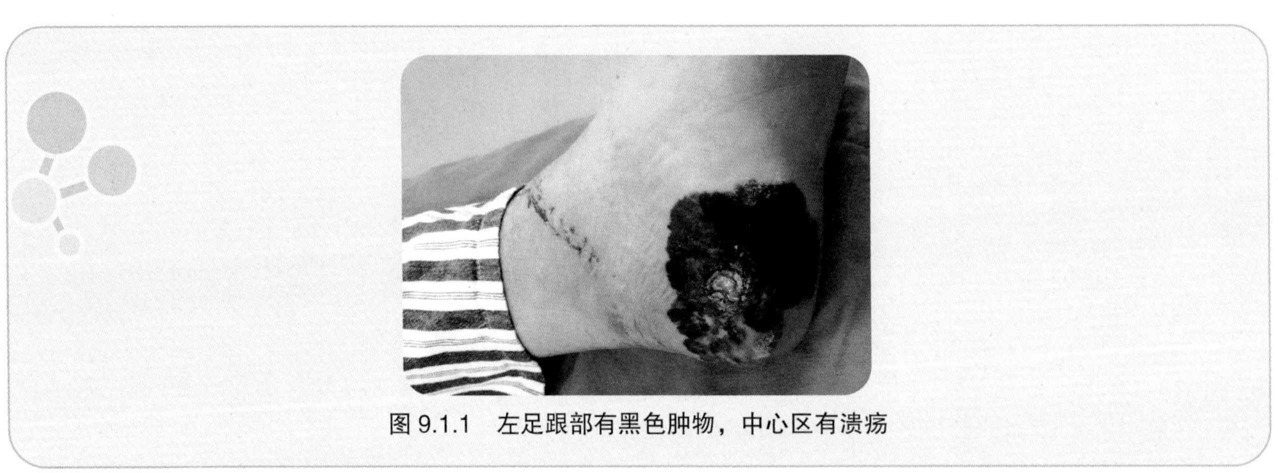

图 9.1.1　左足跟部有黑色肿物，中心区有溃疡

◆ 治疗方案

1. 入院后局部病理组织切片为恶性黑色素瘤。

2. 全身各器官检查未见转移灶。

3. 全麻下行足部肿物切除，局部肿物边缘 1 cm、深度为皮下脂肪层，电凝彻底止血。于右侧下腹部切取全厚皮肤移植于足跟部，创面喷洒重组人碱性成纤维细胞生长因子，植皮边缘间断缝合（图 9.1.2 ~ 图 9.1.5）。植皮区油纱布加压包扎，同侧髂腹股沟淋巴结活检。7 天后病理报告未发现转移病变。

4. 肿物边缘多个切缘送检未发现肿瘤细胞，深部活检未发现肿瘤细胞，同侧淋巴结活检未发现肿瘤转移。

5. 术后 12 天拆线，局部植皮完全成活。术后 3 年来院复诊，足部植皮皮肤恢复良好。

Case 1 Malignant melanoma in the heel area

◆ Cause of illness

The patient, a 42-year-old male, was born with black spots the size of corn kernels on the skin of his heel. As he grew older, the spots gradually increased and covered the entire heel. In the past 5 years, the central area has been worn out, unhealed, painful, and he is afraid to bear weight, with mucous like exudation. Healing occurs from time to time, but walking once again wears out the bleeding.

◆ Signs and symptoms

There is a 6 cm × 7 cm square black mass on the left heel, slightly protruding with an uneven surface. There is a 1 cm circular ulcer in the central area, with a concave ulcer, purulent discharge, no redness or swelling locally, mild tenderness, low skin temperature, hard texture, and clear boundaries (Figure 9.1.1). There is no enlargement of superficial lymph nodes throughout the body.

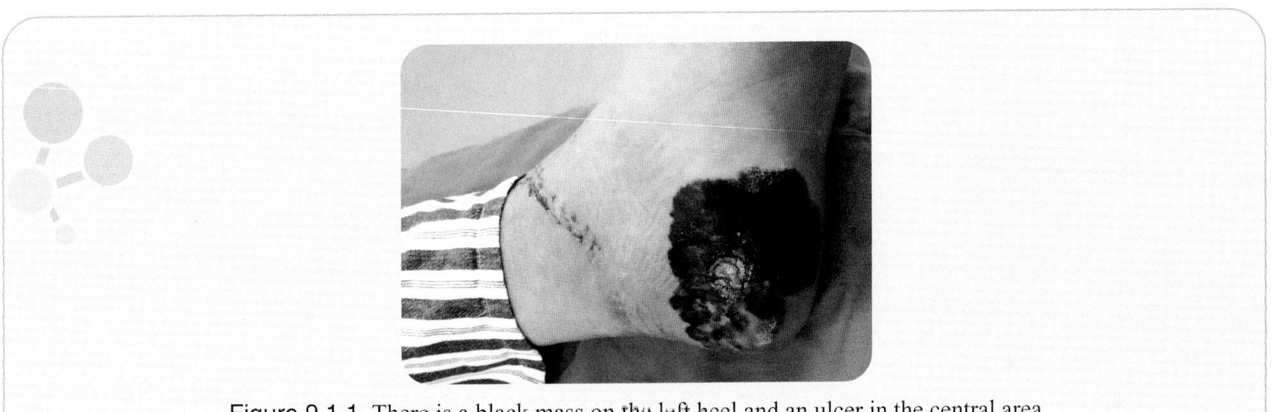

Figure 9.1.1 There is a black mass on the left heel and an ulcer in the central area

◆ Treatment plan

1. After admission, the local pathological tissue section showed malignant melanoma.

2. No metastases were found during the examination of all organs in the body.

3. Under general anesthesia, the foot mass is removed, with a local mass edge of 1 cm and a depth of subcutaneous fat layer. Electrocoagulation is used to completely stop the bleeding. Cut full thickness skin from the lower right abdomen and transplant it onto the heel. Spray recombinant human basic fibroblast growth factor onto the wound, and intermittently suture the edge of the skin graft (Figure 9.1.2- Figure 9.1.5). Apply pressure bandage with oil gauze in the skin grafting area, and perform lymph node biopsy on the same side of the ilioinguinal region. After 7 days, no metastatic lesions were found in the pathological report.

4. Multiple incisions at the edge of the tumor were examined and no tumor cells were found. Deep biopsy did not detect tumor cells, and ipsilateral lymph node biopsy did not detect tumor metastasis.

5. After 12 days of surgery, the stitches were removed and the local skin graft completely survived. Follow up at the hospital 3 years after surgery, and the skin graft on the foot has recovered well.

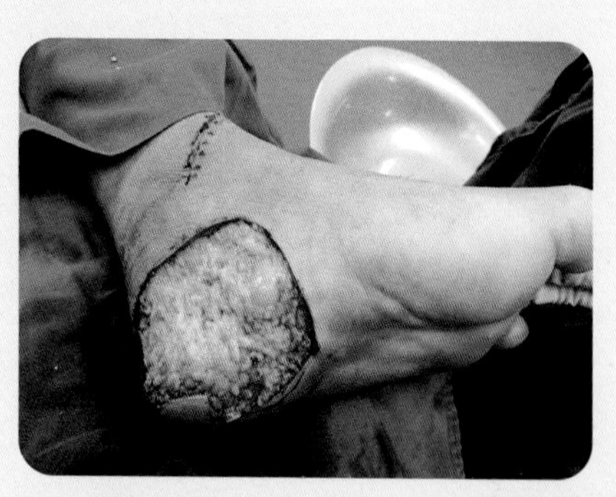
图 9.1.2　黑色肿物完全切除、基底部裸露脂肪

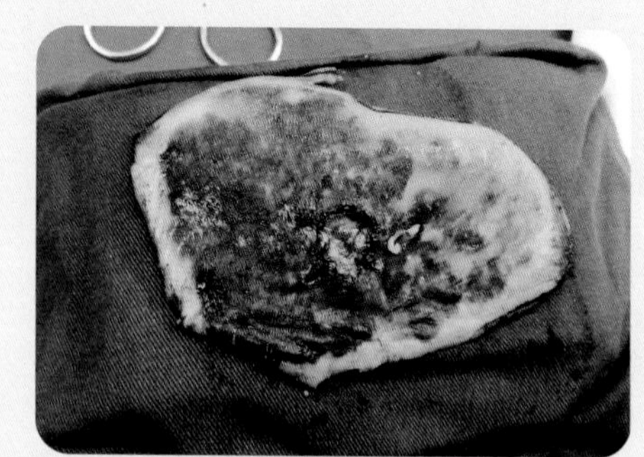
图 9.1.3　据黑色肿物边缘 0.5 cm 扩大切除

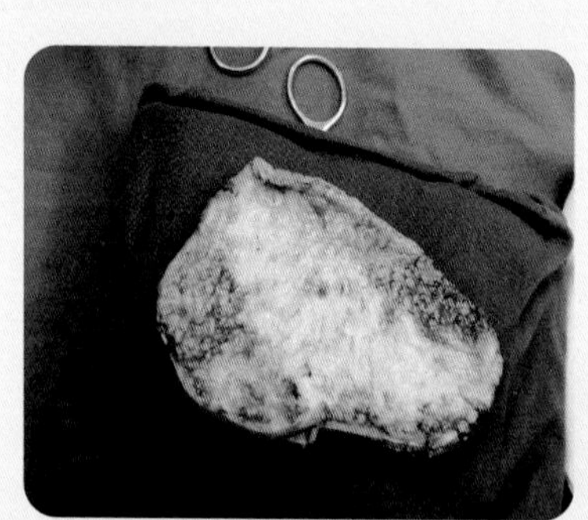
图 9.1.4　肿物基底部未见恶性浸润

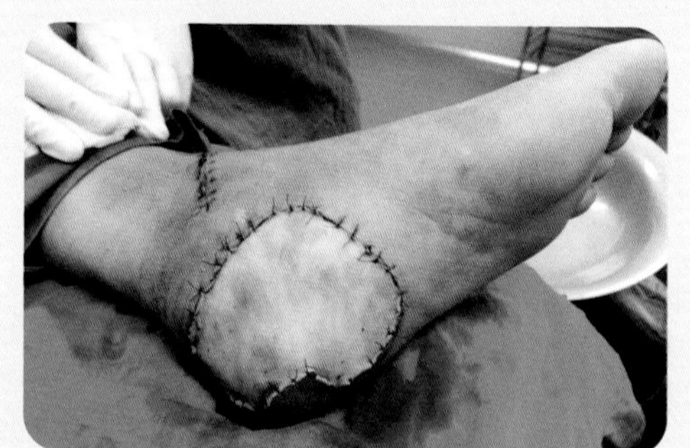
图 9.1.5　全厚皮肤游离移植

（陈善亮）

案例二　头皮巨大鳞癌溃疡

◆ 致病原因

患者，男性，81 岁，头顶拇指大小包块 5 年，碰破流血不止，于当地医院行肿物切除，术后病理切片确诊为鳞癌，切口没有愈合，逐渐扩大流脓水。

◆ 症状与体征

头部剧痛难忍，每天呻吟不止，因疼痛不能入眠，溃疡味恶臭。头顶部有 12 cm × 10 cm 凹陷溃疡，局部散发恶臭气味，有蛆虫蠕动，皮缘硬化红肿，触之出血活跃，溃疡有大量坏死组织，中心区颅骨内外板破坏缺损，硬脑膜外露，可见基底部动脉搏动（图 9.2.1）。触痛明显，左侧额顶部有 1 cm 圆形突起菜花样

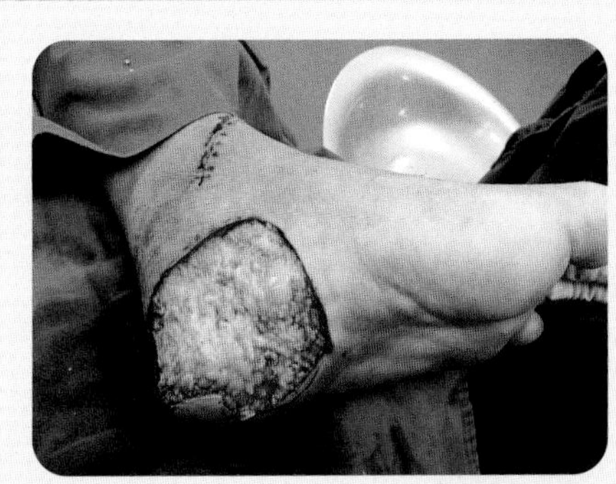
Figure 9.1.2 Complete resection of black mass with exposed fat at the base

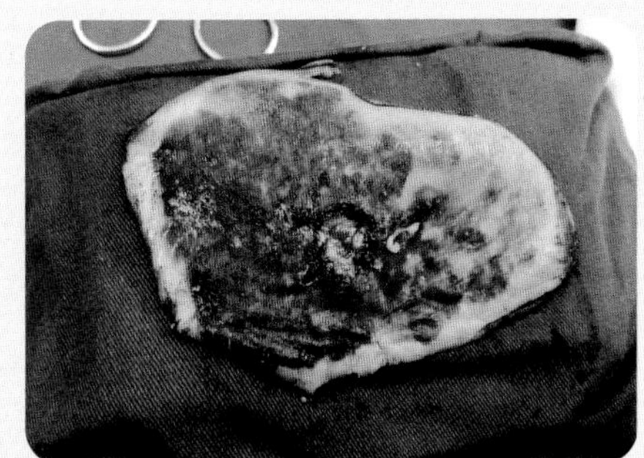
Figure 9.1.3 Enlarged resection based on the edge of the black mass by 0.5 cm

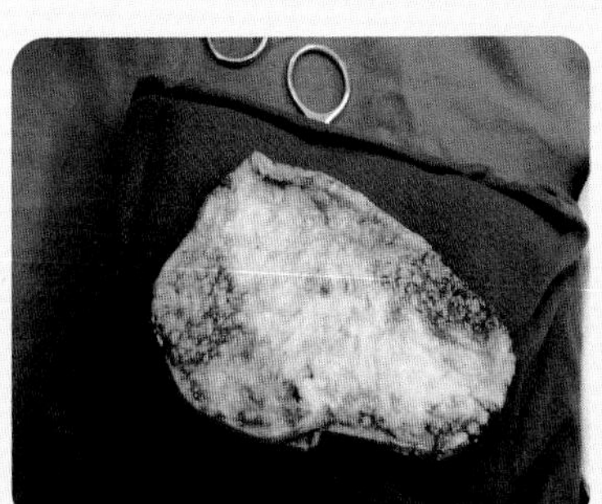
Figure 9.1.4 No malignant infiltration observed at the base of the tumor

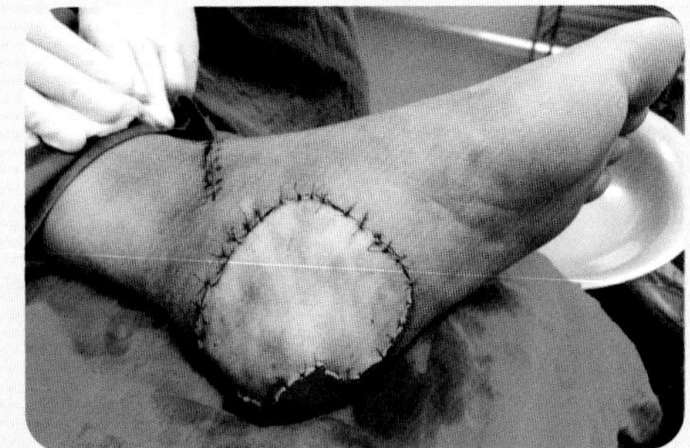
Figure 9.1.5 Full thickness skin free transplantation

(Chen Shanliang)

Case 2 Giant squamous cell carcinoma ulcer on the scalp

◆ Cause of illness

The patient is an 81-year-old male with a thumb sized lump on the top of his head that has been bleeding continuously for 5 years. He underwent tumor resection at a local hospital and was diagnosed with squamous cell carcinoma by pathological examination after surgery. The incision did not heal and gradually expanded with pus and water.

◆ Signs and symptoms

The severe pain in the head is unbearable, and I moan incessantly every day. I cannot sleep due to the pain, and the smell of ulcers is foul. There is a 12 cm × 10 cm concave ulcer on the top of the head, emitting a foul odor locally, with maggots wriggling, hardened and red skin edges, active bleeding upon contact, and a large amount of necrotic tissue in the ulcer. The central area of the skull has internal and external plate damage and defects, with the dura mater exposed. Arterial pulsations can be seen at the base (Figure 9.2.1). Significant tenderness, with a 1 cm circular cauliflower like nodule protruding from the top of the left forehead. Hard lymph nodes the size of walnuts

结节。双侧颌下可触及核桃大小硬性淋巴结，触痛明显。皮温增高。体态消瘦，痛苦面容。

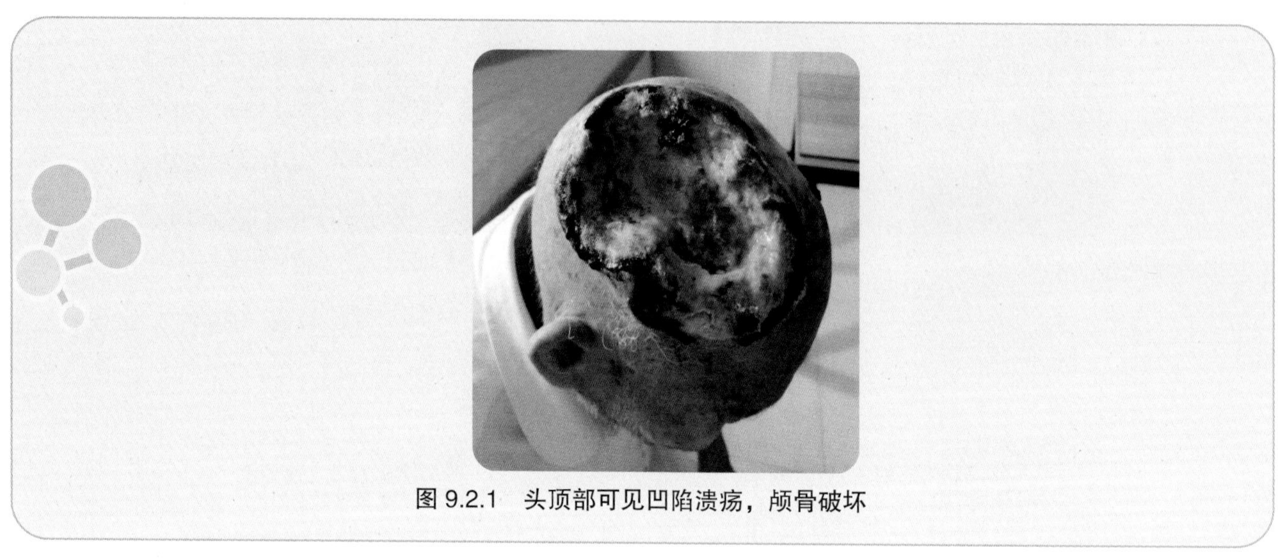

图 9.2.1 头顶部可见凹陷溃疡，颅骨破坏

◆ 治疗方案

1. 高龄老人、恶性肿瘤晚期，全身多器官转移。

2. 治疗以临终关怀治疗为主，解决头部巨大创面换药问题。生命体征支持治疗。

3. 镇痛治疗，减轻疼痛，原则为大痛转为中痛，中痛转为小痛，小痛转为不痛；有效促进睡眠，提高生活质量（图 9.2.2、图 9.2.3）。

4. 保持头部溃疡消毒洁净，驱除蛆虫，控制感染。用柔软胶原蛋白敷料保护创面，防止溃疡深部血管破溃引发大出血。

5. 全流饮食、保持大便通畅软化，预防大便干燥，防止便秘增加脑压。预防因颅内压增高引发溃疡出血。

6. 住院解决癌性疼痛问题。

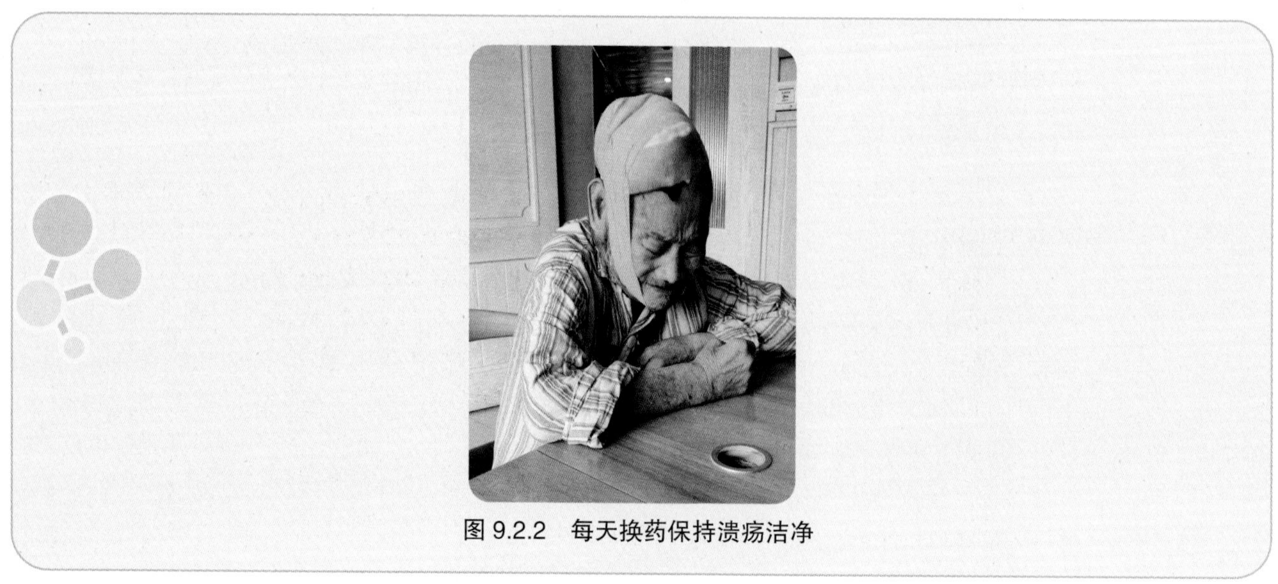

图 9.2.2 每天换药保持溃疡洁净

can be palpated under both jaws, with obvious tenderness. Skin temperature increases. Thin and emaciated, with a painful expression.

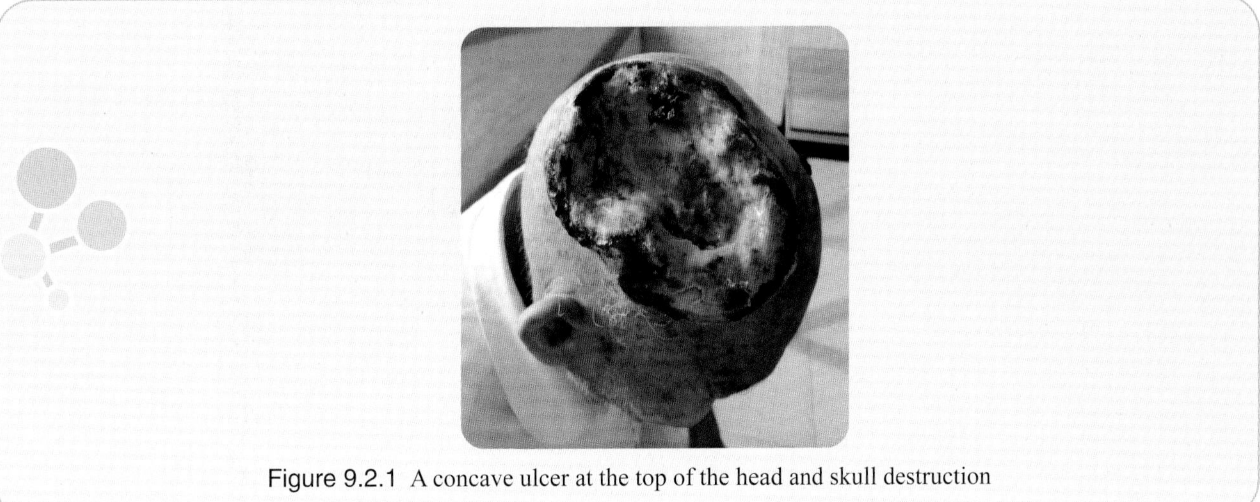

Figure 9.2.1 A concave ulcer at the top of the head and skull destruction

◆ Treatment plan

1. Elderly individuals with advanced malignant tumors and multiple organ metastases throughout the body.

2. The treatment mainly focuses on end-of-life care, solving the problem of changing dressings for large head wounds. Vital signs support treatment.

3. Analgesic treatment to alleviate pain, with the principle of converting severe pain into moderate pain, moderate pain into minor pain, and minor pain into no pain; Effectively promote sleep and improve quality of life (Figure 9.2.2, Figure 9.2.3).

4. Keep the head ulcer disinfected and clean, eliminate maggots, and control infections. Protect the wound with a soft collagen dressing to prevent deep blood vessel rupture and heavy bleeding caused by ulcers.

5. Maintain a full flow diet, keep bowel movements smooth and soft, prevent dry stools, and prevent constipation from increasing brain pressure. Prevent ulcer bleeding caused by increased intracranial pressure.

6. Hospitalization to address cancer pain issues.

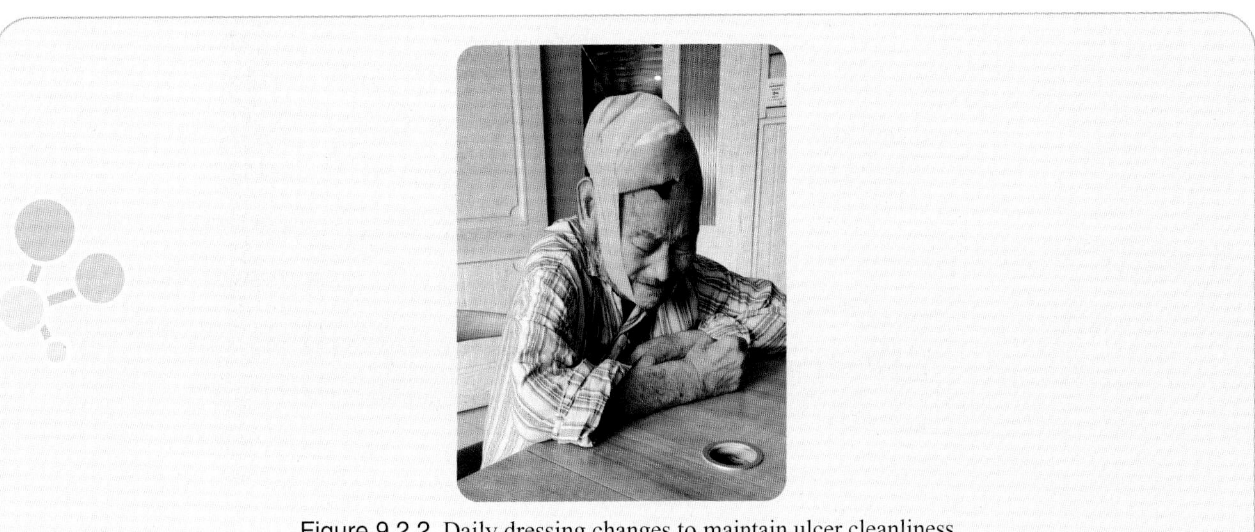

Figure 9.2.2 Daily dressing changes to maintain ulcer cleanliness

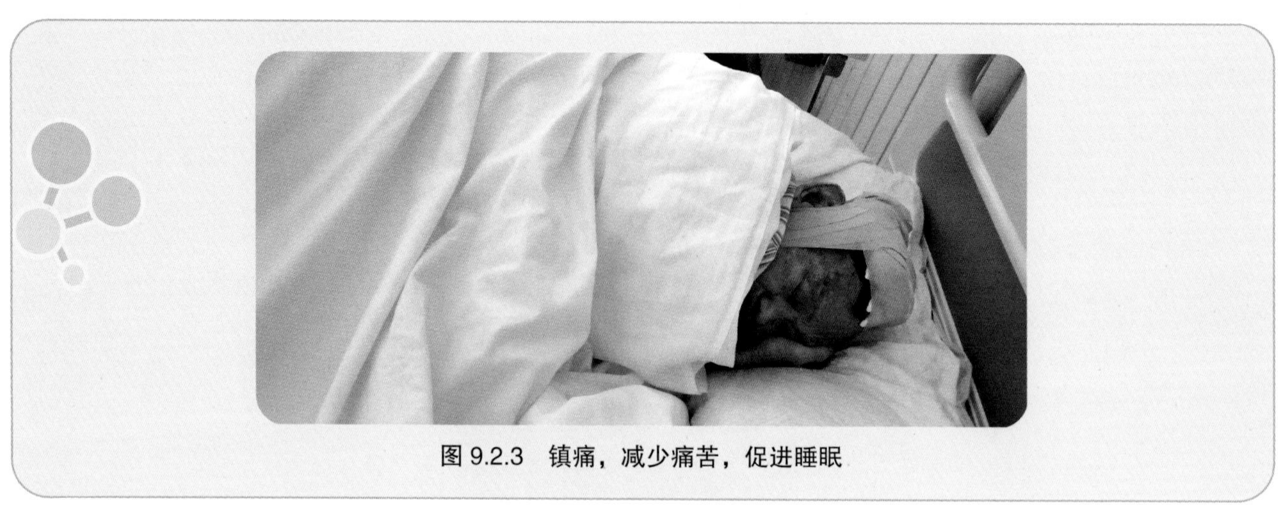

图 9.2.3　镇痛，减少痛苦，促进睡眠

（陈善亮）

案例三　小腿骨肉瘤

◆ 致病原因

患者，男性，47 岁。3 年前发现左侧小腿深部出现一肿物，并逐渐增大，并出现多个肿物，胀痛，足趾麻木，走路瘸行。

◆ 症状与体征

左侧小腿中段偏外侧后侧有明显突起肿物，局部质地较硬凹凸不平，膨隆行外突，无波动，无红肿，触痛明显，多个肿物连成一团（图 9.3.1）。踝关节活动良好，足背动脉波动消失，足趾屈趾活动良好，伸趾功能减弱，足底感觉正常，足背感觉减退，小腿前外侧色沉。左侧髂腹股沟淋巴结未触及肿大和压痛。

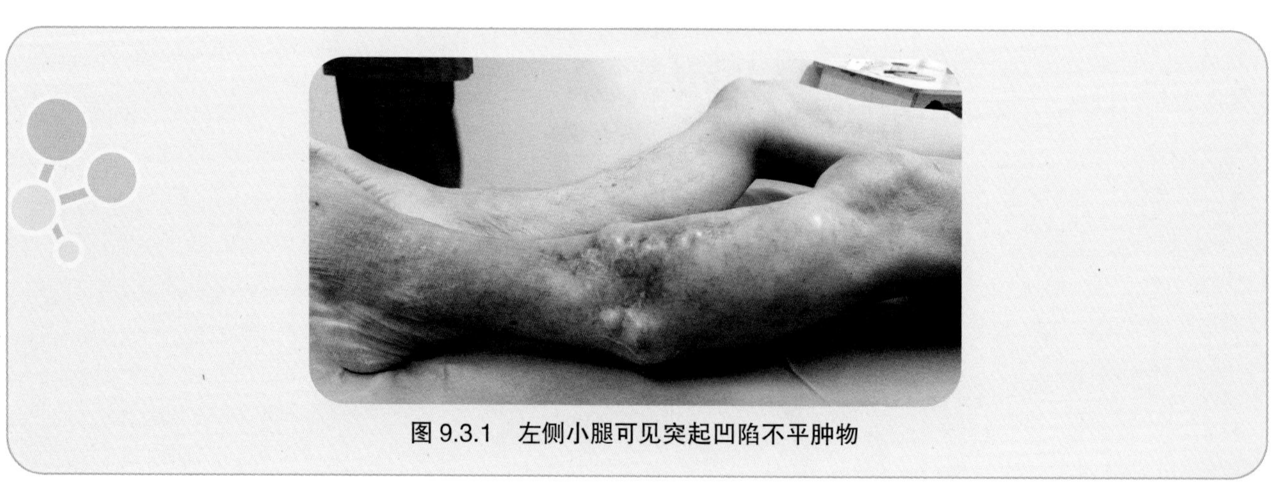

图 9.3.1　左侧小腿可见突起凹陷不平肿物

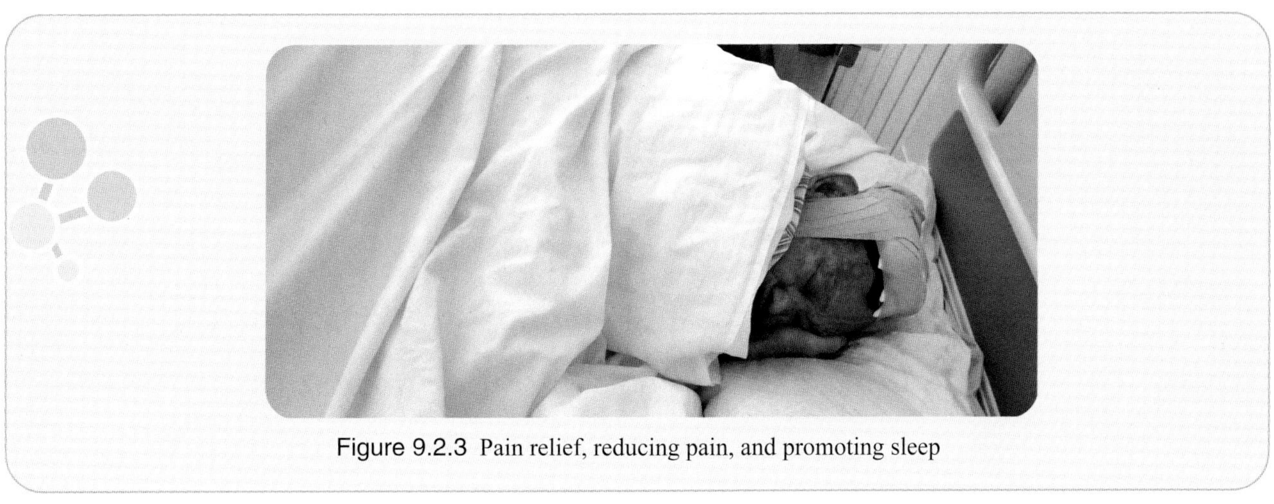

Figure 9.2.3 Pain relief, reducing pain, and promoting sleep

(Chen Shanliang)

Case 3 Osteosarcoma of the lower leg

◆ Cause of illness

Patient, male, 47 years old. Three years ago, a mass was discovered in the deep part of the left calf, which gradually increased in size and presented with multiple lumps, swelling and pain, numbness in the toes, and walking disability.

◆ Signs and symptoms

There is a significant protruding mass on the lateral posterior side of the middle section of the left calf, with a locally hard and uneven texture, bulging outward without fluctuations or redness, and obvious tenderness. Multiple masses are connected together (Figure 9.3.1). Ankle joint activity is good, the fluctuation of the dorsalis pedis artery disappears, the toe flexion activity is good, the toe extension function is weakened, the plantar sensation is normal, the dorsalis pedis sensation is reduced, and the color of the anterior lateral side of the calf is dull. There is no palpable swelling or tenderness in the left iliac inguinal lymph nodes.

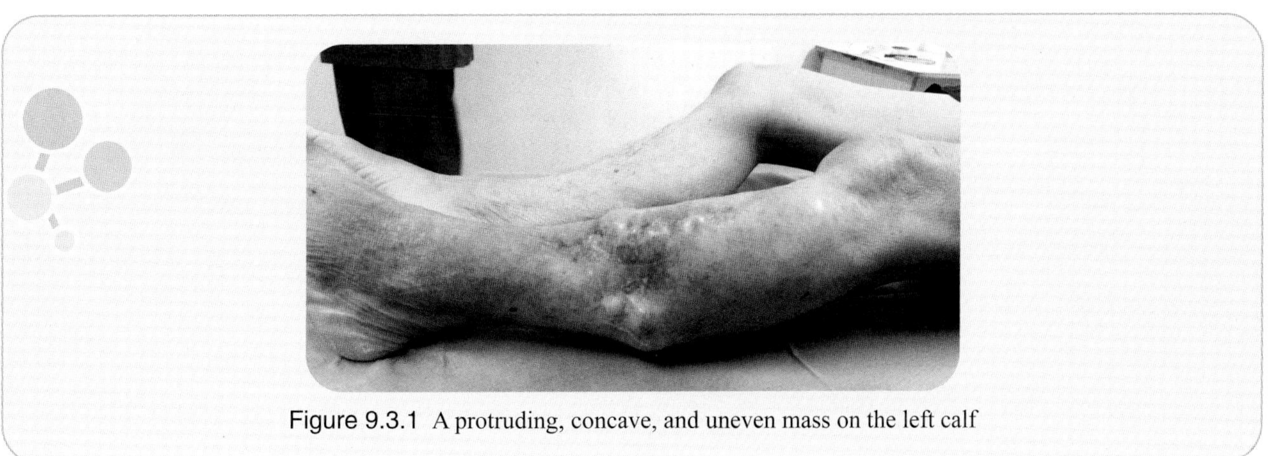

Figure 9.3.1 A protruding, concave, and uneven mass on the left calf

◆ 治疗方案

1. 全身辅助检查未发现肿瘤转移。DR 局部显示腓骨破坏伴缺损，胫骨骨膜增生，超声显示小腿多个实性包块，边界模糊不清，胫前动脉静脉闭塞（图 9.3.2）。

2. 术中病理切片考虑为恶性肿瘤，倾向骨肉瘤，髂腹股沟淋巴结活检未见转移。局部姑息治疗，术中见肿瘤浸润波及胫前肌组织，腓骨中段虫蚀样变并有 6 cm 破坏缺损。切除软组织肿瘤和腓骨破坏段，局部彻底止血，深部防止负压引流管（图 9.3.3 ～图 9.3.5）。

3. 术后抗炎对症治疗，术后 2 周切口甲级愈合。去肿瘤科辅以化疗等综合抗肿瘤治疗。

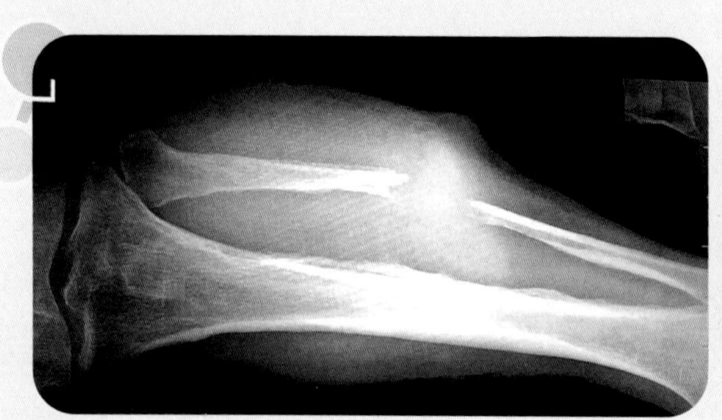

图 9.3.2 DR 显示腓骨破坏缺损，胫骨骨膜增生和软组织增大影

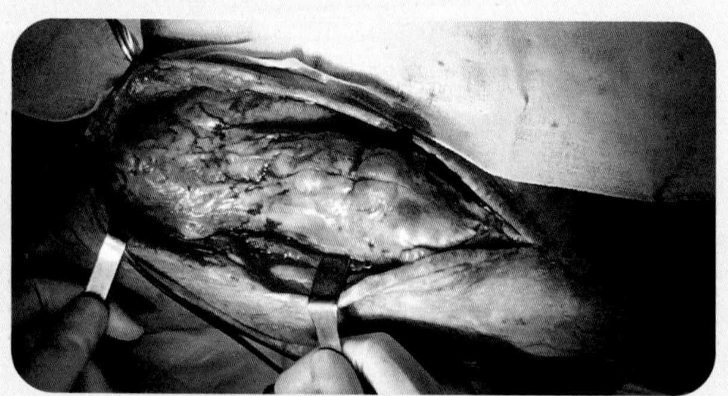

图 9.3.3 术中见多个肿瘤融合成团

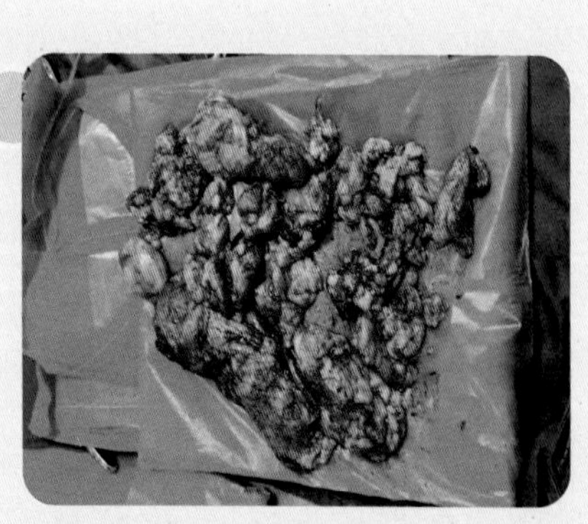

图 9.3.4 肉眼见到肿瘤完全切除

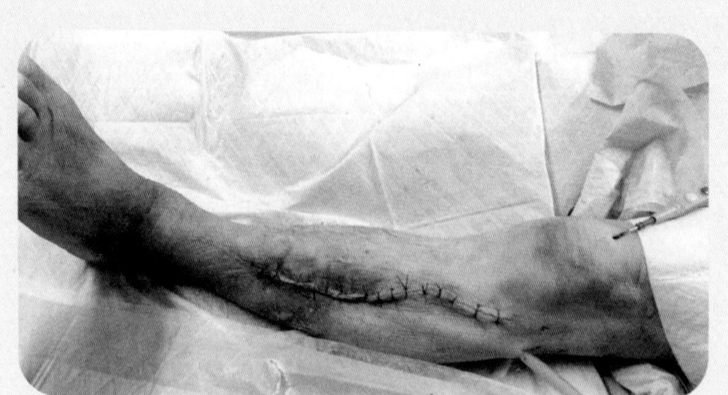

图 9.3.5 肿瘤和破坏段腓骨切除

（陈善亮）

◆ Treatment plan

1. No tumor metastasis was found during whole-body auxiliary examination. DR shows local destruction of the fibula with defects, tibial periosteum hyperplasia, and ultrasound shows multiple solid masses in the lower leg with blurred boundaries and occlusion of the anterior tibial artery and vein (Figure 9.3.2).

2. Intraoperative pathological section suggests malignant tumor, with a tendency towards osteosarcoma. No metastasis was found in the iliac inguinal lymph node biopsy. Local palliative treatment was performed, and during the operation, tumor infiltration was observed affecting the tibialis anterior muscle tissue, with a worm like lesion in the middle of the fibula and a 6 cm damaged defect. Remove the soft tissue tumor and the damaged segment of the fibula, completely stop bleeding locally, and prevent negative pressure drainage in the deep part (Figure 9.3.3-Figure 9.3.5).

3. Postoperative anti-inflammatory and symptomatic treatment, with Grade A wound healing 2 weeks after surgery. Go to the oncology department and receive comprehensive anti-tumor treatment such as chemotherapy.

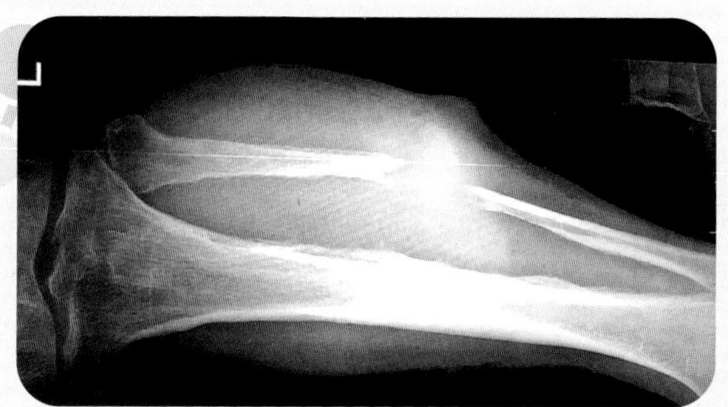

Figure 9.3.2 DR shows fibular destruction defect, tibial periosteum hyperplasia, and soft tissue enlargement shadow

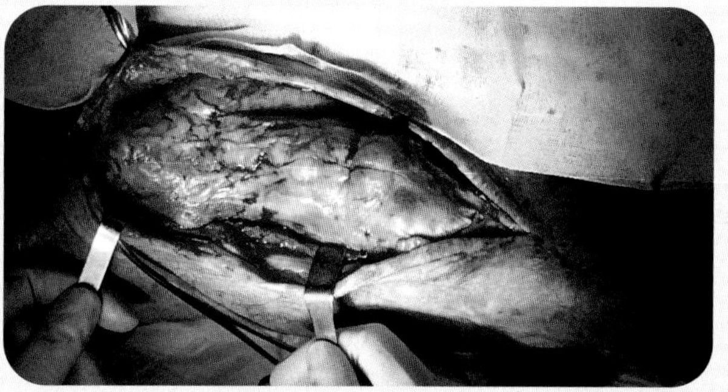

Figure 9.3.3 Multiple tumors fused into clusters during surgery

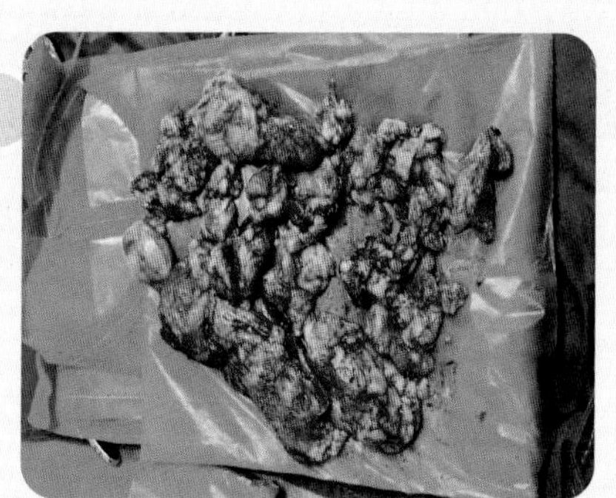

Figure 9.3.4 Visible complete tumor resection with naked eye

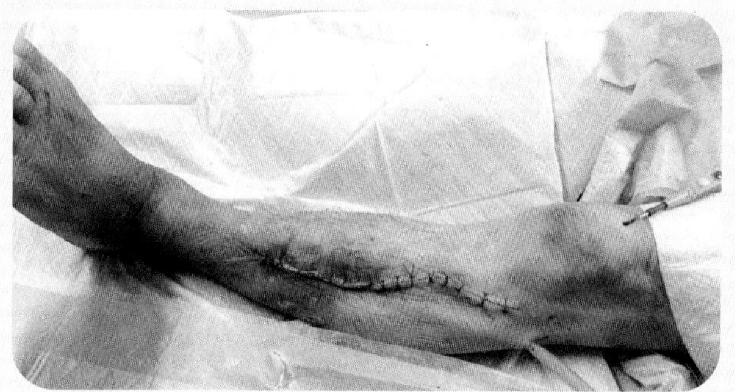

Figure 9.3.5 Tumor and destruction segment fibular resection

(Chen Shanliang)

案例四 左下肢骨巨细胞瘤

◆ 致病原因

患者，男性，54 岁。15 年前，跌伤致左侧股骨干下段骨折，在当地医院行骨折复位钢板内固定术，术后局部逐渐肿大，膝关节出现僵硬，不能屈伸活动，短缩，走路瘸行，之后左下肢因短缩不能行走，扶拐行走，肿瘤无疼痛，无胀痛感，下肢无明显麻木。

◆ 症状与体征

体态消瘦，左侧膝关节部见巨大椭圆形肿物，有 42 cm 长，周径 41 cm；环绕膝关节，波及大腿中下方，小腿上方，局部质地较硬，膨隆样生长，表面布满扩张浅静脉，反流增快，皮温不高，边界模糊不清，外侧色素沉着，皮革样改变，大腿和小腿肌肉明显萎缩，肢体短缩 7 cm；X 线检查，股骨中下段可见巨大膨隆样肿瘤，可见钢板固定其中（图 9.4.1 ~ 图 9.4.5）。足踝活动良好，足底感觉减退，足背动脉和足踝部胫后动脉搏动良好。髂腹股沟淋巴结无明显肿大和压痛。

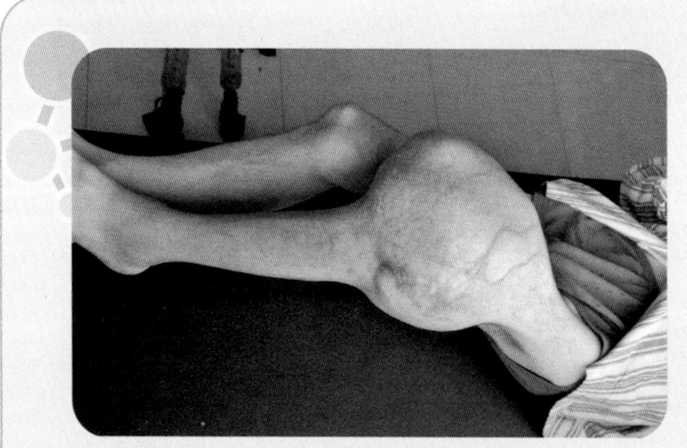
图 9.4.1 左侧下肢外侧可见巨大肿块

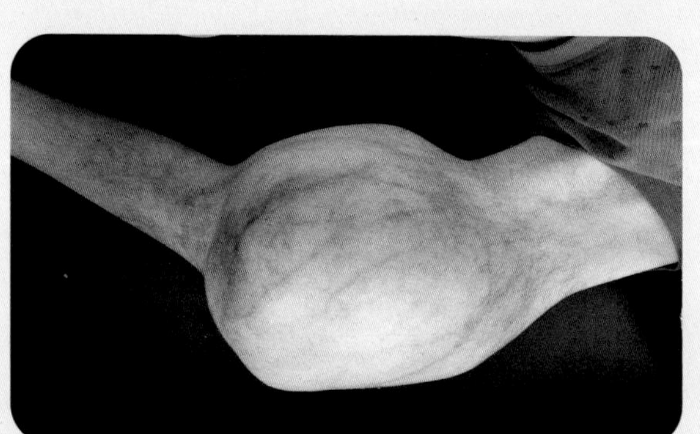
图 9.4.2 肿物表面布满扩张血管

Case 4 Giant cell tumor of left lower limb bone

◆ Cause of illness

Patient, male, 54 years old. 15 years ago, a fall injury caused a fracture of the lower segment of the left femoral shaft. The patient underwent fracture reduction and steel plate internal fixation surgery at a local hospital. After the surgery, the local area gradually swelled, and the knee joint became stiff, unable to bend and extend, shortened, and walked with a limp. Later, the left lower limb was unable to walk due to shortening, and the patient was able to walk with crutches. The tumor did not cause pain or swelling, and there was no obvious numbness in the lower limb.

◆ Signs and symptoms

Body emaciated, with a large oval mass on the left knee joint, measuring 42 cm in length and 41 cm in circumference; Surrounding the knee joint, affecting the middle and lower thighs, and the upper part of the calf, the local texture is relatively hard, with bulging growth, covered with dilated superficial veins on the surface, increased reflux, low skin temperature, blurred boundaries, lateral pigmentation, leather like changes, significant atrophy of thigh and calf muscles, and limb shortening of 7 cm; X-ray examination shows a huge bulging tumor in the middle and lower segments of the femur, which can be fixed with steel plates (Figure 9.4.1-Figure 9.4.5). Good ankle movement, reduced plantar sensation, and good pulsation of the dorsalis pedis artery and posterior tibial artery in the ankle. There is no significant swelling or tenderness in the ilioinguinal lymph nodes.

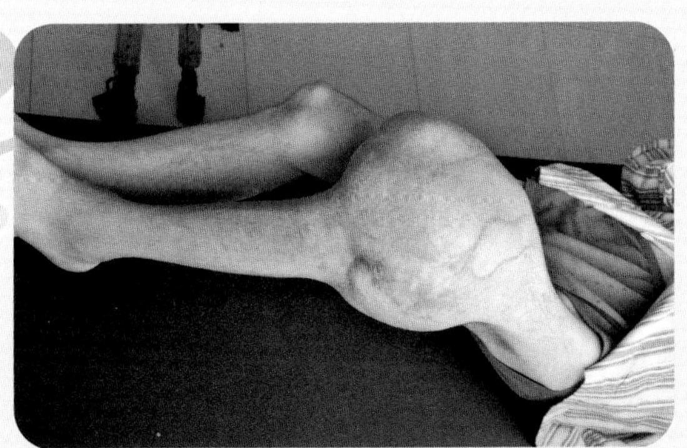

Figure 9.4.1 Large mass visible on the lateral side of the left lower limb

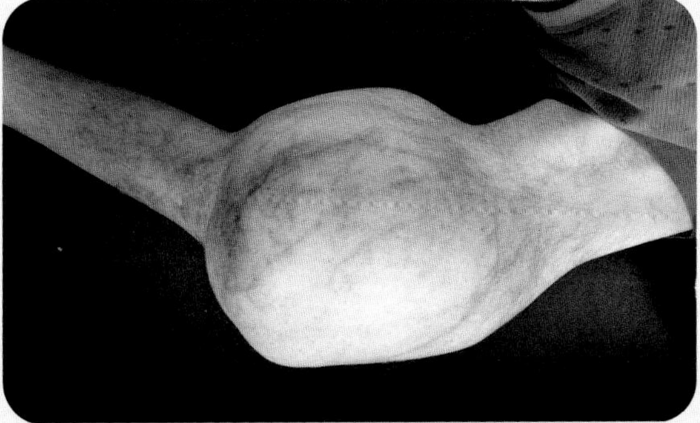

Figure 9.4.2 The surface of the tumor is covered with dilated blood vessels

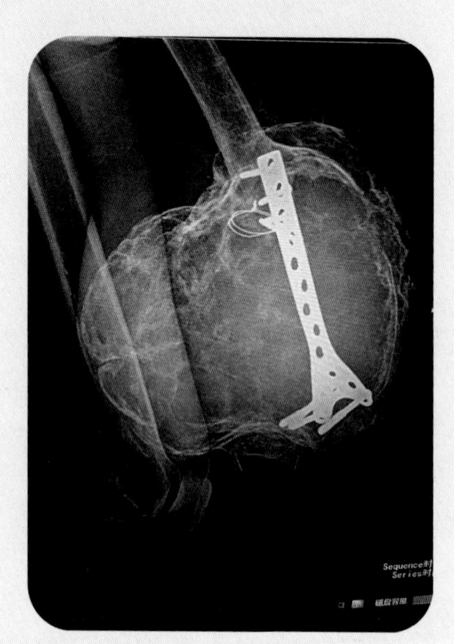

图 9.4.3 股骨中下段可见巨大膨隆样肿瘤

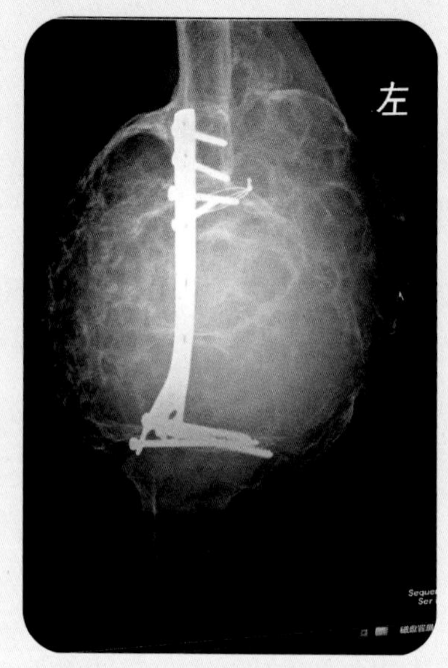

图 9.4.4 可见钢板固定其中

图 9.4.5 平时生活状态，体态消瘦

◆ 治疗方案

1. 入院后全身排查未发现其他脏器肿瘤病灶。

2. 考虑肿瘤巨大，骨关节和周围软组织破坏严重，膝关节功能缺失，肢体短缩 7 cm 和患者意愿，采用截肢方案。

3. 全麻下，于大腿上段高位截肢，术中髂腹股沟淋巴结病理活检未发现肿瘤细胞。肿瘤组织病理活检倾向骨巨细胞肿瘤。

4. 术后 2 周拆线，去肿瘤科抗肿瘤综合治疗。术后 3 个月安装假肢并逐渐去拐行走，系统康复训练（图 9.4.6）。

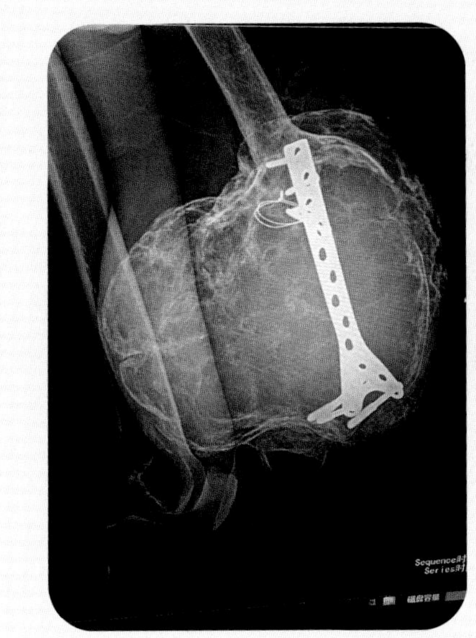

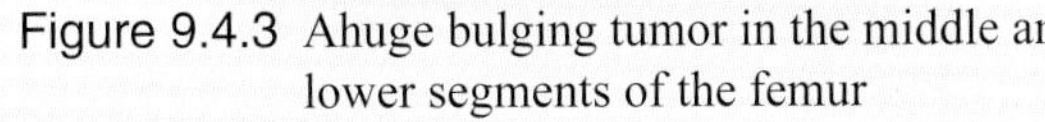

Figure 9.4.3 Ahuge bulging tumor in the middle and lower segments of the femur

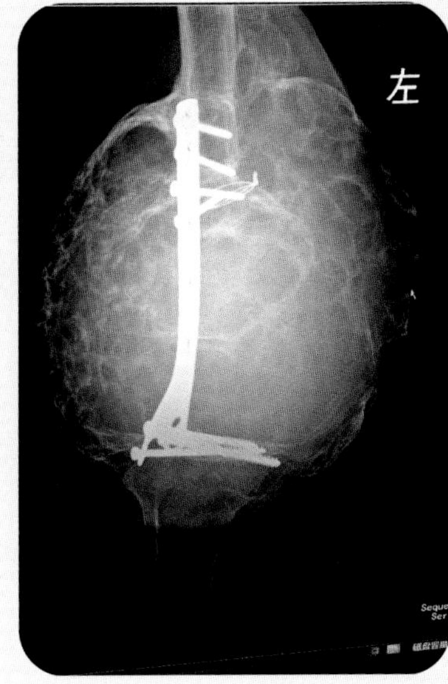

Figure 9.4.4 The steel plate is fixed in place

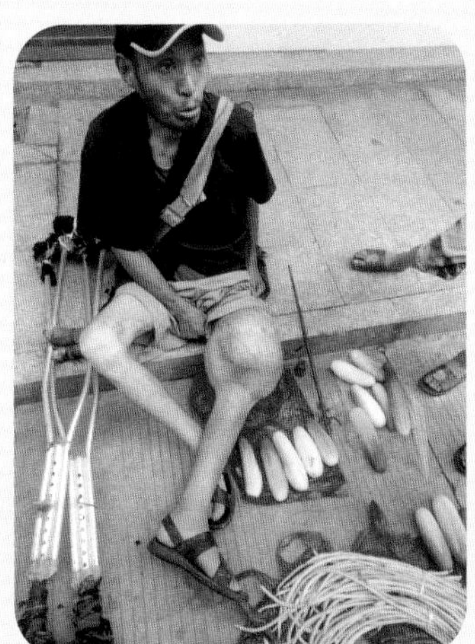

Figure 9.4.5 Daily life status, emaciated body shape

◆ Treatment plan

1. After admission, no other organ tumor lesions were found during the whole-body examination.

2. Considering the huge tumor, severe damage to bone joints and surrounding soft tissues, loss of knee joint function, limb shortening of 7 cm, and the patient's wishes, amputation is adopted.

3. Under general anesthesia, a high amputation was performed on the upper thigh, and no tumor cells were found in the pathological biopsy of the ilioinguinal lymph nodes during the operation. Pathological biopsy of tumor tissue tends to favor giant cell tumors of bone.

4. Two weeks after surgery, remove the stitches and go to the oncology department for comprehensive anti-tumor treatment. Three months after surgery, prosthetics were installed and gradually reduced to crutch walking, followed by systematic rehabilitation training (Figure 9.4.6).

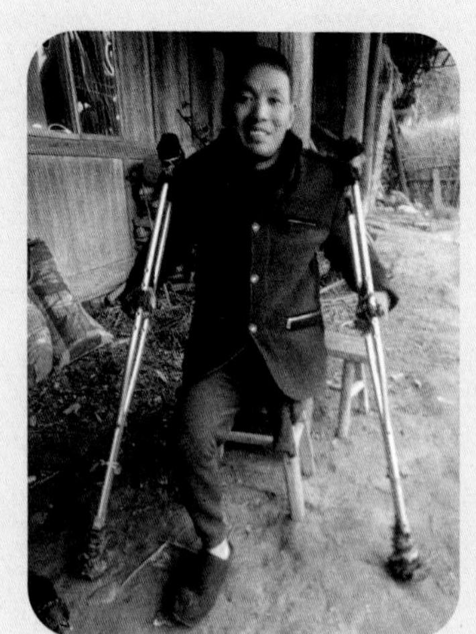

图 9.4.6　大腿上段截肢后，未安装假肢前，和术前对比胖了很多

（陈善亮）

案例五　癌性溃疡、腹壁坏死性肌筋膜炎

◆ 致病原因

患者，男性，68 岁，糖尿病史 21 年，发现肝癌肠转移 2 年。突发剧烈腹痛 2 天，在当地医院行开腹探查肠造瘘姑息手术治疗，腹壁减张，引流术。疑为肠癌穿孔，粪便漏入腹腔，致泛发性腹壁坏死性筋膜炎。

◆ 症状与体征

腹壁正中有 30 cm 纵行切口瘢痕，未拆线，左侧中腹部有造瘘口，携带粪便收纳袋，右侧中腹部有腹腔硅胶引流管，下腹部有 8 个大小不一减张缝合伤口，并有数条橡皮条减张引流，中下腹部创口红肿明显，伤口有大量炎性渗出，皮下潜行游离，创面污秽不清，体态消瘦，贫血貌，恶抑质体态，精神萎靡，走路蹒跚（图 9.5.1、图 9.5.2）。

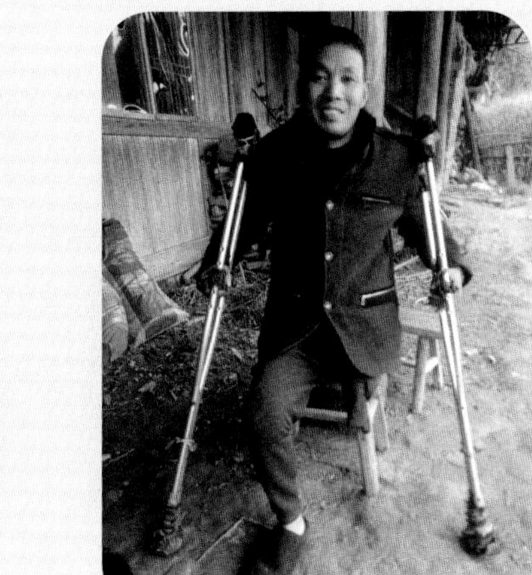

Figure 9.4.6 After amputation of the upper thigh, before the installation of prosthetics, there was a significant increase in weight compared to before surgery

(Chen Shanliang)

Case 5 Cancer ulcer and necrotizing fasciitis of the abdominal wall

◆ Cause of illness

A 68-year-old male patient with 21 years history of diabetes found intestinal metastasis of liver cancer for 2 years. Sudden severe abdominal pain for 2 days, underwent open abdominal exploration and intestinal fistula palliative surgery at a local hospital, abdominal wall dilation reduction, and drainage surgery. Suspected perforation of colon cancer, fecal leakage into the abdominal cavity, causing generalized necrotizing fasciitis of the abdominal wall.

◆ Signs and symptoms

There is a 30 cm longitudinal incision scar in the center of the abdominal wall, with no stitches removed. There is a fistula opening in the left middle abdomen, carrying a fecal storage bag. There is a silicone drainage tube in the right middle abdomen, and there are 8 varying sizes of tension reducing sutured wounds in the lower abdomen, with several rubber strips for tension reducing drainage. The incision in the middle and lower abdomen is significantly red and swollen, with a large amount of inflammatory exudate. The subcutaneous area is free, the wound is dirty and unclear, the body is thin, the appearance is anemic, the body is depressed, the spirit is weak, and the walking is unsteady (Figure 9.5.1, Figure 9.5.2).

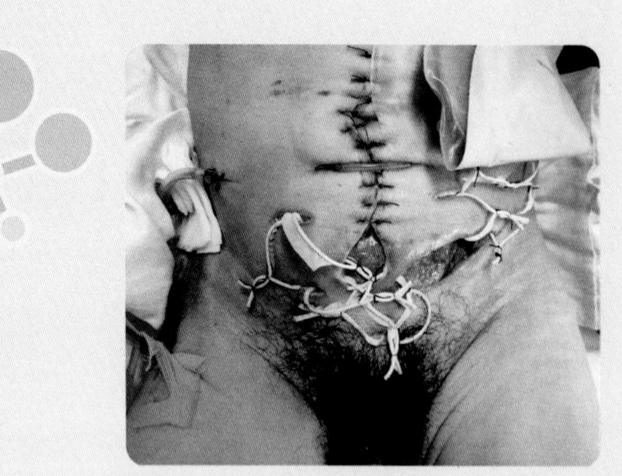

图 9.5.1　腹壁显露造瘘，多处不愈合溃疡

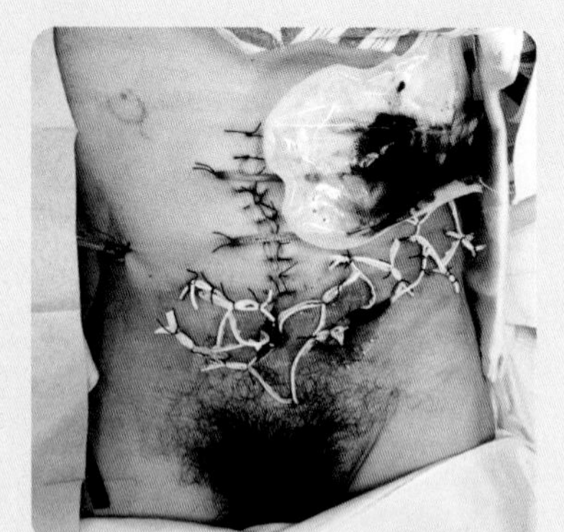

图 9.5.2　腹壁溃疡有大量炎性渗出，脓液稀薄

◆ 治疗方案

1. 全身基础疾病较多，肝癌全身多器官转移，生命支持疗法为主，全流饮食。

2. 严重贫血，血红蛋白 54 g/L；低蛋白血症，白蛋白 22 g/L。根据贫血和低蛋白情况，输入红细胞和白蛋白，营养支持治疗，提高免疫力，纠正贫血和低蛋白血症是治疗创面愈合重要手段之一。

3. 腹壁肠道造瘘护理，腹壁多发溃疡换药治疗，逐渐拆除多处缝线和引流条，局部填塞纱布创面敷料引流，减少缝线和橡皮条异物刺激，刮除坏死筋膜和不新鲜组织，局部喷洒生长因子促进肉芽组织新鲜加速伤口愈合。

4. 经过 2 周全身基础疾病纠正，血红蛋白提升至 96 g/L，白蛋白提升至 42 g/L。腹部创面逐渐新鲜渗血活跃。与全麻下行腹壁清创术缝合术，下腹壁局部转移皮瓣移植减张缝合，深部放两枚橡皮条引流，预防皮瓣下积液，弹力腹带环绕腹部包扎。2 天拔出引流，10 天拆线，腹壁创面完全愈合而出院，转肿瘤科抗癌治疗（图 9.5.3 ~图 9.5.6）。

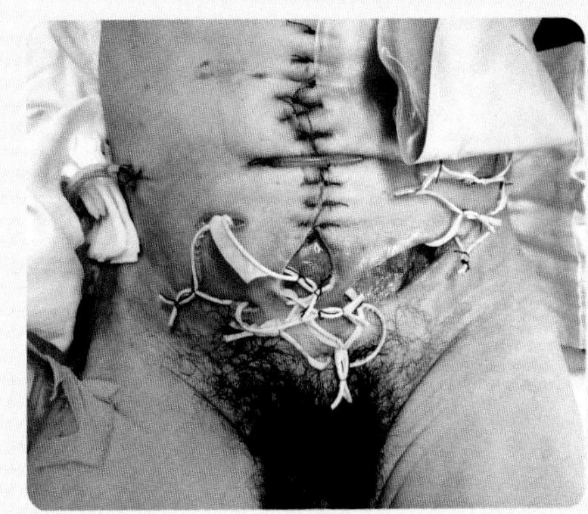

Figure 9.5.1 Abdominal wall exposed fistula, multiple non healing ulcers

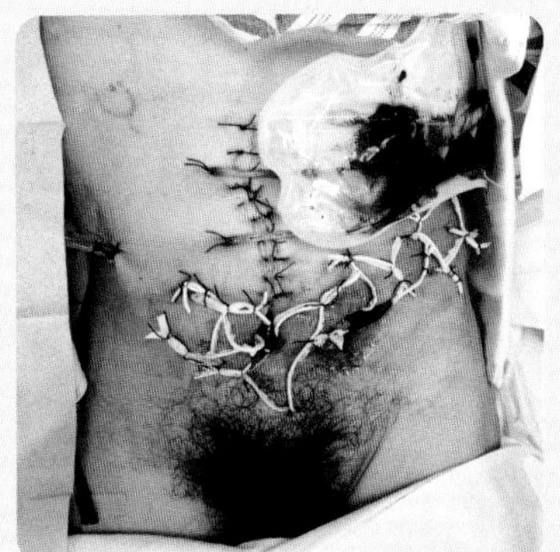

Figure 9.5.2 Abdominal wall ulcer has a large amount of inflammatory exudate and thin pus

◆ Treatment plan

1. There are many underlying diseases throughout the body, such as liver cancer with multiple organ metastases. Life support therapy is the main approach, and a full flow diet is recommended.

2. Severe anemia, hemoglobin 54 g/L; Hypoproteinemia, albumin 22 g/L. According to the anemia and hypoalbuminemia conditions, inputting red blood cells and albumin, nutritional support therapy, improving immunity, and correcting anemia and hypoalbuminemia are important means of treating wound healing.

3. Abdominal wall intestinal fistula care, dressing change treatment for multiple abdominal wall ulcers, gradually removing multiple sutures and drainage strips, locally filling the wound with gauze dressing for drainage, reducing foreign body stimulation from sutures and rubber strips, scraping off necrotic fascia and stale tissue, locally spraying growth factors to promote fresh granulation tissue and accelerate wound healing.

4. After 2 weeks of systemic disease correction, hemoglobin increased to 96 g/L and albumin increased to 42 g/L. The abdominal wound gradually shows fresh and active bleeding. Under general anesthesia, abdominal wall debridement and suturing were performed, and a local transfer skin flap was transplanted and sutured to reduce tension in the lower abdominal wall. Two rubber strips were placed deep to prevent fluid accumulation under the skin flap, and an elastic abdominal band was wrapped around the abdomen for bandaging. After 2 days of drainage and 10 days of suture removal, the abdominal wall wound completely healed and the patient was discharged, and transferred to the oncology department for anti-cancer treatment (Figure 9.5.3- Figure 9.5.6).

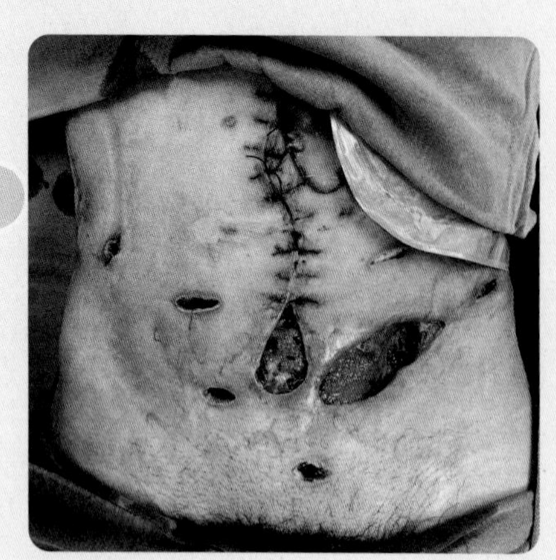
图 9.5.3　腹壁清创，把引流管全部取出

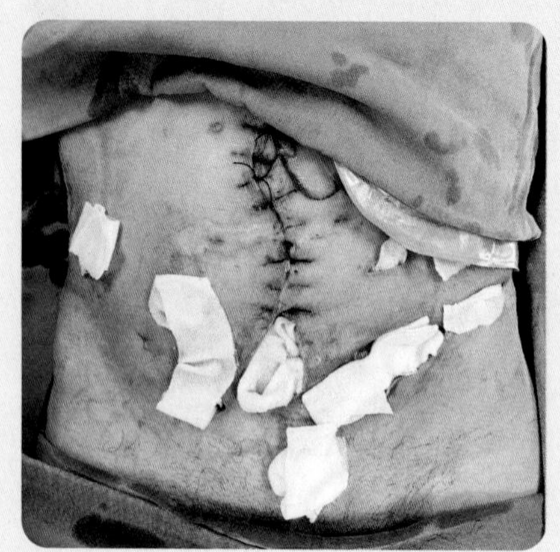
图 9.5.4　改用伤口纱布创面敷料引流，换药

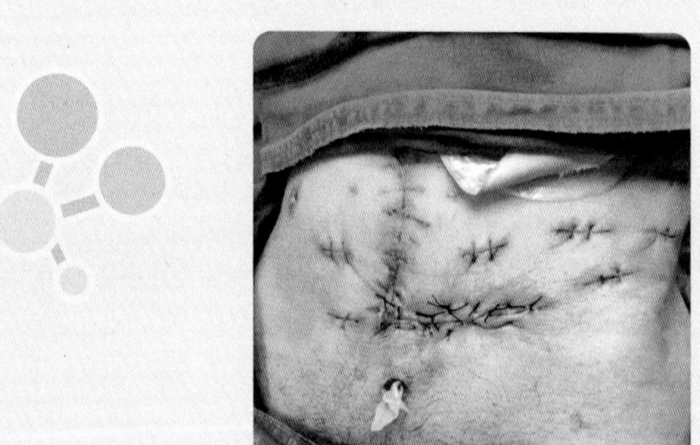
图 9.5.5　换药后、创面新鲜，局部皮瓣，减张缝合，深部放置引流

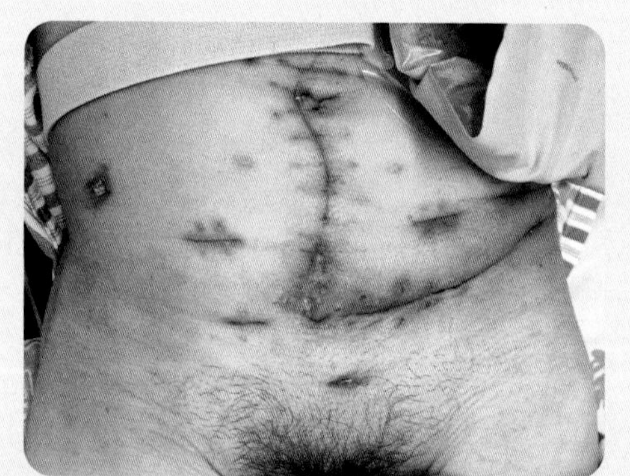
图 9.5.6　术后 12 天腹壁溃疡完全愈合

（陈善亮）

案例六　艾滋病性溃疡

◆ 致病原因

患者，男性，76 岁，发现获得性免疫缺陷综合征（简称艾滋病）32 年，右下肢破溃经久不愈合 28 年，长期抗艾滋病药物治疗，曾在本地医院清创植皮 2 次，植皮不久后继续溃烂。

◆ 症状与体征

右侧小腿胫前有 8 cm × 6 cm 溃疡，局部肉芽组织污秽不清，表面散在脓苔，红肿（图 9.6.1）。味臭，

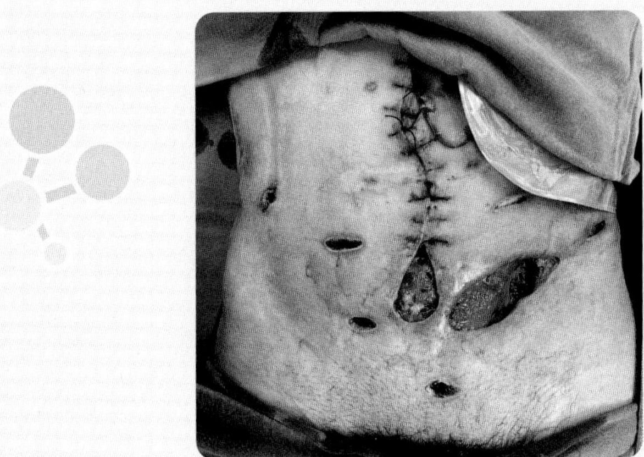

Figure 9.5.3 Abdominal wall debridement, remove all drainage tubes

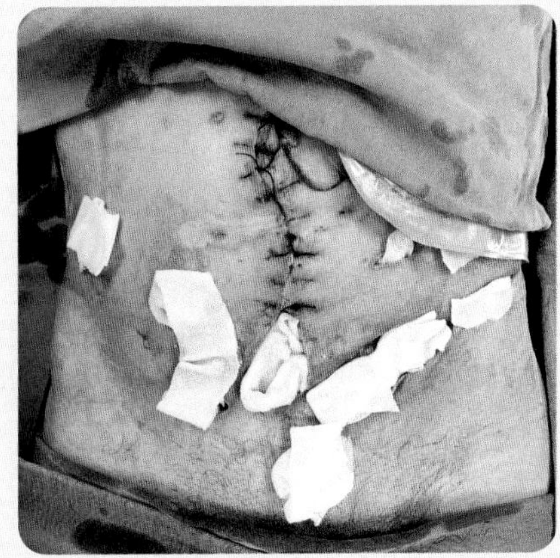

Figure 9.5.4 Switching to wound gauze and wound dressing for drainage and dressing change

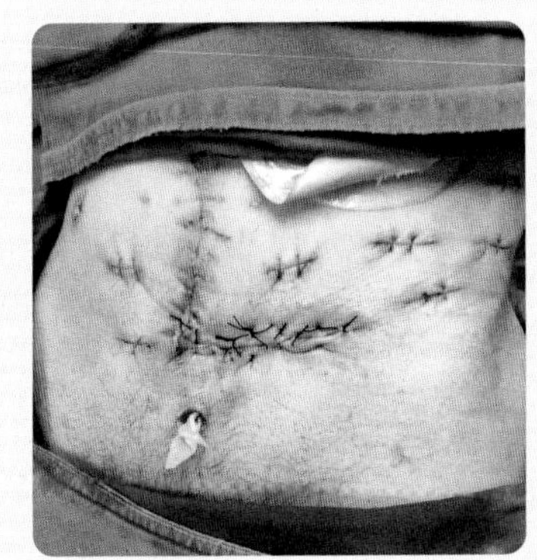

Figure 9.5.5 After dressing change, fresh wound, local skin flap, reduced tension suture, deep drainage placement

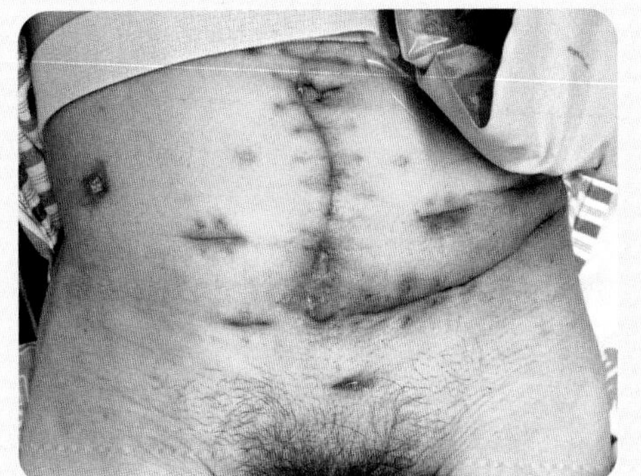

Figure 9.5.6 Complete healing of abdominal wall ulcer 12 days after surgery

(Chen Shanliang)

Case 6 AIDS ulcer

◆ Cause of illness

The patient, a 76-year-old male, was found to have acquired immune deficiency syndrome (AIDS for short) for 32 years, and his right lower limb had been broken for 28 years without healing. He had been treated with anti AIDS drugs for a long time. He had debridement and skin grafting twice in the local hospital, and the skin graft continued to fester soon after.

◆ Signs and symptoms

There is an 8 cm × 6 cm ulcer in front of the tibia on the right calf, with unclear granulation tissue and scattered pus coating on the surface, causing redness and swelling (Figure 9.6.1). Stinky odor, large areas of darkened skin

创面周边皮肤大面积色沉，瘢痕硬化、边缘内陷，触之不出血，膝关节踝关节足趾关节活动良好，足背动脉搏动有力，足趾感觉良好。

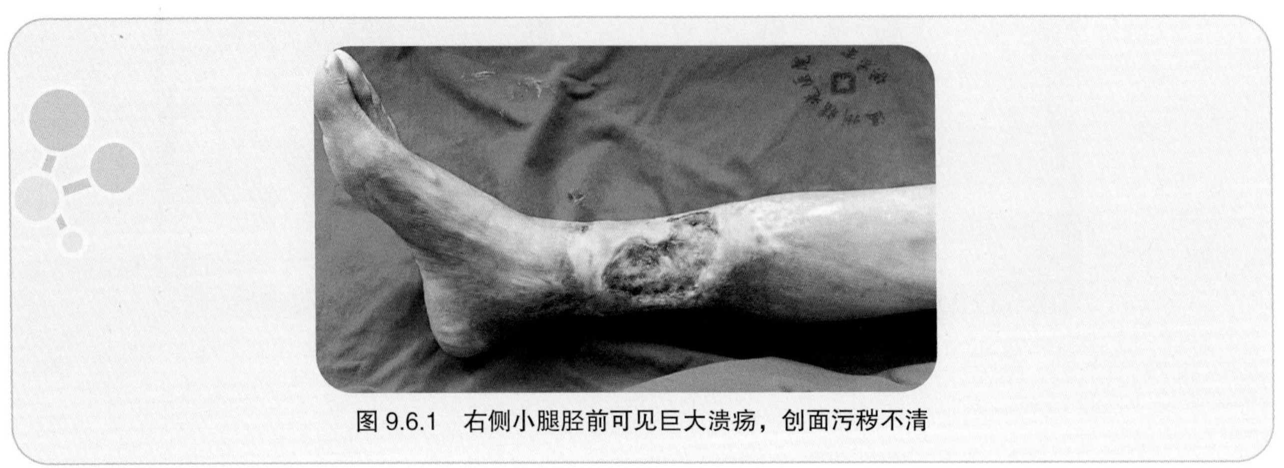

图 9.6.1 右侧小腿胫前可见巨大溃疡，创面污秽不清

◆ 治疗方案

1. 入院后完善各项检验指标，胫骨拍片显示硬化性骨髓炎，考虑局部慢性感染引起的增生性骨感染，心肺功能良好。

2. 细菌培养 + 药物敏感试验，给予敏感抗菌药物。局部换药治疗。

3. 全麻下行内陷皮缘坏死增生肉芽组织切除，纤维板增厚硬化，无血运，采用电钻硬化纤维板打孔，打孔至胫骨髓腔，至活跃出血为止，然后人工真皮覆盖创面，待肉芽组织活跃后取下（图 9.6.2 ~ 图 9.6.4）。

4. 术后 3 周，观察人工真皮下肉芽组织红润新鲜，取下硅胶模后，肉芽组织出血活跃，可以植皮。全麻下，在大腿前侧切取中厚皮肤，游离移植于创面，皮肤打孔后，油纱覆盖并加压包扎（图 9.6.5 ~ 图 9.6.7）。

5. 术后 7 天，换药见植皮完全成活，边缘散在少许创面，经换药后愈合（图 9.6.8）。

6. 此类难愈合案例少见，术后加强宣教，授意患者保护创面意识，防止再次破溃。

around the wound, hardened scars, and sunken edges, no bleeding when touched, good movement of knee, ankle, and toe joints, strong pulsation of dorsalis pedis arteries, and good toe sensation.

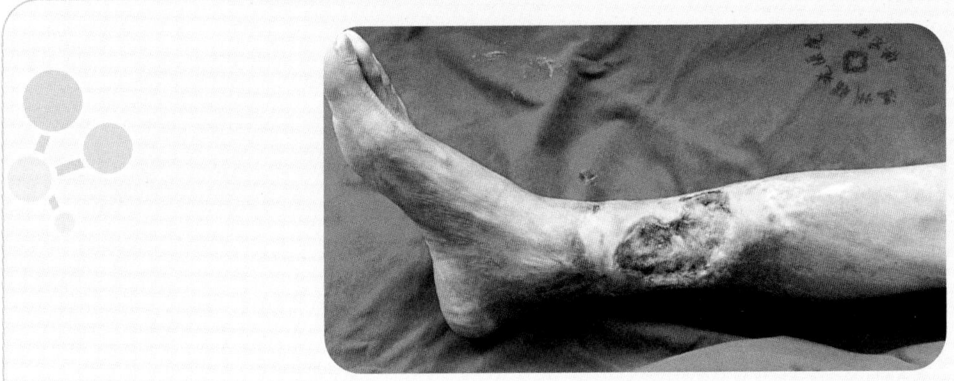

Figure 9.6.1 A huge ulcer can be seen in the anterior tibia of the right calf, and the wound is dirty and unclear

◆ Treatment plan

1. After admission, various test indicators were improved, and the tibial X-ray showed sclerosing osteomyelitis, suggesting proliferative bone infection caused by local chronic infection, with good cardiovascular and pulmonary function.

2. Bacterial culture + drug sensitivity test, administering sensitive antibiotics. Local dressing change treatment.

3. Under general anesthesia, the necrotic and hypertrophic granulation tissue of the invaginated skin margin is removed, and the fibrous plate thickens and hardens without blood circulation. An electric drill is used to harden the fibrous plate and drill holes until the tibial medullary cavity becomes active and bleeding occurs. Then, artificial dermis is used to cover the wound, and the granulation tissue is removed after it becomes active (Figure 9.6.2-Figure 9.6.4).

4. Three weeks after surgery, observe that the artificial subcutaneous granulation tissue is red and fresh. After removing the silicone mold, the granulation tissue bleeds actively and can be transplanted with skin. Under general anesthesia, a medium thick skin was cut from the front of the thigh and transplanted onto the wound. After punching holes in the skin, it was covered with oil gauze and pressure bandaged (Figure 9.6.5- Figure 9.6.7).

5. After 7 days of surgery, the skin graft was found to be completely alive with a few scattered wounds at the edges after dressing change, and healed after dressing change (Figure 9.6.8).

6. Such cases of difficult healing are rare, and postoperative education should be strengthened to educate patients on the importance of protecting the wound and prevent further rupture.

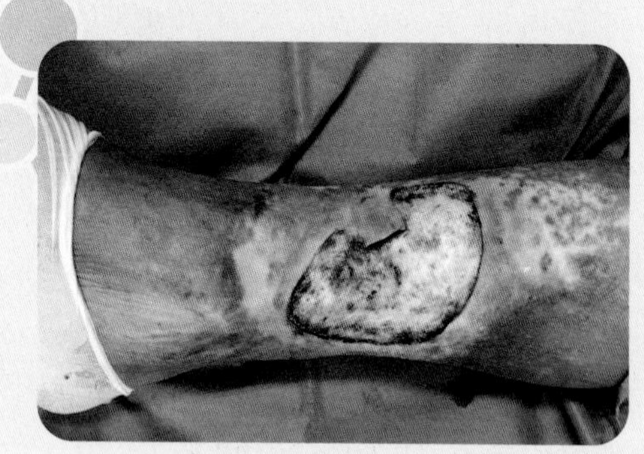
图 9.6.2 内陷皮缘坏死增生肉芽组织切除

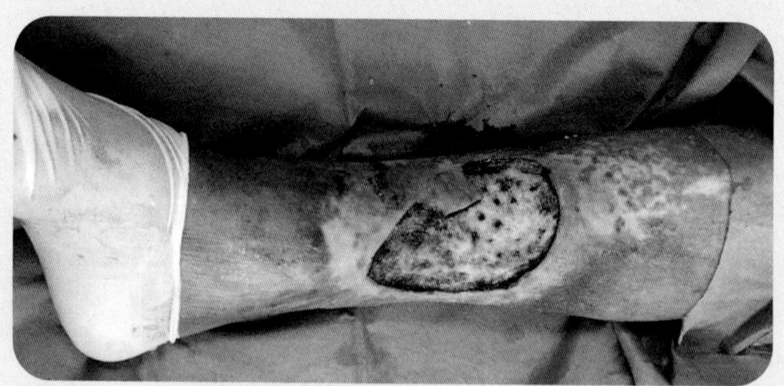
图 9.6.3 采用电钻硬化纤维板打孔，打孔至胫骨髓腔

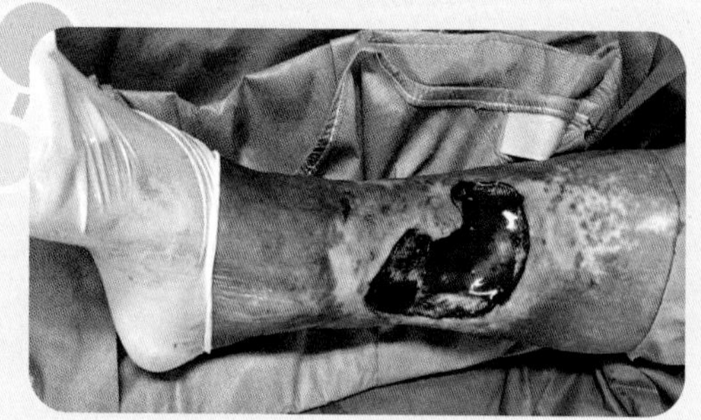
图 9.6.4 人工双层真皮覆盖

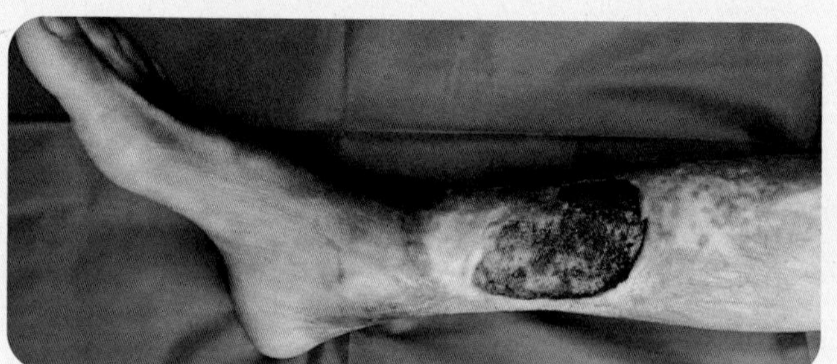
图 9.6.5 3 周后，人工真皮拆除，创面肉芽组织新鲜、呈颗粒样增生，触之出血活跃

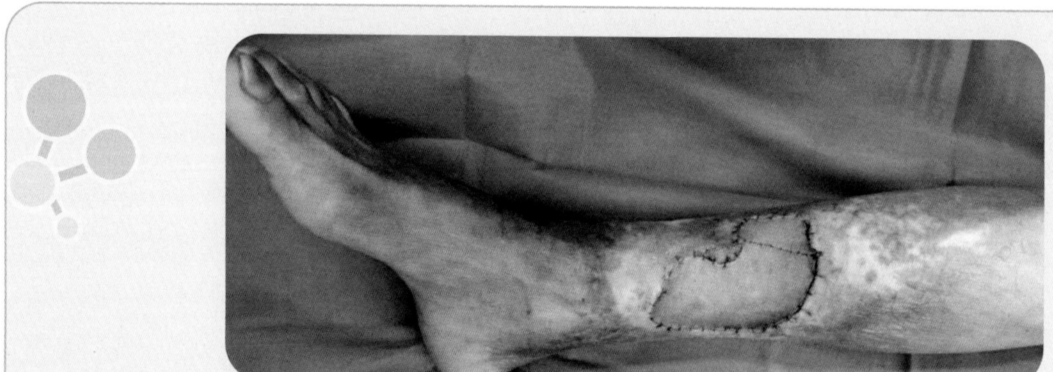
图 9.6.6 中厚游离皮肤移植

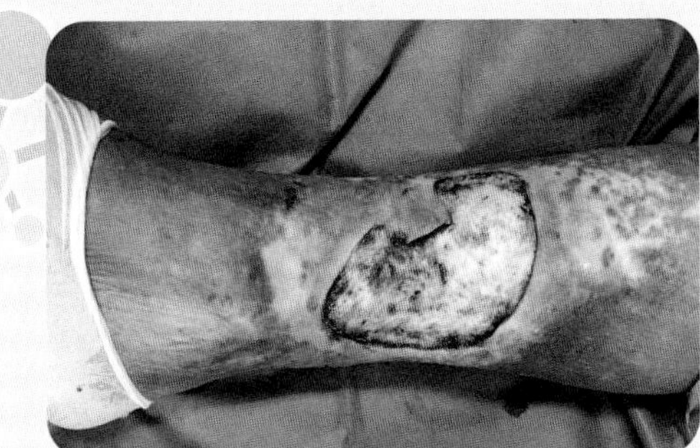

Figure 9.6.2 Removal of necrotic and hypertrophic granulation tissue at the edge of the sunken skin

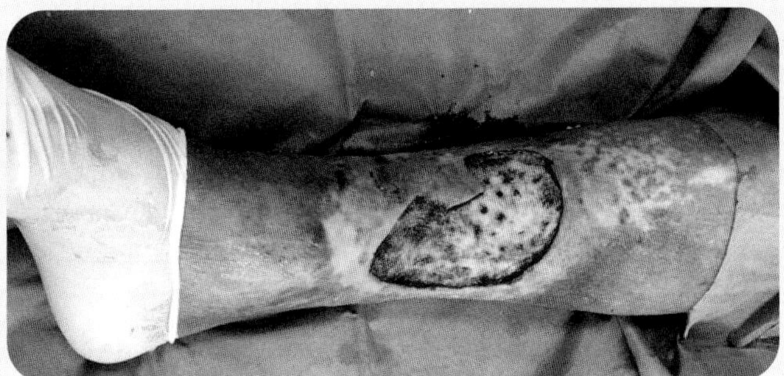

Figure 9.6.3 Using an electric drill to harden fiberboard and drill holes into the tibial medullary cavity

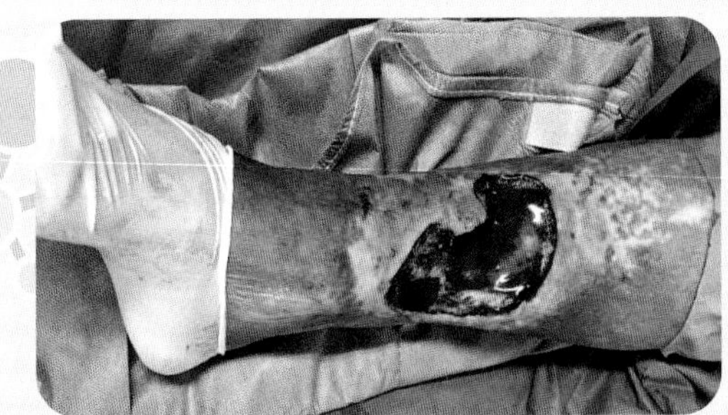

Figure 9.6.4 Artificial double-layer leather cover

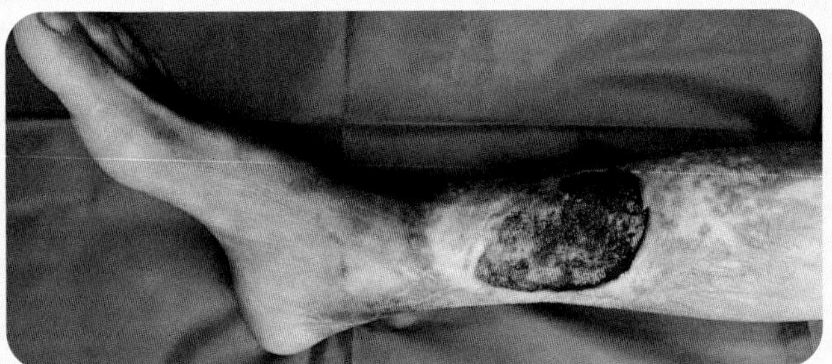

Figure 9.6.5 After 3 weeks, the artificial dermis was removed, and the granulation tissue on the wound was fresh and had granular proliferation, with active bleeding upon contact

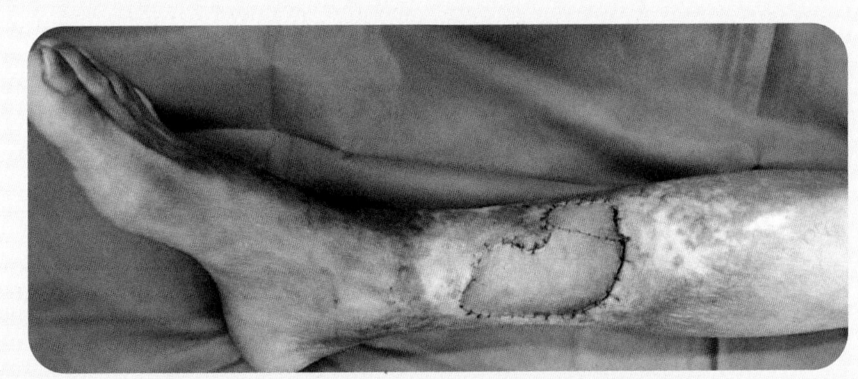

Figure 9.6.6 Medium thickness free skin transplantation

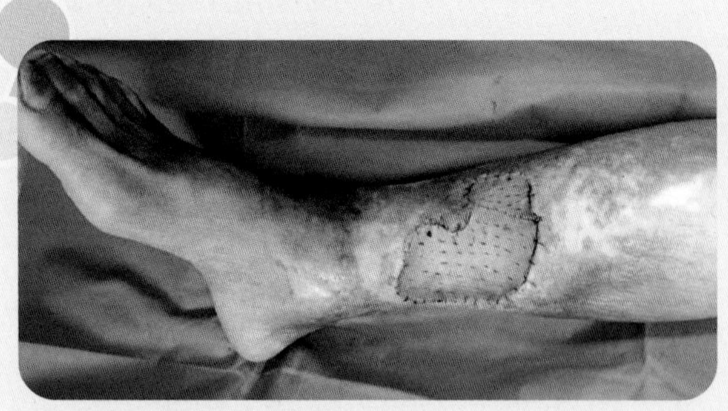

图 9.6.7　游离皮肤打孔，利于皮下积液渗出，防止积液将皮肤浮起

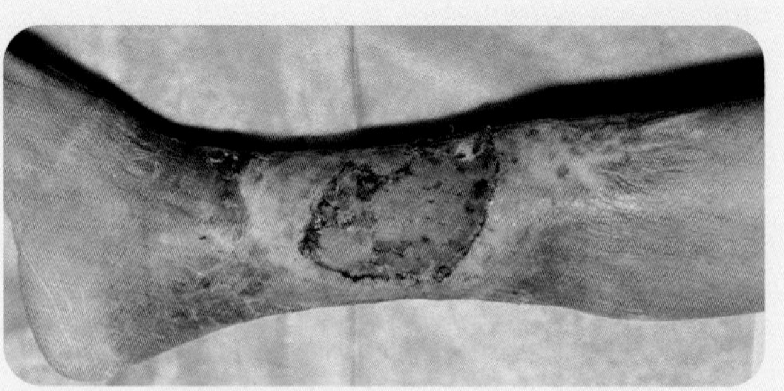

图 9.6.8　1 周后植皮完全成活，散在少许创面，换药后愈合

（陈善亮）

案例七　背部巨大神经纤维瘤切除修复

◆ 致病原因

患儿因 17 号染色体基因异常，致常染色体显性遗传病 I 型神经纤维瘤病，背部巨大皮肤肿物。

◆ 症状与体征

自述背部异物感，尤以躺卧时明显。皮肤呈黑褐色，呈现 I 型神经纤维瘤病特有“咖啡牛奶斑”，皮肤增厚粗糙，上覆盖茂密体毛，可触及一范围约 37 cm × 20 cm 大小肿物，质软（图 9.7.1）。

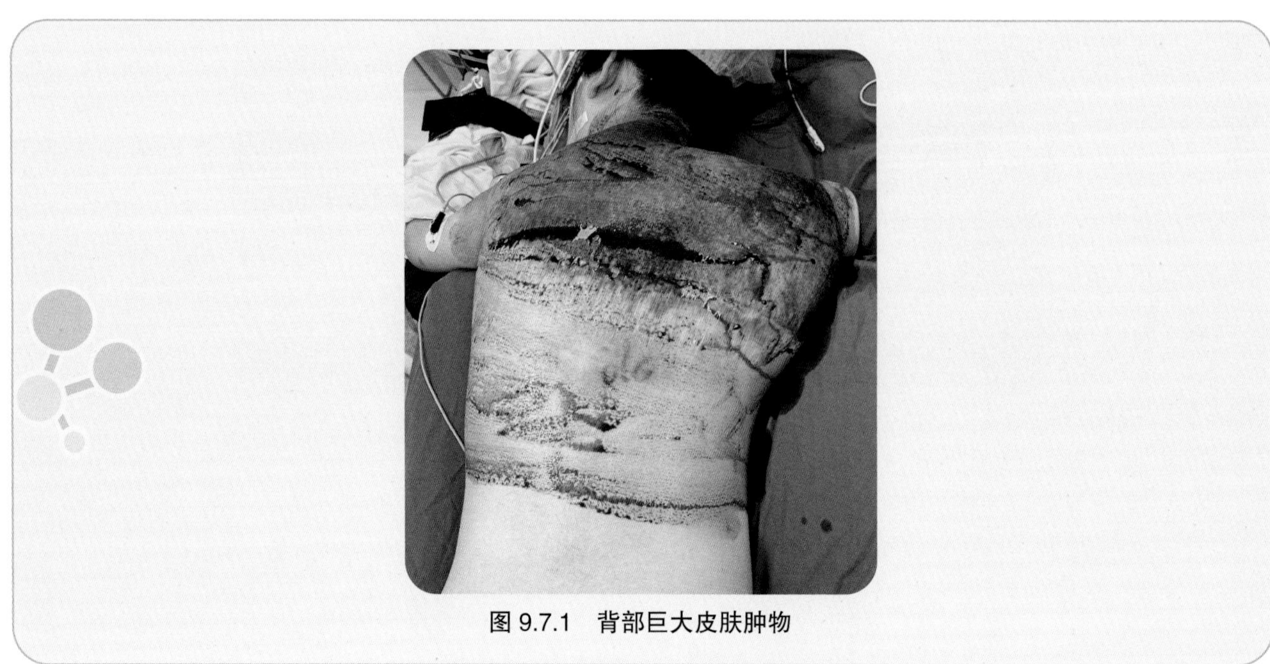

图 9.7.1　背部巨大皮肤肿物

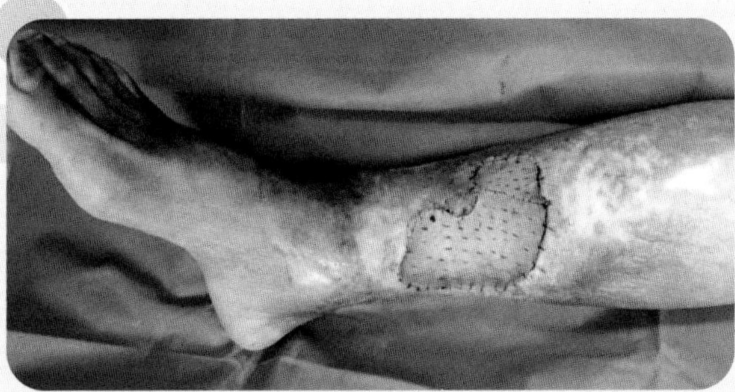

Figure 9.6.7 Free skin perforation facilitates subcutaneous fluid leakage and prevents fluid from floating the skin

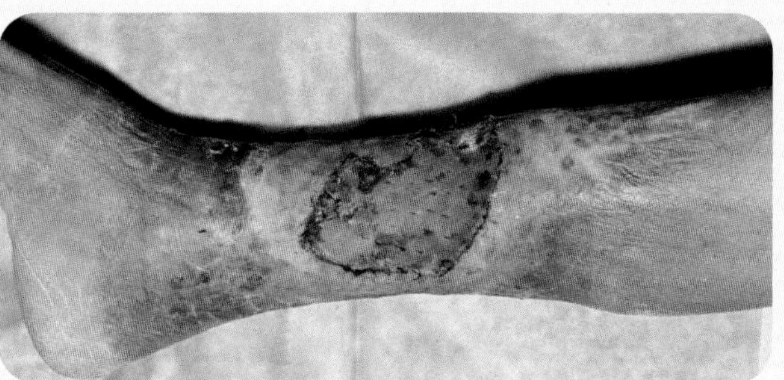

Figure 9.6.8 After one week, the skin graft completely survived and scattered on a few wounds, which healed after dressing change

(Chen Shanliang)

Case 7 Removal and repair of a giant neurofibroma in the back

◆ Cause of illness

The child has an autosomal dominant inherited disease type I neurofibromatosis and a huge skin mass on the back due to genetic abnormalities in chromosome 17.

◆ Signs and symptoms

Self reported feeling of foreign body in the back, especially noticeable when lying down. The skin is dark brown and presents the characteristic coffee milk spots of type I neurofibromatosis. The skin is thickened and rough, covered with dense body hair, and a soft mass of about 37 cm × 20 cm in size can be palpated (Figure 9.7.1).

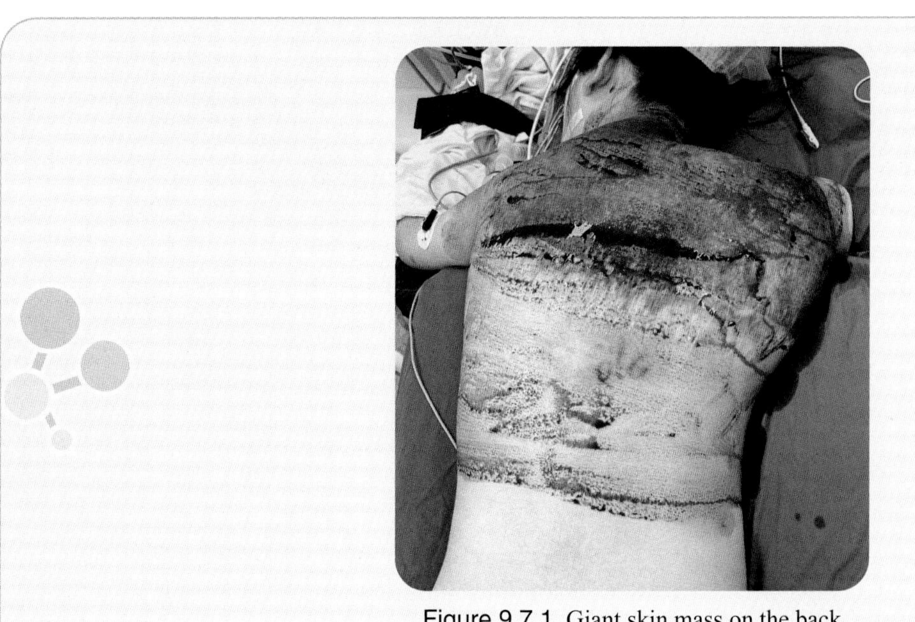

Figure 9.7.1 Giant skin mass on the back

◆ 治疗方案

鉴于患儿年龄较小、皮肤肿物巨大，设计分期切除肿物＋创面修复，避免术中失血过多，降低手术风险。

1. 术前B超、CT均提示肩背部广泛皮下占位，最厚处约50 mm，内部血流丰富。术前备血。

2. 俯卧位下全身麻醉。

3. 因背部肿物切除后创面较大，一期手术切除肩背部大部肿物，确切止血，给予异体皮覆盖可有效保护创面，有利于创面新生血管形成和肉芽组织增生，为二期自体皮移植提供良好的创基；二期手术头皮取皮术＋真皮支架＋自体皮移植术，手术切取患儿自体头皮移植修复创面，未见明显瘢痕及脱发，肩胛间区给予异体真皮支架自体刃厚皮复合移植修复，减少瘢痕形成（图9.7.2～图9.7.5）。

4. 创面外用生长因子辅助使用VSD，有效缩短创面愈合时间，提高手术成功率（图9.7.6）。

5. 术后病理提示神经纤维瘤病。关注血红蛋白量，及时输血。加强术后护理，避免创面受压。

6. 门诊随诊，植皮区及供皮区愈合良好，未见明显瘢痕及脱发；遗留颈部及右侧肩背部皮肤肿物（图9.7.7）。

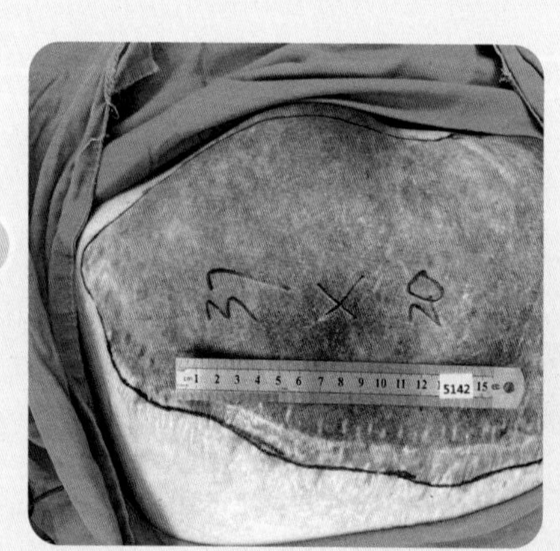

图9.7.2 背部皮肤肿物切除准备，测量大小约37 cm×20 cm

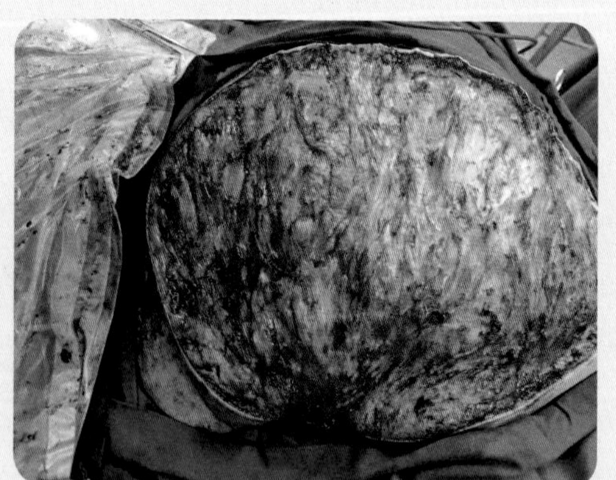

图9.7.3 一期手术切除背部肿物后创面，基底深达浅筋膜（脂肪层）

◆ Treatment plan

Considering the young age of the patient and the large size of the skin mass, staged excision of the mass and wound repair are designed to avoid excessive intraoperative blood loss and reduce surgical risks.

1. Preoperative ultrasound and CT both showed extensive subcutaneous mass in the shoulder and back, with the thickest part being about 50 mm and abundant internal blood flow. Preoperative blood preparation.

2. General anesthesia in prone position.

3. Due to the large size of the wound after the removal of the back mass, the first stage surgery involves the removal of most of the shoulder and back mass, precise hemostasis, and coverage with allogeneic skin to effectively protect the wound. This is beneficial for the formation of new blood vessels and granulation tissue proliferation in the wound, providing a good foundation for the second stage autologous skin transplantation; The second stage surgery involved scalp peeling, dermal stent, and autologous skin transplantation. The patient underwent autologous scalp transplantation to repair the wound, and no obvious scars or hair loss were observed. The scapular area was repaired with allogeneic dermal stent and autologous thick skin composite transplantation to reduce scar formation (Figure 9.7.2- Figure 9.7.5).

4. External application of growth factors to assist VSD can effectively shorten wound healing time and improve surgical success rate (Figure 9.7.6).

5. Postoperative pathology suggests neurofibromatosis. Pay attention to hemoglobin levels and receive timely blood transfusions. Strengthen postoperative care to avoid pressure on the wound.

6. Outpatient follow-up showed good healing in the skin graft and donor areas, with no obvious scars or hair loss observed; Remaining skin masses on the neck and right shoulder back (Figure 9.7.7).

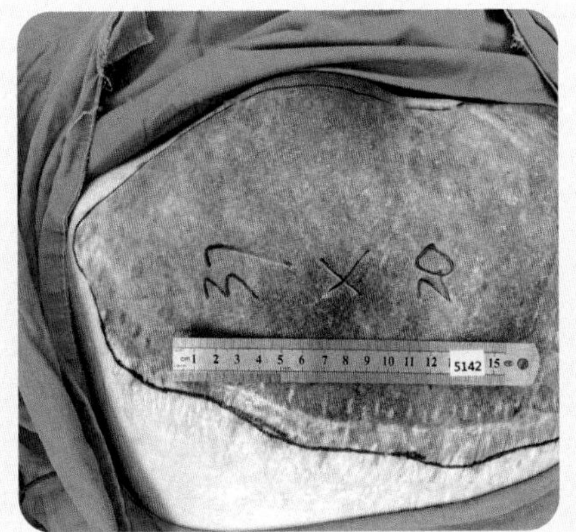

Figure 9.7.2 Preparation for resection of back skin mass, measuring approximately 37 cm × 20 cm in size

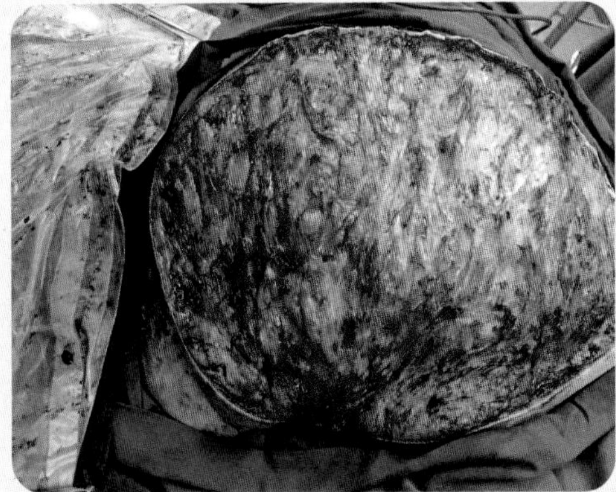

Figure 9.7.3 After the first stage surgical resection of a back mass, the wound surface extends deep into the superficial fascia (fat layer) at the base

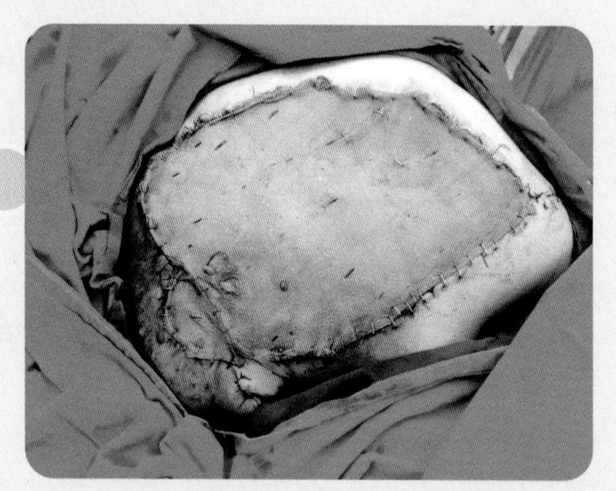
图 9.7.4　异体生物敷料外敷建立临时创面生理屏障

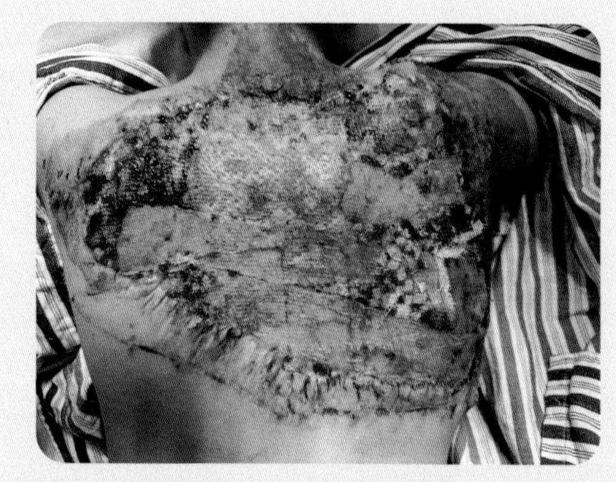
图 9.7.5　二期手术，采用头皮取皮 + 大张皮片 / 邮票状皮片移植修复创面

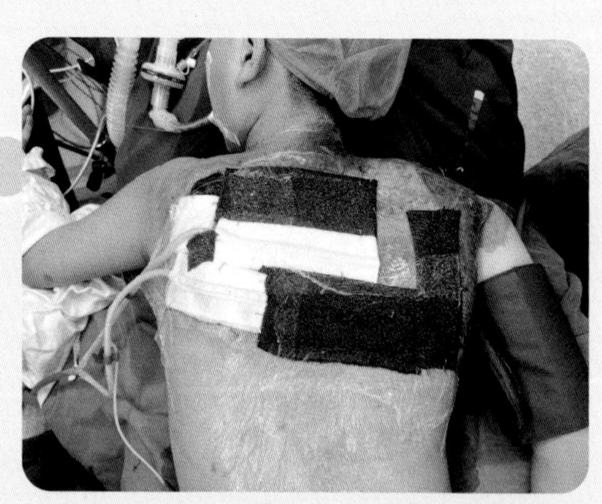
图 9.7.6　创面外用生长因子辅助使用 VSD

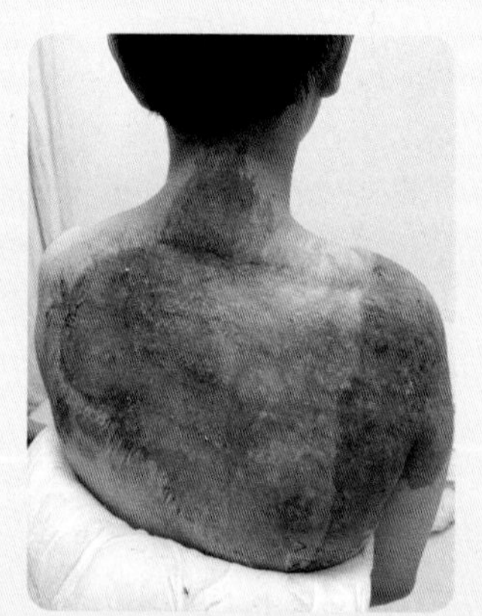
图 9.7.7　门诊随诊，植皮区及供皮区愈合良好，未见明显瘢痕及脱发；遗留颈部及右侧肩背部皮肤肿物

（林　才　尹翼虎）

案例八　乳腺癌术后切口感染

◆ 致病原因

患者既往有糖尿病史，行胸部左乳癌改良根治术，术后切口感染。

◆ 症状与体征

左侧锁骨下有胀痛感，皮温升高，左侧切口近腋侧有胀感。

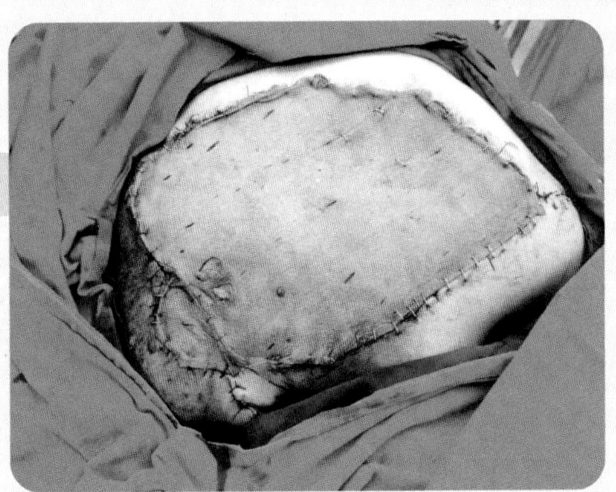

Figure 9.7.4 Establishment of temporary wound physiological barrier by external application of allogeneic biological dressing

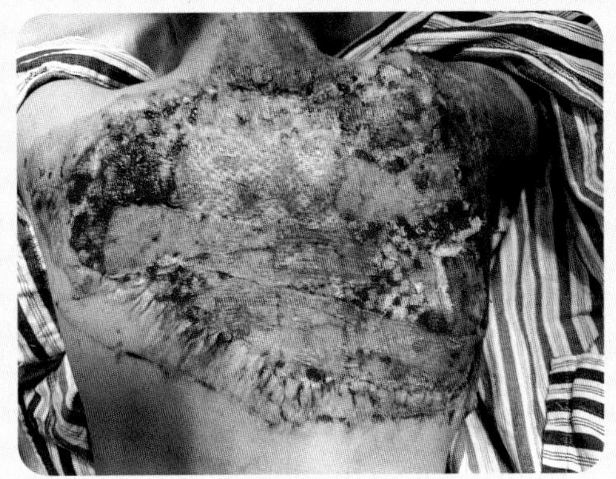

Figure 9.7.5 Second stage surgery, using scalp peeling+large skin grafts/stamp shaped skin grafts to repair wounds

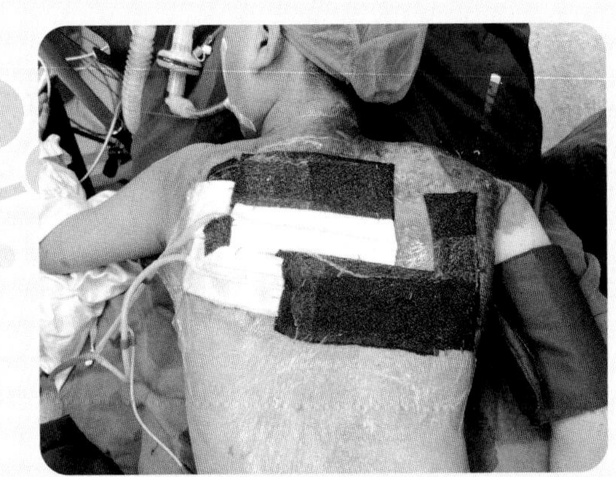

Figure 9.7.6 External application of growth factor assisted VSD on wounds

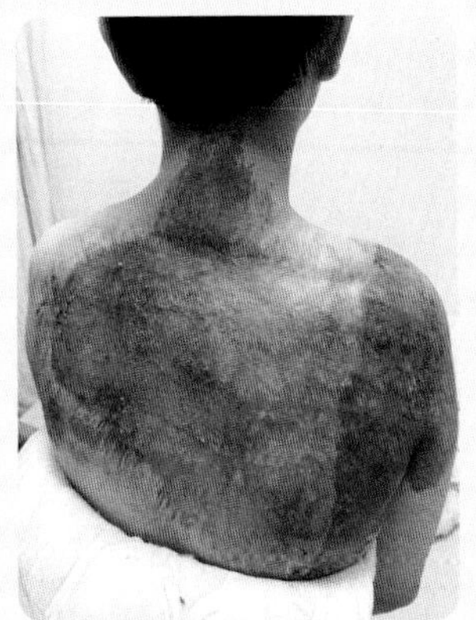

Figure 9.7.7 Outpatient follow-up shows good healing of the skin graft and donor areas, with no obvious scars or hair loss observed; Remaining skin mass on the neck and right shoulder and back

(Lin Cai, Yin Yihu)

Case 8 Postoperative incision infection of breast cancer

◆ Cause of illness

The patient had a history of diabetes, and underwent modified radical mastectomy for left breast cancer, with postoperative incision infection.

◆ Signs and symptoms

There is swelling and pain under the left clavicle, with elevated skin temperature, and swelling near the axilla of the left incision.

◆ 治疗方案

1. 患者糖尿病史，血糖控制，加强营养。给予大清创 + 伤口分泌物培养。

2. 清创后用简易 VSD，促进伤口愈合。

2.1 第一次清创后，创面 13 cm × 5 cm × 0.5 cm，75% 红色，25% 黄黑色，创周皮肤略红，切口 2 ~ 5 点方向潜行 2.8 ~ 7 cm，9 点潜行 2.8 cm，床边锐器清创 + 伤口清洁液 + 自制简易负压治疗（图 9.8.1）。

2.2 第二次清创后，创面 14 cm × 4.4 cm × 0.5 cm，100% 红色，2 ~ 5 点方向潜行 1 ~ 3 cm，9 点潜行 1 cm，加用造口底盘拉合伤口（图 9.8.2）。

2.3 第三次清创后，创面 13.8 cm × 3.5 cm × 0.5 cm，100% 红色，5 点方向潜行 2.5 cm，9 点潜行 0.5 cm（图 9.8.3）。

3. 换药，伤口清洁液及硫酸银敷料局部抗感染，使用创面拉合技术缩小创面。

4. 第三次清创术后 4 天，采用游离皮瓣移植术，缩短创面愈合时间（图 9.8.4）。

5. 游离皮瓣移植术后使用生长因子及脂质水胶体敷料促进表皮爬行，完成创面愈合；游离皮瓣移植术后 2 周，创面愈合（图 9.8.5）。

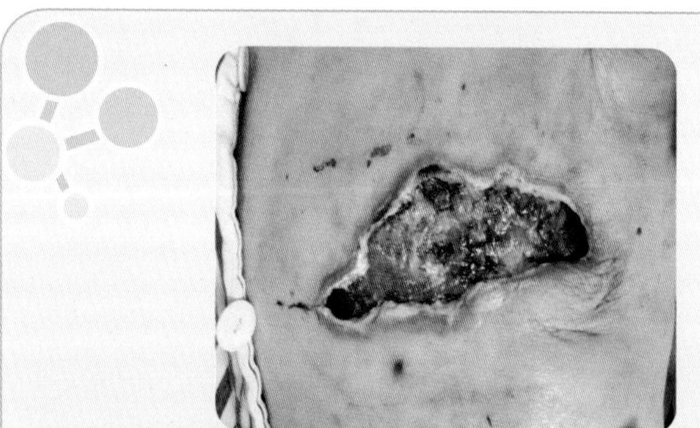

图 9.8.1　第一次清创后，创面 13 cm × 5 cm × 0.5 cm

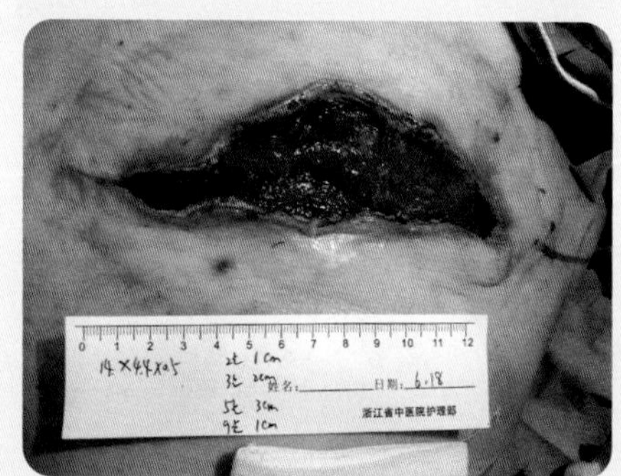

图 9.8.2　第二次清创后，创面 14 cm × 4.4 cm × 0.5 cm

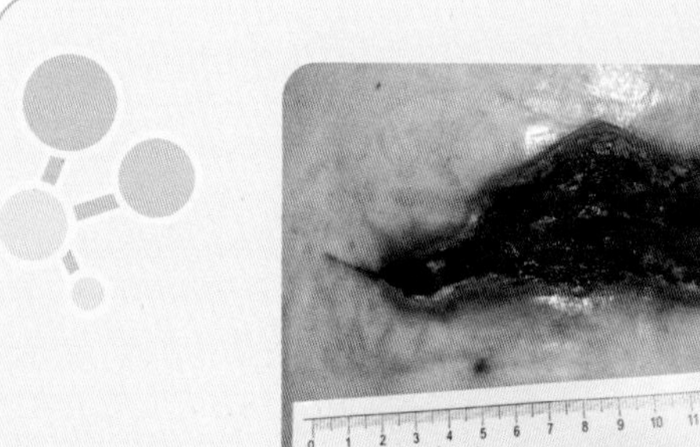

图 9.8.3　第三次清创后，创面 13.8 cm × 3.5 cm × 0.5 cm

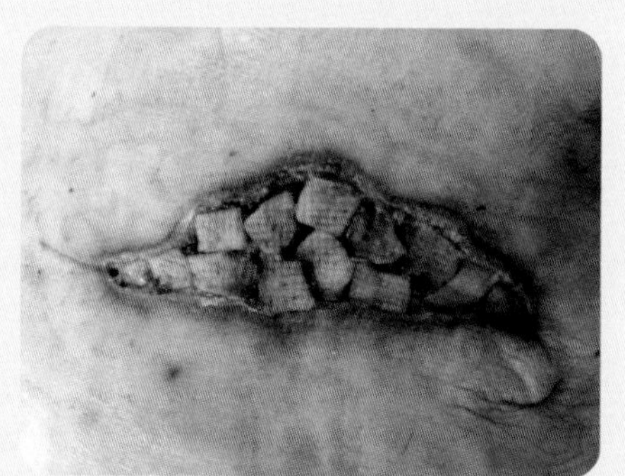

图 9.8.4　游离皮移植术，生长因子 + 脂质水胶体敷料促进爬皮

◆ Treatment plan

1. The patient's diabetes history, blood sugar control, and nutrition enhancement. Provide Daqing Chuang with wound secretion cultivation.

2. Use a simple VSD after debridement to promote wound healing.

2.1 After the first debridement, the wound was 13 cm × 5 cm × 0.5 cm, 75% red, 25% yellow black, and the skin around the wound was slightly red. The incision had a depth of 2.8-7 cm in the 2-5 o'clock direction and a depth of 2.8 cm at 9 o'clock. Bedside sharp instrument debridement, wound cleaning solution, and self-made simple negative pressure treatment were performed (Figure 9.8.1).

2.2 After the second debridement, the wound was 14 cm × 4.4 cm × 0.5 cm, 100% red, and had a depth of 1-3 cm in the 2-5 o'clock direction and 1 cm at 9 o'clock. The wound was then closed with an ostomy base (Figure 9.8.2).

2.3 After the third debridement, the wound was 13.8 cm × 3.5 cm × 0.5 cm, 100% red, with a depth of 2.5 cm in the 5-point direction and 0.5 cm at the 9-point direction (Figure 9.8.3).

3. Change dressing, use wound cleaning solution and silver sulfate dressing for local anti infection, and use wound closure technique to shrink the wound.

4. Four days after the third debridement surgery, free skin flap transplantation was performed to shorten the wound healing time (Figure 9.8.4).

5. After free skin flap transplantation, use growth factors and lipid hydrogel dressings to promote epidermal crawling and complete wound healing; Two weeks after free flap transplantation, the wound healed (Figure 9.8.5).

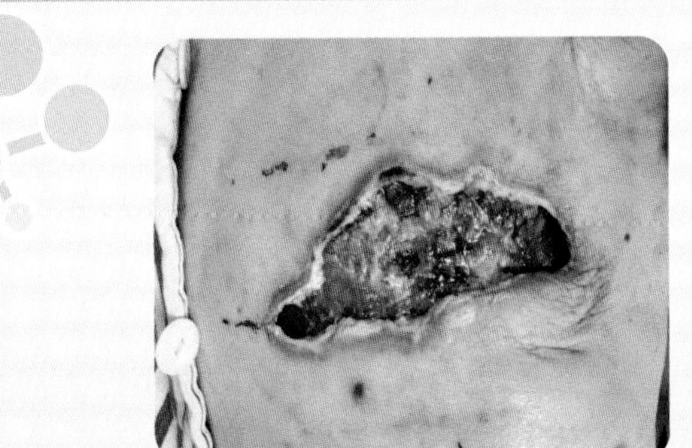

Figure 9.8.1 After the first debridement, the wound is 13 cm × 5 cm × 0.5 cm

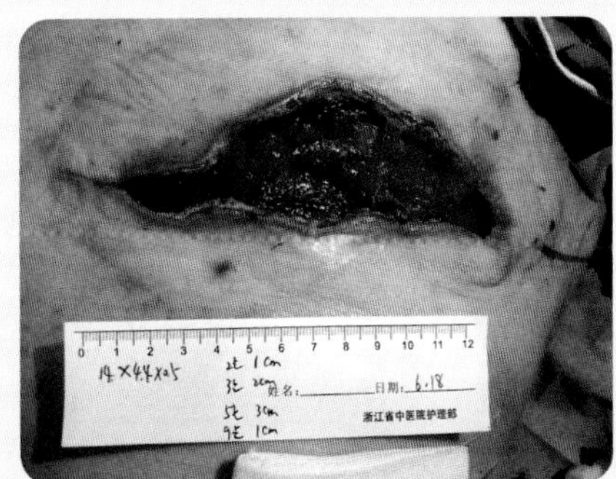

Figure 9.8.2 After the second debridement, the wound size is 14 cm × 4.4 cm × 0.5 cm

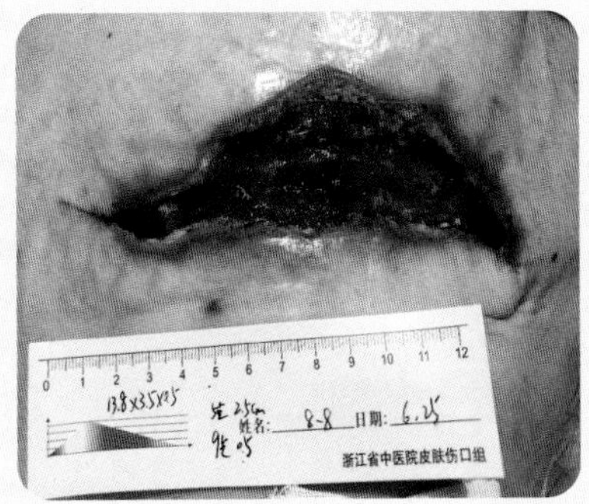

Figure 9.8.3 After the third debridement, the wound size is 13.8 cm × 3.5 cm × 0.5 cm

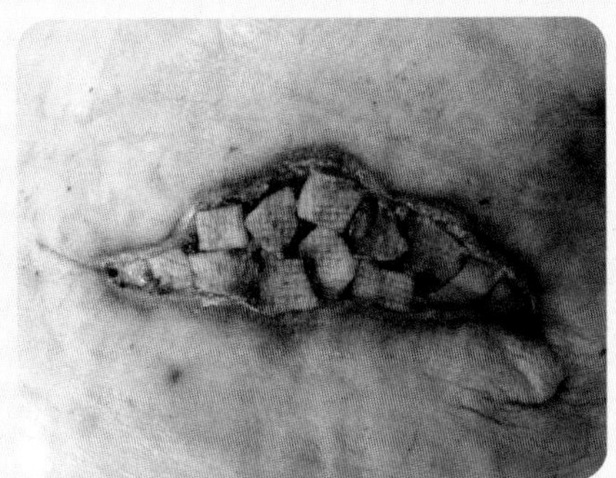

Figure 9.8.4 Free skin transplantation, growth factor + lipid hydrogel dressing promotes skin crawling

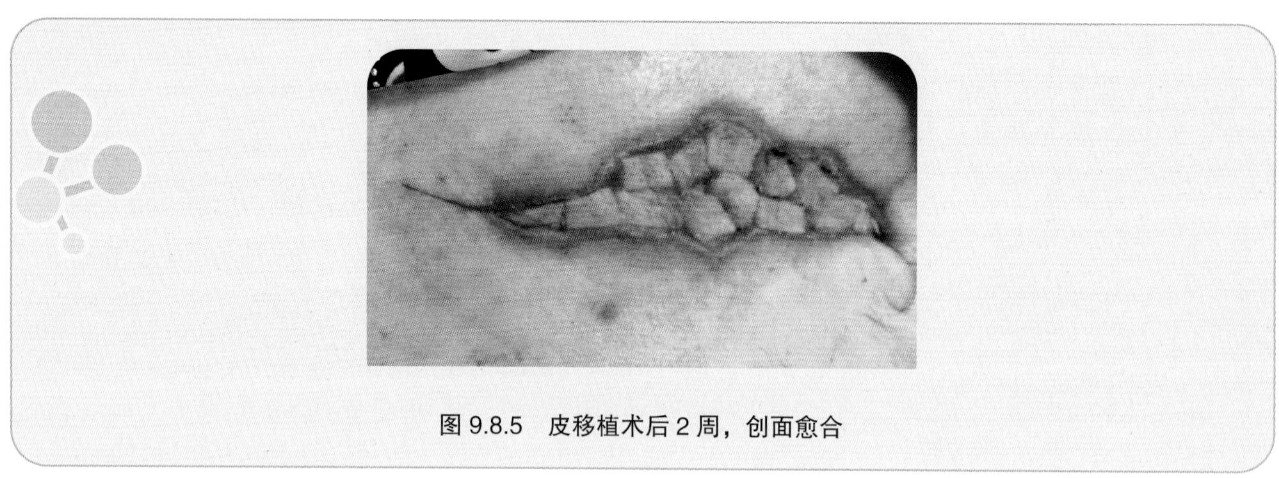
图 9.8.5　皮移植术后 2 周，创面愈合

（邱巧如　王永高）

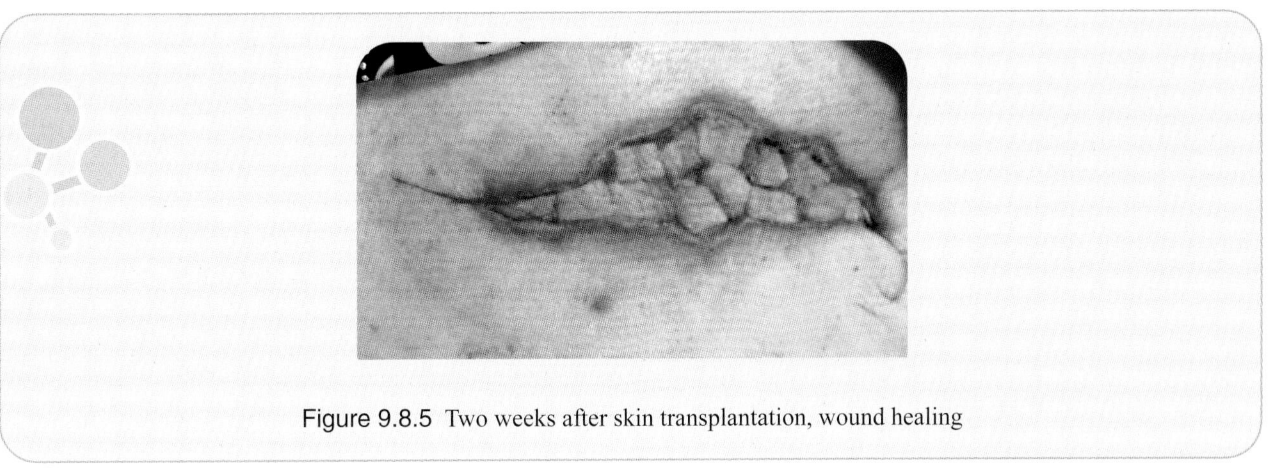

Figure 9.8.5 Two weeks after skin transplantation, wound healing

(Qiu Qiaoru, Wang Yonggao)

第 10 章
Chapter 10

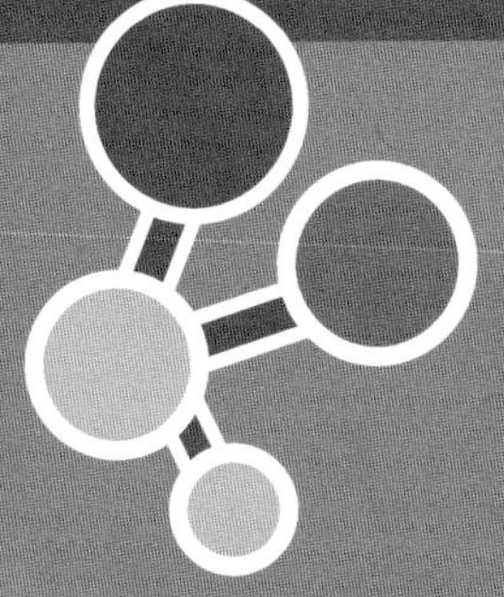

烧烫伤创面修复
Repair of Burn and Scald Wounds

案例一　双足浅二度烫伤

◆ 致病原因

患者，男性，56 岁。穿水靴工作时，不慎将开水倒入水靴中，慌忙中 3 分钟后才脱下水靴，致双足浅二度烫伤。

◆ 症状与体征

双足散在巨大张力性水疱，疱皮较厚，触痛不明显，局部无红肿，疱皮无破溃，肿胀明显，足趾活动良好，皮温不高（图 10.1.1）。

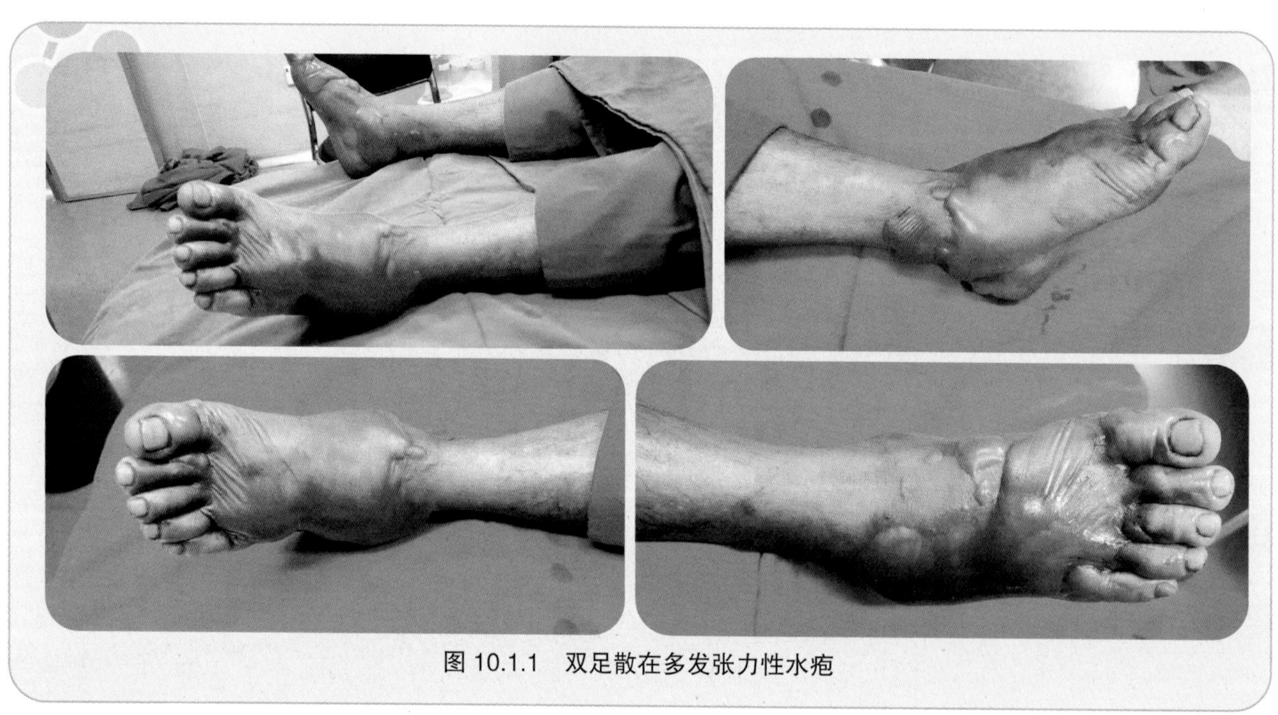

图 10.1.1　双足散在多发张力性水疱

◆ 治疗方案

1. 急诊入院后完善手术前准备。

2. 碘伏常规消毒后，将疱皮切取数个空洞，并保证疱皮完整性，安装 VSD 装置，持续负压吸引，并使用生长因子滴注冲洗创面（图 10.1.2）。

3. 7 天后取下 VSD 装置，修建脱落疱皮，创面覆盖 S-100 止血绫纱布加厚棉垫包扎。

4. 3 周后打开包扎敷料，创面完全愈合（图 10.1.3）。

Case 1 Shallow second degree burns on both feet

◆ Cause of illness

Patient, male, 56 years old. When wearing water boots to work, accidentally pouring boiling water into the boots and taking them off in a panic for 3 minutes, causing shallow second degree burns to both feet.

◆ Signs and symptoms

There are large tension blisters scattered on both feet, with thick blister skin, no obvious tenderness, no local redness or swelling, no ulceration of blister skin, obvious swelling, good toe movement, and low skin temperature (Figure 10.1.1).

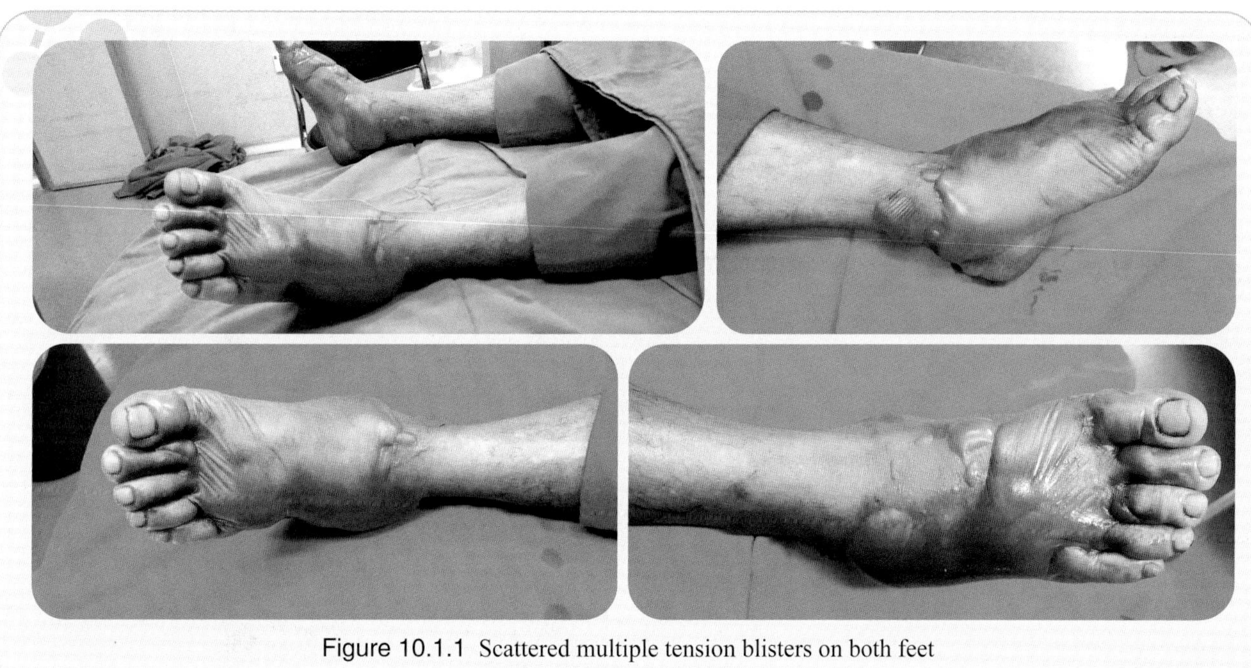

Figure 10.1.1 Scattered multiple tension blisters on both feet

◆ Treatment plan

1. Complete preoperative preparation after emergency admission.
2. After routine disinfection with iodine, cut several cavities into the blister skin and ensure its integrity. Install a VSD device, continue negative pressure suction, and use growth factor infusion to flush the wound (Figure 10.1.2).
3. After 7 days, remove the VSD device, construct a detached blister skin, and cover the wound with S-100 hemostatic gauze and thickened cotton pad for bandaging.
4. After 3 weeks, the dressing was opened and the wound was completely healed (Figure 10.1.3).

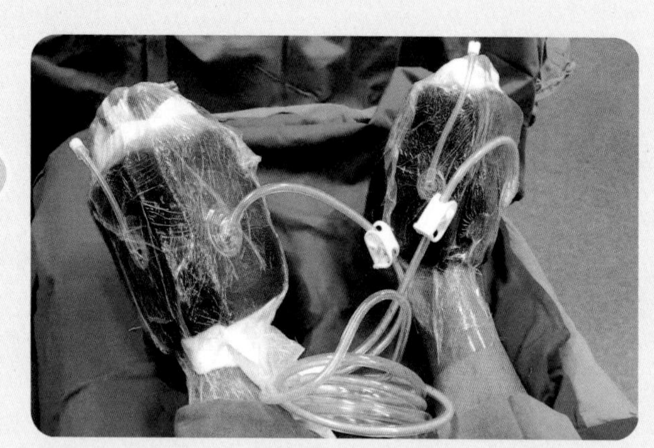
图 10.1.2 在水疱表面剪开数个空洞，利于渗出，并用 VSD 吸引 + 生长因子

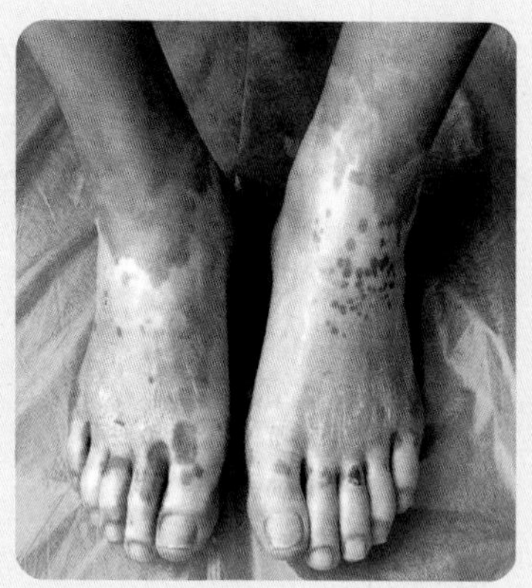
图 10.1.3 3 周后创面完全愈合

（陈善亮）

案例二 下肢烧伤瘢痕大面积挛缩（陈旧性）

◆ 致病原因

患者，女性，45 岁。2 岁时，不慎掉入火盆烧伤右大腿，致右大腿腘窝区大面积烧伤。

◆ 症状与体征

走路跛行，右膝关节疼痛，不能伸直走路。右大腿、腘窝区、小腿上段有大面积瘢痕，局部瘢痕增生伴硬化，纤维板增厚，膝关节屈曲挛缩，伸直活动受限，小腿肌肉萎缩，足部感觉运动良好，足背动脉搏动良好（图 10.2.1 ~图 10.2.3）。骨盆倾斜畸形，脊柱侧弯畸形。

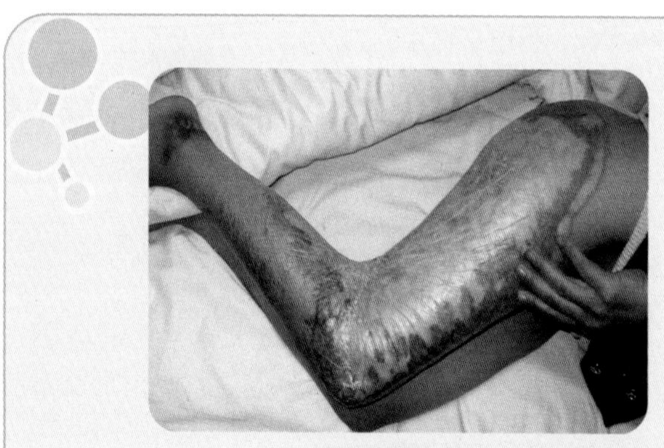
图 10.2.1 右大腿后侧大面积瘢痕

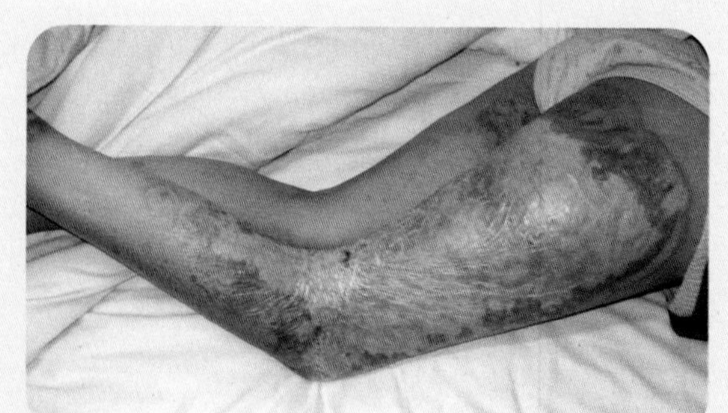
图 10.2.2 右腿腘窝区可见大面积瘢痕挛缩

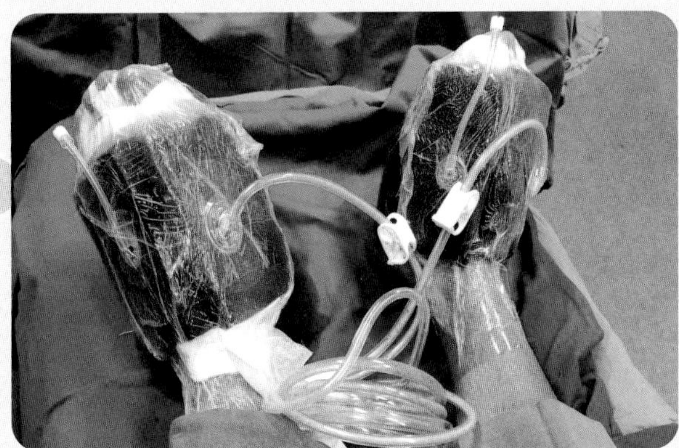

Figure 10.1.2 Cut several cavities on the surface of the blister to facilitate exudation, and use VSD to attract growth factors

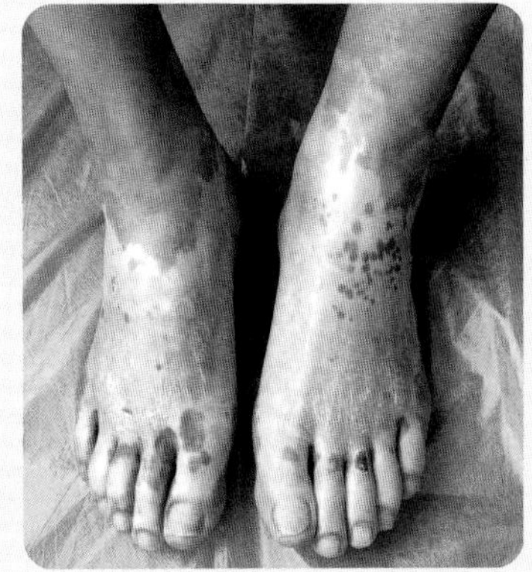

Figure 10.1.3 Complete wound healing after 3 weeks

(Chen Shanliang)

Case 2 Large area contracture of lower limb burn scars (old)

◆ Cause of illness

Patient, female, 45 years old. At the age of 2, accidentally fell into a brazier and burned the right thigh, causing extensive burns in the popliteal area of the right thigh.

◆ Signs and symptoms

Limping while walking, pain in the right knee joint, and inability to walk straight. There are large areas of scars on the right thigh, popliteal area, and upper leg, with local scar hyperplasia accompanied by hardening, thickening of the fibrous plate, knee joint flexion contracture, limited extension movement, leg muscle atrophy, good foot sensation and movement, and good dorsal artery pulsation (Figure 10.2.1-Figure 10.2.3). Pelvic tilt deformity and scoliosis deformity.

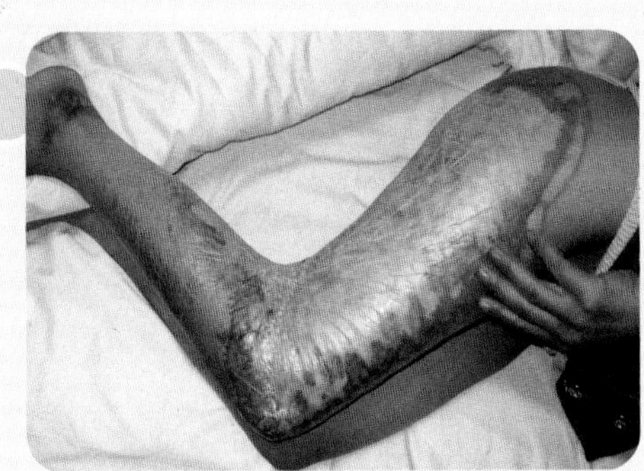

Figure 10.2.1 Large area scar on the back of the right thigh

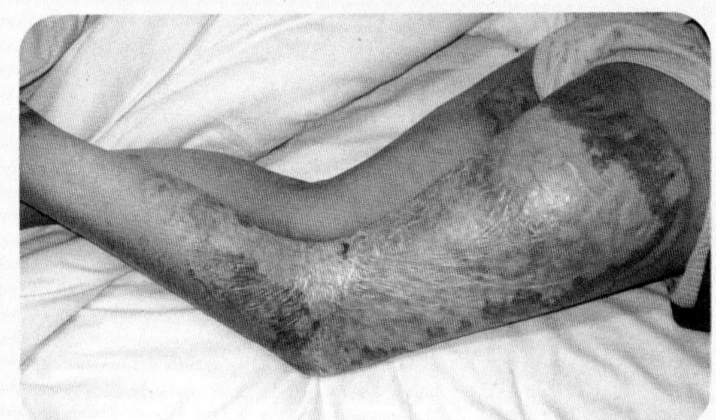

Figure 10.2.2 Large area scar contracture visible in the right leg popliteal fossa area

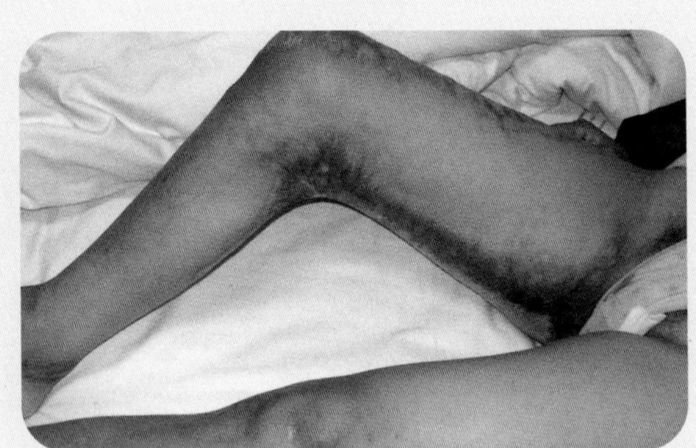

图 10.2.3　右膝关节屈曲畸形

◆ 治疗方案

1. 手术方案首选，切除腘窝区巨大硬化瘢痕，松解挛缩组织结构。

2. 选择全身麻醉，膝关节后侧严重瘢痕挛缩，制约膝关节伸直困难，将增生肥厚纤维板等瘢痕组织彻底切除，瘢痕切除后形成巨大创面，切取全厚皮肤移植于腘窝后创面，覆盖凡士林纱布，加厚敷料覆盖伤口（图 10.2.4 ~ 图 10.2.7）。

3. 腘窝区瘢痕切除后，膝关节可以伸直，植皮区放置两枚橡皮条引流，2 天后拔出引流条。

4. 术后 12 天拆线，植皮完全成活，下肢长腿石膏固定 3 周。3 周去除石膏固定并进行膝关节功能训练。

5. 术后 3 天给予抗菌药物，预防感染。

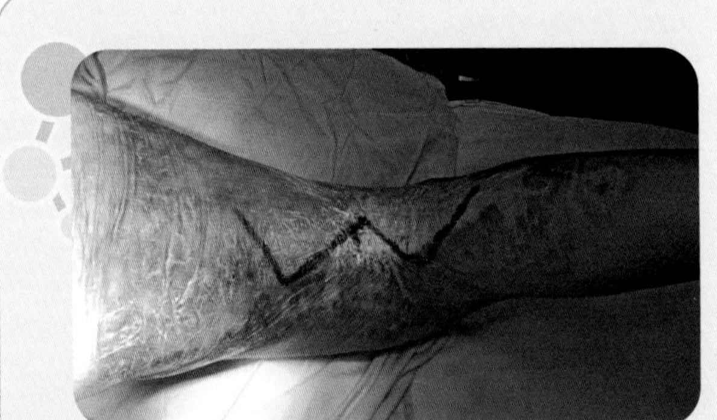

图 10.2.4　腘窝处设计 W 切口

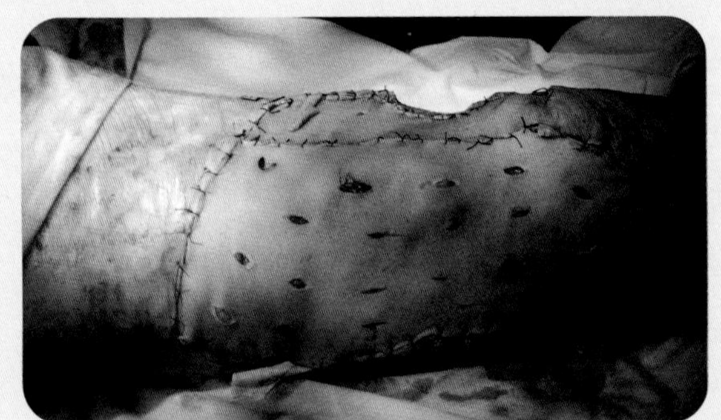

图 10.2.5　切除腘窝大面积挛缩瘢痕，腘绳肌松解

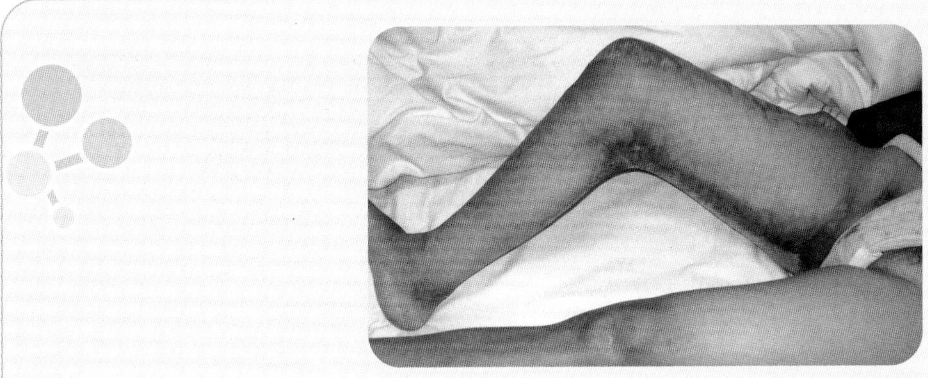

Figure 10.2.3 Right knee joint flexion deformity

◆ Treatment plan

1. The preferred surgical plan is to remove the huge hardened scar in the popliteal area and release the contracted tissue structure.

2. General anesthesia was chosen to treat severe scar contractures on the posterior side of the knee joint, which hindered the extension of the knee joint. The hypertrophic fibrous plate and other scar tissues were completely removed, forming a huge wound after scar removal. Full thickness skin was cut and transplanted onto the wound behind the popliteal fossa, covered with Vaseline gauze, and thickened dressings were applied to cover the wound (Figure 10.2.4- Figure 10.2.7).

3. After scar removal in the popliteal area, the knee joint can be straightened, and two rubber strips are placed in the skin graft area for drainage. Two days later, the drainage strips are removed.

4. The stitches were removed 12 days after surgery, and the skin graft survived completely. The lower limbs and long legs were fixed with plaster for 3 weeks. Remove the plaster fixation for 3 weeks and perform knee joint function training.

5. Administer antibiotics 3 days after surgery to prevent infection.

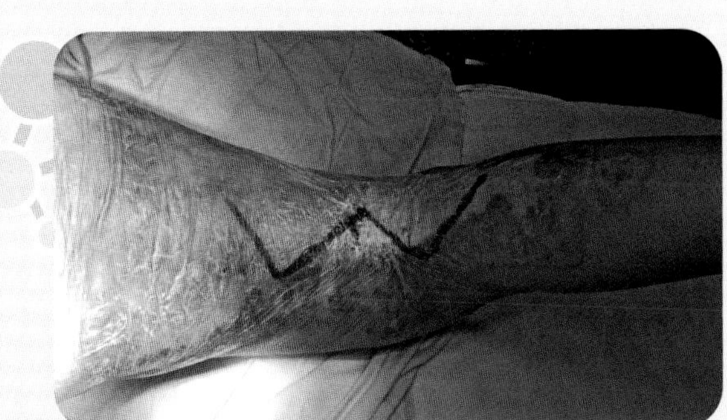

Figure 10.2.4 Design of W incision at popliteal fossa

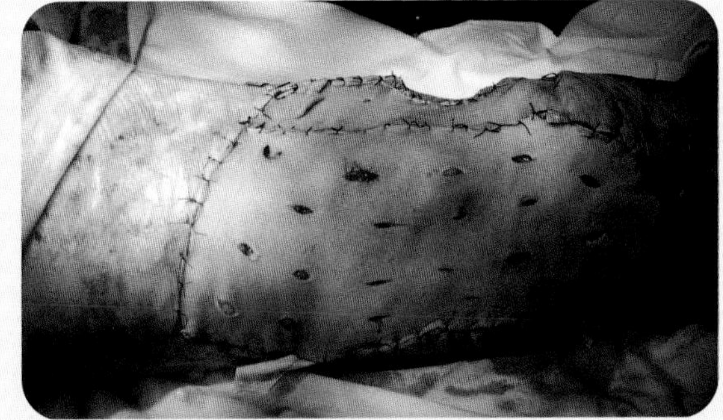

Figure 10.2.5 Removal of large area contracture scar in the popliteal fossa, release of hamstring muscle

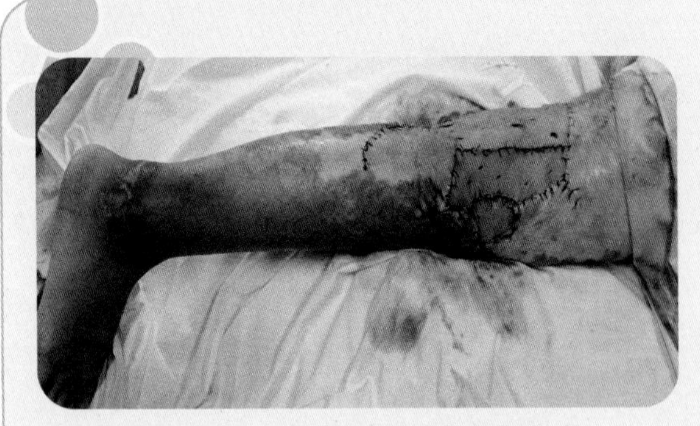
图 10.2.6 松解后膝关节完全伸直

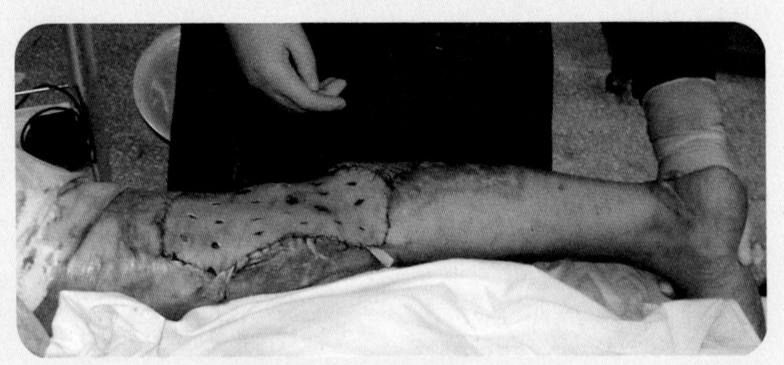
图 10.2.7 全厚皮肤移植

（陈善亮　张振伟）

案例三　双手高压电弧灼伤

◆ 致病原因

患者，男性，59 岁，被 380 V 高压电弧灼伤双手。

◆ 症状与体征

双手剧痛难忍，肿胀并逐渐加重，双手屈伸活动受限。双手肿胀明显，局部手掌手指皮肤烧焦皮革样改变，局部皮温增高，触痛明显，皮肤皮革样影响手指屈伸活动，指端感觉减退，手指指端血液反流迟缓，手背部散在张力性水疱，疱皮破溃并有大量渗出液，全身其他部位无损伤，无心悸气促，无头晕乏力（图 10.3.1）。

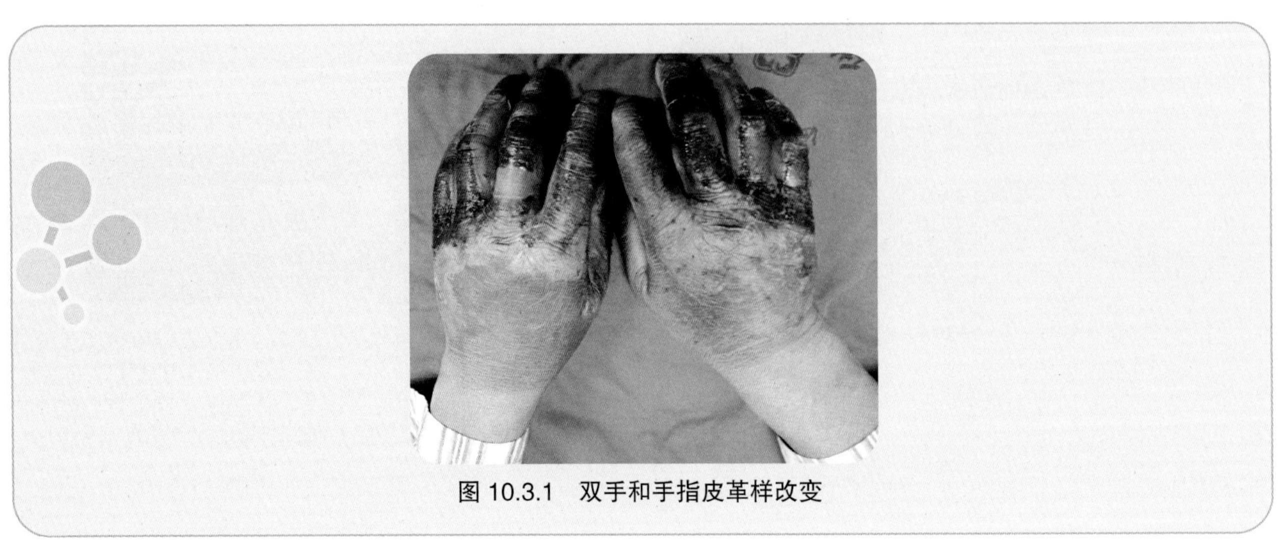
图 10.3.1　双手和手指皮革样改变

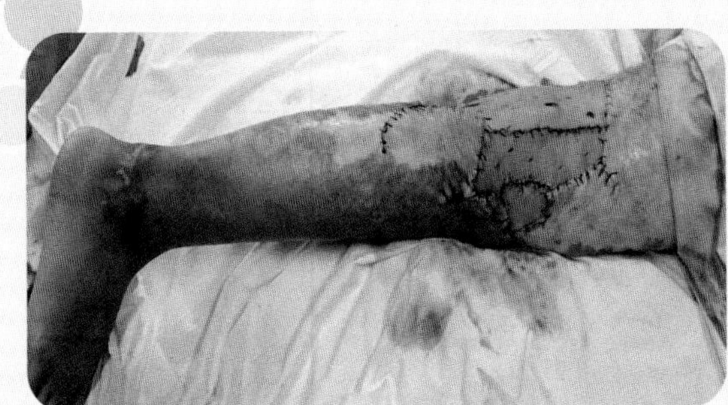

Figure 10.2.6 Complete extension of knee joint after release

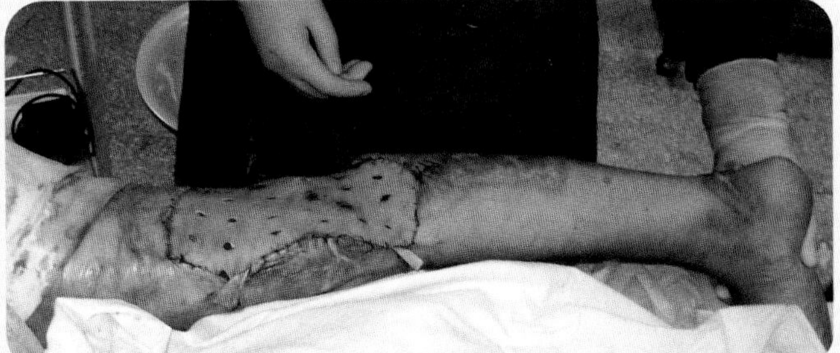

Figure 10.2.7 Full thickness skin transplantation

(Chen Shanliang, Zhang Zhenwei)

Case 3 High voltage arc burns on both hands

◆ Cause of illness

Patient, male, 59 years old, had his hands burned by a 380 V high-voltage arc.

◆ Signs and symptoms

The pain in both hands is unbearable, swelling and gradually worsening, and the movement of both hands is restricted. There is obvious swelling in both hands, with locally burnt leather like changes in the skin of the palm and fingers, increased local skin temperature, and obvious tenderness. The leather like skin affects the flexion and extension of the fingers, and the sensation at the fingertips decreases. The blood reflux at the fingertips is slow, and there are scattered tension blisters on the back of the hand. The blister skin is ruptured and has a large amount of exudate. There is no damage to other parts of the body, no palpitations or shortness of breath, and no dizziness or fatigue (Figure 10.3.1).

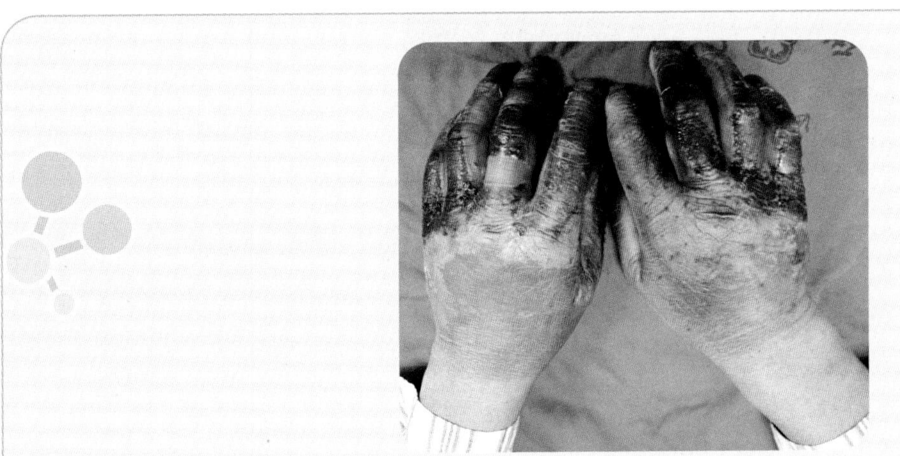

Figure 10.3.1 Leather like changes in hands and fingers

◆ 治疗方案

1. 入院后完善各项检查，评估是否有心脏心肌损害，给予镇痛药和抗菌药物，预防组织水肿和皮肤坏死等药物治疗。

2. 急诊进行坏死焦皮及污染物清除，手部新鲜创面应用重组人碱性成纤维细胞生长因子 + 胶原蛋白海绵敷料贴贴敷，凡士林纱布覆盖厚棉垫分指包扎（图 10.3.2）。

3. 3 天内抬高患肢，局部冰敷。3 天后抬高患肢，红外线理疗，治疗期间，手部创面敷料渗透，及时更换敷料。

4. 3 周后，去除敷料，创面完全愈合，并常规涂抹创肤宁液体伤口敷料保护新生嫩皮，促进上皮角化（图 10.3.3）。

5. 常规关节松动，促进手指关节功能恢复。

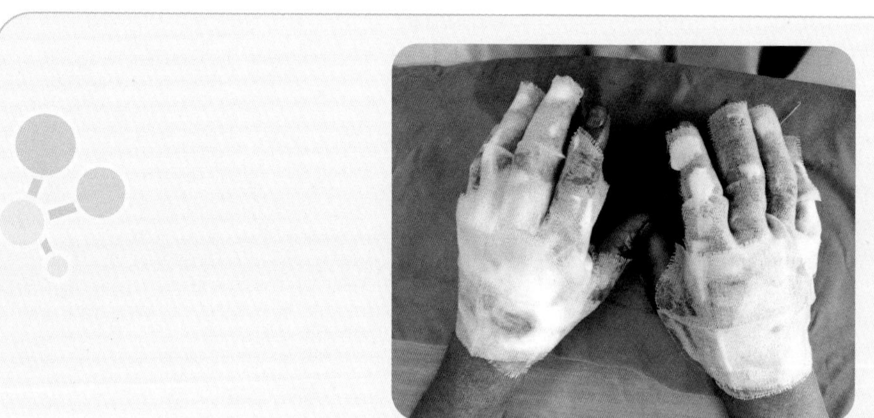

图 10.3.2 清洁消毒后去除焦皮，胶原蛋白油纱敷料包扎

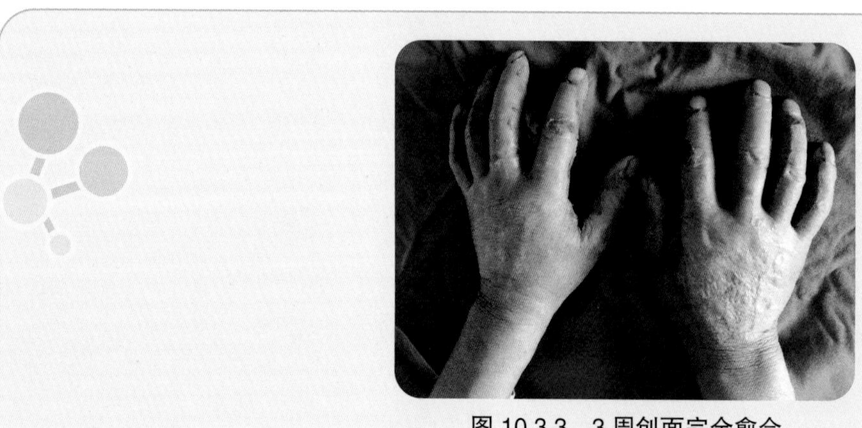

图 10.3.3 3 周创面完全愈合

（陈善亮 高士强）

◆ Treatment plan

1. After admission, complete various examinations to evaluate whether there is cardiac and myocardial damage, administer analgesics and antibiotics, and prevent drug treatment such as tissue edema and skin necrosis.

2. In the emergency department, necrotic skin and pollutants should be removed. Fresh wounds on the hands should be treated with recombinant human basic fibroblast growth factor and collagen sponge dressing, and covered with Vaseline gauze and thick cotton pads for finger wrapping (Figure 10.3.2).

3. Raise the affected limb and apply local ice within 3 days. Three days later, raise the affected limb and undergo infrared therapy. During the treatment period, the wound dressing on the hand should be infiltrated and replaced promptly.

4. After 3 weeks, the dressing was removed and the wound was completely healed. The wound dressing with Chuangfuning liquid was routinely applied to protect the newly formed tender skin and promote epithelial keratinization (Figure 10.3.3).

5. Conventional joint loosening promotes the recovery of finger joint function.

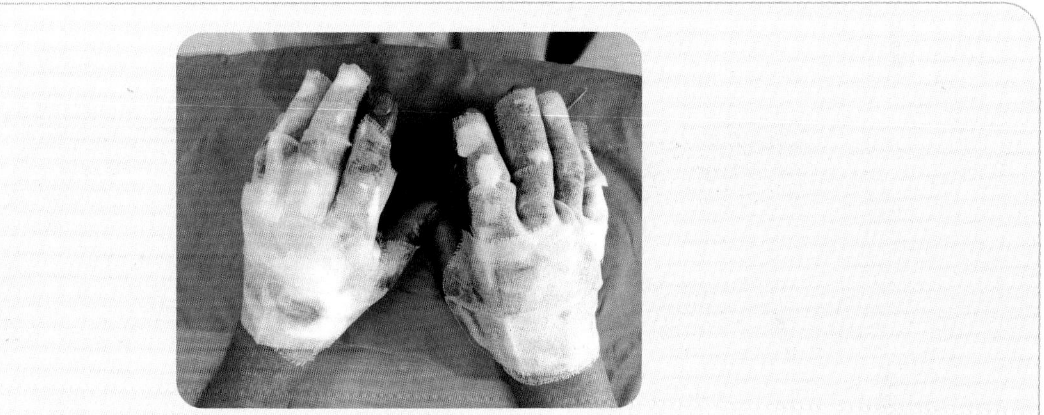

Figure 10.3.2 Removing burnt skin after cleaning and disinfection, wrapping with collagen oil gauze dressing

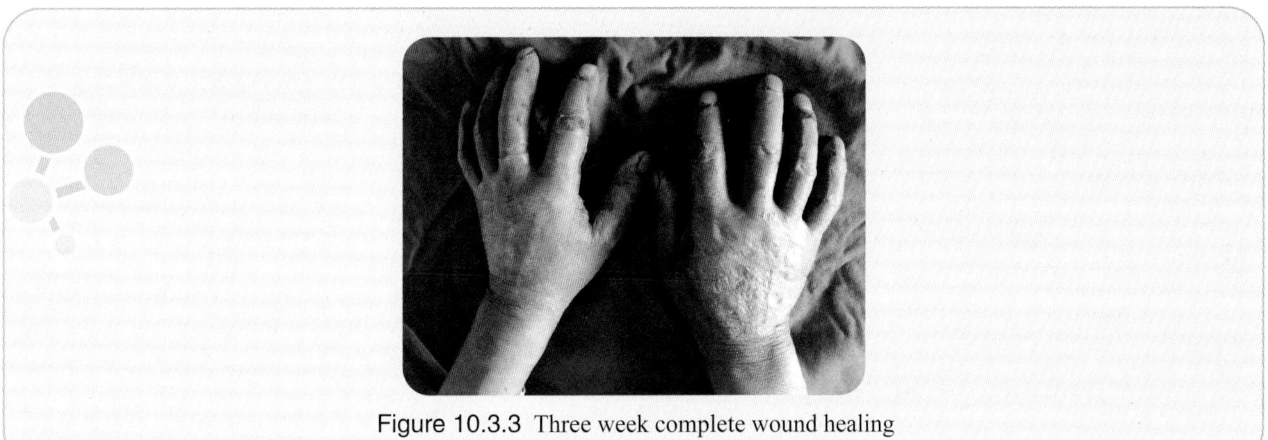

Figure 10.3.3 Three week complete wound healing

(Chen Shanliang, Gao Shiqiang)

案例四　双足开水烫伤

◆ 致病原因

患儿，女性，1.5 岁，不慎踏入开水盆中，烫伤双足。

◆ 症状与体征

双足烫伤后剧痛难忍，哭闹不止，家属在家脱袜子时疱皮大面积脱落，足趾水疱疱皮未脱落，双足肿胀明显，创面红润，有大量炎性渗出，部分趾甲脱落，局部皮温不高，髂腹股沟淋巴结无肿（图 10.4.1、图 10.4.2）。

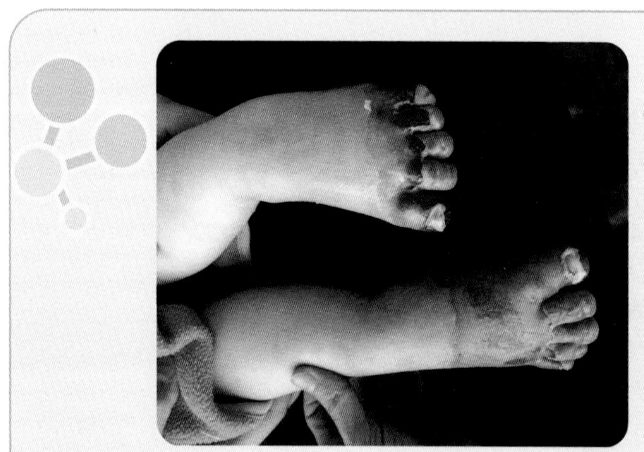

图 10.4.1　双足足背创面

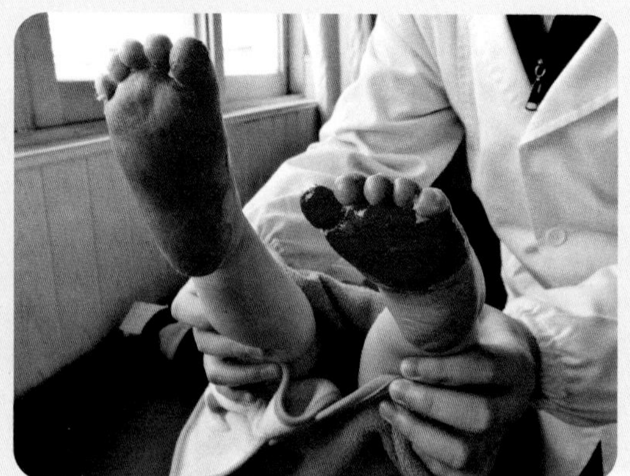

图 10.4.2　双足足底创面

◆ 治疗方案

1. 入院后完善各项手术前检查，禁食水。给予静脉麻醉后清创包扎，由于儿童恐惧哭闹，不能安静配合清创包扎，必须在麻醉下处置。

2. 将脱落残留疱皮完全清创干净，采用重组人碱性成纤维细胞生长因子和油纱分趾包扎覆盖创面，厚棉垫加压包扎，由于儿童配合程度有限，包扎固定要牢固，定时检查敷料松动情况，有渗出时及时换药。

3. 及时观察体温变化，预防和控制创面感染情况，原则不给予抗菌药物治疗。

4. 2 周后打开基层敷料，创面完全愈合（图 10.4.3）。

Case 4 Foot scald caused by boiling water

◆ Cause of illness

Child, female, 1.5 years old, accidentally stepped into a boiling water basin and burned both feet.

◆ Signs and symptoms

After being burned on both feet, the pain was unbearable and there was constant crying. When the family members took off their socks at home, a large area of blister skin fell off, but the blister skin on the toes did not fall off. The feet were swollen significantly, and the wounds were red with a large amount of inflammatory exudate. Some toenails fell off, and the local skin temperature was not high. There was no swelling in the iliac and inguinal lymph nodes (Figure 10.4.1, Figure 10.4.2).

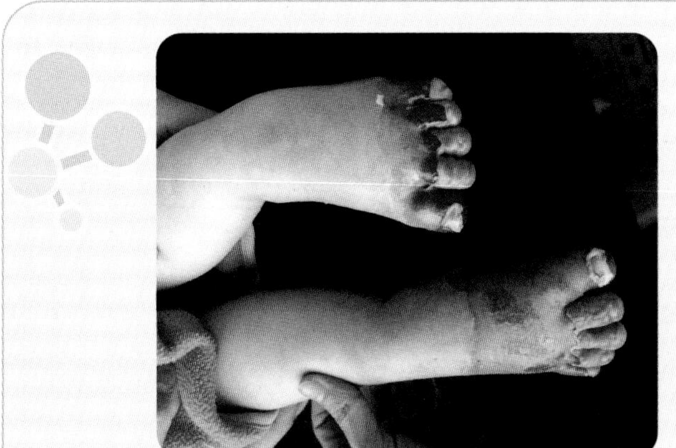

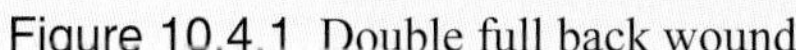

Figure 10.4.1 Double full back wound

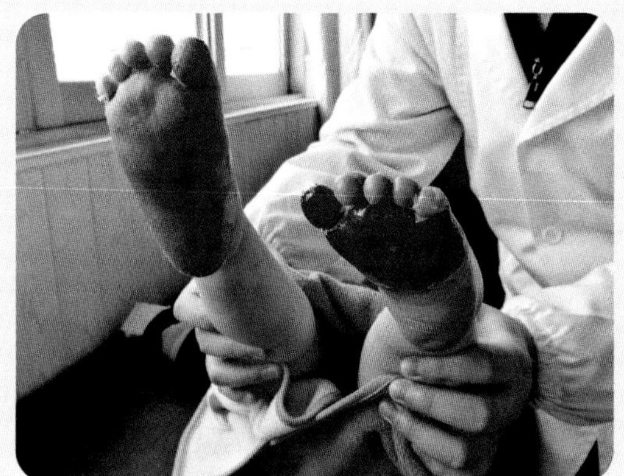

Figure 10.4.2 Foot sole wounds on both feet

◆ Treatment plan

1. After admission, complete all preoperative examinations and refrain from drinking water. After intravenous anesthesia, debridement and bandaging were performed. Due to the child's fear of crying, they were unable to cooperate with the debridement and bandaging quietly and must be treated under anesthesia.

2. Completely clean the remaining blister skin that has fallen off, use recombinant human alkaline fibroblast growth factor and oil gauze to cover the wound with toe dressing, and apply thick cotton pads for pressure dressing. Due to the limited cooperation of children, the dressing should be firmly fixed, and the looseness of the dressing should be checked regularly. If there is leakage, the dressing should be changed in a timely manner.

3. Timely observe changes in body temperature, prevent and control wound infections, and generally do not administer antibiotic treatment.

4. After 2 weeks, the base dressing was opened and the wound fully healed (Figure 10.4.3).

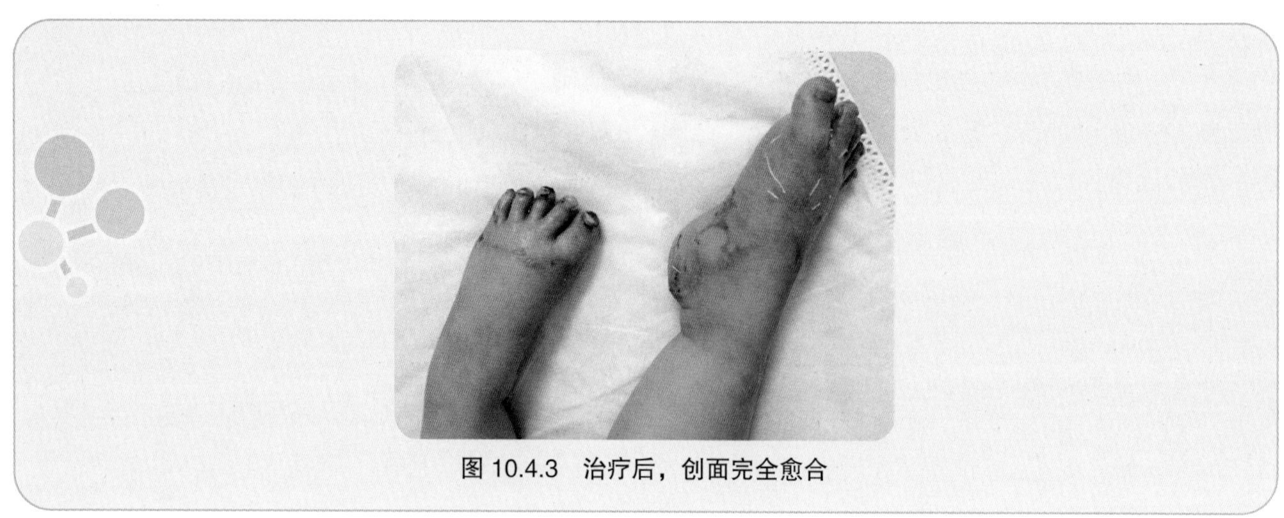

图 10.4.3　治疗后，创面完全愈合

（陈善亮　杨艳行）

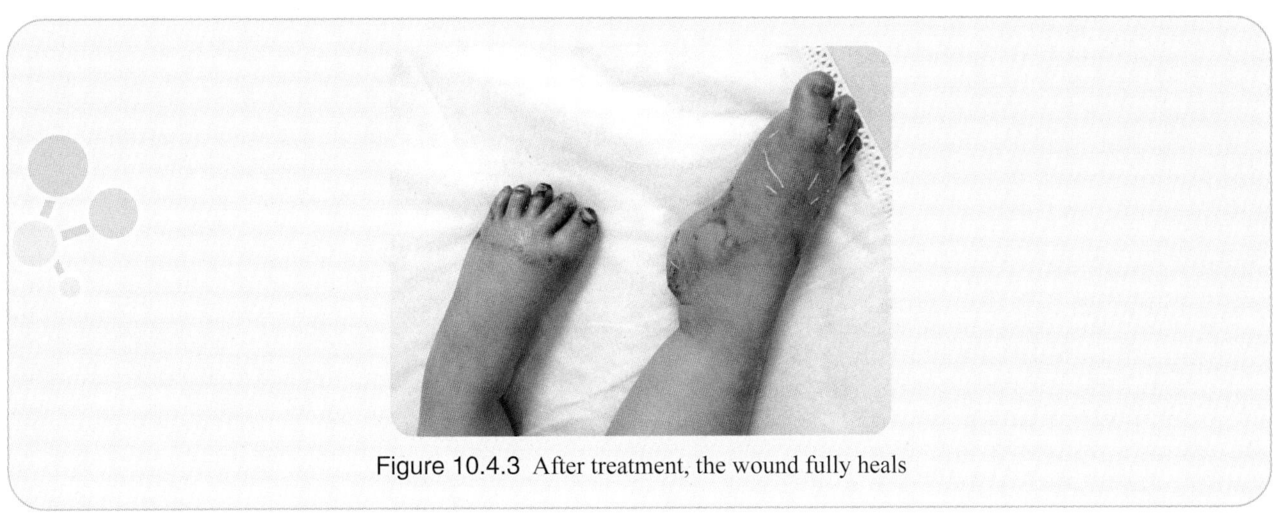

Figure 10.4.3 After treatment, the wound fully heals

(Chen Shanliang, Yang Yanxing)

第 11 章
Chapter 11

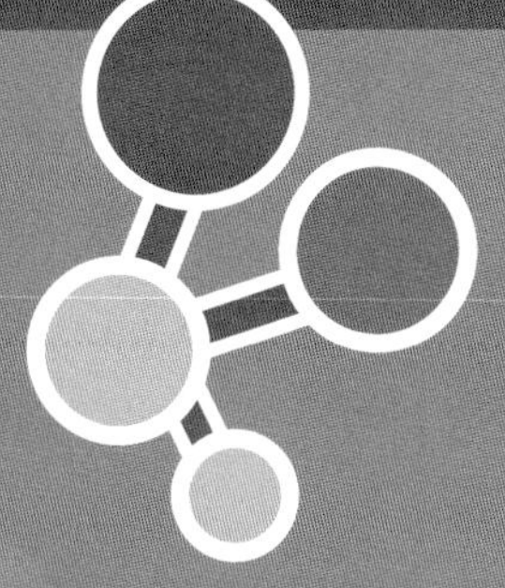

创面修复的镇痛管理
Pain Management for Wound Repair

创面损伤的常见症状之一是疼痛，按持续时间可分为急性创面疼痛和慢性创面疼痛。对于各类创面而言，在随后的愈合过程中，疼痛管理具有重要意义。

绝大多数的急性疼痛是可控的，随着手术方式的改良、微创手术的广泛应用以及多模式镇痛、预防性镇痛等理念的实践，术后急性疼痛管理水平近些年已明显提高。

第一节　术后慢性疼痛的基础认识

慢性疼痛是一种从急性状态发展为慢性状态的症状，持续到愈合过程之外。术后慢性疼痛（CPSP），不仅严重影响患者的康复及生活质量，还会显著增加抑郁、焦虑、失眠等疾病的发病率，给患者带来了巨大的病痛折磨，造成了数以亿计的医疗支出和社会负担。

大量临床研究表明，外科术后 15% ~ 60% 的患者可能经历 CPSP。虽然 CPSP 属于比较常见的慢性疼痛，但是，由于对 CPSP 的危险因素、发病机制、严重程度缺乏足够的认识，目前仍缺乏有效的早期识别手段和防治措施，很少被诊断和治疗，这也使得 CPSP 成为临床上亟待解决的难题之一。

疼痛机制

◆ 神经损伤

大部分 CPSP 源于手术时神经损伤，手术区域大多有神经分布，神经全部或部分损伤，从而导致 CPSP。例如，开胸术后疼痛综合征（PTPS），又称开胸术后慢性疼痛是开胸手术后常见的并发症，常与扩开肋骨时直接或者间接损伤肋间神经密切相关。一项对 24 例开胸术后患者的观察研究发现，术后 1 个月，肋间神经损伤风险程度高的患者发生开胸术后疼痛的比例更高。腹股沟疝修补手术中，部分或全部切断神经，与异物接触（如神经被粘入网片间隙中，网片被纤维物质粘连后收缩引起神经扭结等）、瘢痕组织压迫神经、形成神经瘤等是出现 CPSP 的常见原因。

◆ 炎症反应

手术创伤后，组织损伤部位的修复主要包括 3 个时期：炎性反应期、炎性细胞浸润期及组织重塑期。炎性介质的释放和来自损伤部位 C 神经纤维神经激肽 A（NKA）的释放，都是神经系统重塑过程中的重要启动因子。炎性介质的释放与神经损伤导致的神经系统重塑是相互促进的过程。创面修复不佳时，手术损伤部位的慢性炎性反应可以持续存在，从而导致 CPSP 的发生。慢性炎症还可能通过重塑脊髓背角神经而放大疼痛信号，导致中枢敏化而产生慢性疼痛。

One of the common symptoms of wound injury is pain, which can be divided into acute wound pain and chronic wound pain according to duration. For various types of wounds, pain management is of great significance in the subsequent healing process.

The vast majority of acute pain is controllable. With the improvement of surgical methods, the widespread application of minimally invasive surgery, and the practice of multimodal analgesia, preventive analgesia, and other concepts, the level of postoperative acute pain management has significantly improved in recent years.

Section 1 Basic understanding of postoperative chronic pain

Chronic pain is a symptom that develops from an acute state to a chronic state and persists beyond the healing process. Postoperative chronic pain (CPSP) not only seriously affects the rehabilitation and quality of life of patients, but also significantly increases the incidence rate of depression, anxiety, insomnia and other diseases, which brings huge pain to patients, causing hundreds of millions of medical expenditure and social burden.

Numerous clinical studies have shown that 15% to 60% of patients after surgery may experience CPSP. Although CPSP is a relatively common chronic pain, due to a lack of sufficient understanding of its risk factors, pathogenesis, and severity, there is still a lack of effective early identification and prevention measures, and it is rarely diagnosed and treated. This also makes CPSP one of the urgent challenges to be solved in clinical practice.

Pain mechanism

◆ Neurological damage

Most CPSP originates from nerve damage during surgery, with nerve distribution in the surgical area, resulting in complete or partial nerve damage, leading to CPSP. For example, Post thoracotomy Pain Syndrome (PTPS), also known as chronic pain after thoracotomy, is a common complication after thoracotomy, often closely related to direct or indirect damage to intercostal nerves during rib expansion. A observational study of 24 patients after thoracotomy found that one month after surgery, patients with a higher risk of intercostal nerve injury had a higher proportion of postoperative pain. During inguinal hernia repair surgery, partial or complete nerve cutting, contact with foreign objects (such as nerves being stuck in the mesh gap, mesh being adhered by fibrous material and contracting, causing nerve tangles, etc.), scar tissue compressing nerves, and the formation of neuromas are common causes of CPSP.

◆ Inflammatory response

After surgical trauma, the repair of tissue damage mainly includes three stages: inflammatory response stage, inflammatory cell infiltration stage, and tissue remodeling stage. The release of inflammatory mediators and the release of neurokinin-A (NKA) from nerve fibers at the site of injury are important initiating factors in the process of neural remodeling. The release of inflammatory mediators and the remodeling of the nervous system caused by nerve damage are mutually reinforcing processes. When the wound repair is poor, chronic inflammatory reactions at the surgical site can persist, leading to the occurrence of CPSP. Chronic inflammation may also amplify pain signals by reshaping the spinal dorsal horn nerve, leading to central sensitization and chronic pain.

◆ 周围神经和中枢神经敏化

CPSP 主要表现为神经病理性疼痛，是继发于神经或感觉传导系统损伤的疼痛，其机制包括周围神经敏感化和中枢神经敏感化过程。研究提示，周围神经、背根神经节及脊髓中的促炎细胞因子、趋化因子、生长因子等炎性介质在慢性疼痛的发生与维持中具有重要作用。神经胶质细胞可通过分泌神经递质、炎症介质作用于对应受体，导致躯体感觉神经元异常兴奋，同时伴有突触可塑性的增强，从而诱发中枢神经敏化现象。目前神经炎症介导慢性疼痛的发病机制研究以中枢神经敏化为主，而对围绕周围神经敏化机制的研究展开不足。

危险因素

◆ 手术因素

1. 手术部位、方式和时间长短等因素均可能影响 CPSP 的发生。CPSP 发生率在不同手术类型间存在很大差异，如胆囊切除术约为 3%，而截肢手术则超过 80%。一项纳入 187 项研究的荟萃分析显示，同样是乳腺癌手术，行前哨淋巴结活检者较行腋窝淋巴结切除者 CPSP 风险降低 17%。研究显示，剖宫产术后慢性疼痛与手术时间长有关，这是术后 3 个月 CPSP 的重要影响因素。

2. 术后是否行局部放射治疗、带有神经毒性的化学治疗也会影响慢性术后疼痛出现。研究表明，乳腺癌的放射治疗和化学治疗可能引起乳腺癌术后疼痛综合征（PMPS）。放射治疗同时可以使肋间神经进一步损伤，从而使 PMPS 恶化。

◆ 患者因素

1. 患者心理因素如焦虑、抑郁是术后疼痛的危险因素。有研究发现，术前焦虑状态是术后 6 个月后发生慢性疼痛的独立危险因素，术前抑郁、焦虑过度会提升疼痛发生率。Hetmann 等发现，术前具有焦虑或抑郁状态可升高开胸手术CPSP的发生率。术前焦虑和术前暗示也是甲状腺手术后发生慢性疼痛的危险因素。

2. 大量研究表明，CPSP 可能与患者的生理因素如性别、年龄、体重指数、术前合并的基础疾病和个体特异性等各项因素有关。心脏手术后胸骨慢性疼痛发生率术后 3 个月为 43%，危险因素包括女性、年轻、体重指数大、冠脉搭桥、既往手术史等。同时，多篇研究报告患者术前疼痛与 CPSP 发病率呈正相关，一项纳入 33 项研究 (n=53 362) 的荟萃分析数据显示，术前疼痛的患者 CPSP 风险增加 21%，而疼痛程度较重而需要药物治疗的患者，CPSP 风险增加 54%。

◆ 麻醉因素

1. 麻醉药物种类和剂量对 CPSP 的影响尚无明确定论。目前尚未发现手术中使用的麻醉药物（地氟醚、七氟醚和丙泊酚）与手术后急性疼痛的发生有关。但是，有研究表明，在亚洲人群中，吸入麻醉联合一氧

◆ Peripheral and central nervous system sensitization

CPSP is mainly manifested as neuropathic pain, which is secondary to nerve or sensory conduction system damage. Its mechanism includes peripheral nerve sensitization and central nerve sensitization processes. Research suggests that pro-inflammatory cytokines, chemokines, growth factors, and other inflammatory mediators in peripheral nerves, dorsal root ganglia, and spinal cord play important roles in the occurrence and maintenance of chronic pain. Glial cells can act on corresponding receptors by secreting neurotransmitters and inflammatory mediators, leading to abnormal excitation of somatic sensory neurons and enhanced synaptic plasticity, thereby inducing central nervous system sensitization. At present, the research on the pathogenesis of chronic pain mediated by neuroinflammation mainly focuses on central nervous system sensitization, while there is insufficient research on the mechanism of peripheral nervous system sensitization.

Risk factors

◆ Surgical factors

1. Factors such as surgical site, method, and duration may all affect the occurrence of CPSP. The incidence of CPSP varies greatly among different surgical types, with cholecystectomy accounting for about 3% and amputation surgery exceeding 80%. A meta-analysis of 187 studies showed that those who performed sentinel lymph node biopsy for breast cancer surgery also had a 17% lower risk of CPSP than those who performed axillary lymph node resection. Research has shown that chronic pain after cesarean section is related to the length of surgery, which is an important influencing factor for CPSP at 3 months after surgery.

2. Whether to undergo local radiation therapy or chemotherapy with neurotoxicity after surgery can also affect the occurrence of chronic postoperative pain. Research shows that radiotherapy and chemotherapy for breast cancer may cause postoperative pain syndrome (PMPS) of breast cancer. Radiation therapy can further damage the intercostal nerves and worsen PMPS.

◆ Patient factors

1. Psychological factors such as anxiety and depression are risk factors for postoperative pain in patients. A study has found that preoperative anxiety is an independent risk factor for chronic pain 6 months after surgery, and excessive preoperative depression and anxiety can increase the incidence of pain. Hetmann et al. found that preoperative anxiety or depression can increase the incidence of CPSP in open chest surgery. Preoperative anxiety and suggestion are also risk factors for chronic pain after thyroid surgery.

2. Numerous studies have shown that CPSP may be related to various physiological factors of patients, such as gender, age, body mass index, preoperative comorbidities, and individual specificity. The incidence of chronic sternal pain after cardiac surgery is 43% at 3 months post surgery, with risk factors including female gender, youth, high body mass index, coronary artery bypass grafting, and previous surgical history. At the same time, many studies reported that preoperative pain was positively correlated with the incidence rate of CPSP. A meta-analysis of 33 studies (n=53 362) showed that the risk of CPSP in patients with preoperative pain increased by 21%, while the risk of CPSP in patients with severe pain requiring drug treatment increased by 54%.

◆ Anesthesia factors

1. There is no definitive theory on the impact of the type and dosage of anesthetic drugs on CPSP. At present, no association has been found between the use of anesthesia drugs (desflurane, sevoflurane, and propofol) during surgery and the occurrence of acute pain after surgery. However, studies have shown that in Asian populations, inhalation anesthesia combined with nitrous oxide can reduce CPSP by 30%; However, more studies have shown

化二氮能使 CPSP 降低 30%；而更多研究表明，一氧化二氮对 CPSP 的影响尚未明确，且有报道指出其可能存在的毒性反应限制了目前的临床应用。在临床上全身麻醉时大量阿片类药物的使用会使得术后痛觉敏化的发生率大大提高，不仅增加了术后镇痛所需要的阿片类药物，同时增加 CPSP 发生率。

2 . 麻醉方式对慢性术后疼痛的影响目前亦无明确定论。但在某些手术中，麻醉方式的合理选择对慢性术后疼痛有缓解作用。开胸或开腹手术中应用区域麻醉技术，能明显降低 CPSP 发生率。在 Brandsborg 的子宫切除术相关研究中，脊髓麻醉患者中仅有 14.5% 发生子宫切除术后慢性疼痛，显著低于全麻患者的 33.6%。然而在同一研究中，硬膜外麻醉并未降低 CPHP 的发生率。

◆ 术后急性疼痛

Katz 等于 1996 年首次提供了明确的证据，证实术后急性疼痛及其发展与慢性疼痛之间的显著相关性，指出术后急性疼痛可能是发生慢性疼痛的预示。短暂的术后急性疼痛是对损伤发生的一种适应性反应，而 CPSP 则是非适应性反应，严重或持久的应激，尤其是慢性应激可引起生理或精神稳态的改变，而这是 CPSP 的高危因素。有研究发现，应激小鼠术后机械痛痛阈的恢复时间明显延长，且更易发生痛觉敏化，证明了慢性应激诱发术后急性疼痛的慢性化。而慢性应激诱发术后急性疼痛慢性化的具体机制尚不明确。

术后急性期疼痛控制不佳是 CPSP 发生的重要危险因素，美国的一项研究调查了膝关节和髋关节置换术后 1 年慢性疼痛的发生率，分别为 53% 和 38%，术后急性疼痛控制不佳是其独立危险因素之一。

症状和体征 》》

与术后急性疼痛不同，CPSP 有其自身特点：①其疼痛主诉与其在常规体检和诊断的结果的严重程度不成比例，常常存在手术刀口已愈合、局部炎症已消失的情况下患者仍有疼痛主诉；②疼痛主诉的时间超过预期恢复时间；③客观上存在一定程度的功能障碍或功能减退；④患者常有抑郁或焦虑性的心理问题。

有学者认为，大部分的 CPSP 均与术中周围神经组织损伤有关。神经损伤是形成神经病理性疼痛的必要前提，神经病理性疼痛具有持续性、难以治疗的特点，与伤害性疼痛、炎症性疼痛有很大不同。在开胸术后，患者对非损伤性刺激感到疼痛（异常性痛觉），或轻微的疼痛刺激会感到剧烈的疼痛（痛觉过敏），尤其是伴有麻木感觉，可以考虑是周围神经损伤导致神经继发炎症所引起的神经病理性疼痛，这些疼痛症状常常分布于肋间神经支配区域。

疼痛的性质随着不同手术部位而改变。胸科术后慢性疼痛的性质呈现出一种“电击样”或者“烧灼样”刺痛，常会伴有手术同侧肩部疼痛。截肢手术后的慢性疼痛也十分突出，患者常常存在十分严重的幻觉和幻肢痛，据报道可达 51% ~ 85%，残肢痛的发生率达 45% ~ 74%。

CPSP 通常伴随着社会心理问题、睡眠障碍、躯体功能障碍等。一项纳入 14 831 例非心脏手术患者的国际多中心前瞻性队列研究的数据显示，在发生 CPSP 的患者中，高达 60% 的患者认为 CPSP 影响了情

that the effect of nitrous oxide on CPSP is not yet clear, and there are reports indicating that its possible toxic reactions limit its current clinical application. The extensive use of opioid drugs during general anesthesia in clinical practice greatly increases the incidence of postoperative pain sensitization, not only increasing the need for opioid drugs for postoperative analgesia, but also increasing the incidence of CPSP.

2. The impact of anesthesia methods on chronic postoperative pain is currently uncertain. However, in some surgeries, the reasonable choice of anesthesia can alleviate chronic postoperative pain. The application of regional anesthesia techniques during open chest or abdominal surgery can significantly reduce the incidence of CPSP. In Brandsborg's hysterectomy related study, only 14.5% of spinal anesthesia patients experienced chronic pain after hysterectomy, significantly lower than the 33.6% of general anesthesia patients. However, in the same study, epidural anesthesia did not reduce the incidence of CPHP.

◆ Postoperative acute pain

Katz provided clear evidence for the first time in 1996, confirming a significant correlation between postoperative acute pain and its development with chronic pain, suggesting that postoperative acute pain may be a predictor of chronic pain. Transient postoperative acute pain is an adaptive response to injury, while CPSP is a non adaptive response. Severe or persistent stress, especially chronic stress, can cause changes in physiological or mental homeostasis, which is a high-risk factor for CPSP. A study has found that the recovery time of mechanical pain threshold in stressed mice after surgery is significantly prolonged, and they are more prone to pain sensitization, demonstrating the chronicity of acute postoperative pain induced by chronic stress. The specific mechanism by which chronic stress induces the chronicity of postoperative acute pain is not yet clear.

Poor postoperative acute pain control is an important risk factor for CPSP. A study in the United States investigated the incidence of chronic pain one year after knee and hip replacement surgery, which was 53% and 38%, respectively. Poor postoperative acute pain control is one of its independent risk factors.

Symptoms and signs

Unlike postoperative acute pain, CPSP has its own characteristics: The severity of pain complaints is not proportional to the results of routine physical examination and diagnosis, and patients often have pain complaints even after the surgical incision has healed and local inflammation has disappeared. The duration of pain complaints exceeds the expected recovery time. Objectively, there is a certain degree of functional impairment or decline in function. Patients often have psychological problems such as depression or anxiety.

Some scholars believe that most CPSPs are related to intraoperative peripheral nerve tissue damage. Neurological injury is a necessary prerequisite for the formation of neuropathic pain, which has the characteristics of persistence and difficulty in treatment, and is very different from nociceptive pain and inflammatory pain. After thoracotomy, patients may experience pain from non-invasive stimuli (allodynia), or mild pain stimuli may cause severe pain (hyperalgesia), especially accompanied by numbness. This can be considered as neuropathological pain caused by secondary inflammation of the nerves due to peripheral nerve injury, and these pain symptoms are often distributed in the intercostal nerve innervation area.

The nature of pain varies with different surgical sites. The nature of chronic pain after thoracic surgery presents a "shock like" or "burn like" stabbing sensation, often accompanied by pain in the shoulder on the same side of the surgery. The chronic pain after amputation surgery is also very prominent, and patients often experience severe hallucinations and phantom limb pain, which has been reported to reach 51% to 85%. The incidence of residual limb pain is 45% to 74%.

CPSP is usually accompanied by social and psychological problems, sleep disorders, physical dysfunction, and so on. According to data from an international multicenter prospective cohort study involving 14 831 non cardiac

绪和日常生活，41.5% 的患者认为 CPSP 影响了个人社交活动，甚至 10% 的患者出现自杀倾向。一项纳入 14 000 多例非心脏手术患者的多中心前瞻性队列研究数据则显示，CPSP 患者出现睡眠障碍的比率高达 60%。研究表明，CPSP 会影响患者的睡眠，同时睡眠障碍可能会降低疼痛阈值从而增加 CPSP 发生率，二者可能是共病关系。

第二节　疼痛的管理

围手术期疼痛管理

◆ 与麻醉有关的疼痛管理

1. 完善术前访视，识别高危人群。麻醉医生应在术前与患者充分沟通交流，告知术后疼痛的发生情况，这可能有助于减轻患者焦虑情绪，提高其对术后疼痛治疗的满意度。对于术前已经存在慢性疼痛或者阿片类药物耐受的患者来说，发生 CPSP 的风险明显升高。术前对药物进行干预或调整可能有利于提高围手术期疼痛管理质量。多项临床研究表明，围手术期使用加巴喷丁有利于降低术后神经病理性疼痛的发生率，并能减少术中阿片类药物使用量。

2. 合理选择麻醉镇痛药物与方法

2.1 制订完善的术中镇痛计划：临床研究发现，手术期间应用阿片类镇痛药物可能激活 N- 甲基 -D- 天冬氨酸 (NMDA) 受体和 / 或胶质细胞，使疼痛评分升高，进而增加阿片类药物的使用量，导致更高的术后急性痛觉敏化。术中应尽量减少阿片类镇痛药物的使用对 CPSP 的防治具有积极作用。值得注意的是，氯胺酮是一种非竞争性 NMDA 谷氨酸受体拮抗剂，常被用作全麻和短效镇痛药。有研究表明，鞘内给予可乐定或硬膜外给予氯胺酮，会降低切口周围机械性刺激的痛觉敏感。一项关于乳腺癌切除术的临床前瞻性研究发现，术中小剂量氯胺酮干预可以显著降低术后 3 个月内持续性术后疼痛的发生率。同时，随着超声技术的发展，术中使用神经阻滞越来越常见，有效减少 CPSP 的发生。荟萃分析发现，在乳腺手术中给予利多卡因静脉注射虽然并没有改变急性疼痛评分，但显著减少了术后早期镇痛药的消耗，并轻微降低了术后持续疼痛的发生。在乳腺癌手术中，杜海云等研究了超声引导下的肋间神经阻滞复合全麻与单纯全麻在乳腺癌改良根治术中的应用，结果发现，术后镇痛效果神经阻滞组优于单纯全麻组，而不论是在不良反应发生率还是术后镇痛药物使用率上都是肋间神经复合全麻组更低。开胸或开腹手术中应用区域麻醉技术，亦能明显降低 CPSP 发生率。

2.2 静脉镇痛：是常见的术后镇痛方法之一。其中患者自控静脉镇痛（PCIA）最为常见。目前常用的

surgery patients, up to 60% of patients who experienced CPSP believed that CPSP affected their emotions and daily life, 41.5% believed that CPSP affected personal social activities, and even 10% of patients showed suicidal tendencies. A multicenter prospective cohort study involving over 14 000 non cardiac surgery patients showed that the incidence of sleep disorders in CPSP patients was as high as 60%. Research has shown that CPSP can affect patients' sleep, and sleep disorders may lower pain thresholds and increase the incidence of CPSP, which may be a comorbidity.

Section 2 Pain management

Perioperative pain management

◆ Pain management related to anesthesia

1. Improve preoperative visits and identify high-risk populations. Anesthesiologists should communicate fully with patients before surgery, informing them of the occurrence of postoperative pain, which may help alleviate patients' anxiety and improve their satisfaction with postoperative pain treatment. For patients who already have chronic pain or opioid tolerance before surgery, the risk of developing CPSP is significantly increased. Preoperative intervention or adjustment of medication may be beneficial for improving the quality of perioperative pain management. Multiple clinical studies have shown that the use of gabapentin during the perioperative period is beneficial in reducing the incidence of postoperative neuropathic pain and can also reduce the use of opioid drugs during surgery.

2. Reasonable selection of anesthetic and analgesic drugs and methods

2.1 Developing a comprehensive intraoperative analgesia plan: Clinical studies have found that the use of opioid analgesics during surgery may activate N-methyl-D-aspartate (NMDA) receptors and/or glial cells, leading to an increase in pain scores and an increase in opioid use, resulting in higher postoperative acute pain sensitization. Minimizing the use of opioid analgesics during surgery has a positive effect on the prevention and treatment of CPSP. It is worth noting that ketamine is a non competitive NMDA glutamate receptor antagonist commonly used as a general anesthesia and short acting analgesic. Studies have shown that intrathecal administration of clonidine or epidural administration of ketamine can reduce pain sensitivity to mechanical stimuli around the incision site. A clinical prospective study on breast cancer resection found that small and medium dose ketamine intervention could significantly reduce the incidence of persistent postoperative pain within 3 months after surgery. Meanwhile, with the development of ultrasound technology, the use of nerve block during surgery has become increasingly common, effectively reducing the occurrence of CPSP. Meta analysis found that intravenous injection of lidocaine during breast surgery did not change acute pain scores, but significantly reduced the consumption of early postoperative analgesics and slightly reduced the occurrence of persistent postoperative pain. In the operation of breast cancer, Du Haiyun and others studied the application of intercostal nerve block combined general anesthesia and simple general anesthesia guided by ultrasound in the modified radical mastectomy for breast cancer. The results showed that the postoperative analgesia effect of nerve block group was better than that of simple general anesthesia group, while the incidence of adverse reactions and the use rate of postoperative analgesic drugs were lower in intercostal nerve combined general anesthesia group. The application of regional anesthesia techniques during open chest or abdominal surgery can also significantly reduce the incidence of CPSP.

2.2 Intravenous analgesia is one of the common postoperative pain relief methods. Patient controlled

术后静脉镇痛药物还是以阿片类药物为主。手术后的疼痛尤其是急性疼痛多与手术创伤所导致的炎症反应有关，同时非甾体抗炎药没有阿片类药物的成瘾性、呼吸抑制性等缺点，因此常常作为术后镇痛药的首选用药。李春光在临床试验中给予一组患者氟比洛芬酯 100 mg+ 舒芬太尼 100 μg+ 托烷司琼 8 mg，另一组舒芬太尼 150 μg+ 托烷司琼 8 mg，均用生理盐水稀释至 50 mL，连接自控镇痛泵（图 11.2.1），进行静脉患者自控镇痛。发现使用氟比洛芬酯在降低不良反应发生率的同时还能减少阿片类药物的用量。此外，硬膜外镇痛，通过阻滞脊神经后根纤维的神经传导，从而阻断躯体和内脏的疼痛刺激传入，被认为是上腹部手术术后镇痛的金标准。有研究显示，与 PCIA 相比，使用硬膜外镇痛可以缩短术后首次排气排便时间，减少术后胃肠道功能恢复时间。

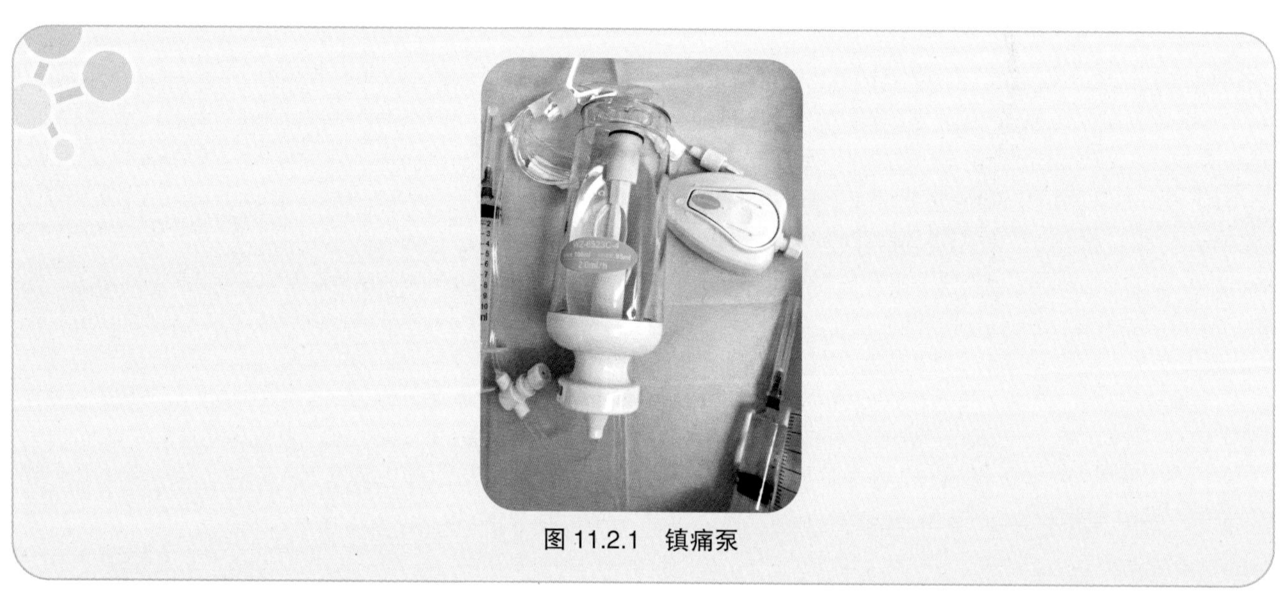

图 11.2.1　镇痛泵

2.3 局部浸润麻醉：在减轻 CPSP 发生率也发挥一定的作用。其主要是将局部麻醉药物直接作用于切口周围的神经，阻断钠离子内流，阻断神经冲动传递，从而减轻患者的痛苦。一项关于罗哌卡因切口周围局部浸润对大鼠慢性术后疼痛影响的实验表明，在行皮肤 / 肌肉切开牵拉模型的大鼠中，切口周围予以罗哌卡因局部浸润相对于对照组（等容积生理盐水局部浸润）而言，机械缩足反射阈值升高，表明术中罗哌卡因切口周围局部浸润可以抑制术后疼痛。

2.4 区域阻滞预防慢性术后疼痛：是多模式镇痛中的重要组成部分。多种神经阻滞方式在术后长期镇痛效果、操作简化、安全性等方面展现出各自的优势，持续的神经阻滞可以阻断周围神经伤害和炎症向中枢神经系统的传输。例如，臂丛神经通过胸外侧神经、胸内侧神经、胸长神经和胸背神经支配乳房的感觉。锁骨下入路和肌间沟入路的臂丛神经阻滞均能应用于乳腺癌术后镇痛，锁骨下入路的效果更完全，且能提供腋窝镇痛，但在加大给药剂量时，单纯应用肌间沟入路也能达到较好效果（图 11.2.2、图 11.2.3）。在老

intravenous analgesia (PCIA) is the most common among them. Currently, the commonly used postoperative intravenous analgesics are mainly opioid drugs. The pain after surgery, especially acute pain, is often related to the inflammatory response caused by surgical trauma. At the same time, nonsteroidal anti-inflammatory drugs do not have the addictive and respiratory inhibitory disadvantages of opioid drugs, so they are often used as the first choice for postoperative analgesics. In a clinical trial, Li Chunguang administered 100 mg of flurbiprofen axetil, 100 μg of sufentanil, and 8 mg of tropisetron to one group of patients, and 150 μg of sufentanil and 8 mg of tropisetron to another group. Both groups were diluted with physiological saline to 50 mL and connected to a patient-controlled analgesia pump for intravenous patient-controlled analgesia (Figure 11.2.1). It was found that the use of flurbiprofen axetil can reduce the incidence of adverse reactions while also reducing the dosage of opioid drugs. In addition, epidural analgesia, which blocks the nerve conduction of the posterior root fibers of the spinal nerve, thereby blocking the transmission of pain stimuli from the body and organs, is considered the gold standard for postoperative analgesia in upper abdominal surgery. Studies have shown that compared to PCIA, the use of epidural analgesia can shorten the time for the first bowel movement after surgery and reduce the time for postoperative gastrointestinal function recovery.

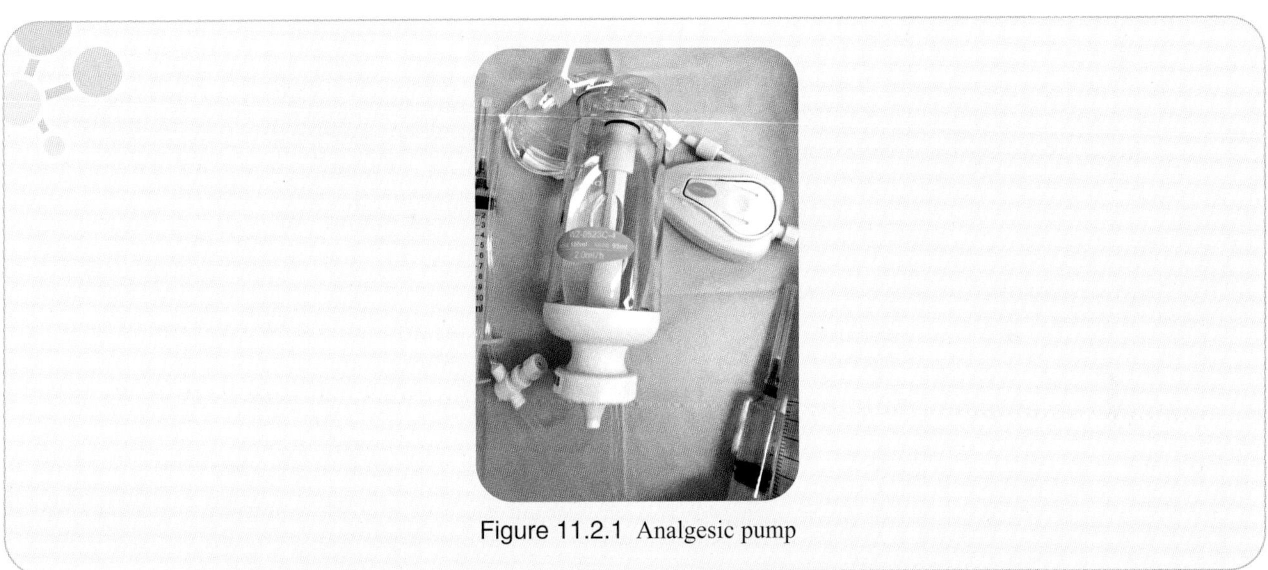

Figure 11.2.1 Analgesic pump

2.3 Local infiltration anesthesia: also plays a certain role in reducing the incidence of CPSP. It mainly involves directly applying local anesthetic drugs to the nerves around the incision, blocking the influx of sodium ions and the transmission of nerve impulses, thereby reducing the patient's pain. An experiment on the effect of local infiltration around the incision with ropivacaine on chronic postoperative pain in rats showed that in a skin/muscle incision traction model, compared to the control group (equal volume saline local infiltration), the mechanical foot contraction reflex threshold was increased when ropivacaine was locally infiltrated around the incision, indicating that intraoperative local infiltration around the incision with ropivacaine can suppress postoperative pain.

2.4 Regional blockade for preventing chronic postoperative pain is an important component of multimodal analgesia. Multiple nerve block methods have demonstrated their respective advantages in long-term postoperative pain relief, simplified operation, and safety. Continuous nerve block can block the transmission of peripheral nerve damage and inflammation to the central nervous system. For example, the brachial plexus nerve innervates the sensation of the breast through the lateral thoracic nerve, medial thoracic nerve, thoracic long nerve, and thoracic dorsal nerve. Brachial plexus block via subclavian approach and intermuscular sulcus approach can be used for postoperative analgesia of breast cancer. The effect of subclavian approach is more complete and can provide axillary analgesia, but when the dosage is increased, the application of intermuscular sulcus approach alone can

年患者膝关节置换术术后，有研究表明超声引导下连续股神经阻滞与自控静脉镇痛组相比，在术后 25 小时内静息和持续运动状态下的镇痛效果明显存在优势，不良反应发生率低（图 11.2.4）。并且 Paul 等通过前瞻性随机对照研究表明，将持续坐骨神经阻滞用于控制足踝部术后疼痛的控制，发现可明显缓解疼痛并减少术后镇痛药物的使用，提高患者的满意度（图 11.2.5）。针对疝修补术带来的术后疼痛，对于一般症状较轻，呈间歇性疼痛的患者多采用非甾体抗炎药物镇痛治疗配合理疗；针对神经受累的患者，需采用局部神经阻滞，在受累神经周围，主要是髂腹下、髂腹股沟和生殖股神经，注射局麻药加类固醇混合剂。

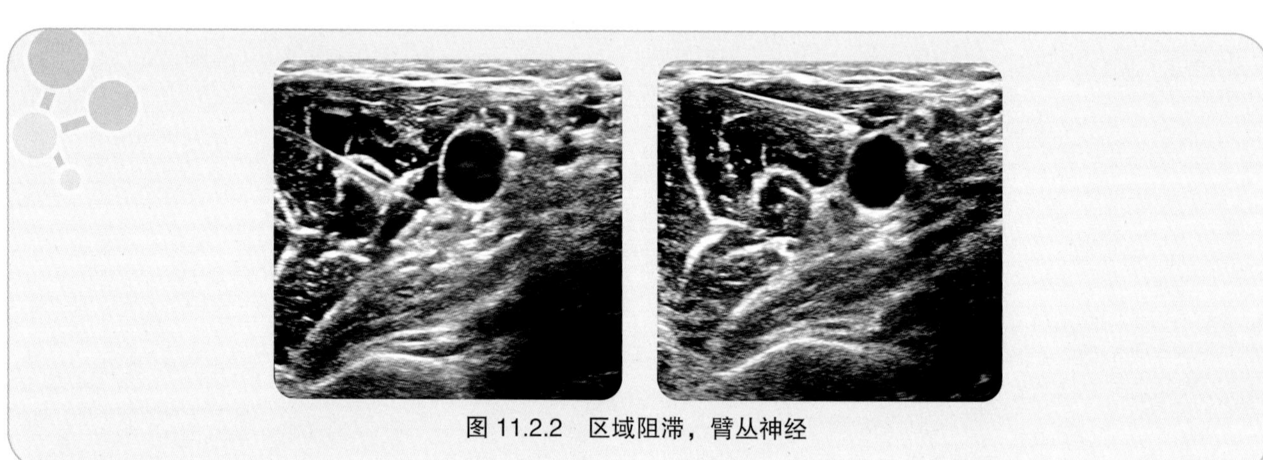

图 11.2.2　区域阻滞，臂丛神经

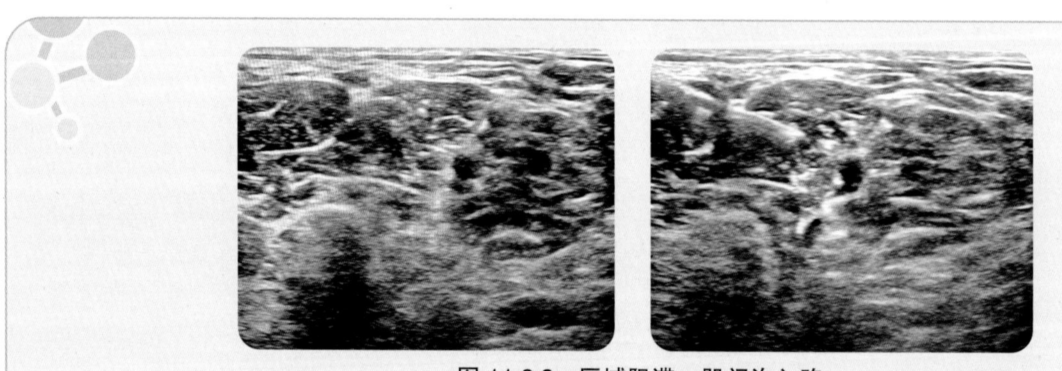

图 11.2.3　区域阻滞，肌间沟入路

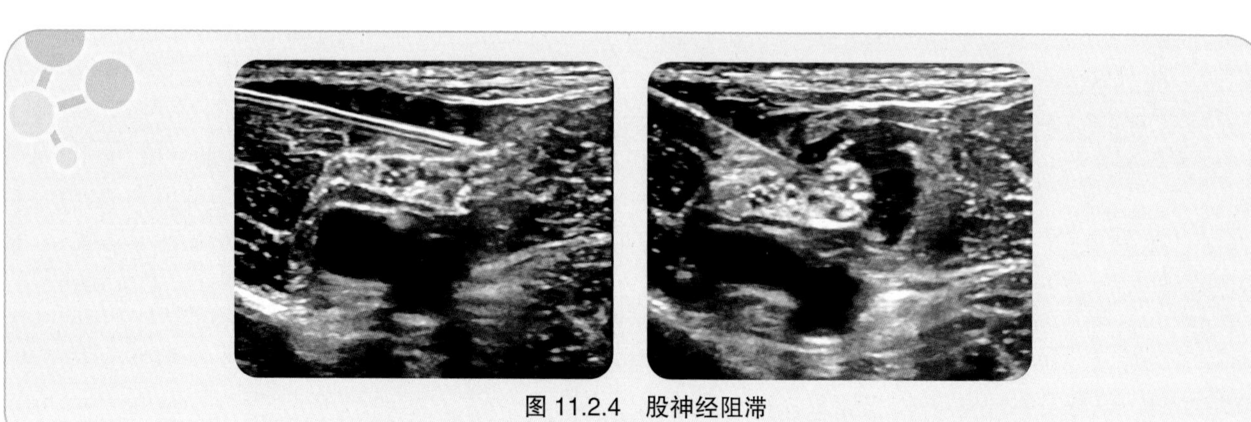

图 11.2.4　股神经阻滞

also achieve better results (Figure 11.2.2, Figure 11.2.3). After knee replacement surgery in elderly patients, studies have shown that continuous femoral nerve block under ultrasound guidance has a significant advantage in pain relief compared to the self controlled intravenous analgesia group, with a lower incidence of adverse reactions within 25 hours of rest and continuous exercise (Figure 11.2.4). And Paul et al. demonstrated through a prospective randomized controlled study that using continuous sciatic nerve block for controlling postoperative pain in the ankle region can significantly alleviate pain and reduce the use of postoperative analgesics, improving patient satisfaction (Figure 11.2.5). For patients with mild symptoms and intermittent pain caused by hernia repair surgery, nonsteroidal anti-inflammatory drugs are often used in combination with physical therapy for pain relief; For patients with nerve involvement, local nerve block is required. Local anesthetics and steroid mixtures are injected around the affected nerves, mainly the iliopsoas, ilioinguinal, and genitofemoral nerves.

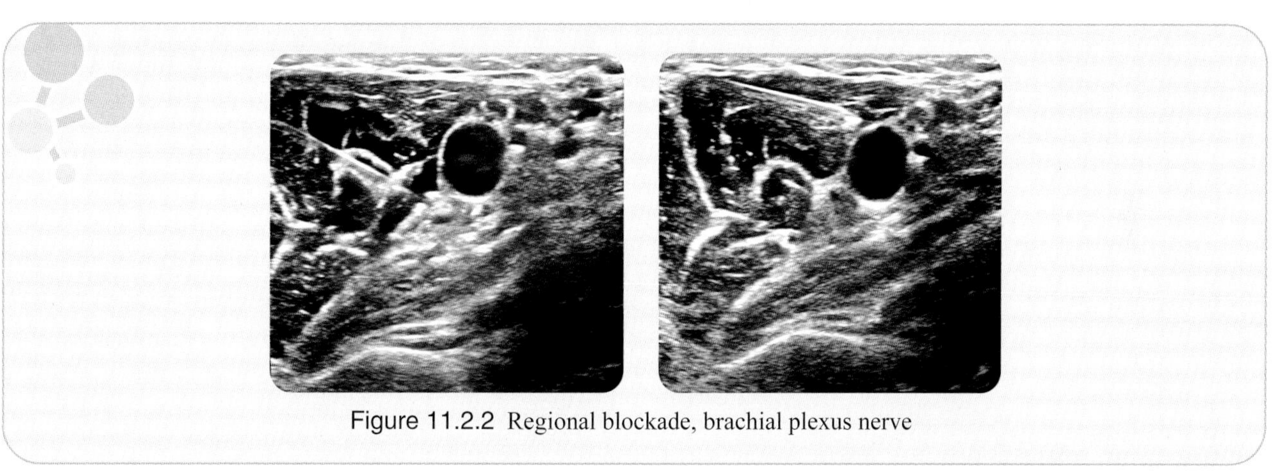

Figure 11.2.2 Regional blockade, brachial plexus nerve

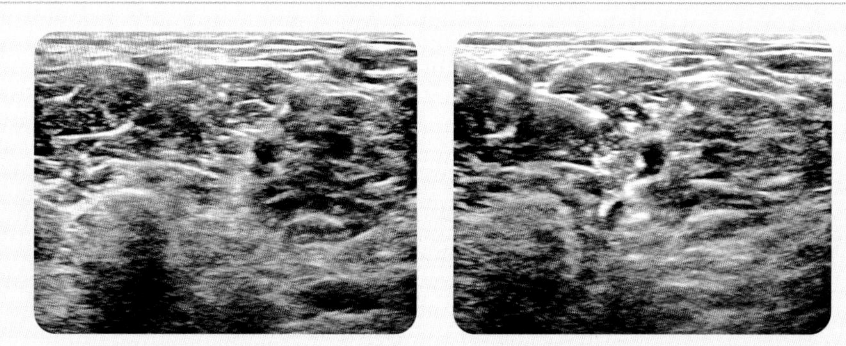

Figure 11.2.3 Regional blockade, intermuscular groove approach

Figure 11.2.4 Femoral nerve block

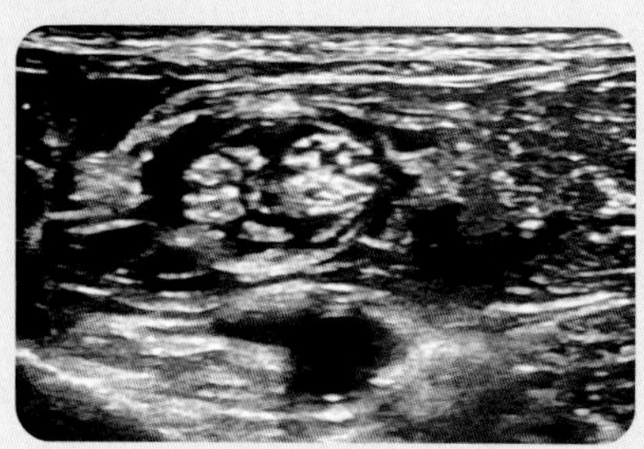
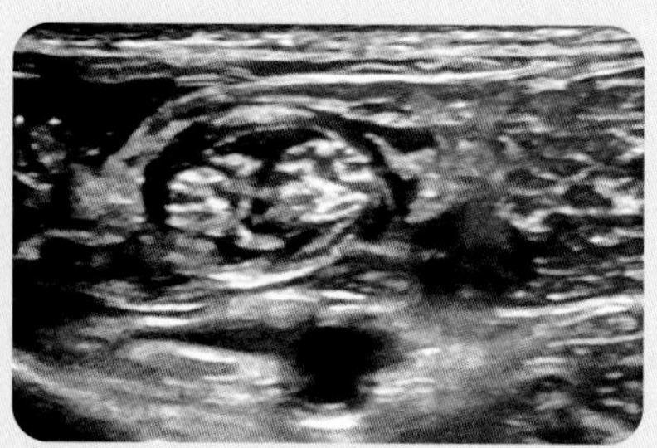

图 11.2.5　坐骨神经阻滞

3. 运用超前镇痛、预防性镇痛、多模式镇痛理念

3.1 超前镇痛：20 世纪初，美国外科医生 Crile 首次提出“超前镇痛”的概念，指出外科手术切皮之前给予一定药物治疗措施，以阻断伤害性刺激传入大脑，从而降低术中疼痛和预防术后疼痛。目前认为超前镇痛是在手术切口前或组织损伤前给予镇痛治疗，这个概念的提出是建立在公认的外科疼痛病理生理基础上的，即周围神经及中枢神经的敏化作用。大量动物实验研究表明，超前镇痛具有较好的预防和抑制周围神经和中枢神经敏化现象的作用。但超前镇痛的临床有效性具有一定的争议，临床研究中众多的结果并不完全相同，同时也难以达到有效性和一致性的完美统一。值得注意的是，多篇研究报告术前疼痛与 CPSP 相关。一项纳入 33 项研究（n=53 362）的荟萃分析数据显示，术前疼痛的患者 CPSP 风险增加 21%，而疼痛程度较重且需要药物治疗的患者，CPSP 风险增加 54%。因此，术前及时治疗已有疼痛对减少 CPSP 可能是有效的。超前镇痛的方式有硬膜外麻醉、切口局部浸润及使用非甾体抗炎药。

3.2 预防性镇痛：随着麻醉与镇痛研究的不断深入，超前镇痛的概念和内涵也在不断更新和修正。2000 年 Dionne 等对超前镇痛相关研究进行了综述并提出“预防性镇痛”的概念，主张镇痛治疗应贯穿整个围手术期，而非仅限于手术之前，其关注重点是减轻围手术期有害刺激的影响，降低周围神经和中枢神经敏化，从而降低术后疼痛强度。预防性镇痛具有两个特征：①与其他治疗相比，能够降低术后疼痛程度和 / 或镇痛药物消耗量；②干预效果的持续时间超过了目标药物的临床作用持续时间。手术区域局部浸润、使用非甾体抗炎药或环氧合酶 -2 抑制剂是常用的预防性镇痛方式，但临床使用需考虑到可能出现心脏、胃肠道的不良反应。

3.3 多模式镇痛：强调在围手术期应用不同的镇痛药物及方式，有助于降低 CPSP 的发生，包括非阿片类药物、局部浸润镇痛、区域阻滞等，在提供有效镇痛的同时最小化阿片类药物使用，减少不良反应，促进患者快速康复。氯胺酮、普瑞巴林和加巴喷丁是目前研究报告可能有效预防 CPSP 的药物。有研究表明，在神经受损之后，钙离子通道的 $\alpha 2\delta$ 亚单位表达也会明显上调，加巴喷丁和普瑞巴林可与该亚单位结合，从而抑制中枢敏化，可能减少慢性疼痛的发生。氯胺酮为 NMDA 受体拮抗剂，可抑制中枢敏化，有研究

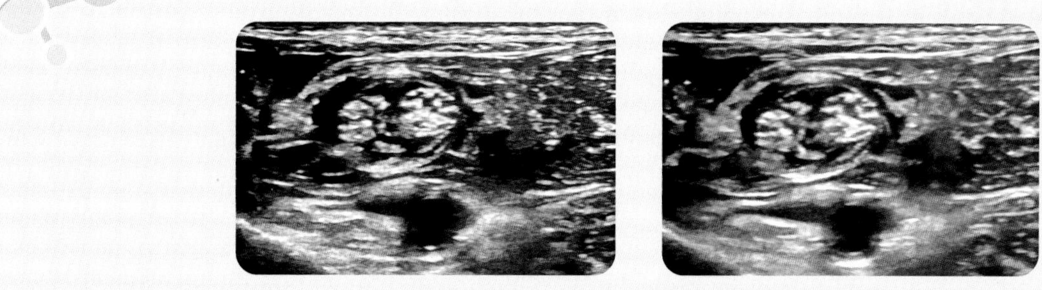

Figure 11.2.5 Sciatic nerve block

3. Apply the concepts of preemptive analgesia, preventive analgesia, and multimodal analgesia

3.1 Advanced analgesia: In the early 20th century, American surgeon Crile first proposed the concept of "advanced analgesia", which pointed out that certain drug treatment measures should be given before surgical skin cutting to block the transmission of harmful stimuli to the brain, thereby reducing intraoperative pain and preventing postoperative pain. At present, it is believed that preemptive analgesia is administered before surgical incision or tissue injury, and this concept is based on the recognized pathological and physiological basis of surgical pain, namely the sensitization of peripheral and central nervous systems. A large number of animal experiments have shown that preemptive analgesia has a good preventive and inhibitory effect on peripheral and central nervous system sensitization. However, the clinical effectiveness of preemptive analgesia is somewhat controversial, as numerous results in clinical studies are not completely consistent, and it is also difficult to achieve a perfect unity of effectiveness and consistency. It is worth noting that multiple studies have reported a correlation between preoperative pain and CPSP. A meta-analysis of 33 studies (n=53 362) showed that patients with preoperative pain had a 21% increased risk of CPSP, while patients with severe pain requiring medication had a 54% increased risk of CPSP. Therefore, timely treatment of pre-existing pain before surgery may be effective in reducing CPSP. The methods of preemptive analgesia include epidural anesthesia, local incision infiltration, and the use of nonsteroidal anti-inflammatory drugs.

3.2 Preventive analgesia: With the continuous deepening of anesthesia and analgesia research, the concept and connotation of preemptive analgesia are also constantly updated and revised. In 2000, Dionne et al. reviewed the research on preemptive analgesia and proposed the concept of "preventive analgesia", advocating that analgesic treatment should be carried out throughout the entire perioperative period, not just before surgery. The focus is on reducing the impact of harmful stimuli during the perioperative period, reducing peripheral and central nervous system sensitization, and thus reducing postoperative pain intensity. Preventive analgesia has two characteristics: ① it can reduce postoperative pain and/or analgesic drug consumption compared to other treatments; ② The duration of intervention effect exceeds the clinical duration of the target drug. Local infiltration in the surgical area and the use of nonsteroidal anti-inflammatory drugs or cyclooxygenase-2 inhibitors are commonly used preventive analgesic methods, but clinical use should consider the possibility of adverse reactions in the heart and gastrointestinal tract.

3.3 Multimodal analgesia: Emphasizing the use of different analgesic drugs and methods during the perioperative period can help reduce the occurrence of CPSP, including non opioid drugs, local infiltration analgesia, regional blockade, etc. While providing effective analgesia, it minimizes the use of opioid drugs, reduces adverse reactions, and promotes rapid recovery of patients. Ketamine, pregabalin, and gabapentin are currently reported to be drugs that may effectively prevent CPSP. Studies have shown that after nerve damage, the expression of the $\alpha 2 \delta$ subunit of calcium ion channels is significantly upregulated. Gabapentin and pregabalin can bind to this subunit, thereby inhibiting central sensitization and potentially reducing the occurrence of chronic pain. Ketamine is an

表明，鞘内给予可乐定或硬膜外给予氯胺酮，会降低切口周围机械性刺激的痛觉敏感。一项纳入 39 项研究（*n*=3027）的系统评价显示，与单纯全麻比较，全麻复合区域阻滞的乳腺癌手术患者 CPSP 风险降低了 57%。对于存在 CPSP 高危因素的患者，应制订个体化的用药方案，并在术后 3 个月内加强随访。然而，80% 的患者在术后最初 3 个月内的持续性疼痛并没有得到及时有效的干预措施，从而导致疼痛的慢性化。因此我们强调，应建立完善的过渡期疼痛治疗服务，早发现、早治疗，以预防或减少 CPSP 的发生。

◆ 与手术有关的疼痛管理

1. 选择合适的手术方式、手术操作精细化可能有助于降低 CPSP 的发生。例如，从避免损伤腹股沟神经、选择合适的术式和补片、预防感染等，可能有助于降低腹股沟疝修补术后慢性疼痛的发生率。乳腺癌手术时，清扫腋窝淋巴结时注意保留神经也可能有助于降低 CPSP。各种微创手术及治疗的发展可能也有助于降低术后疼痛的发生率。

2. 在某些手术中，如果已尝试各种保守治疗方法，患者疼痛仍持续存在，则可考虑采取手术方法。例如，在腹股沟疝术后，可通过术中探查疼痛原因所在，若发现神经被缝扎，应松解相关神经；若因补片刺激神经，则需切除相应的补片，这样对症治疗，术后疼痛往往能缓解。

◆ 与患者有关的疼痛管理

1. 进行社会心理干预。如前所述，心理因素与 CPSP 相互影响。Yang 等在一项纳入 33 项研究 (*n*=53 362) 的荟萃分析中报告，抑郁和焦虑患者发生 CPSP 的风险分别增加 71% 和 22%。另有一项纳入 3528 例患者的观察性研究显示，即使没有发生焦虑、抑郁，仅仅是术前有消极心理预期的患者，CPSP 发生率增加 56%。因此，对 CPSP 患者进行综合的心理社会治疗，包括及时的疼痛知识的宣教，帮助患者认识并缓解焦虑、恐惧，是有意义的。

2. 改善睡眠。如前所述，睡眠障碍与 CPSP 存在共病关系。荟萃分析显示，睡眠障碍是 CPSP 的重要预测因素，且随着时间的累加，可能产生更为严重的后果。早期认识和发现睡眠障碍可以更有针对性地进行干预，从而有利于更好地进行疼痛管理。

术后长期疼痛管理

◆ 药物治疗

阿片类药物是最经典、镇痛作用最强的镇痛用药。有研究认为，手术患者术后发生 CPSP 可能需长期使用阿片类药物，但是这类患者可能出现一系列药物不良反应，包括恶心、呕吐、瘙痒、镇静、呼吸抑制、免疫抑制，甚至呼吸、心搏骤停等。此外，有研究（*n*=5146）显示，术后阿片类药物长期使用患者新发抑

NMDA receptor antagonist that can inhibit central sensitization. Studies have shown that intrathecal administration of clonidine or epidural administration of ketamine can reduce pain sensitivity to mechanical stimuli around the incision site. A systematic evaluation involving 39 studies (n=3027) showed that compared with general anesthesia alone, the risk of CPSP in breast cancer patients undergoing surgery under general anesthesia combined with regional anesthesia was reduced by 57%. For patients with high-risk factors for CPSP, individualized medication plans should be developed and follow-up should be strengthened within 3 months after surgery. However, 80% of patients do not receive timely and effective intervention measures for persistent pain within the first 3 months after surgery, leading to the chronicity of pain. Therefore, we emphasize the need to establish comprehensive transitional pain treatment services, early detection and treatment, in order to prevent or reduce the occurrence of CPSP.

◆ Pain management related to surgery

1. Choosing appropriate surgical methods and refining surgical procedures may help reduce the occurrence of CPSP. For example, avoiding damage to the inguinal nerve, selecting appropriate surgical procedures and patches, and preventing infections may help reduce the incidence of chronic pain after inguinal hernia repair surgery. During the operation of breast cancer, attention should be paid to the preservation of nerves during axillary lymph node dissection, which may also help to reduce CPSP. The development of various minimally invasive surgeries and treatments may also help reduce the incidence of postoperative pain.

2. In some surgeries, if various conservative treatment methods have been attempted and the patient's pain persists, surgical methods may be considered. For example, after inguinal hernia surgery, the cause of pain can be explored during the operation. If nerve sutures are found, the relevant nerves should be loosened; If the nerve is stimulated by the patch, the corresponding patch needs to be removed for symptomatic treatment, and postoperative pain can often be relieved.

◆ Pain management related to patients

1. Conduct social and psychological interventions. As mentioned earlier, psychological factors interact with CPSP. Yang et al. reported in a meta-analysis of 33 studies (n=53 362) that patients with depression and anxiety had a 71% and 22% increased risk of developing CPSP, respectively. Another observational study involving 3528 patients showed that even without experiencing anxiety or depression, patients with only negative psychological expectations before surgery had a 56% increase in CPSP incidence. Therefore, it is meaningful to provide comprehensive psychological and social treatment for CPSP patients, including timely pain knowledge education, to help patients recognize and alleviate anxiety and fear.

2. Improve sleep. As mentioned earlier, there is a comorbidity between sleep disorders and CPSP. Meta analysis shows that sleep disorders are an important predictor of CPSP, and over time, they may lead to more severe consequences. Early recognition and detection of sleep disorders can lead to more targeted interventions, which can facilitate better pain management.

Long term postoperative pain management

◆ Drug therapy

Opioids are the most classic and potent analgesic drugs. Some studies suggest that postoperative CPSP in surgical patients may require long-term use of opioid drugs, but such patients may experience a range of adverse drug reactions, including nausea, vomiting, itching, sedation, respiratory depression, immune suppression, and even respiratory and cardiac arrest. In addition, studies (n=5146) have shown that long-term use of opioid drugs after surgery increases the risk of developing new onset depression, which is related to medication frequency. Increasing

郁症风险增加，且与用药频率相关，增加用药频率后新发抑郁症风险可增加高达 40%。术后阿片类药物长期使用还可能影响患者生存率，一项纳入逾 5 万例肺癌术后患者的回顾性研究发现，术后阿片类药物长期使用患者的 2 年全因死亡率风险增加 40%。

抗惊厥药物如加巴喷丁和普瑞巴林等，被广泛用于治疗神经病理性疼痛，可降低疼痛评分和减少阿片类药物的使用。目前对于抗惊厥药物在 CPSP 防治中的作用仍缺乏统一结论，尤其是考虑到部分患者在用药过程中会出现过度镇静、头晕和视力障碍等不良反应，多数临床医师不将此类药物作为 CPSP 防治的首选，因此，在临床应用中应仔细评估患者病情，谨慎使用此类药物。

糖皮质激素药理作用广泛，在疼痛治疗中主要利用其抗炎和免疫抑制作用。目前主要用于治疗炎症及创伤后疼痛、神经根病变引起的疼痛、癌痛以及一些复杂区域疼痛综合征。安全、有效使用糖皮质激素，应严格掌握其在 CPSP 治疗中的药物剂型、剂量和给药方法。

◆ 微创介入治疗

射频治疗可用于治疗神经病理性疼痛，有研究显示，超声引导下射频消融治疗能有效缓解腹股沟疝无张力修补术后慢性疼痛，临床疗效显著，并发症较少，是一种有效安全的治疗方法。一组明确诊断为 PTPS 的 47 例患者，经背根节脉冲射频治疗后，视觉模拟评分法（VAS）评分在术后第 1 天即出现明显降低，在术后 12 个月时随访，仍显示良好效果。同时，患者镇痛药服用量大大减少，药物相关副作用也相应降低，且未见明显手术相关并发症发生，说明胸背根节脉冲射频是治疗 PTPS 的一种安全且有效的方法。

在 2021 年，樊碧发等在中疼痛医学杂志中发表的《脊髓电刺激治疗慢性疼痛专家共识》指出，脊髓电刺激适应证包括但不仅限于腰椎术后疼痛综合征、周围神经损伤性疼痛、慢性神经根性疼痛、放化疗引起的痛性神经病变、癌性疼痛等。

◆ 其他治疗方法

物理治疗中目前常用的方法有微波治疗、局部热敷、针灸等，前两者是通过热效应与生物效应促进局部血液循环及炎性因子的消退，从而减轻术后疼痛；后者则可通过干预多种信号通路抑制免疫细胞释放组胺、5- 羟色胺等炎性介质，从而阻遏周围神经的痛觉敏化。随着针灸的发展，出现了温针灸、微针、电针、小针刀等方式，也受到越来越多关注。例如，电针可以通过抑制 Toll 样受体 2（TLR2）的信号传导，使 TNF-α、IL-1β、IL-6 等炎性细胞因子的表达下调，抑制炎性疼痛的产生。另外，经皮神经电刺激疗法（通过皮肤将特定的低频脉冲电流输入人体治疗疼痛的电疗方法）也取得了不错的效果。超激光照射瞬间可产生较高强度的辐射波，穿透力好，对局部疼痛区域或神经干进行照射疼痛，可以有效缓解慢性疼痛，促进

medication frequency can increase the risk of developing new onset depression by up to 40%. Long term use of postoperative opioid drugs may also affect patient survival rates. A retrospective study involving over 50 000 postoperative lung cancer patients found that the risk of 2-year all-cause mortality increased by 40% in patients with long-term use of postoperative opioid drugs.

Anticonvulsant drugs such as gabapentin and pregabalin are widely used to treat neuropathic pain, which can reduce pain scores and decrease the use of opioid drugs. At present, there is still a lack of unified conclusion on the role of anticonvulsant drugs in the prevention and treatment of CPSP, especially considering that some patients may experience adverse reactions such as excessive sedation, dizziness, and visual impairment during medication. Most clinical physicians do not consider such drugs as the first choice for the prevention and treatment of CPSP. Therefore, in clinical application, patients' conditions should be carefully evaluated and such drugs should be used with caution.

Corticosteroids have a wide range of pharmacological effects, mainly utilizing their anti-inflammatory and immunosuppressive effects in pain treatment. At present, it is mainly used to treat inflammation and post-traumatic pain, pain caused by nerve root lesions, cancer pain, and some complex regional pain syndromes. The safe and effective use of glucocorticoids should strictly control their drug formulation, dosage, and administration method in CPSP treatment.

◆ Minimally invasive interventional therapy

Radiofrequency therapy can be used to treat neuropathic pain. Studies have shown that ultrasound-guided radiofrequency ablation can effectively alleviate chronic pain after tension-free repair of inguinal hernia, with significant clinical efficacy and few complications. It is an effective and safe treatment method. A group of 47 patients diagnosed with PTPS showed a significant decrease in Visual Analog Scale (VAS) scores on the first postoperative day after dorsal root ganglion pulsed radiofrequency treatment. Follow up at 12 months after surgery showed good results. At the same time, the amount of analgesics taken by patients has been greatly reduced, and the drug-related side effects have also been correspondingly reduced. No significant surgical related complications have been observed, indicating that thoracic dorsal root ganglion pulsed radiofrequency is a safe and effective method for treating PTPS.

In 2021, Fan Bifa et al. published the *Expert Consensus on Spinal Cord Electrical Stimulation Therapy for Chronic Pain* in the Chinese Journal of Pain Medicine, which pointed out that the indications for spinal cord electrical stimulation include but are not limited to postoperative pain syndrome of lumbar spine, peripheral nerve injury pain, chronic radicular pain, painful neuropathy caused by radiotherapy and chemotherapy, cancer pain, etc.

◆ Other treatment methods

At present, the commonly used methods in physical therapy include microwave therapy, local hot compress, acupuncture and moxibustion, etc. The first two are to promote local blood circulation and the elimination of inflammatory factors through thermal and biological effects, so as to reduce postoperative pain; The latter can inhibit the release of inflammatory mediators such as histamine and serotonin by immune cells by intervening in various signaling pathways, thereby suppressing peripheral nerve pain sensitization. With the development of acupuncture and moxibustion, warm acupuncture and moxibustion, micro acupuncture, electroacupuncture, small needle knife and other methods have emerged, which have also attracted more and more attention. For example, electroacupuncture can suppress the signaling of Toll like receptor 2 (TLR2), downregulate the expression of inflammatory cytokines such as TNF-α, IL-1β, IL-6, and inhibit the production of inflammatory pain. In addition, transcutaneous nerve electrical stimulation therapy (an electrical therapy method that uses specific low-frequency pulse currents input into the human body through the skin to treat pain) has also achieved good results. Ultra laser

神经功能恢复。

针对不同的心理状态，疼痛的感觉或阈值也不相同，当患者出现术后疼痛时，可进行适当的心理治疗，采用转移注意力法，通过看电视、讲故事、看报、相互交谈等多种方式分散注意力，起到减轻疼痛的作用，同时可配合医务人员的解释、家人的鼓励与安慰等手段，帮助患者消除焦虑和恐惧等不良心理因素，提高患者疼痛阈值，增强机体抗病痛的能力。此外，还有催眠与暗示疗法、认知疗法、生物反馈疗法等。

对于创面损伤来说，疼痛管理的目标在于缓解疼痛、促进康复、预防疼痛的复发，使患者在治疗过程中保持良好的身体和心理状态。

（耿武军　张文静）

irradiation can instantly generate high-intensity radiation waves with good penetration, which can effectively alleviate chronic pain and promote nerve function recovery by irradiating pain areas or nerve trunks.

According to different psychological states, the feeling or threshold of pain also varies. When patients experience postoperative pain, appropriate psychological treatment can be carried out, using the method of shifting attention. By watching TV, telling stories, reading newspapers, talking to each other and other ways to distract attention, it can reduce pain. At the same time, it can be accompanied by explanations from medical staff, encouragement and comfort from family members, and other means to help patients eliminate negative psychological factors such as anxiety and fear, improve the patient's pain threshold, and enhance the body's ability to resist pain. In addition, there are hypnosis and suggestion therapy, cognitive therapy, biofeedback therapy, and so on.

For wound injuries, the goal of pain management is to alleviate pain, promote recovery, prevent pain recurrence, and maintain a good physical and psychological state for patients during the treatment process.

(Geng Wujun, Zhang Wenjing)

第三部分
Part 3

附录
Appendix

科技惠民　大爱肤生
——打造中国最有温度的科技医疗慈善品牌

由中国工程院院士、温州医科大学校长李校堃院士发起的“肤生工程”项目，是温州医科大学、温州市慈善总会、温州都市报以及温州曙光医院等单位共同主办，项目利用全国义工志愿者平台，建立救助网络，用院士团队的科技成果惠泽百姓，为深受创面问题困扰的人群提供慈善救助服务，避免“因病返贫”现象发生，服务乡村振兴战略，为浙江高质量发展、建设共同富裕示范区贡献力量。项目开展以来，在社会各界的支持下，秉承“内抓管理，外树形象”“勇担职责、务实创新”的基本原则，培育了“千村千点救助站”“藏区医疗公益行”“百年红、肤生行”“肤生浙里行”“肤生海西行”等活动品牌，建立了辐射浙、闽、陕、青、藏的救助网络，开启了“一带一路”远程救助新模式，并探索公益慈善品牌助力共同富裕的道路上，努力打造“医疗、教育、科技、慈善、志愿服务”于一体的新时代慈善公益品牌。“肤生工程”还获得浙江慈善奖、温州慈善奖、感动温州十大人物集体奖等荣誉。

温州医科大学在创伤修复领域有深厚的研究基础，李校堃院士团队深耕创伤修复的理论和实践研究三十来年，基于生长因子的创伤修复研究处于国际领先地位，在世界上率先开发成功促组织损伤与再生修复的一类新药和三类载药医疗器械等，广泛应用于烧伤、难愈性溃疡、糖尿病和老年病并发症、重大灾害性创伤、国防战伤救治。研究成果曾获得国家科学技术进步奖一等奖、国家科学技术进步奖二等奖、光华工程科技奖、转化医学杰出贡献奖等，培养了一批医药人才。

李校堃院士及其团队不仅取得了该项研究领域的“制高点”，也使我国成为世界上第一个把细胞生长因子开发为创面修复药物的国家。2020 年 1 月，李校堃院士牵头成立了“浙江创面修复与转化应用中心暨温州医科大学创伤修复与再生医学中心”，致力于引领创面修复基础与转化研究，争创该领域的中国温州模式。李校堃院士担任该中心主任。李校堃院士说，“肤生工程”将以温州的创面修复成果，致力于解决广大糖尿病、老年病并发症等慢性难愈合创面患者的病痛，提高患者的生活品质，降低医疗费用，减轻患者的负担。这对于国家推进健康扶贫，实现 2020 年脱贫攻坚目标具有重要意义。

“肤生工程”惠及抗疫医务工作者

“肤生工程”是一个科技为民、服务社会的慈善公益项目，惠民项目以院士团队长期从事创面修复与组织再生相关药物研究成果为基础。该项目正式启动于 2020 年全国上下抗击新型冠状病毒感染疫情之时，

Technology benefits the people and loves skin care – Build the most warm technology medical charity brand in China

The "F&S CHARITY" , initiated by Li Xiaokun, an academician of the CAE Member and president of Wenzhou Medical University, is co sponsored by Wenzhou Medical University, Wenzhou Charity Federation, Wenzhou Metropolis Daily, Wenzhou Dawn Hospital and other units. The project uses the national volunteer platform to establish a relief network, benefit the people with the scientific and technological achievements of the academician team, provide charity relief services for people suffering from wounds, avoid "returning to poverty due to illness", serve the rural revitalization strategy, and contribute to the high-quality development of Zhejiang and the construction of a common prosperity demonstration area. Since the launch of the project, with the support of all sectors of society, adhering to the basic principles of "internal management, external image", "brave responsibility, pragmatic innovation", the project has fostered "1000 villages and 1000 points rescue station", "Tibetan Medical Public Welfare Tour", "Centennial Red, Skin Health line", "Skin Health Tour in Zhejiang", "Skin Health Tour in the West" and other activity brands, established a rescue network radiating to Zhejiang, Fujian, Shaanxi, Qinghai, and Tibet, opened a new model of "the Belt and Road" remote rescue, explored the path of public welfare brands to help common prosperity, and worked hard to create a new era charity brand integrating "medical, education, science and technology, charity, and voluntary services". The "F&S CHARITY" has also won honors such as the Zhejiang Charity Award, Wenzhou Charity Award, and the Wenzhou Top Ten Touching Figures Collective Award.

Wenzhou Medical University has a deep research foundation in the field of wound repair. Academician Li Xiaokun's team has been deeply engaged in the theoretical and practical research of wound repair for more than three decades. The research on wound repair based on growth factors is in the leading position in the world, and it is the first in the world to successfully develop a class of new drugs and class III drug carrying medical devices that promote tissue damage and regenerative repair, which are widely used in the treatment of burns, refractory ulcers, complications of diabetes and geriatrics, major catastrophic trauma, and national defense war wounds. The research results have won the first prize of the National Science and Technology Progress Award, the second prize of the National Science and Technology Progress Award, the Guanghua Engineering Science and Technology Award, and the Outstanding Contribution Award for Translational Medicine, cultivating a group of pharmaceutical talents.

Academician Li Xiaokun and his team not only achieved the "high ground" in this research field, but also made China the first country in the world to develop cell growth factors as wound repair drugs. In January 2020, Academician Li Xiaokun led the establishment of the "Zhejiang Wound Repair and Transformation Application Center and Wenzhou Medical University Trauma Repair and Regenerative Medicine Center", dedicated to leading basic and translational research in wound repair and striving to create the Wenzhou model in this field in China. Academician Li Xiaokun serves as the director of the center. Academician Li Xiaokun said that the "F&S CHARITY" will use the wound repair achievements in Wenzhou to solve the pain of the majority of patients with chronic refractory wounds such as diabetes and senile complications, improve the quality of life of patients, reduce medical costs and reduce the burden of patients. This is of great significance for the country to promote healthy poverty alleviation and achieve the 2020 poverty alleviation goals.

The "F&S CHARITY" benefits anti epidemic medical workers

The "F&S CHARITY" is a charity and public welfare project that uses technology to serve the people and society. The Huimin project is based on the long-term research achievements of the academician team in wound repair and tissue regeneration related drugs. The project was officially launched in 2020 when the whole country was fighting against the COVID-19. When medical personnel from all over the country threw themselves into the fight against the epidemic without hesitation, the pressure skin injuries caused by the first-line anti epidemic medical

当全国各地医务人员义无反顾地投身到这场抗击疫情的战斗时，抗疫一线医护人员因长时间佩戴防护装备造成的压力性皮肤损伤时见报道，牵动着全国人民的心。

国有难，操戈披甲；人有危，众士争先。“肤生工程”发起“关爱医务人员、抚平天使印记”爱心活动，得到温州爱心单位和爱心人士的大力支持，纷纷捐赠善款；浙江、上海、安徽等地多家生物制药公司的捐赠支持，共同“守护最美逆行者”。抗击疫情一线医疗人员在隔离病房工作期间因为长期、反复使用护目镜、防护服、胶皮手套等而导致的颜面部压力性破溃、压疮、过敏性皮炎、汗疹等，出现了“天使印记”。为此，李校堃院士团队联合温州都市报陈忠慈善工作室、温州曙光医院等单位设立“肤生”慈善公益项目——预防医用防护装备损伤爱心包计划。

“天使印记”我们来抚平
“肤生”慈善工程-防护爱心包驰援武汉战“疫”捐赠仪式

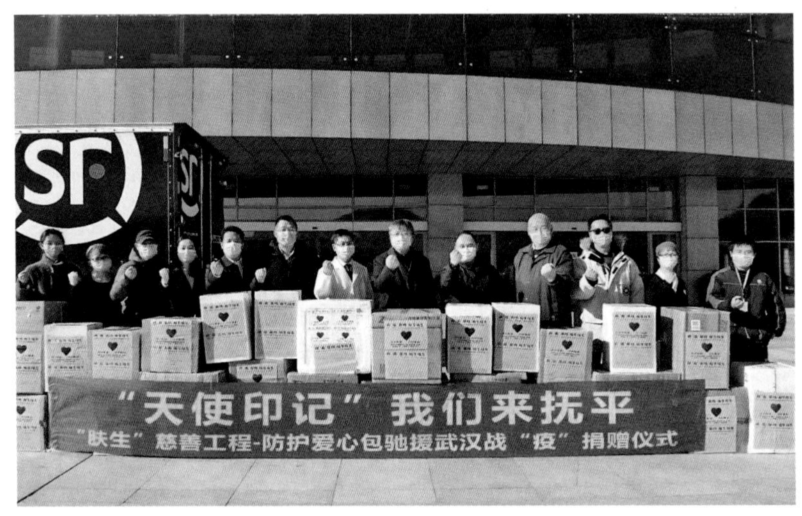

附图 1　“肤生”慈善工程 – 防护爱心包捐赠仪式

李校堃院士团队利用他们长期在创面修复方向的研发积累，提高一线医护人员防护水平，预防穿戴医用防护装备导致的各种损伤，最大限度降低医源性感染风险，保护战“疫”医务人员生命安全，促进损伤皮肤再生，保证医务人员强大的战斗力，不惧生死，守护新型冠状病毒性肺炎患者生命与健康。李校堃院士亲自开出“处方”，在捐赠的“肤生”爱心包里配备生长因子喷剂、水胶体敷料及神洁、丹皮软膏等药物和敷料。其中，细胞生长因子系列促组织再生与创面修复的高科技产品，是皮肤创面愈合不可缺少的蛋白。在交通封闭、物资短缺的情况下，2020 年 2 月 19 日，首批 1000 个防护爱心包从温州启运，尔后，“肤生工程”向武汉华中科技大学同济医学院附属协和医院、武汉科技大学附属天佑医院、武汉市第四医院以及温州各医院的一线医务人员送上 1516 个、价值近百万元的预防医用防护装备损伤爱心包，关爱医护人员，抚平天使印记，新华社播发《温州“肤生”爱心包抚平“天使印记”》一文予以点赞。

personnel wearing protective equipment for a long time were reported, which touched the hearts of the people all over the country.

In times of national crisis, one must engage in military tactics and armor; When people are in danger, the people rush forward. The "F&S CHARITY" launched the "Care for Medical Personnel, Smooth the Angel Mark" charity activity, which received strong support from Wenzhou charity units and individuals, who donated funds one after another; Donations and support from multiple biopharmaceutical companies in Zhejiang, Shanghai, Anhui, and other regions jointly "safeguard the most beautiful traitors". Frontline medical personnel fighting against the epidemic have developed "angel marks" due to long-term and repeated use of goggles, protective clothing, rubber gloves, etc. during their work in isolation wards, resulting in facial pressure ulcers, pressure sores, allergic dermatitis, sweat rashes, etc. To this end, the team of Academician Li Xiaokun, together with Wenzhou Urban Daily Chen Zhong Charity Studio, Wenzhou Shuguang Hospital and other units, established the "Skin Life" charity public welfare project - Prevention of Medical Protective Equipment Damage Love Package Plan.

“天使印记” 我们来抚平
“肤生”慈善工程-防护爱心包驰援武汉战“疫”捐赠仪式

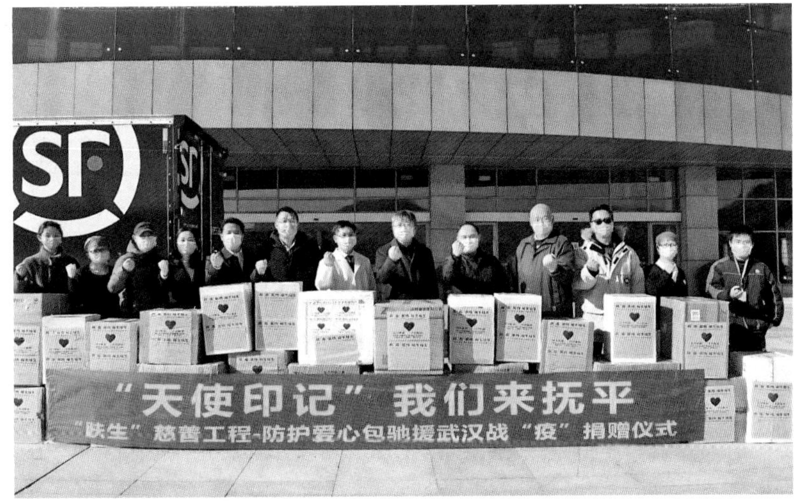

Figure 1 "Skin Life" Charity Project - Donation ceremony for protective love packages

Academician Li Xiaokun's team made use of their long-term research and development accumulation in the direction of wound repair to improve the protection level of front-line medical staff, prevent various injuries caused by wearing medical protective equipment, minimize the risk of iatrogenic infection, protect the life safety of medical staff fighting "epidemic", promote the regeneration of damaged skin, ensure the strong combat effectiveness of medical staff, fear life and death, and protect the life and health of patients with novel coronavirus pneumonia. Academician Li Xiaokun personally issued a "prescription" to equip the donated "Fusheng" love package with growth factor spray, hydrogel dressing, as well as drugs and dressings such as Shenjie and Danpi ointment. Among them, the high-tech products of the cell growth factor series that promote tissue regeneration and wound repair are essential proteins for skin wound healing. In the context of traffic closure and material shortage, on February 19, 2020, the first batch of 1000 protective love packages were shipped from Wenzhou. Subsequently, the "F&S CHARITY" sent 1516 protective equipment damage prevention love packages worth nearly one million yuan to frontline medical staff at Tongji Medical College Affiliated Union Hospital of Huazhong University of Science and Technology in Wuhan, Tianyou Hospital Affiliated to Wuhan University of Science and Technology, Wuhan Fourth Hospital, and various hospitals in Wenzhou, caring for medical staff and smoothing out the "angel mark". Xinhua News Agency praised the article *Wenzhou Skin Life " love package smoothing out the " angel mark* .

破解创面之殇，“肤生工程”启动仪式

2020 年 5 月 17 日，由中国工程院院士、温州医科大学校长李校堃院士发起的“肤生工程”在温启动。该项目旨在为全国深受创面问题困扰的弱势人群提供慈善救助服务，同时培养造血型的创面修复人才，以温州的创面修复成果引领全国、服务大众。

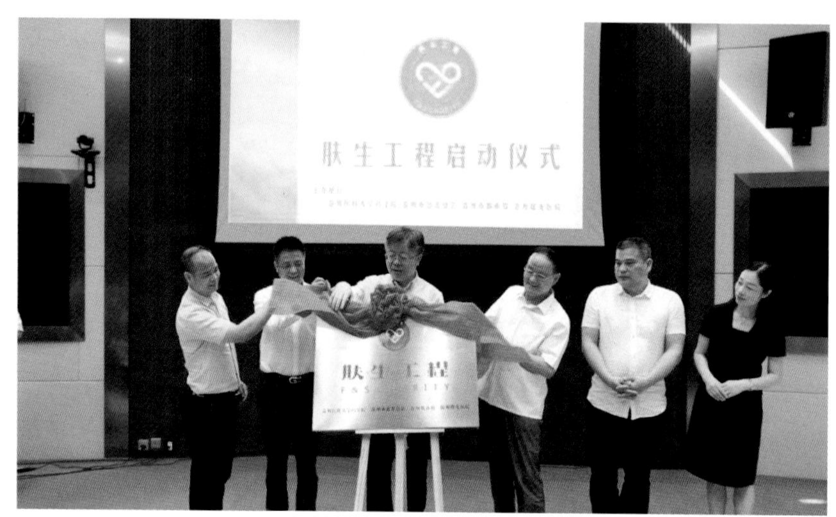

附图 2　“肤生工程”温州启动仪式

据统计，全球约 1% 的人口被持续性的创面问题所困扰，约 5% 的医疗费用花费在创面修复上。目前我国由糖尿病、老年病等临床常见病和多发病引起的难愈合创面病例越来越多，而每年需要创面治疗的患者约 1 亿人次，其中严重患者约 3000 万人次，糖尿病引发的溃疡创伤从十年前的 4.9% 上升到 35%。在深受创面之痛的人群中，低保、低收入等弱势群体又占了相当大比例。

为此，温州医科大学、温州市慈善总会、温州都市报、温州曙光医院等单位联合主办“肤生工程”，立足温州，面向全国，开展精准健康帮扶。

“肤生工程”每年将组织多次全国大型公益活动，结对医院，对患者进行救助；利用全国义工志愿者平台，建立救助网络，精准帮扶、长期跟踪，解决基层贫困患者创面问题；结对养老机构护理人员、社区家庭医生，开展慢性创面护理培训；在温州医科大学附属医院等建立创面修复专科和人才培养，聘请全国一批创面修复领域专家入库，参与创面修复的大型慈善活动和临床指导研究工作，培养创面修复人才；布局“千村千点”开展精准健康帮扶，让偏远地区患者在家门口享受创面修复医疗服务；启动高原地区创面救助援藏医疗项目等。

Cracking the tragedy of wounds, launching ceremony of "F&S CHARITY"

On May 17, 2020, the "F&S CHARITY" initiated by Li Xiaokun, academician of the CAE Member and president of Wenzhou Medical University, was launched in Wenzhou. The project aims to provide charitable assistance services to vulnerable groups across the country who are deeply troubled by wound problems, while cultivating blood type wound repair talents, leading the country and serving the public with Wenzhou's wound repair achievements.

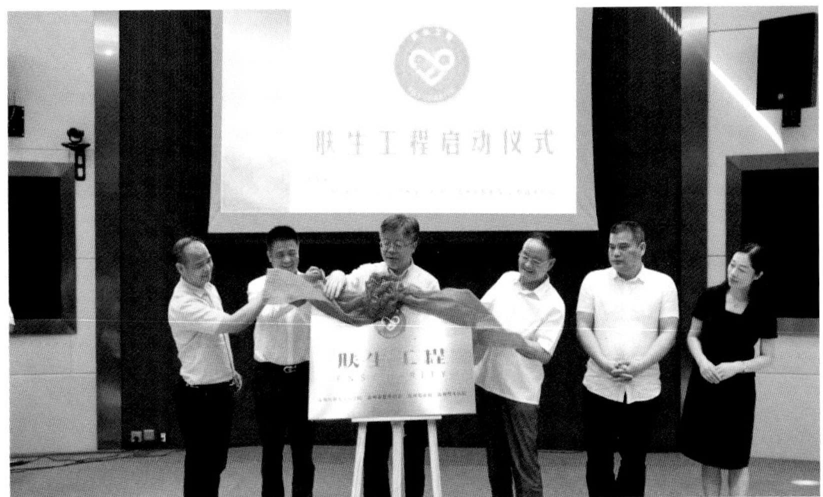

Figure 2 Launch ceremony of the "F&S CHARITY" in Wenzhou

According to statistics, about 1% of the global population is troubled by persistent wound problems, and about 5% of medical expenses are spent on wound repair. At present, there are more and more cases of difficult to heal wounds caused by clinical common diseases and frequently occurring diseases such as diabetes and geriatrics in China. Every year, about 100 million patients need wound treatment, including about 30 million serious patients. Ulcerative wounds caused by diabetes have risen from 4.9% ten years ago to 35%. Among the people who suffer from the pain of wounds, vulnerable groups such as low-income and low-income families account for a considerable proportion.

To this end, Wenzhou Medical University, Wenzhou Charity Federation, Wenzhou Urban Daily, Wenzhou Shuguang Hospital and other units jointly organized the "F&S CHARITY", based in Wenzhou and facing the whole country, to carry out precise health assistance.

The "F&S CHARITY" will organize multiple large-scale national public welfare activities every year, pairing hospitals to provide assistance to patients; Utilize the national volunteer platform to establish a rescue network, provide precise assistance and long-term tracking, and solve the wound problems of impoverished patients at the grassroots level; Pair up nursing staff in elderly care institutions and community family doctors to conduct training on chronic wound care; Establishing wound repair specialties and talent training at affiliated hospitals of Wenzhou Medical University, hiring a group of experts in the field of wound repair from across the country to participate in large-scale charity activities and clinical guidance research on wound repair, and cultivating wound repair talents; Layout "Thousand Villages and Thousand Points" to carry out precise health assistance, allowing patients in remote areas to enjoy wound repair medical services at their doorstep; Initiate medical projects for wound relief and aid to Tibet in high-altitude areas.

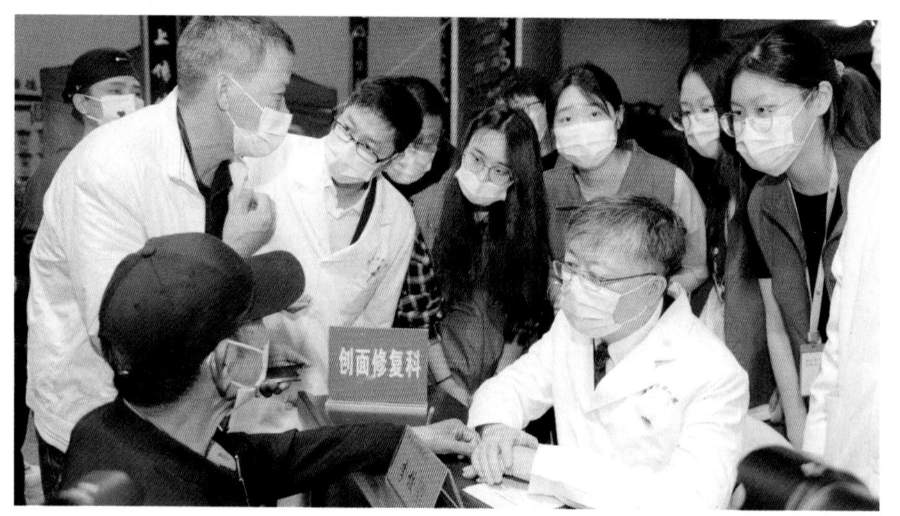

附图 3　开展精准健康帮扶

当天的启动仪式上进行了首批 6 个“肤生工程”示范点授牌、首批 10 支义工队授旗。义工队将寻找贫困难愈合慢性创面患者，并提供救助和志愿服务。温州护士学校藏族学生益西卓玛、三郎乓等 10 人成为首批藏族志愿者，他们将为藏族地区开展志愿服务。当天，首批 1 名藏族贫困慢性难愈合性创面患者接到温州治疗。温州曙光医院副院长陈善亮分享了“肤生工程”一次救助的感动故事。

温州市援藏工作组组长、浙江省援藏指挥部副指挥、嘉黎县委常务副书记周建清出席启动仪式，他点赞“肤生工程”是极寒高原最温暖的阳光，给嘉黎患者带来希望。市慈善总会秘书长肖国庆说，“肤生工程”是面向全国的大型慈善救助项目，主要为深受创面问题困扰的弱势人群提供救助，体现了面向群众、面向基层扶贫济困的特色。

院士藏区医疗公益行

海拔 4500 多米的“世界屋脊”西藏那曲市嘉黎县，2020 年 8 月 3 日，迎来温州医科大学李校堃院士西藏医疗公益行，给当地送上公益医疗大礼：温州医科大学“肤生工程”创面修复救助基地、生长因子与复杂创面高原临床基地、儿童先天性心脏病救助项目基地等八大基地落户嘉黎并授牌，造福高原地区百姓。

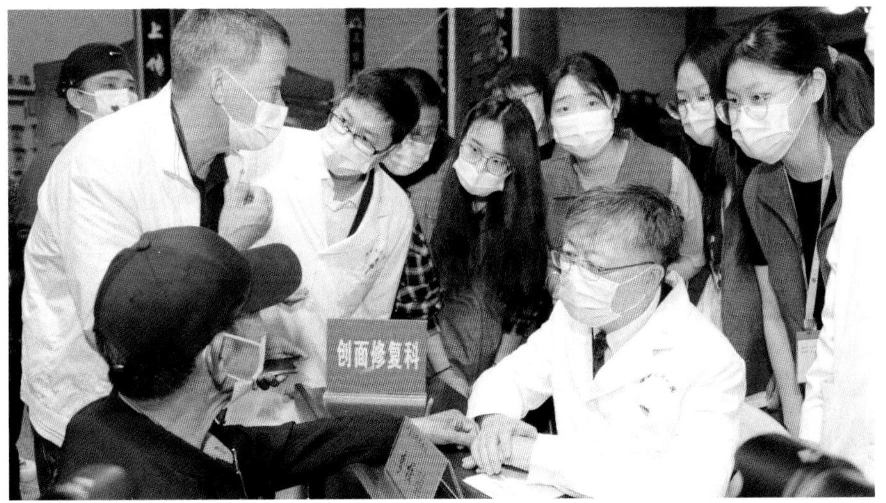

Figure 3 Implementing precise health assistance

At the launch ceremony on that day, the first batch of 6 "F&S CHARITY" demonstration sites were awarded plaques, and the first batch of 10 volunteer teams were awarded flags. The volunteer team will search for impoverished patients with difficult to heal chronic wounds and provide assistance and volunteer services. Ten Tibetan students including Yixi Zhuoma and Sanlangping from Wenzhou Nursing School have become the first batch of Tibetan volunteers, who will provide volunteer services to Tibetan areas. On that day, the first batch of impoverished Tibetan patients with chronic difficult to heal wounds received treatment in Wenzhou. Chen Shanliang, Vice President of Wenzhou Shuguang Hospital, shared the touching story of a rescue project called "F&S CHARITY".

Zhou Jianqing, the leader of the Wenzhou Aid Tibet Work Group, deputy commander of the Zhejiang Aid Tibet Command, and executive deputy secretary of the Jiali County Committee, attended the launch ceremony and praised the "F&S CHARITY" as the warmest sunshine on the extremely cold plateau, bringing hope to Jiali patients. Xiao Guoqing, Secretary General of the Municipal Charity Federation, said that the "F&S CHARITY" is a large-scale charity assistance project aimed at the whole country, mainly providing assistance to vulnerable groups who are deeply troubled by wound problems, reflecting the characteristics of poverty alleviation and assistance for the masses and grassroots.

Academician Tibetan Medical Public Welfare Tour

On August 3, 2020, Jiali County, Naqu City, Xizang, the "roof of the world" with an altitude of more than 4500 meters, welcomed academician Li Xiaokun of Wenzhou Medical University to Xizang Medical Public Welfare Trip, and gave the local public welfare medical gifts: eight major bases, including the "F&S CHARITY" wound repair and rescue base of Wenzhou Medical University, the growth factor and complex wound plateau clinical base, and the children's congenital heart disease relief project base, were settled in Jiali and awarded medals, benefiting the people in the plateau area.

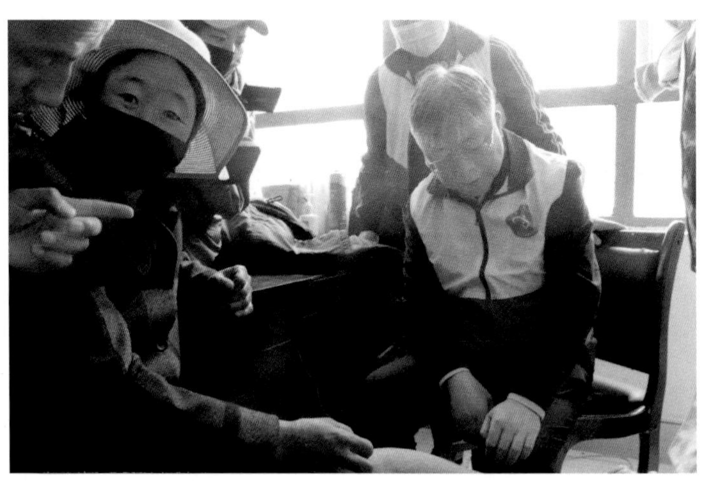

附图 4　院士藏区医疗公益行

◆ 精准医疗帮扶，造福高原地区百姓

在当天举行的温州医科大学一嘉黎县考察交流工作会上，八大公益医疗基地落户嘉黎县。温州医科大学药学院整合医药研究院成立了生长因子与复杂创面高原临床基地，该院党委书记肖健、院长林丽为嘉黎基地授牌。

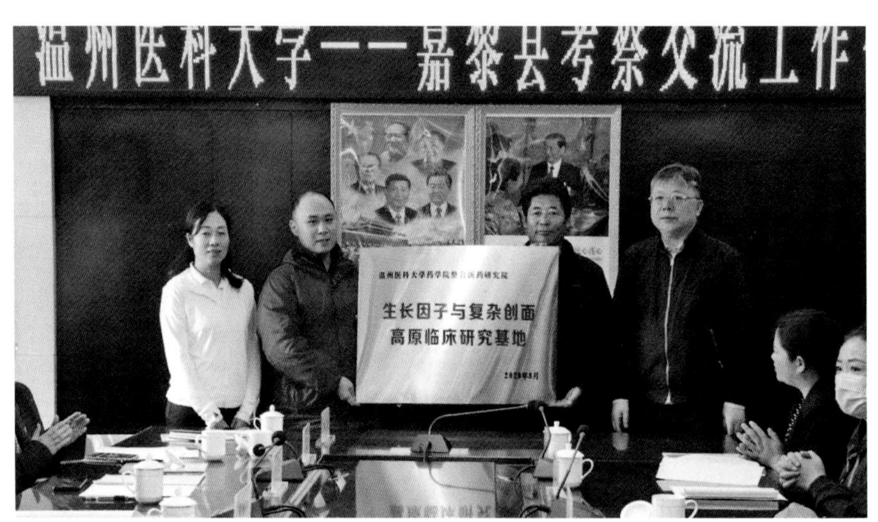

附图 5　生长因子与复杂创面高原临床基地授牌

温州医科大学附属眼视光医院在嘉黎县人民医院成立角膜救助项目基地，用于救助嘉黎县乃至那曲市贫困角膜病患者，2 日下午，该院副院长陈蔚在那曲市人民医院开展了当地首台角膜移植手术，为 52 岁藏族同胞央加实施角膜手术，使他重见光明。

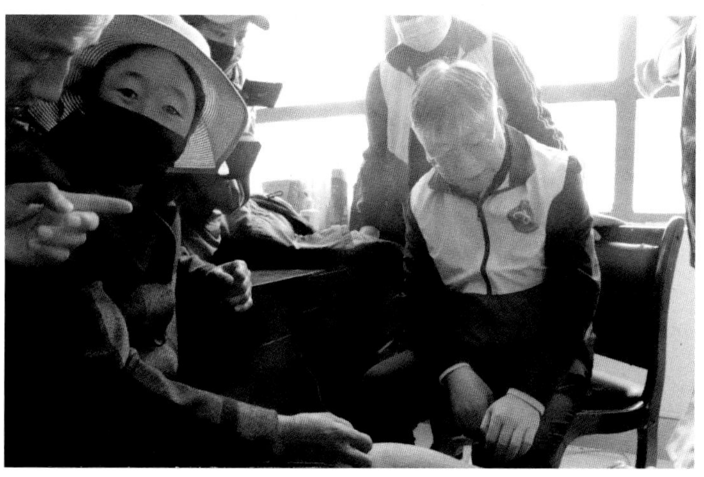

Figure 4 Academician Tibetan Medical Public Welfare Tour

◆ Precision medical assistance, benefiting the people in high-altitude areas

At the inspection and exchange work meeting of Wenzhou Medical University in Jiali County held on the same day, the eight major public welfare medical bases were settled in Jiali County. The School of Pharmacy at Wenzhou Medical University has established a high-altitude clinical base for growth factors and complex wounds through the integration of pharmaceutical research institutes. The hospital's Party Secretary, Xiao Jian, and Dean, Lin Li, have awarded the Jiali base.

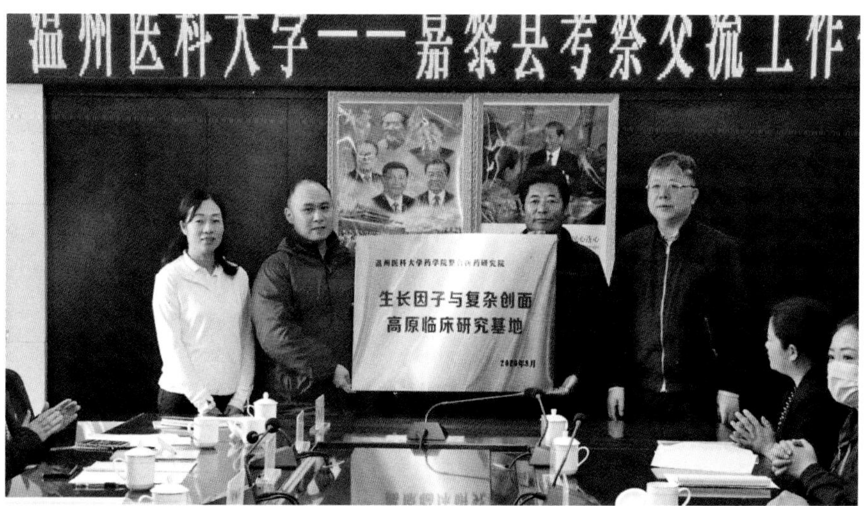

Figure 5 Awarding of Growth Factors and Complex Wound Plateau Clinical Base

Wenzhou Medical University Affiliated Eye and Vision Hospital has established a corneal rescue project base at Jiali County People's Hospital to assist impoverished corneal disease patients in Jiali County and even Nagqu City. On the afternoon of the 2nd, Chen Wei, the vice president of the hospital, carried out the first corneal transplant surgery in Nagqu City People's Hospital, performing corneal surgery for a 52-year-old Tibetan compatriot, allowing him to see the light again.

第三部分 附录

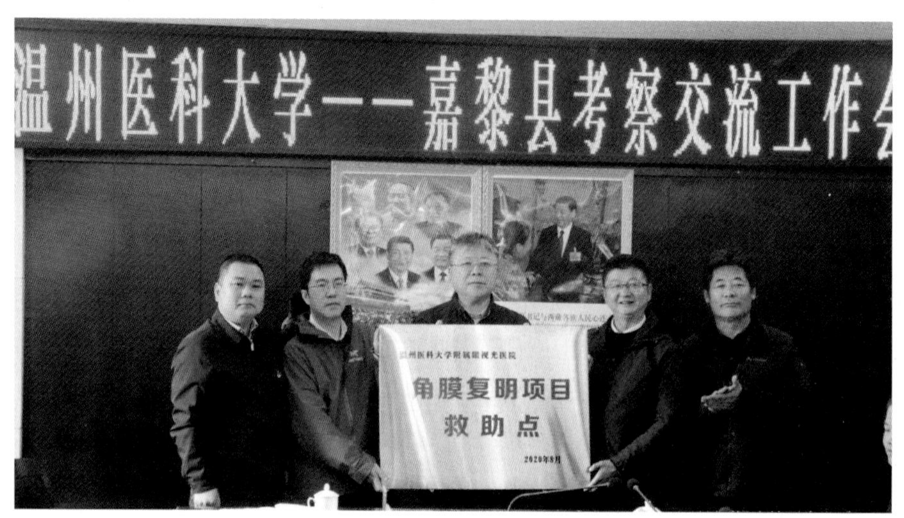

附图 6　角膜复明项目救助点授牌

温州医科大学附属第二医院、育英儿童医院党委书记褚茂平将该院儿童先天性心脏病救助项目基地授予嘉黎县，长期对当地儿童先天性心病进行救助。褚茂平率儿童心血管科主任吴蓉洲、医生仇慧仙，从温州带来 200 多万元的心脏彩超机，为当地 20 多名儿童做心超检查，检查发现其中半数儿童有心脏疾病，其中一名 6 岁藏族男孩患有房缺先天性心脏病，将把他接到温州免费治疗。

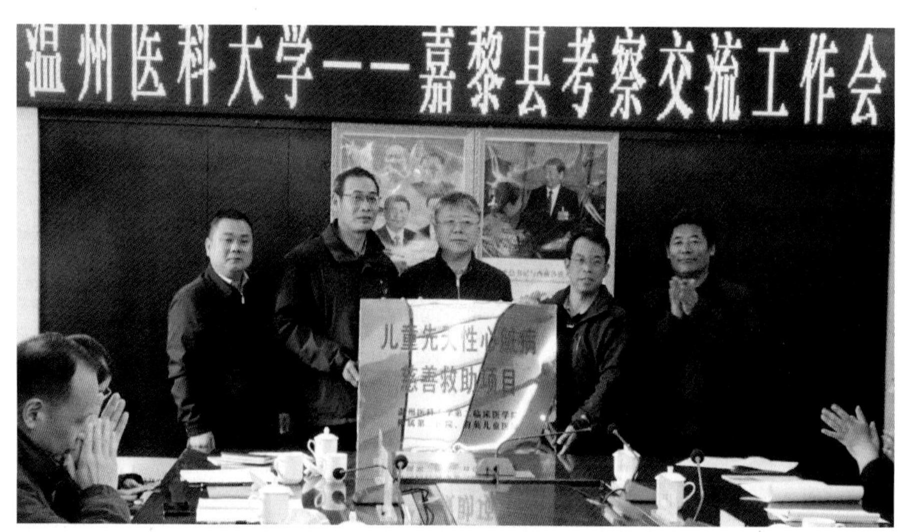

附图 7　儿童先天性心脏病慈善救助项目基地授牌

温州医科大学附属口腔医院党委书记麻健丰将微笑工程协力医院的牌子授给嘉黎县人民医院，今后，微笑工程将派专家到当地做手术，或把患者接到温州治疗。当天，麻健丰与该院医务科副科长刘登峰为当

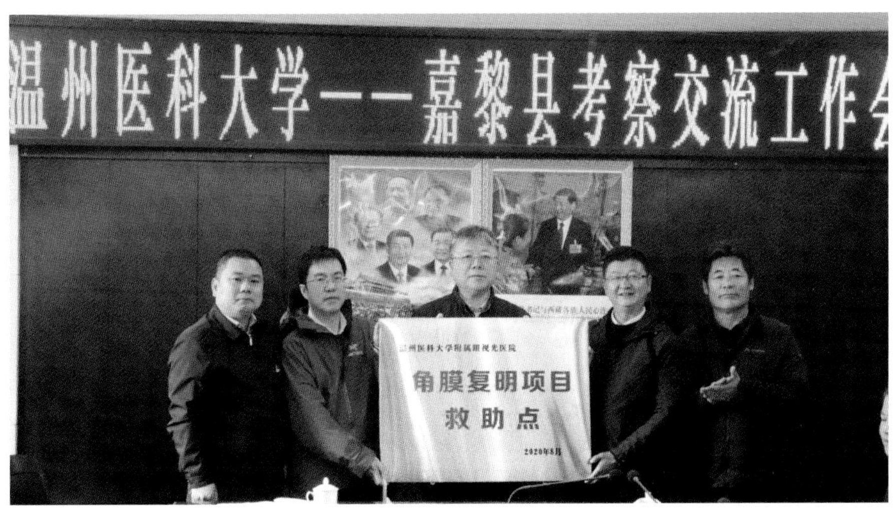

Figure 6 Awarding of Corneal Brightening Project Rescue Points

Chu Maoping, Secretary of the Party Committee of the Second Affiliated Hospital of Wenzhou Medical University and Yuying Children's Hospital, awarded the hospital's Children's Congenital Heart Disease Rescue Project Base to Jiali County, providing long-term assistance to local children with congenital heart disease. Chu Maoping led the director of the pediatric cardiovascular department, Wu Rongzhou, and doctor, Qiu Huixian, to bring over 2 million yuan worth of cardiac ultrasound machines from Wenzhou to conduct cardiac ultrasound examinations for more than 20 local children. The examination found that half of the children had heart disease, including a 6-year-old Tibetan boy with congenital heart disease caused by atrial septal defect. He will be taken to Wenzhou for free treatment.

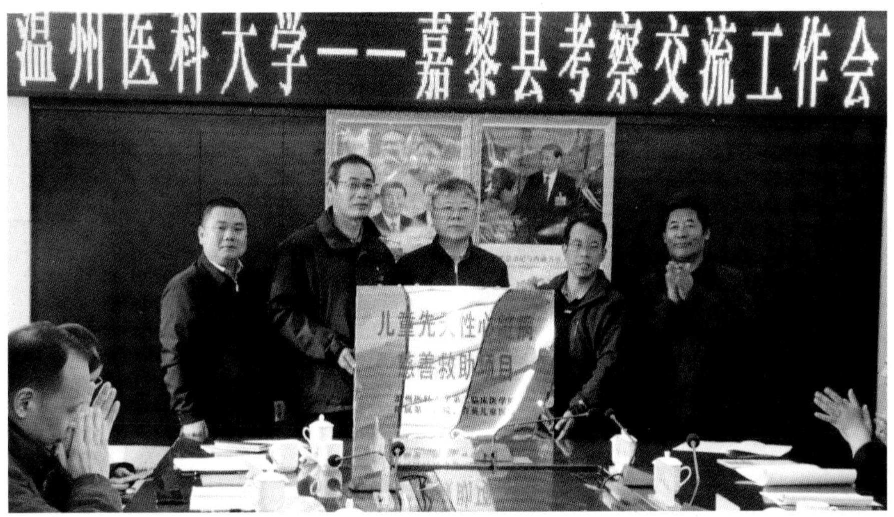

Figure 7 Awarding of Charity Assistance Project Base for Children with Congenital Heart Disease

Ma Jianfeng, Secretary of the Party Committee of the Affiliated Stomatological Hospital of Wenzhou Medical University, awarded the brand of Smile Project Cooperation Hospital to Jiali County People's Hospital. In the future, Smile Project will send experts to the local area for surgery or send patients to Wenzhou for treatment. On that day, Ma Jianfeng and Liu Dengfeng, the deputy director of the medical department of the hospital, conducted screening and postoperative follow-up examinations for dozens of children with cleft lip and palate in the local area. Children

地数十名儿童进行辱腭裂筛选和手术后的复查，对于符合条件的唇腭裂儿童患者将接到温州免费治疗。

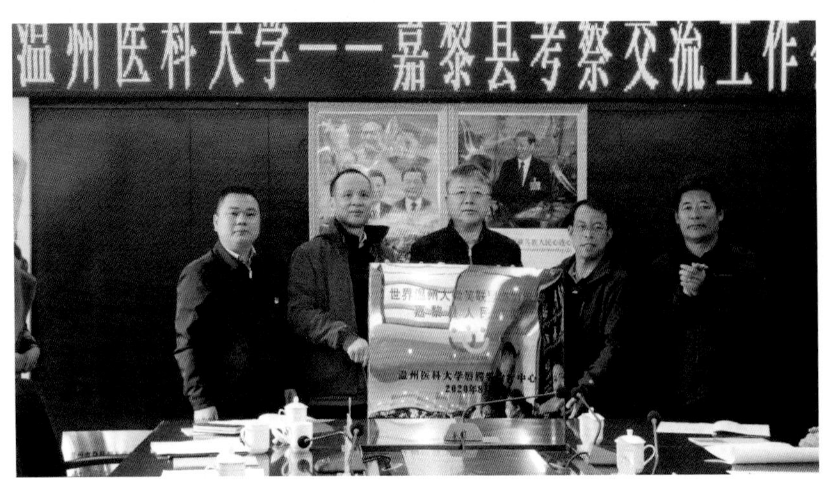

附图 8　微笑工程协力医院授牌

温州曙光医院院长金叶道参加李校堃院士西藏医疗公益行，为西藏温州商会的企业家和员工开展义诊活动。

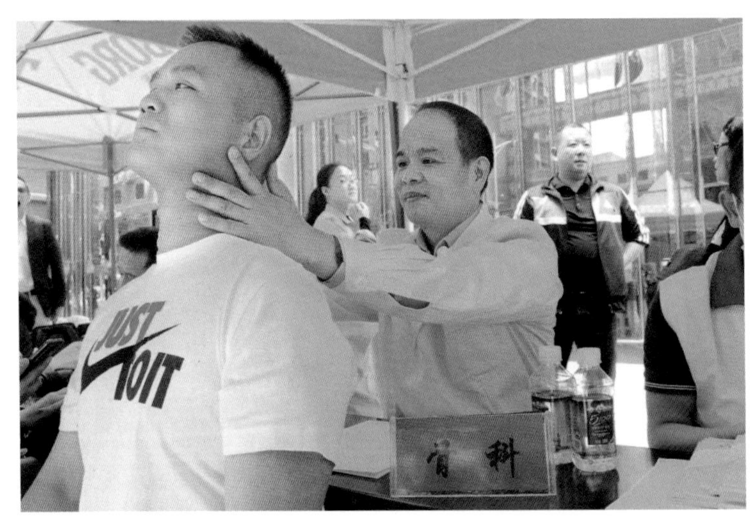

附图 9　开展义诊活动

当天，温州医科大学附属第一医院手外科主任王健和温州曙光医院副院长陈善亮在嘉黎县人民医院开展手术，为 2 名难愈合创面伤患者实施手术，这是当地首次开展这样的手术。当天，李校堃院士将“肤生工程”创面修复救助基地牌子授给嘉黎县委副书记、县长吾金才塔，启动“肤生工程”高原救助项目，长期救助难愈合创面患者。他还与陈善亮等“肤生工程”团队专家为嘉黎县 60 多名患者做检查，筛查出多名难愈合创面伤患者，将把他们接到温州治疗。

with cleft lip and palate who meet the conditions will receive free treatment in Wenzhou.

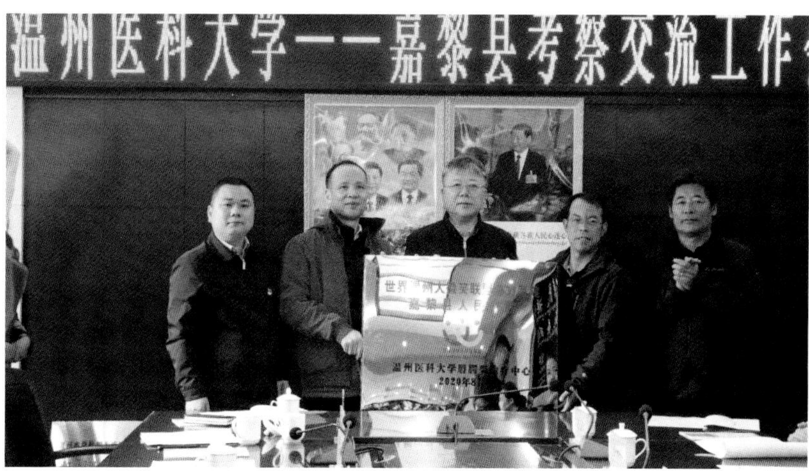

Figure 8 Smiling Project Cooperation Hospital awarded plaque

Jin Yedao, president of Wenzhou Shuguang Hospital, participated in the Xizang Medical Charity Walk of Academician Li Xiaokun, and carried out free clinic activities for entrepreneurs and employees of Xizang Wenzhou Chamber of Commerce.

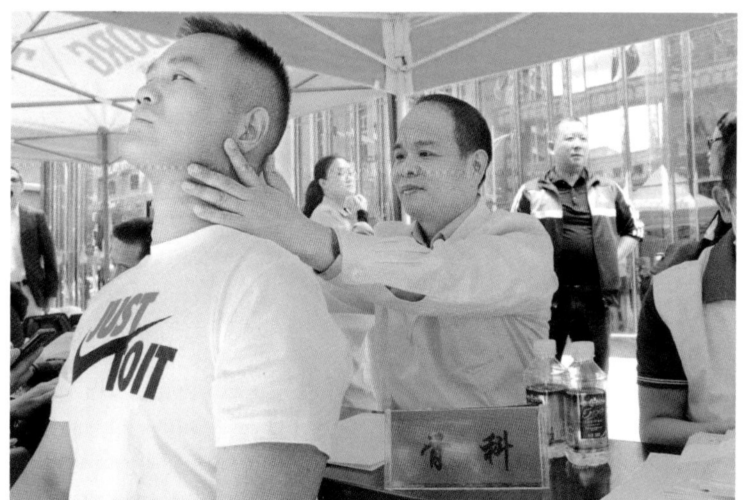

Figure 9 Conducting free clinic activities

On that day, Wang Jian, Director of the Department of Hand Surgery at the First Affiliated Hospital of Wenzhou Medical University, and Chen Shanliang, Vice President of Wenzhou Shuguang Hospital, performed surgery at Jiali County People's Hospital for two patients with difficult to heal wounds. This was the first time such surgery had been carried out in the local area. On that day, Academician Li Xiaokun awarded the brand of "F&S CHARITY" Wound Repair and Rescue Base to Wu Jincai Tower, Deputy Secretary of Jiali County Committee and County Mayor, and launched the "F&S CHARITY" high-altitude rescue project to provide long-term assistance to patients with difficult to heal wounds. He also conducted examinations for more than 60 patients in Jiali County with experts from the "F&S CHARITY" team such as Chen Shanliang, screened out multiple patients with difficult to heal wounds, and will send them to Wenzhou for treatment.

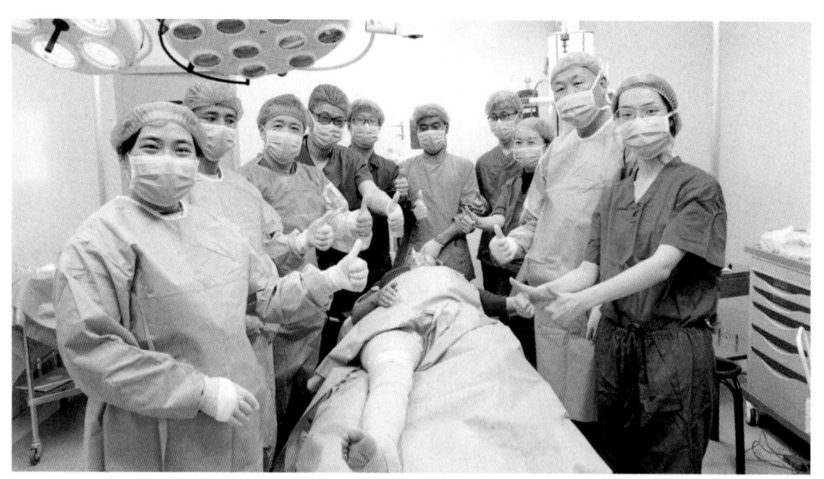

附图 10　在嘉黎县人民医院开展手术

“肤生工程”项目启动时，把嘉黎县一名难愈合创面伤患者强曲旺姆接到温州曙光医院免费治疗。

李校堃院士西藏医疗公益行，社会各界为嘉黎县捐赠物资 130 多万元，其中包括温州医科大学附属第一医院骨科党支部和温州曙光医院为 2 名患者捐出 4800 元和 1 万元的手术费。

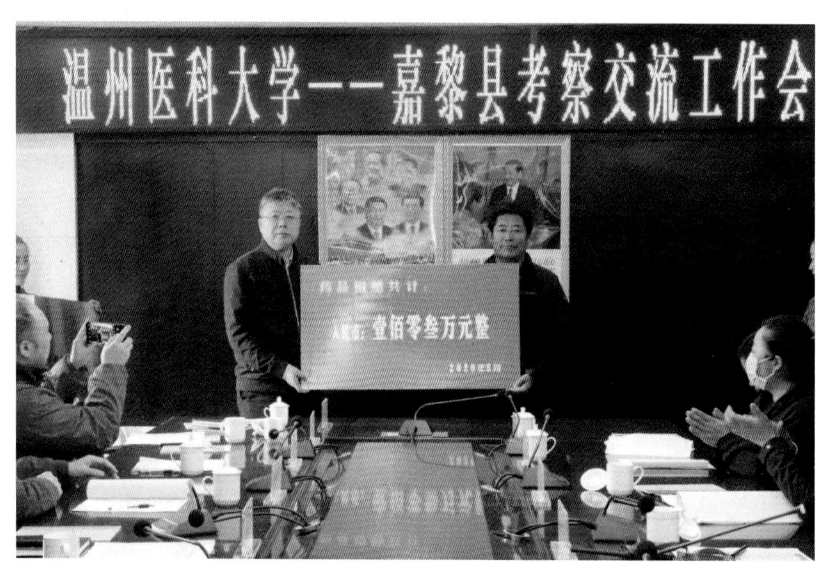

附图 11　捐赠物资

意尔康股份有限公司董事长单志敏得知这次公益行活动后，捐款 20 万元给“肤生工程”，用于嘉黎难愈合创面伤的贫困患者。他说，他们会尽力帮助需要帮助的人。多次参加温都陈忠慈善工作室慈善活动的鹿城区一位 90 岁老人和上海市洋泾菊园实验学校学生张梦颖分别捐出 1 万元和 7500 元。此前，两人还为李校堃院士为武汉等地抗疫一线肤生爱心包捐赠善款。温州三禾生物医药有限公司每年资助嘉黎县人民医院一名医护人员短期培训，连续 3 年。在赴嘉黎途中，李校堃院士还专程赶赴那曲，看望该校在那曲市人

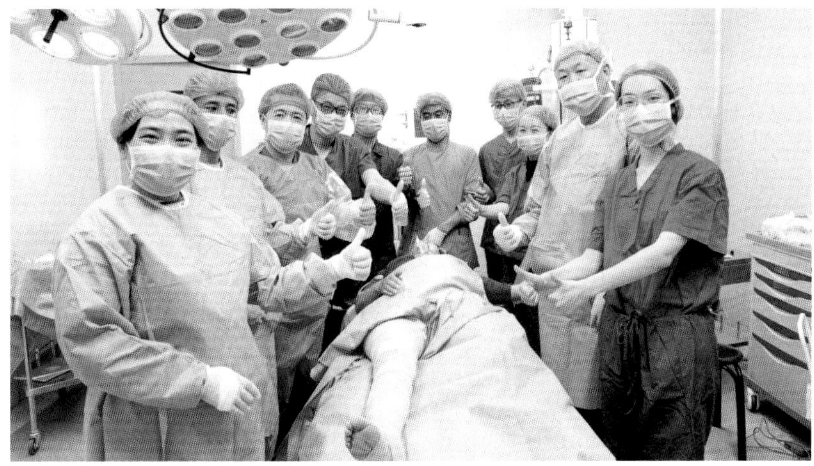

Figure 10 Surgery conducted at Jiali County People's Hospital

When the "F&S CHARITY" was launched, Qiang Quwangmu, a difficult to heal wound patient from Jiali County, was taken to Wenzhou Shuguang Hospital for free treatment.

Academician Li Xiaokun donated more than 1.3 million yuan of materials to Jiali County for the Xizang Medical Charity Walk, including 4800 yuan and 10 000 yuan of surgical fees for two patients from the orthopedic party branch of the First Affiliated Hospital of Wenzhou Medical University and Wenzhou Shuguang Hospital.

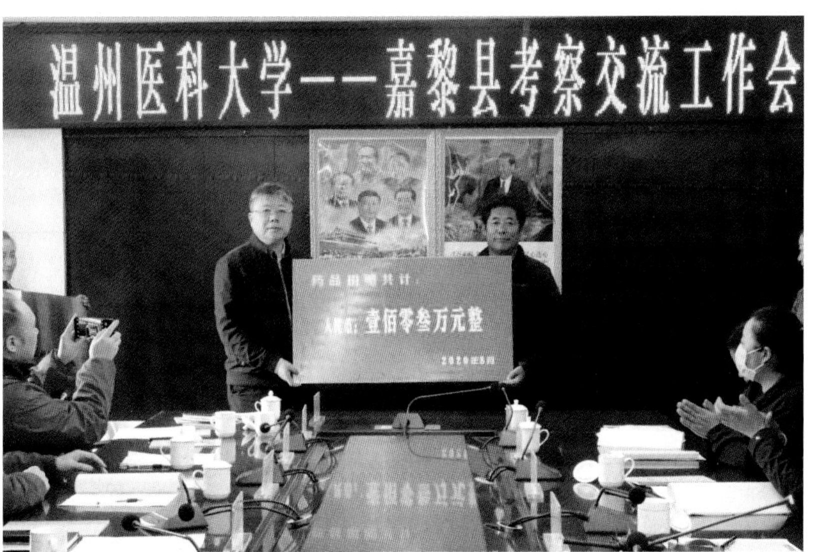

Figure 11 Donated materials

After learning about this charity event, Shan Zhimin, Chairman of Yierkang Co., Ltd., donated 200 000 yuan to the "F&S CHARITY" for impoverished patients with difficult to heal wounds in Jiali. He said they will do their best to help those in need. A 90 year old man from Lucheng District and Zhang Mengying, a student from Shanghai Yangjing Juyuan Experimental School who has participated in the charity activities of Wendu Chenzhong Charity Studio multiple times, donated 10 000 yuan and 7500 yuan respectively. Previously, the two also donated funds for Academician Li Xiaokun's skin care package for frontline anti epidemic workers in Wuhan and other places. Wenzhou Sanhe Biopharmaceutical Co., Ltd. provides annual funding for short-term training of one medical staff member at Jiali County People's Hospital for three consecutive years. On the way to Jiali, Academician Li Xiaokun

民医院工作的2018届仁济临床专业毕业生卓典典，鼓励他充分利用在校所学知识，用医者仁心，为西藏百姓的健康做贡献。

参与此次西藏医疗公益行的专家和志愿者大多出现头痛、呕吐、坏肚子、失眠等严重的高原反应，他们一一克服，还坐大巴车来回20多个小时，奔赴海拔4500多米嘉黎县，为当地百姓做医疗检查并开展手术。一些受益的藏族同胞拖家带口从乡下赶来，给专家献上哈达致谢。这次，最年轻志愿者是90后的黄文婷等人，他们还是高校在读生，随同专家一起走进手术室和筛查现场提供志愿服务。浙江省援藏指挥部副指挥长、嘉黎县常务副书记周建清说，温州援建那曲嘉黎县已派九批46名援藏干部，促进了嘉黎县各项事业发展，这届援藏把医疗援藏作为重点来做，邀请李校堃院士西藏医疗公益行，把温州医科大学优质的医疗资源和公益品牌带到嘉黎县，以全面提升当地医疗卫生事业，造福当地百姓。嘉黎县委副书记、县长吾金才塔说，嘉黎县医疗资源缺乏，原先群众看病难，患者要到那曲和拉萨看病，在温州援藏25周年，群众看病难有所改善，这次李院士组团来支援嘉黎医疗卫生事业，充分体现了藏汉一家亲。

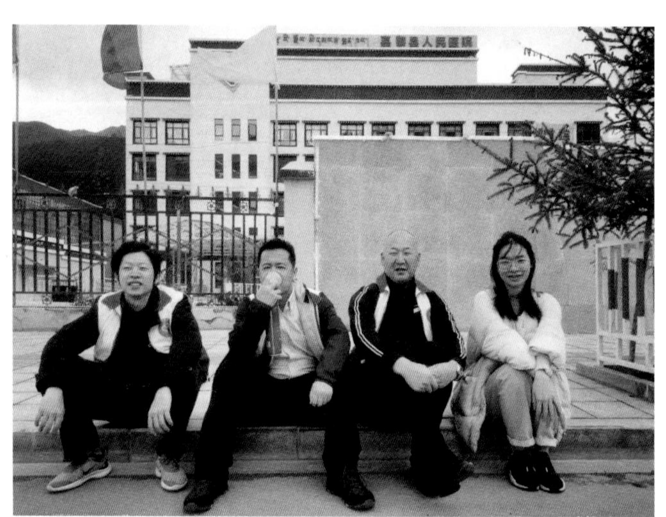

附图12 参与西藏医疗公益行的专家和志愿者

浙江省第九批援藏指挥部指挥长、西藏那曲市委副书记、常务副市长苗伟伦，那曲市委副书记、嘉黎县委书记索朗嘎瓦对李校堃院士西藏医疗公益行给予高度评价。

李校堃院士表示，温州医科大学作为浙江省属医科院校，素来重视学生的品德教育，培育了很多具有影响力的医疗公益慈善品牌项目，关心支援边区老区百姓。学校将长期坚持把各类医疗援助项目带到雪域

also made a special trip to Naqu to visit Zhuo Diandian, the 2018 Renji clinical graduates who worked in Naqu People's Hospital, and encouraged him to make full use of the knowledge he learned at school and the kindness of the medical users to contribute to the health of the people of Xizang.

Most of the experts and volunteers who participated in the Xizang medical public service trip experienced severe altitude reactions such as headache, vomiting, bad stomach, insomnia, etc. They overcame them one by one, and went back and forth by bus for more than 20 hours to Jiali County, more than 4500 meters above sea level, to do medical examination and surgery for the local people. Some Tibetan compatriots who benefited came from the countryside with their families to offer Hada thanks to the experts. This time, the youngest volunteers are Huang Wenting and others born in the 1990s. They are still college students and went into the operating room and screening site with experts to provide volunteer services. Zhou Jianqing, Deputy Commander of the Tibet Assistance Headquarters of Zhejiang Province and Executive Deputy Secretary of Jiali County, said that Wenzhou's assistance to the construction of Naqu Jiali County has sent nine batches of 46 Tibetan aid cadres, which has promoted the development of various undertakings in Jiali County. This Tibetan aid focused on medical aid to Tibet. Academician Li Xiaokun was invited to participate in the Xizang Medical Public Service, bringing the high-quality medical resources and public service brands of Wenzhou Medical University to Jiali County to comprehensively improve the local medical and health undertakings and benefit the local people. Wu Jinchaita, Deputy Secretary of Jiali County Party Committee and County Mayor, said that Jiali County lacks medical resources. Previously, it was difficult for the masses to see a doctor, and patients had to go to Nagqu and Lhasa for treatment. However, after the 25th anniversary of Wenzhou's aid to Tibet, the difficulty of seeing a doctor has improved. This time, Academician Li's group came to support Jiali's medical and health care industry, fully reflecting the unity of Tibetan and Han families.

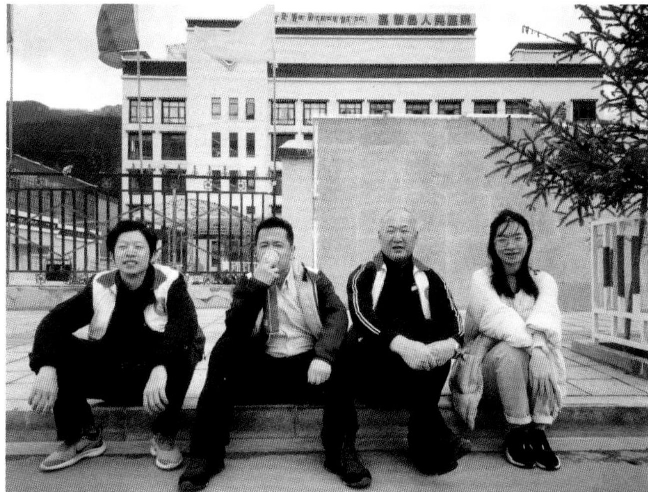

Figure 12 Experts and volunteers participating in Xizang's medical public welfare activities

Miao Weilun, the commander of the ninth batch of Tibet aid headquarters in Zhejiang Province, deputy secretary of Naqu Municipal Party Committee and executive vice mayor of Xizang, and Sorang Gawa, deputy secretary of Naqu Municipal Party Committee and secretary of Jiali County Party Committee, spoke highly of Academician Li Xiaokun's Xizang medical charity.

Academician Li Xiaokun stated that Wenzhou Medical University, as a medical institution under the jurisdiction of Zhejiang Province, has always attached great importance to students' moral education, cultivated many influential medical public welfare and charity brand projects, and cared for and supported the people in the border areas. The school will persist in bringing all kinds of medical assistance projects to the snow covered plateau for a long time.

高原，针对高原地区百姓的实际需求，用医者仁心，真正为西藏百姓服务，把大爱写在祖国大地上。

高原地区创面救助项目启动以来，将近十位难愈合性创面藏族同胞接到温州免费治疗。其中，6 年前全身严重烫伤的青海玉树州拉吾尕藏族小学 7 岁藏族女孩，下半身创面巨大，共需要 10 多次手术才能完全治愈。在此期间，肤生团队免费为其提供生长因子药物，助力创面修复和愈合，从长远上帮助她解决今后的治疗药物、费用等后顾之忧。

公益活动每到一处都致力为当地培养医疗力量，以远程帮扶与来温实地培训相结合的方式，提升当地学科建设水平，变“输血”为“造血”，用优质的创面修复技术为各地培养“带不走的医生”。经帮扶培训，培养出格桑平措等一批当地优秀的创面修复医生。西藏嘉黎县人民医院于去年成功实施了由当地医生主刀的首例静脉曲张手术，公益医疗成果真正在高原“落地生根”。长期以来，温州医科大学不仅组织公益医疗团队为藏区患者提供优质的医疗服务，更一直注重提升藏区的“造血”能力，为藏区培养优秀医学生和培训医务人员。学校先后接受四批 78 名西藏住院医师进行规范化培训，并为他们提供最好的师资力量，量身定制培训计划，学员执业医师考试通过率达 100%。多次来温州医科大学附属第一医院学习的嘉黎人民医院的格桑平措已经担任副院长，索朗扎西也成为医院医务科科长。目前温州医科大学还有西藏在校生 20 余人，学校还鼓励优秀毕业生积极参加”西部计划”，在祖国最需要的地方建功立业，先后已有 20 多名学生到西藏日喀则、那曲、林芝等地区的医疗系统工作，很多人已经成为医院的骨干，在雪域高原上守护人民健康。

肤生海西行 >>>

“学党史、守初心、担使命，喜迎建党 100 周年”肤生海西行 2021 年 5 月 9 日首站走进福鼎市柏洋村，温州医科大学附二院、眼视光医院、口腔医院以及红日亭、温州曙光医院、宁德市温州商会、温州都市报陈忠慈善工作室等单位的公益团队为当地群众送医送药送健康送名小吃，并为 10 名老党员送上慰问品和慰问金。

◆ “童心筑梦”永远在路上，让爱传播更广

温州医科大学附二院、育英儿童医院儿童心内科“童心筑梦”志愿服务公益团队阵容强大，由该院儿内科党总支书记、儿童心内科主任吴蓉洲带队，儿童心内科主任医师项如莲、副主任医师荣星 3 位专家领衔 6 人医疗团队，另有“童心筑梦”学生志愿者若干，为柏洋村的儿童提供义诊服务及健康宣教，还带上了 200 万元的便携式心脏彩超机。

In view of the actual needs of the people in the plateau area, the medical users will be kind, truly serve the people in Xizang, and write the great love on the motherland.

Since the launch of the high-altitude wound rescue project, nearly ten Tibetan compatriots with difficult to heal wounds have received free treatment in Wenzhou. Among them, a 7-year-old Tibetan girl from Lawuga Tibetan Primary School in Yushu Prefecture, Qinghai, who suffered severe burns all over her body 6 years ago, had a huge wound on her lower body and required more than 10 surgeries to fully recover. During this period, the Fusheng team provided her with free growth factor drugs to assist in wound repair and healing, helping her solve future concerns such as treatment drugs and costs in the long run.

Every public welfare activity is dedicated to cultivating medical talents for the local area. By combining remote assistance with on-site training in Wenzhou, we aim to improve the level of local discipline construction, transform "blood transfusion" into "hematopoiesis", and use high-quality wound repair techniques to cultivate "doctors who cannot be taken away" for various regions. Through assistance and training, we have trained a group of excellent local wound repair doctors such as Gesangpingcuo. Last year, the People's Hospital of Jiali County, Xizang, successfully performed the first varicose surgery operated by local doctors, and the achievements of public health care really took root on the plateau. For a long time, Wenzhou Medical University has not only organized a public welfare medical team to provide high-quality medical services for patients in Tibetan areas, but also focused on improving the "hematopoietic" ability of Tibetan areas, cultivating excellent medical students and training medical personnel for Tibetan areas. The school has received four batches of 78 Xizang residents for standardized training, and provided them with the best teachers. The training plan was tailored to meet the needs of the students. The passing rate of the licensed physician exam reached 100%. Gesangpingcuo, who has come to study at the First Affiliated Hospital of Wenzhou Medical University multiple times, has become the vice president of Jiali People's Hospital, and Sorangzhaxi has also become the head of the hospital's medical department. At present, Wenzhou Medical University has more than 20 students in Xizang. The university also encourages outstanding graduates to actively participate in the "Western Plan" and make contributions to the places where the motherland needs most. More than 20 students have worked in the medical system in Shigatse, Naqu, Linzhi and other regions of Xizang. Many have become the backbone of hospitals, protecting people's health on the snowy plateau.

Skin Health Tour in the West

On May 9, 2021, during the "Learning Party History, Adhering to the Original Aspiration, Shouldering the Mission, and Celebrating the 100th Anniversary of the Founding of the Party" journey, the first stop of the "Skin Health Tour in the West" was Baoyang Village in Fuding City. Public welfare teams from Wenzhou Medical University Affiliated Second Hospital, Eye and Vision Hospital, Stomatological Hospital, as well as Hongri Pavilion, Wenzhou Shuguang Hospital, Ningde Wenzhou Chamber of Commerce, Wenzhou Urban Daily Chen Zhong Charity Studio and other units delivered medical supplies, medicines, healthy snacks, and 10 old party members with condolence gifts and money to the local people.

◆ "Childhood builds dreams" is always on the road, spreading love more widely

Wenzhou Medical University Affiliated Second Hospital and Yuying Children's Hospital have a strong team of volunteer service public welfare teams for the "Childhood Dream Building" program in the Department of Pediatric Cardiology. Led by Wu Rongzhou, Secretary of the Party Branch of the Department of Pediatric Cardiology and Director of the Department of Pediatric Cardiology, the medical team consists of six experts, including Chief Physician Xiang Rulian and Deputy Chief Physician Rong Xing. In addition, there are several student volunteers for the "Childhood Dream Building" program, providing free medical services and health education for children in Baiyang Village. They also brought a portable heart ultrasound machine worth 2 million yuan.

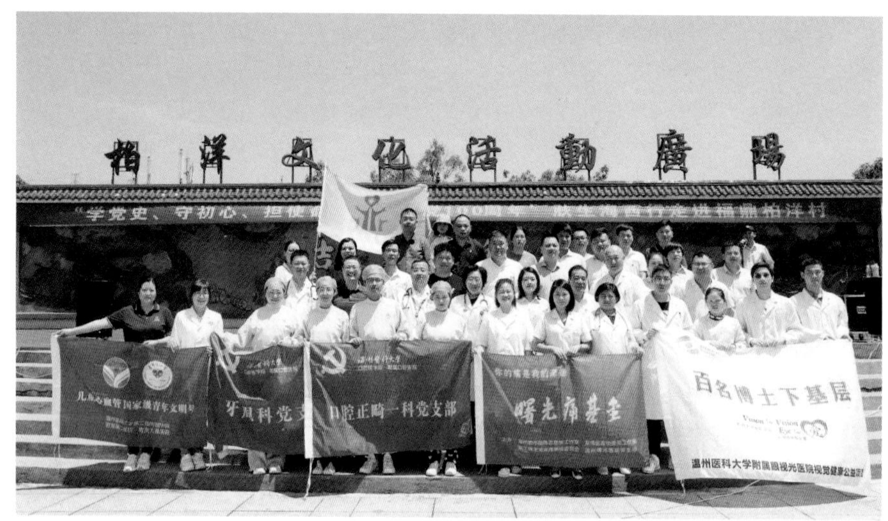

附图 13　肤生海西行参与团队

老专家项如莲忙得不亦乐乎。当地 53 岁的郑阿婆找到项主任，说自己甲状腺疾病很严重，已经是五级了，要不要做手术？项主任耐心询问了郑阿姨的情况，郑阿姨已经出现了乏力等症状，项主任告诉郑阿姨去医院好好验血，再决定做手术。

义诊现场，“主任，我的宝宝晚上总是睡不安，您能不能给他看看是什么原因呢？”一位 8 个月小男孩的妈妈焦急地向项主任问道。“主任，我感觉我的孩子心跳总是偏快，您能给她听听看吗？”一位 10 岁小女孩的妈妈来向荣主任求助了。诸如此类的儿童还有很多，而该院的医护人员也是尽心竭力地对待每一位前来就诊的患儿和家属。活动现场，专家们细致地询问病史，一丝不苟地对儿童们进行查体，悉心地指导喂养，对于发育落后的宝宝们提出了一系列训练方法，家长们也一一认真记录。

除此之外，团队负责人夏天和主治医师耐心地为在场患儿免费进行了心超检查。对于检查过程中发现异常，怀疑有先天性心脏病且需要手术的患儿，吴蓉洲建议家属带患儿至他们医院进一步评估，并可通过“童心筑梦”工程提供必要的帮助。现场还分发了先天性心脏病宣传册，让家长们增加对它的认识。

吴蓉洲说，“童心筑梦”永远在路上，为更多儿童先天性心脏病患者服务。

◆ 中老年口腔健康意识差，口腔医院逐个检查

这次，温州医科大学附属口腔医院牙周科护士长吴园园与正畸科护士长廖雪妙、吴国省、徐倩 4 名医务人员来到现场义诊。今年 77 岁的陈阿婆牙周炎很严重，还有缺牙，徐倩细心给阿婆检查，并告诉陈阿婆及时把缺牙补上，还有的 50 多岁的人连智齿牙也没有拔掉。而吴园园拿着牙齿模型耐心地教当地群众正确刷牙的办法。

义诊现场有很多来检查的中老年人口腔卫生不佳，牙龈出血牙齿松动的情况多见，牙周炎患病率较高。

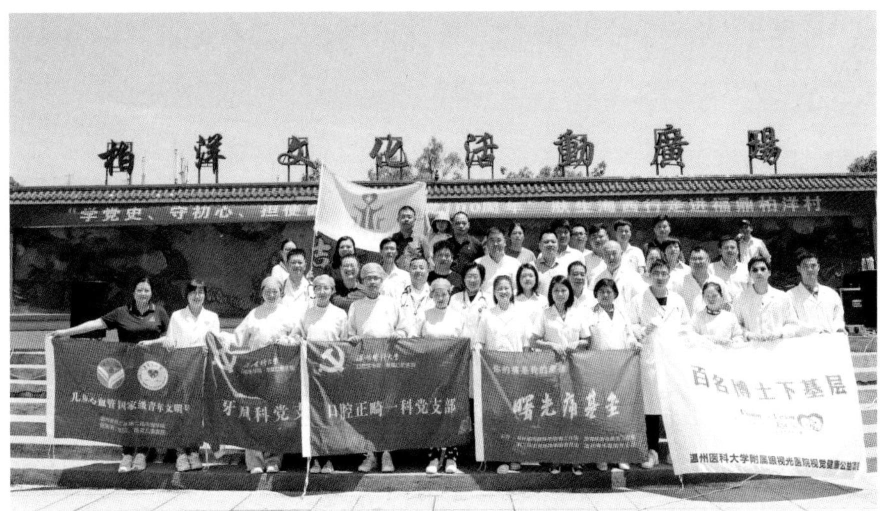

Figure 13 Participating team of Skin Health Tour in the West

Old expert Xiang Rulian is very busy. Local 53 years old Grandma Zheng approached Director Xiang and said that her thyroid gland was very serious, already at level five. Should she undergo surgery? Director Xiang patiently inquired about Aunt Zheng's condition, and she had already shown symptoms such as fatigue. Director Xiang told Aunt Zheng to go to the hospital for a good blood test before deciding to undergo surgery.

At the free clinic, "Director, my baby always sleeps restless at night. Can you show him the reason?" An 8-month-old boy's mother anxiously asked Director Xiang. "Director, I feel that my child's heartbeat is always too fast. Can you listen to it for her? "The mother of a 10-year-old girl came to Director Rong for help. There are many children like this, and the medical staff at the hospital are also doing their best to treat every child and family member who comes for treatment. At the event site, experts meticulously inquired about the medical history of the children, conducted thorough physical examinations, provided careful guidance on feeding, and proposed a series of training methods for babies with developmental delays. Parents also carefully recorded each method.

In addition, the team leader Xia Xia and the attending physician patiently conducted free cardiac ultrasound examinations for the children present. For children who are suspected of having congenital heart disease and require surgery due to abnormalities found during the examination process, Wu Rongzhou suggests that family members take the child to their hospital for further evaluation and provide necessary assistance through the "Childhood Dream Building" project. A brochure on congenital heart disease was also distributed on site to increase parents' awareness of it.

Wu Rongzhou said that "building dreams with childlike innocence" is always on the road, serving more children with congenital heart disease.

◆ Middle aged and elderly people have poor awareness of oral health, and dental hospitals check them one by one

This time, four medical staff including Wu Yuanyuan, the head nurse of the periodontal department, Liao Xuemiao, the head nurse of the orthodontic department, Wu Guosheng, and Xu Qian from the Affiliated Stomatological Hospital of Wenzhou Medical University came to the site for free consultation. Mrs. Chen, who is 77 years old this year, has severe periodontitis and missing teeth. Xu Qian carefully examined her and told her to promptly fill in the missing teeth. Some people in their 50s have not even had their wisdom teeth removed. And Wu Yuanyuan patiently taught the local people the correct way to brush their teeth with a dental model.

There are many middle-aged and elderly people who come to the free clinic for examination, with poor oral

他们都认为口腔问题都是小毛病，有点问题就熬着不愿意去医院，殊不知熬到最后都成了大问题，不仅治疗难度增加，治疗费用更是翻番。基层口腔卫生宣教，普及口腔预防知识还有很长的路要走。口腔医院医务人员还给前来义诊的群众赠送了牙膏、牙刷等。

◆ “医生，我眼睛流眼泪怎么办？”眼视光医生传经送宝

温州医科大学附属眼视光医院防盲治盲办公益医务人员孙方舟、董良才、李广丽、王宇舟为村民检查眼睛。

眼视光团队的眼健康义诊活动刚刚开始，前来咨询和检查眼睛的群众络绎不绝，其中翼状胬肉和干眼症、泪道阻塞患者占了大多数，很多老人觉得这些小毛病不值得去大医院就诊，病程拖了很久，医生都相应给了他们治疗的建议和绿色通道。

王阿公说近年来看不清东西，初步诊断他患了白内障，医生提醒他早日到医院眼部检查并治疗。一名阿公原先做过白内障手术，如今看不清了，还流眼泪，经过孙方舟检查这名阿公患上了干眼症，需要到医院做进一步检查和治疗。在当天的眼健康义诊中，发现不少患上了干眼症，一名阿姨说，“医生，我眼睛流眼泪怎么办”经过初步检查，她患上了干眼症，干眼症主要是手机等电子产品使用频繁，医生建议少用电子产品或不能持续用眼时间太长。

◆ 温州曙光医院为患者“解痛”，并把一名烂腿患者接来治疗

温州曙光医院由 7 名医务人员组成的医疗团队开展义诊，该院党支部书记周鹏、副院长陈善亮带队。

刚开始，温州曙光医院的义诊摊位被团团围住，现场来了不少“痛和臭”患者，陈善亮逐个仔细检查，给有的患者贴上膏药。其中，59 岁柏洋村村民叶大叔，左眼角边长了颗很大的肿块，已经有 2 年的时间造成眼、脸部不适，又影响美观。当他得知温州医疗专家要来到柏洋村开展义诊活动后，早早地就过来等候检查。在经过陈善亮仔细检查后，确认这是皮脂腺囊肿，建议尽快做手术去除。叶大叔开心地说：“好好好，拿掉、拿掉，谢谢医生，你们辛苦了”。

今年 73 岁的周阿公双腿溃烂已经 20 多年，尤其右腿烂得很厉害，周阿公苦不堪言，福鼎爱心接力志愿者协会义工卓耐已经帮助了周阿公五六年时间，但是周阿公烂腿的事一直解决不了，听说柏洋村来了温州专家，他把周阿公从沿州村接来看病，经过陈善亮会诊，周阿公的烂腿可以通过治疗解除病痛，决定帮助周阿公，当天，周阿公被接到温州曙光医院免费治疗。5 月 11 日，经过治疗周阿公的烂腿不臭了，也不痛了，他说，非常感谢温州医生和志愿者。

hygiene, gum bleeding and loose teeth, and a high incidence of periodontitis. They all think that oral problems are minor issues, and if there are some problems, they will endure and refuse to go to the hospital, but little do they know that in the end, it has become a big problem, not only increasing the difficulty of treatment, but also doubling the cost of treatment. Grassroots oral health education and popularization of oral prevention knowledge still have a long way to go. The medical staff of the dental hospital also gave away toothpaste, toothbrushes, and other items to the people who came for free consultations.

◆ "Doctor, what should I do if my eyes shed tears? "Said the optometrist, passing on his teachings

Sun Fangzhou, Dong Liangcai, Li Guangli, and Wang Yuzhou, public welfare medical staff from the Eye and Vision Hospital affiliated with Wenzhou Medical University, conducted eye examinations for villagers.

The eye health consultation activity of the optometry team has just begun, and there is a continuous stream of people who come to consult and check their eyes. Among them, patients with pterygium, dry eye syndrome, and lacrimal duct obstruction account for the majority. Many elderly people feel that these small problems are not worth seeking medical treatment in large hospitals, and the disease has been delayed for a long time. Doctors have given them treatment suggestions and green channels accordingly.

Grandpa Wang said that he couldn't see clearly in recent years and was preliminarily diagnosed with cataracts. The doctor reminded him to go to the hospital for an eye examination and treatment as soon as possible. A grandfather had undergone cataract surgery before, but now he can't see clearly and is shedding tears. After Sun Fangzhou's examination, the grandfather developed dry eye syndrome and needs to go to the hospital for further examination and treatment. During the eye health clinic on that day, it was discovered that many people were suffering from dry eye syndrome. An aunt said, "Doctor, what should I do if my eyes shed tears?" After preliminary examination, she was diagnosed with dry eye syndrome. Dry eye syndrome is mainly caused by frequent use of electronic devices such as mobile phones. The doctor suggested using fewer electronic devices or not using them continuously for too long.

◆ Wenzhou Shuguang Hospital "relieves pain" for patients and brings in a broken leg patient for treatment

Wenzhou Shuguang Hospital has a medical team consisting of 7 medical staff conducting free consultations, led by Zhou Peng, the secretary of the hospital's party branch, and Chen Shanliang, the vice president.

At the beginning, the free clinic booth of Wenzhou Shuguang Hospital was surrounded by many "painful and smelly" patients. Chen Shanliang carefully examined each patient and applied ointment to some of them. Among them, Mr. Ye, a 59 year old resident of Baiyang Village, has a large lump on the edge of his left eye corner, which has been causing discomfort in his eyes and face for 2 years and affecting his appearance. When he learned that Wenzhou medical experts were coming to Baiyang Village to carry out free clinics, he came early to wait for the examination. After careful examination by Chen Shanliang, it was confirmed that this is a sebaceous gland cyst, and it is recommended to undergo surgery to remove it as soon as possible. Uncle Ye said happily, 'Okay, okay, remove, remove. Thank you, doctor. You've worked hard."

Mr. Zhou, who is 73 years old this year, has been suffering from leg ulcers for more than 20 years, especially in his right leg. Mr. Zhou is in unbearable pain. Volunteer Zhuo Nai from the Fuding Love Relay Volunteer Association has been helping Mr. Zhou for five or six years, but he has been unable to solve his leg problem. It is said that a Wenzhou expert came to Baiyang Village and brought Mr. Zhou from Yanzhou Village for medical treatment. After consultation with Chen Shanliang, Mr. Zhou's leg can be treated to relieve the pain. He decided to help Mr. Zhou. On the same day, Mr. Zhou was taken to Shuguang Hospital in Wenzhou for free treatment. On May 11th, after treatment, Grandpa Zhou's rotten leg no longer smelled or hurt. He said he was very grateful to the doctors and volunteers in Wenzhou.

该院医务人员王娇、刘德哲、金玲丽、林秀娟、李正英也忙着为市民看病、测血糖、量血压等，并做好登记。目前，“肤生工程”已经救助福鼎难愈合创面伤患者，资助善款20多万元。

◆ 红日亭送名小吃，慰问当地10名老党员

“乡亲们，我们为大家准备了些温州名小吃，有炒粉干、凉粉、葱油蛋饼，大家检查好后过来品尝”。在当地义诊现场，红日亭的义工们在吆喝温州的名小吃。

大家说，真的好吃，第一次在家门口吃到爱心温州名小吃，在柏洋村办企业的温商也尝到温州名小吃。

红日亭义工提前一天准备食材，活动当天，她们上午7时从温州出发前往福鼎柏洋村，红日亭孙兰香、蔡艳、石秀琴、王金元、张晓萍、沙定友、金光龙、姜皋8名义工不停地忙碌着，现场送出名小吃各300多份。

孙兰香说，这是红日亭第一次走出温州来到福鼎市柏洋村，能为当地百姓做点实实在在的事情，送一份温暖，忙点、累点都是开心的。

当天，温州都市报陈忠慈善工作室联合红日亭慰问当地10名老党员，红日亭送上慰问品和慰问金。今年79岁黄日容和82岁的黄日团均是有50多年党龄的老党员，黄日容是在20世纪60年代当兵时入党，而黄日团是在村里入党的，他们入党后为村民办实事，他们说，很感谢你们献爱心。

当天，主办单位还举办“肤生工程”千村千点创面修复救助点和志愿协作体（柏洋站）授予柏洋村。福鼎市医保局许明令邀请福鼎市微爱行动志愿者协会10多名志愿者开展现场布置和帮助专家翻译等志愿服务。温州医学院药学院的“肤生工程”志愿者也参与志愿服，鹿城区慈善总会义工分会秘书长陈招乐也参与了志愿服务。义诊后，这次公益团成员参观了柏洋村乡村振兴展示馆。

这次公益活动得到了宁德市温州商会的大力支持，该会会长王岩豪说，该村作为全国先进基层党组织，在今年迎来建党100周年前，肤生海西行走进该村特别有意义，学党史明哲理，为民服务，同时温商也在这里创办了多家企业，也是对该村的感谢。

宁德福鼎市的柏洋村只用了20多年，让这个曾经村民年收入不足600元、村财政负债43万元的“赤贫村”，一跃成为远近闻名的“小康明星村”，如今柏洋村农民人均可支配收入超3万元。该村党委书记王周齐说，全靠党的好政策，他们村早就开始新农村建设和建设全面小康社会。

值此中国共产党百年华诞之际，“肤生工程”开展“百年红 肤生行”健康中国行大型公益活动，“百

The medical staff of the hospital, including Wang Jiao, Liu Dezhe, Jin Lingli, Lin Xiujuan, and Li Zhengying, are also busy treating citizens, measuring blood sugar, blood pressure, and keeping records. At present, the "F&S CHARITY" has assisted patients with difficult to heal wounds in Fuding, with a donation of over 200 000 yuan.

◆ Red Sun Pavilion delivers famous snacks and expresses condolences to 10 local veteran party members

"Villagers, we have prepared some famous Wenzhou snacks for you, including fried rice noodles, bean jelly, and onion oil Egg cakes. Come and taste them after you check them." At the local free clinic site, volunteers from Hongri Pavilion were shouting out famous snacks from Wenzhou.

Everyone said it's really delicious. It's the first time I've had a heartwarming Wenzhou snack at my doorstep, and the Wenzhou merchants who run businesses in Baiyang Village have also tasted Wenzhou snacks.

Red Sun Pavilion volunteers prepared ingredients one day in advance. On the day of the event, they departed from Wenzhou at 7am to Baoyang Village in Fuding. Red Sun Pavilion volunteers Sun Lanxiang, Cai Yan, Shi Xiuqin, Wang Jinyuan, Zhang Xiaoping, Sha Dingyou, Jin Guanglong, and Jiang Gao worked tirelessly, delivering over 300 famous snacks each on site.

Sun Lanxiang said that this is the first time that Hongri Pavilion has left Wenzhou to come to Baiyang Village in Fuding City. Being able to do something tangible for the local people, bringing warmth, and being busy or tired brings happiness.

On that day, Wenzhou Urban Daily's Chen Zhong Charity Studio joined forces with the Red Sun Pavilion to offer condolences to 10 local veteran party members. The Red Sun Pavilion presented condolence items and money. 79 year old Huang Rirong and 82 year old Huang Rituan are both veteran party members with over 50 years of party membership. Huang Rirong joined the party in the 1960s while serving in the army, while Huang Rituan joined the party in the village. After joining the party, they worked for the villagers and said, Thank you very much for your love.

On that day, the organizer also held the "F&S CHARITY" Thousand Villages and Thousand Points Wound Repair Rescue Point and Volunteer Collaboration (Baiyang Station) to award to Baiyang Village. Xu Mingling from the Fuding Medical Insurance Bureau invited more than 10 volunteers from the Fuding Weiai Action Volunteer Association to carry out on-site arrangements and assist experts in translation and other volunteer services. Volunteers from the School of Pharmacy at Wenzhou Medical University also participated in volunteer service, and Chen Zhaole, Secretary General of the Volunteer Branch of the Lucheng District Charity Federation, also participated in volunteer service. After the free clinic, members of the public welfare group visited the Baiyang Village Rural Revitalization Exhibition Hall.

This public welfare activity has received strong support from the Wenzhou Chamber of Commerce in Ningde City. Wang Yanhao, the president of the association, said that as an advanced grassroots party organization in China, it is particularly meaningful to visit the village before the 100th anniversary of the founding of the Party this year. We should learn from the history and philosophy of the Party, serve the people, and at the same time, Wenzhou merchants have also founded multiple enterprises here, which is also a gratitude to the village.

In just over 20 years, Baiyang Village in Fuding City, Ningde has transformed from a "poverty-stricken village" where the annual income of villagers was less than 600 yuan and the village's financial debt was 430 000 yuan to a well-known "star village of moderate prosperity". Nowadays, the per capita disposable income of farmers in Baiyang Village exceeds 30 000 yuan. Wang Zhouqi, the secretary of the village party committee, said that thanks to the good policies of the party, their village has long started the construction of new rural areas and the building of a comprehensive well-off society.

On the occasion of the centennial birthday of the CPC, the "F&S CHARITY" launched a large-scale public welfare activity of "One Hundred Year Red Skin Health Walk". "One Hundred Year Red Skin Health Walk", with a

年红肤生行”以“肤生浙里行”结对村帮扶、“肤生中国行”健康公益行、“肤生百年红”宣传教育月等系列子活动为主要载体，联合温州医科大学“明眸皓齿”“童心筑梦”等医疗公益团队，为全国基层及农村群众提供医疗慈善救助服务，继承和发扬党的光荣传统和优良作风，学党史、守初心、担使命，为推进健康中国建设贡献力量！首场公益活动于 3 月 14 日在永嘉县红星社区红十三军旧址举行。

“肤生工程”惠及“一带一路”，构筑中非健康共同体

为更好地开展针对非洲地区的医疗援助，在 2021 世界青年科学家峰会期间，“肤生工程‘一带一路’中非行”公益项目正式启动。该项目将通过捐赠短缺药械、开展远程医疗及培养创面修复人才等方式，帮助中非共和国建立难愈性创面治疗体系与预防体系，满足当地患者在创伤治疗上的需求。温州医科大学附一院还与中非友谊医院签署合作协议，帮助中非友谊医院建设创面感染与修复专科，为中非共和国深受创面问题困扰的人群送去健康，该项目作为国家卫生健康委员会“30 个中非对口医院合作机制”之一，目前已开展医院网络建设、物资捐赠、远程医疗、第一批已经有 3 名中非友谊医院医生来进修等合作，接下去还有 7 名医务人员来温州医科大学附属第一医院进修。目前，这 10 名医务人员全部培训完成，在当地已经发挥很大的作用。

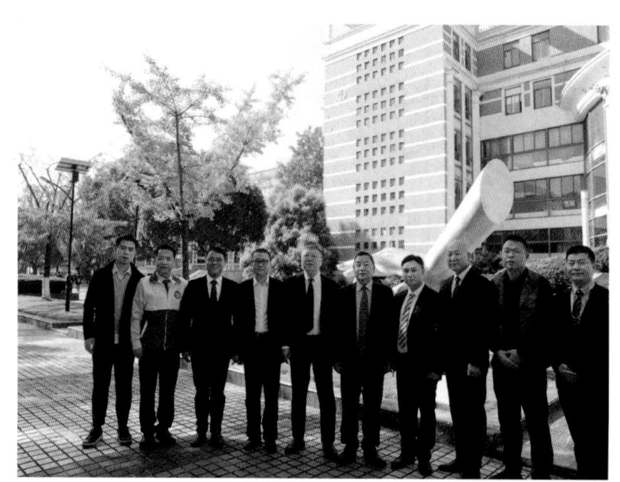

附图 14 “肤生工程‘一带一路’中非行”公益项目正式启动

在携手防疫的基础上，“肤生工程”高度关注非洲基层乡村与部落的医疗问题，尤其是创面修复治疗方面的需求。去年“肤生工程”参与捐赠的医疗物资为综合型全科医药箱，列装常用药械共计 20 多种。捐

series of sub activities such as "Skin Health Zhejiang Trip" paired village support, "Skin Health China Trip" health public welfare walk, "Skin Health One Hundred Year Red" publicity and education month as the main carrier, and with the medical public welfare teams such as "Bright Eyes and Bright Teeth" and "Childlike Dream Building" of Wenzhou Medical University, provides medical charity relief services for the national grass-roots and rural people, inherits and carries forward the glorious tradition and fine style of the Party, learns the history of the Party, adheres to the original intention, assumes the mission, and promotes a healthy China Contribute to the construction! The first public welfare event was held on March 14th at the former site of the Red Tenth Army in Hongxing Community, Yongjia County.

The "F&S CHARITY" benefits the "the Belt and Road" and builds a China Africa health community

In order to better carry out medical assistance for Africa, the public welfare project of "F&S CHARITY' the Belt and Road' China Africa Travel "was officially launched during the 2021 World Summit of Young Scientists. This project will help the Central African Republic establish a treatment and prevention system for difficult to heal wounds by donating scarce medical equipment, conducting remote medical care, and cultivating wound repair talents, in order to meet the needs of local patients in trauma treatment. The First Affiliated Hospital of Wenzhou Medical University has also signed a cooperation agreement with the China Africa Friendship Hospital to assist in the construction of a specialized department for wound infection and repair, providing health care to the population suffering from wound problems in the Central African Republic. As one of the "30 China Africa Matching Hospital Cooperation Mechanisms" of the National Health Commission, this project has carried out cooperation in hospital network construction, material donations, remote medical care, and the first batch of 3 doctors from the China Africa Friendship Hospital have come for further studies. In the future, 7 medical staff will come to the First Affiliated Hospital of Wenzhou Medical University for further studies. At present, all 10 medical personnel have completed their training and have played a significant role in the local area.

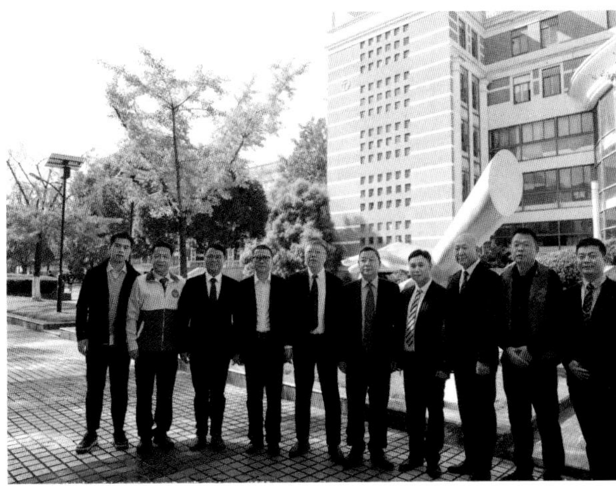

Figure 14 "F&S CHARITY 'the Belt and Road ' China Africa Travel"public welfare project officially launched

On the basis of working together for epidemic prevention, the "F&S CHARITY" attaches great importance to the medical issues of grassroots villages and tribes in Africa, especially the needs for wound repair and treatment. Last year, the "F&S CHARITY" participated in the donation of medical supplies, which were comprehensive general medical kits containing more than 20 commonly used drugs and equipment. Among the donated materials, 700

赠物资中 700 支外用重组人酸性成纤维细胞生长因子由温州医科大学研发、上海腾瑞制药公司生产捐赠，主要用于非洲民众因艾滋病、烧伤、创伤、战伤等导致的各种创面缺损。知名企业意尔康股份有限公司也通过“肤生工程”定向捐赠出医药箱 100 套。“肤生工程”团队还协助使馆筹集采购了另外 600 套医药箱，并组织编译了法语版的“中国 - 中非卫生健康共同体医药箱手册”。此前捐赠的药箱均由时任驻中非共和国大使陈栋亲自转交中非共和国总统。

2022 年 12 月 11 日，2022 世界青年科学家峰会“创面修复与再生医学国际公益论坛”在中国基因药谷举行。“肤生工程”为中非友谊医院捐赠 25 万元善款，并为中非妇女儿童基金会捐赠药箱 50 个，浙江甬誉生物科技有限公司向“肤生工程”捐赠 100 万元。浙商银行与温州医科大学签订“肤生工程”公益帮扶合作协议，“肤生工程”拟发起成立“肤生基金会”，浙商银行作为首发理事捐赠 200 万元，专项用于拥军优属、浙江山区 26 县、东西部协作等创面修复医疗救助项目。

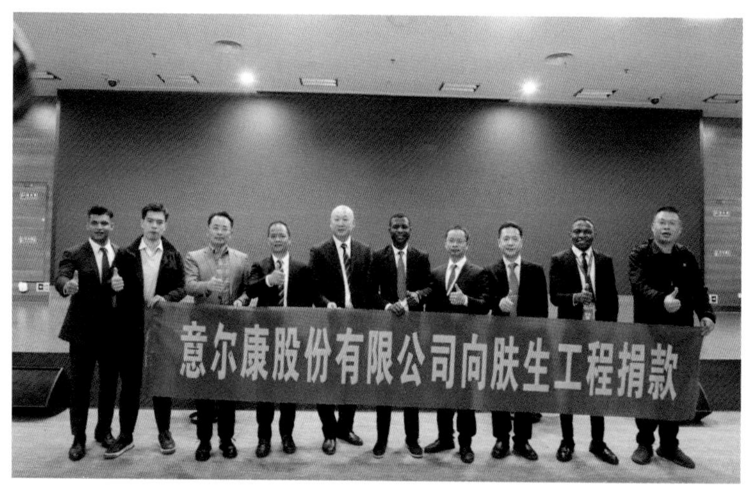

附图 15　意尔康股份有限公司向“肤生工程”捐款

温州市人大常委会副主任徐育斐，温州医科大学校长、中国工程院院士李校堃，浙商银行股份有限公司党委副书记马红，瓯海区委常委、常务副区长林照光，中非共和国班吉友谊医院院长肯特·让·克里索斯托姆出席。浙江省卫生健康委员会合作处、江苏省医学会，温州市民政局、退役军人事务管理局、外办、消防救援支队、青山慈善基金会等相关负责人参加论坛活动。温州医科大学附一院党委书记沈贤致欢迎辞。

externally used recombinant human acidic fibroblast growth factor were developed by Wenzhou Medical University and produced and donated by Shanghai Tengrui Pharmaceutical Company, mainly used for various wound defects caused by AIDS, burns, wounds, war wounds, etc. among African people. Renowned enterprise Yierkang Co., Ltd. also donated 100 sets of medical kits through the "F&S CHARITY". The "F&S CHARITY" team also assisted the embassy in raising funds to purchase an additional 600 sets of medical kits, and organized the compilation of the French version of the "China Central Africa Health Community Medical Kit Handbook". The previously donated medicine boxes were personally handed over to the President of Central Africa Republic by the then Ambassador to Central Africa Republic, Chen Dong.

On December 11, 2022, the "International Public Welfare Forum on Wound Repair and Regenerative Medicine" of the 2022 World Youth Scientists Summit was held at the China Gene Medicine Valley. The "F&S CHARITY" donated 250 000 yuan to the China Africa Friendship Hospital and 50 medicine boxes to the China Africa Women and Children's Foundation. Zhejiang Yongyu Biotechnology Co., Ltd. donated 1 million yuan to the "F&S CHARITY". Zhejiang Commercial Bank and Wenzhou Medical University signed a cooperation agreement for the "F&S CHARITY" public welfare assistance. The "F&S CHARITY" plans to initiate the establishment of the foundation. Zhejiang Commercial Bank, as the first director, donated 2 million yuan, which will be specifically used for wound repair and medical assistance projects such as supporting military families, 26 counties in Zhejiang mountainous areas, and cooperation between the east and west.

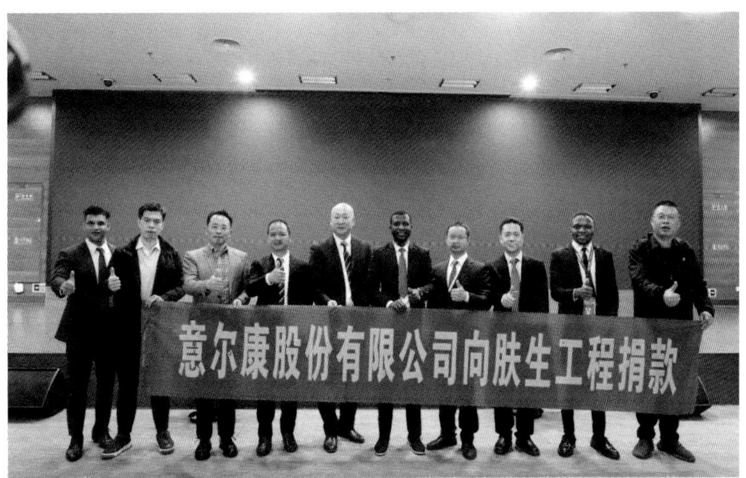

Figure 15 Yierkang Co., Ltd. donates to "F&S CHARITY"

Xu Yufei, Deputy Director of the Standing Committee of Wenzhou Municipal People's Congress, Li Xiaokun, President of Wenzhou Medical University and academician of the CAE Member, Ma Hong, Deputy Secretary of the Party Committee of Zhejiang Merchants Bank Co., Ltd., Lin Zhaoguang, Member of the Standing Committee of Ouhai District Committee and Executive Deputy District Head, and Kent Jean Christostom, President of Bangui Friendship Hospital of the Central African Republic, attended. Officials from the Cooperation Department of Zhejiang Provincial Health Commission, Jiangsu Medical Association, Wenzhou Civil Affairs Bureau, Veterans Affairs Management Bureau, Foreign Affairs Office, Fire Rescue Brigade, Qingshan Charity Foundation and other relevant departments participated in the forum activities. Shen Xian, Secretary of the Party Committee of the First Affiliated Hospital of Wenzhou Medical University, delivered a welcome speech.

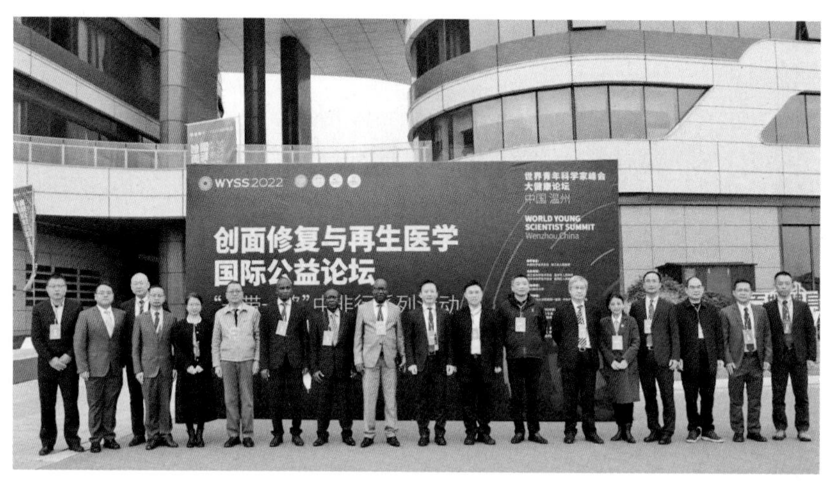

附图 16　创面修复与再生医学国际公益论坛举办

论坛秉承世界青年科学家峰会的愿景目标，围绕“一带一路”医疗卫生国际合作、医疗教育和成果转化、创面修复公益救助等领域开展热烈探讨。论坛由温州医科大学附属第一医院与中非共和国班吉友谊医院共同主办，会议设中国温州主会场及中非共和国班吉友谊医院分会场，300 多位来自多个国家和地区的科学家、院士、援外专家、社会公益组织、30 家中非对口医院合作机制项目负责人通过线上参会。温州医科大学宣传部、研究生院、医院管理处、继续教育学院、药学院、国际教育学院、阿尔伯塔学院等部门与学院相关负责人及中外学生代表，附属第一医院负责人、医护人员代表、援外专家代表，社会媒体、爱心企业，“肤生工程”各救助站负责人、义工志愿者代表等参加论坛。

会议举行了“肤生工程”主题曲《大爱肤生》发布仪式，这首歌曲由“肤生工程”秘书长、温州医科大学阿尔伯塔学院副院长王小尚作词、台湾著名作曲家郭孟雍作曲。“肤生工程”还评出 10 位“最美肤生人”，他们分别是从事医疗、护理、企业、教育、宣传、义工等不同行业的志愿者。温州医科大学校长李校堃院士代表“肤生工程”团队发起“创面修复国际公益救济行动倡议”，在全球广泛开展创面修复国际公益救济行动。

会上，“肤生工程”评出 2022 年“最美肤生人”，他们是温州医科大学阿尔伯塔学院副院长王小尚，温州医科大学附一院创面修复科执行主任王健、医务处副处长暨玲，意尔康股份有限公司执行总裁单尔康，温州曙光医院业务院长陈善亮、护理部主任李正英，福鼎市医保局外伤认定负责人许明令，文成县慈善总会张立亮慈善工作室负责人张立亮，肤生工程志愿者陈银炜、温州都市报陈忠慈善工作室负责人陈忠。

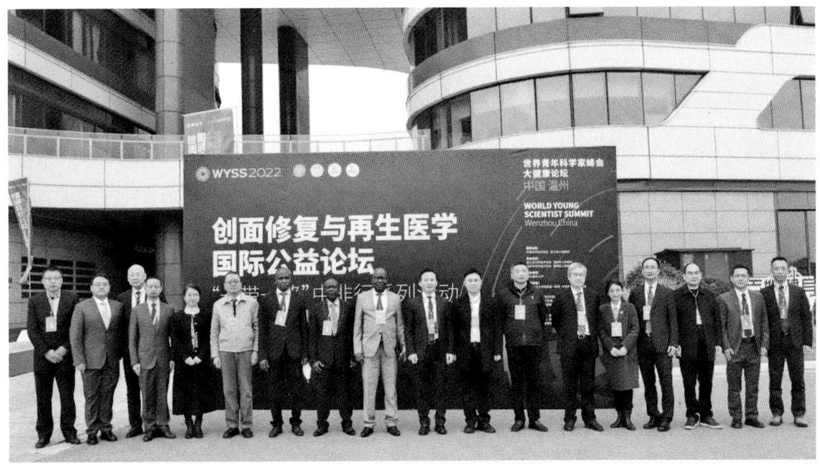

Figure 16 International Public Welfare Forum on Wound Repair and Regenerative Medicine held

Adhering to the vision and goal of the World Summit of Young Scientists, the Forum carried out heated discussions on international cooperation in medical and health care, medical education and achievement transformation, and public welfare assistance for wound repair along the "the Belt and Road". The forum is jointly hosted by the First Affiliated Hospital of Wenzhou Medical University and the Friendship Hospital of Bangui, Central African Republic. The conference has a main venue in Wenzhou, China and a sub venue of the Friendship Hospital of Central Africa. More than 300 scientists, academicians, foreign aid experts, social welfare organizations, and project leaders from 30 China Africa counterpart hospitals from multiple countries and regions participate online. Wenzhou Medical University's Publicity Department, Graduate School, Hospital Management Office, School of Continuing Education, School of Pharmacy, School of International Education, Alberta College, and other relevant departments, as well as representatives of Chinese and foreign students, the head of the First Affiliated Hospital, representatives of medical staff, representatives of foreign aid experts, social media, caring enterprises, leaders of various rescue stations of the "F&S CHARITY", volunteer representatives, etc., participated in the forum.

The conference held a release ceremony for the theme song "Love Skin Life" of the "F&S CHARITY". The song was written by Wang Xiaoshang, Secretary General of the "F&S CHARITY" and Vice Dean of Alberta College of Wenzhou Medical University, and composed by the famous Taiwanese composer Guo Mengyong. The "F&S CHARITY" also selected 10 "Most Beautiful Skin Revitalizers", who are volunteers from different industries such as healthcare, nursing, enterprise, education, publicity, and volunteering. Academician Li Xiaokun, President of Wenzhou Medical University, initiated the "International Public Welfare Relief Action for Wound Repair" on behalf of the "F&S CHARITY" team, and carried out extensive international public welfare relief actions for wound repair worldwide.

At the meeting, the "F&S CHARITY" selected the "Most Beautiful Skin Revitalizers" of 2022. They are Wang Xiaoshang, Vice Dean of Alberta College of Wenzhou Medical University, Wang Jian, Executive Director of the Wound Repair Department and Deputy Director of the Medical Department of Wenzhou Medical University Affiliated First Hospital, Dan Erkang, Executive President of Yierkang Co., Ltd., Chen Shanliang, Business Dean of Wenzhou Shuguang Hospital, Li Zhengying, Director of the Nursing Department, Xu Mingling, Head of Trauma Identification of Fuding Medical Insurance Bureau, Zhang Liliang, Head of Zhang Liliang Charity Studio of Wencheng County Charity Federation, Chen Yinwei, Volunteer of F&S CHARITY, and Chen Zhong, Head of Chen Zhong Charity Studio of Wenzhou Urban Daily.

第三部分 附录

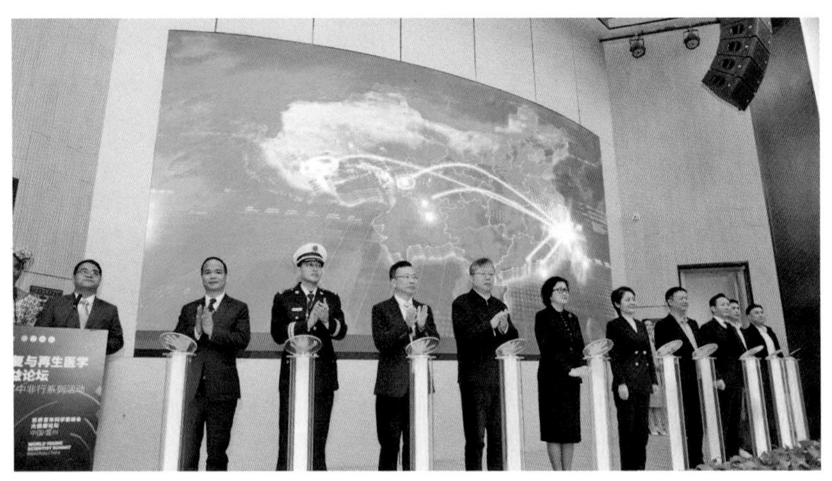

附图 17 “肤生工程”主题曲发布

中非共和国总统夫人、中非妇女儿童基金会创始人布丽吉特·图瓦德拉在视频致辞里表达了对温州医科大学附一院开展创面修复帮扶工作的感谢。她表示，中国政府开展的对口合作机制对于降低创伤、战争等导致皮肤缺损与感染的病痛有着非常积极意义。

中非共和国驻华大使馆代办贝合纳先生线上致辞，对温州医科大学“肤生工程”团队以及温州医科大学附一院提供的物资捐赠、远程网络会诊等表达谢意，希望双方能够在医疗教育、医院建设、医学研究等方面进行深度合作。

中非友谊医院院长肯特·让·克里索斯托姆表达了受邀来华访问并共同举办此次论坛的感激之情。他说，这次论坛在中国与中非卫生合作交流方面具有重要历史意义，希望友谊医院与温州医科大学附属医院在携手抗疫基础上，深入开展创面感染与修复专科联合建设。

温州医科大学附一院党委书记沈贤说，“中非对口医院合作机制”让温州医科大学附一院与中非友谊医院之间的合作更加紧密，医院将继续深入推进远程医疗合作、创面修复学科体系与人才培养等方面的合作交流，深化双方友谊。

李校堃院士表示，“肤生工程”及创面修复学科团队要牢记“科技为民”情怀，以更高标准要求自己，把学科做大做好做强；要响应“一带一路”倡议，继续深化中非合作，用中国温州的创面修复成果，造福世界各地人民；要深入推进实施“精准救助”，做好“千村千点”救治帮扶工作。“我们是一支胸怀爱国报国之志、潜心科技医疗攻关、情系人民群众健康的爱心公益团队。公益爱心事业的脚步绝不能停，而且还要做得更加好，更加有温度，更加有情怀！”李校堃院士说。

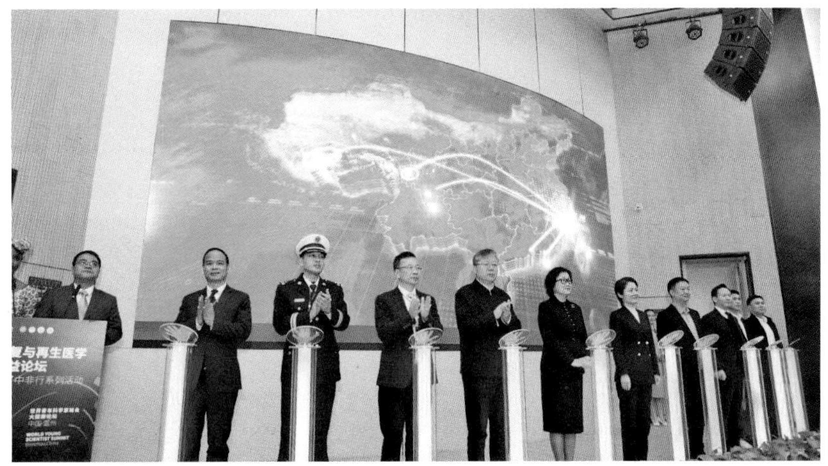

Figure 17 The theme song of "F&S CHARITY" has been released

Bridget Tuwadera, the wife of the President of the Central African Republic and founder of the Central African Women and Children's Foundation, expressed her gratitude to the First Affiliated Hospital of Wenzhou Medical University for carrying out wound repair and assistance work in a video speech. She stated that the Chinese government's targeted cooperation mechanism has a very positive significance in reducing skin defects and infections caused by trauma, war, and other illnesses.

Mr. Beihe Na, the Charg é d'affaires of the Embassy of the Central African Republic in China, delivered an online speech expressing gratitude to the "F&S CHARITY" team of Wenzhou Medical University and the affiliated hospital of Wenzhou Medical University for providing material donations, remote online consultations, etc. He hoped that both sides could deepen cooperation in medical education, hospital construction, medical research, and other areas.

Kent Jean Krissostrom, the director of the China Africa Friendship Hospital, expressed his gratitude for being invited to visit China and cohosting this forum. He said that this forum has significant historical significance in the field of health cooperation and exchange between China and Africa. He hopes that Friendship Hospital and Wenzhou Medical University Affiliated Hospital can deepen the joint construction of wound infection and repair specialties on the basis of working together to fight against the epidemic.

Shen Xian, Secretary of the Party Committee of the First Affiliated Hospital of Wenzhou Medical University, said that the "China Africa Hospital Cooperation Mechanism" has made the cooperation between the First Affiliated Hospital of Wenzhou Medical University and the China Africa Friendship Hospital closer. The hospital will continue to deepen cooperation and exchanges in remote medical cooperation, wound repair discipline system and talent cultivation, and deepen the friendship between the two sides.

Academician Li Xiaokun stated that the teams of the "F&S CHARITY" and wound repair disciplines should always bear in mind the sentiment of "technology for the people", demand higher standards of themselves, and make the discipline bigger, better, and stronger; We should respond to the "the Belt and Road" initiative, continue to deepen China Africa cooperation, and use the wound repair achievements of Wenzhou, China, to benefit people around the world; We need to deepen the implementation of "precision rescue" and do a good job in the "thousands of villages and thousands of points" rescue and assistance work."We are a loving public welfare team with a patriotic and patriotic spirit, dedicated to scientific and technological medical research, and caring for the health of the people. The footsteps of public welfare and love undertakings must not stop, and we must do better, with more warmth and emotion! "Said Academician Li Xiaokun.

肤生健康中国行

2022年8月12—14日，温州医科大学慈善医疗共富行在陕西省渭南市富平县举行，中国工程院院士、温州医科大学校长李校堃院士带领温州医科大学各附属医院，给富平县送上慈善医疗共富大礼：成立富平县四肢难愈性急、慢性创面协作中心，设立富平县创面修复救助站、“童心筑梦”志愿公益服务项目基地、世界温州人微笑联盟协力医院、眼视光诊疗中心等。

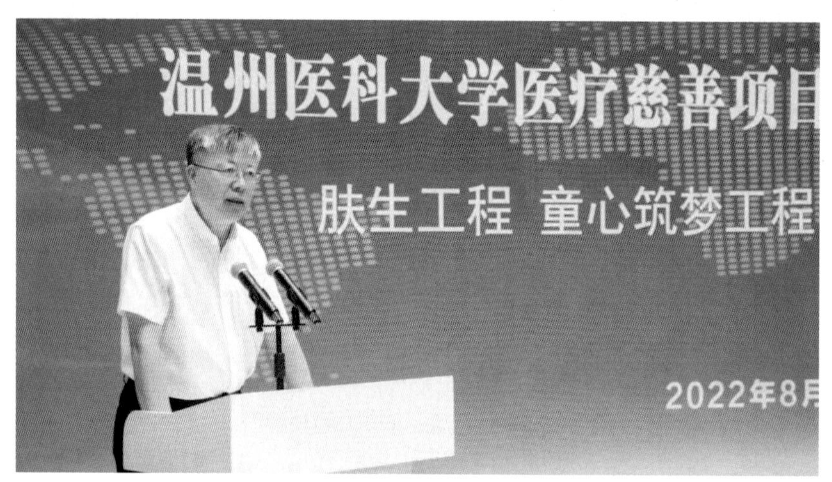

附图18 温州医科大学慈善医疗共富行在陕西省渭南市富平县举行

2020年12月，富平县与温州医科大学签署战略合作框架协议，双方围绕协议目标任务，进行了全面深入的对接沟通，组建成立了富平“院士之家”健康产业协同创新中心，李校堃院士发起的公益慈善项目“肤生工程”，成立了“四肢难愈性急、慢性创面协作中心”“富平县肤生工程创面修复救助站”，同时开展了患者义诊、免费手术及慈善捐赠等活动，让富平老百姓在家门口享受到更多的优质医疗资源。

◆ 为共同富裕贡献科技力量、医疗力量、公益力量

2022年8月14日上午，温州医科大学医疗慈善项目富平公益活动启动仪式在富平县中医院举行。仪式上，渭南市委常委、富平县委书记赵林斌向李校堃院士颁发富平县高端智库专家聘书。温州医科大学医院管理处处长林坚介绍了这次公益活动的相关内容。

Skin Health China Tour

From August 12 to 14, 2022, the Charity Medical Co prosperity Trip of Wenzhou Medical University was held in Fuping County, Weinan City, Shaanxi Province. Academician Li Xiaokun, academician of the CAE Member and president of Wenzhou Medical University, led the affiliated hospitals of Wenzhou Medical University to send a gift of charity medical co prosperity to Fuping County: the Fuping County Wound Repair and Rescue Center for Extremely Healing and Chronic Wounds, the Fuping County Wound Repair and Rescue Station, the "Childhood Dream" voluntary public service project base, the World Wenzhou Smile Alliance Cooperation Hospital, the Eye Optic Diagnosis and Treatment Center, etc.

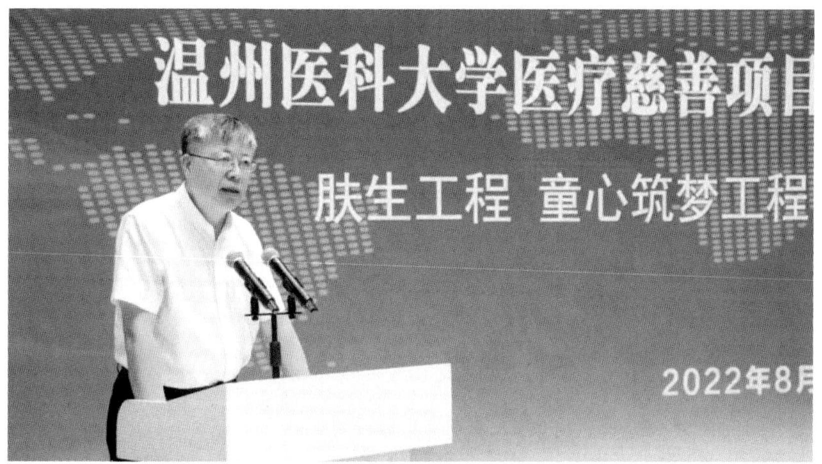

Figure 18 Wenzhou Medical University Charity Medical Co Prosperity Tour held in Fuping County, Weinan City, Shaanxi Province

In December 2020, Fuping County signed a strategic cooperation framework agreement with Wenzhou Medical University. The two sides conducted comprehensive and in-depth communication around the objectives and tasks of the agreement, and established the Fuping "Academician's Home" Health Industry Collaborative Innovation Center. Academician Li Xiaokun initiated the public welfare project "F&S CHARITY", established the "Limb Difficult to heal Acute and Chronic Wound Collaboration Center" and "Fuping County Skin Revitalization Engineering Wound Repair and Rescue Station", and carried out activities such as patient consultations, free surgeries, and charitable donations, allowing Fuping residents to enjoy more high-quality medical resources at their doorstep.

◆ Contribute technological, medical, and public welfare forces to common prosperity

On the morning of August 14, 2022, the launch ceremony of the Fuping Public Welfare Activity of Wenzhou Medical University's medical charity project was held at the Fuping County Traditional Chinese Medicine Hospital. At the ceremony, Zhao Linbin, member of the Standing Committee of Weinan Municipal Party Committee and Secretary of Fuping County Party Committee, presented Academician Li Xiaokun with a letter of appointment as a high-end think tank expert in Fuping County. Lin Jian, Director of the Hospital Management Department of Wenzhou Medical University, introduced the relevant content of this public welfare activity.

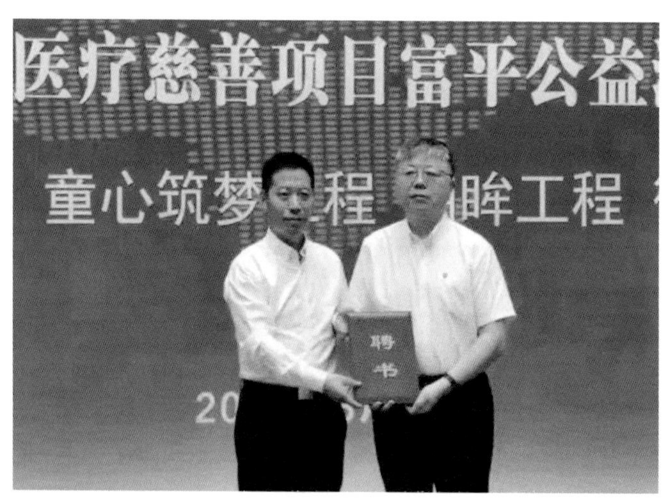

附图 19　李校堃院士接受富平县高端智库专家聘书

温州医科大学附属第一医院党委副书记许慧清与富平县医院院长王武装签订关于成立富平县四肢难愈性急、慢性创面协作中心的协议。许慧清还向富平县医院授牌富平县创面修复救助站；温州医科大学附属第二医院、育英儿童医院副院长张维溪向富平县妇女儿童医院授牌“童心筑梦”志愿公益服务项目基地；温州医科大学附属口腔医院院长潘乙怀向富平县中医院授牌世界温州人微笑联盟协力医院、温州医科大学附属口腔医院（富平）口腔中心、温州医科大学唇腭裂治疗中心；温州医科大学附属眼视光医院副院长陈蔚向富平县第二人民医院授牌陕西省富平县 - 温州医科大学联合眼视光诊疗中心。

李校堃院士说，温州医科大学是近十年来发展最快、最有特色的地方医科大学之一，也是东南沿海 2000 多公里海岸线上最好的医学院校之一，为国家培养了 20 多万优秀医学人才，浙江 70% 的医学人才都是温州医科大学校友。温州医科大学一直致力于大健康教育和公益慈善项目的打造，尤其公益慈善项目走在全国高校前列，多个项目获得中华慈善项目。这次他带队到富平开展医疗公益活动，一方面是想在推动富平医疗卫生和教育事业发展方面再多做些温州医科大学的贡献，另一方面也是希望推动双方的沟通交流更加紧密深入，利用温州医科大学在医疗卫生、健康产业、人才培养、科技成果转化等方面优势资源，助力富平经济社会高质量发展，为推进东西部健康和医疗合作，推动西北地区医疗事业发展，为乡村振兴、共同富裕贡献科技力量、医疗力量、公益力量。

“李院士等专家一行来富开展革命传统教育及公益活动，这是一次红色教育之行，也是一次公益帮扶

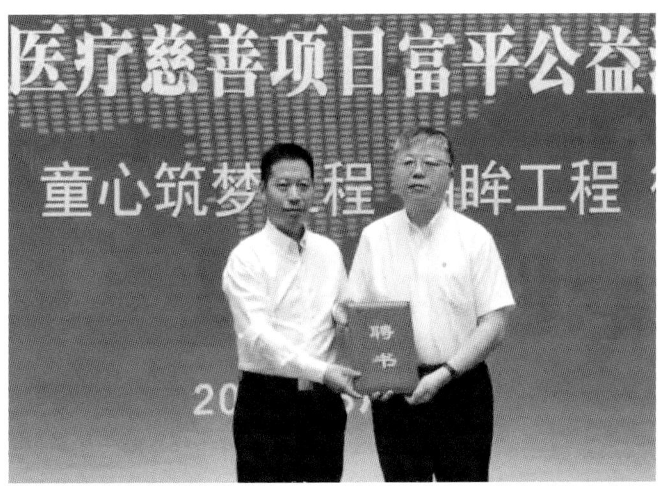

Figure 19 Academician Li Xiaokun accepts the appointment letter as an expert from a high-end think tank in Fuping County

Xu Huiqing, Deputy Secretary of the Party Committee of the First Affiliated Hospital of Wenzhou Medical University, and Wang Armed, President of Fuping County Hospital, signed an agreement to establish the Fuping County Collaborative Center for Limb Difficult to heal Acute and Chronic Wounds. Xu Huiqing also awarded the Fuping County Wound Repair and Rescue Station to the Fuping County Hospital; Zhang Weixi, Vice President of the Second Affiliated Hospital of Wenzhou Medical University and Yuying Children's Hospital, awarded the "Childhood Dream Building" Volunteer Public Welfare Service Project Base to Fuping County Women and Children's Hospital; Pan Yihuai, Dean of the Affiliated Stomatological Hospital of Wenzhou Medical University, awarded the World Wenzhou Smile Alliance Cooperation Hospital, Wenzhou Medical University Affiliated Stomatological Hospital (Fuping) Stomatological Center, and Wenzhou Medical University Cleft Lip and Palate Treatment Center to Fuping County Traditional Chinese Medicine Hospital; Chen Wei, Vice President of Wenzhou Medical University Affiliated Eye and Vision Hospital, awarded the Shaanxi Province Fuping County Wenzhou Medical University Joint Eye and Vision Diagnosis and Treatment Center to the Second People's Hospital of Fuping County.

Academician Li Xiaokun said that Wenzhou Medical University is one of the fastest developing and most distinctive local medical universities in the past decade, and also one of the best medical schools along the more than 2000 kilometer coastline of the southeast coast. It has trained more than 200 000 outstanding medical talents for the country, and 70% of medical talents in Zhejiang are alumni of Wenzhou Medical University. Wenzhou Medical University has always been committed to the development of health education and public welfare and charity projects, especially in the forefront of public welfare and charity projects among universities in China, with multiple projects winning the China Charity Project award. This time, he led the team to Fuping to carry out medical public welfare activities. On the one hand, he wanted to make more contributions to the development of Fuping's medical, health, and education undertakings. On the other hand, he also hoped to promote closer and deeper communication and exchanges between the two sides, utilizing Wenzhou Medical University's advantageous resources in medical and health, health industry, talent cultivation, and technological achievement transformation, to help promote high-quality economic and social development in Fuping, and to contribute scientific and technological strength, medical strength, and public welfare strength to promoting health and medical cooperation between the east and the west, promoting the development of medical undertakings in the northwest region, and contributing to rural revitalization and common prosperity.

"Academician Li and other experts came to Fu to carry out revolutionary traditional education and public welfare activities. This is a red education trip and also a public welfare assistance measure, "Zhao Linbin said.

之举”，赵林斌说，李校堃院士是从富平大地走出去的频阳骄子，从事科教工作20余年，获得了众多国家重要奖项。李院士在个人事业获得巨大成功的同时，一直不忘家乡人民，心系故乡发展，多次回乡考察调研，指导改善医疗卫生事业。这次李院士带领温州医科大学的专家莅临富平，开展慈善项目富平公益活动，充分彰显了李院士对家乡发展的殷殷关切和造福家乡人民的赤子情怀。希望借助温州医科大学的科研资源优势，帮助富平加快“院士之家”建设，促进高端人才资源与产业要素、科技要素等高效融合，打造健康产业集聚发展新高地，推动富平医疗卫生事业迈上新台阶。

◆ 慈善医疗共富行已为当地28名患者实施手术

这次慈善医疗共富行，温州医科大学派出专家在富平县开展白内障、唇腭裂、难愈合创面伤等手术，共为当地28名患者实施手术。

温州医科大学附属第一医院医务处副处长暨玲、手外科主任王健和温州曙光医院副院长陈善亮等“肤生工程”专家，8月13日在富平县医院为3名静脉曲张等患者开展手术。

温州医科大学附属第二医院、育英儿童医院儿童心血管科主任吴蓉洲带领“童心筑梦”工程团队蒋蕾、仇慧仙、吴婷婷、黄静等成员，在富平县妇女儿童医院为当地儿童进行先天性心脏病筛查，从温州专门带来价值100多万元的心脏彩超机，为40多名儿童做心超检查。检查发现其中半数儿童有心脏疾病，其中3名儿童先天性心脏病患者将到温州免费接受手术。

温州医科大学附属眼视光医院角膜临床中心常务副主任郑钦象在富平县第二医院为当地23名白内障患者开展白内障复明手术。该院公益医疗处处长黄象好说，患者的治疗费用由该院资助。

温州医科大学附属口腔医院医务科副科长刘登峰、颌面外科主治医师赵树蕃为当地2名口腔颌骨囊肿、唇腭裂患者实施手术，他们也将带2名唇腭裂患者到温州免费做手术。

8月13日下午，李校堃院士还带领温州医科大学团队参观当地爱国主义教育基地并重温入党誓词，随后带队看望东化村5名光荣在党50年的老党员，为他们送上慰问品和慰问金。

8月14日上午，温州医科大学专家团队还在富平县中医院联合开展义诊。

温州医科大学药学院院长林丽、党委副书记王建波带领团队参加志愿服务，并为慈善医疗共富行提供医疗科技支持。

Academician Li Xiaokun is a proud figure who has been engaged in scientific and educational work for more than 20 years and has won many important national awards. Academician Li, while achieving great success in his personal career, has always remembered the people of his hometown and cared about its development. He has returned to his hometown multiple times for inspection and research, guiding the improvement of medical and health services. This time, Academician Li led experts from Wenzhou Medical University to visit Fuping and carry out a charity project, Fuping Public Welfare Activity, fully demonstrating Academician Li's sincere concern for the development of his hometown and his patriotic sentiment of benefiting the people of his hometown. We hope to leverage the research resource advantages of Wenzhou Medical University to help accelerate the construction of the "Academician's Home" in Fuping, promote the efficient integration of high-end talent resources with industrial and technological elements, create a new highland for the development of the health industry cluster, and promote the medical and health industry in Fuping to a new level.

◆ Charity Medical Co Prosperity Tour has performed surgeries for 28 local patients

This charity medical trip for common prosperity, Wenzhou Medical University sent experts to Fuping County to carry out surgeries such as cataracts, cleft lip and palate, and difficult to heal facial injuries, and performed surgeries for 28 local patients.

On August 13th, Ji Ling, Deputy Director of the Medical Department of the First Affiliated Hospital of Wenzhou Medical University, Wang Jian, Director of the Hand Surgery Department, and Chen Shanliang, Vice President of Wenzhou Shuguang Hospital and other "F&S CHARITY" experts, performed surgeries on three patients with varicose veins and other conditions at Fuping County Hospital.

Wu Rongzhou, director of the Children's Cardiovascular Department at the Second Affiliated Hospital of Wenzhou Medical University and Yuying Children's Hospital, led the "Childhood Dream Building" project team consisting of Jiang Lei, Qiu Huixian, Wu Tingting, Huang Jing, and other members to conduct congenital heart disease screening for local children at the Women's and Children's Hospital in Fuping County. They brought a cardiac ultrasound machine worth over 1 million yuan from Wenzhou to perform cardiac ultrasound examinations for more than 40 children. Half of the children were found to have heart disease during the examination, and three children with congenital heart disease will undergo free surgery in Wenzhou.

Zheng Qinxiang, Executive Deputy Director of the Corneal Clinical Center of Wenzhou Medical University Affiliated Eye and Vision Hospital, performed cataract restoration surgery for 23 local cataract patients at the Second Hospital of Fuping County. Huang Xiang, the director of the Public Welfare Medical Department of the hospital, said that the treatment expenses of patients are funded by the hospital.

Liu Dengfeng, Deputy Director of the Medical Department of Wenzhou Medical University Affiliated Stomatological Hospital, and Zhao Shufan, Chief Physician of Maxillofacial Surgery, will perform surgeries on two local patients with oral and maxillofacial cysts and cleft lip and palate. They will also bring two cleft lip and palate patients to Wenzhou for free surgery.

On the afternoon of August 13th, Academician Li Xiaokun also led a team from Wenzhou Medical University to visit the local patriotic education base and review the oath of joining the Communist Party. Later, he led the team to visit five glorious old party members in Donghua Village who have been with the Party for 50 years, and presented them with condolence gifts and money.

On the morning of August 14th, a team of experts from Wenzhou Medical University jointly conducted a free clinic at Fuping County Traditional Chinese Medicine Hospital.

Lin Li, Dean of the School of Pharmacy at Wenzhou Medical University, and Wang Jianbo, Deputy Secretary of the Party Committee, led a team to participate in volunteer services and provided medical technology support for the charity medical prosperity project.

温州医科大学阿尔伯塔学院副院长王小尚带领白求恩服务社成员尹恬然等人参加志愿服务，并为老党员送上 1 万元慰问金和慰问品。

公益活动仪式结束后，李校堃院士、赵林斌等领导看望受益于微笑工程的 11 岁石同学，给他送上了书籍、文具和水果。李院士鼓励他好好学习，将来为家乡、为国家做贡献。

"肤生工程"延安行

2023 年 9 月 3 日，中国工程院院士、温州医科大学校长李校堃院士带领温州医科大学"肤生工程"等医疗慈善团队赴革命圣地延安开展医疗公益慈善活动。延安市卫生健康委员会二级调研员陈探生、延安市人民医院院长李晖出席仪式。

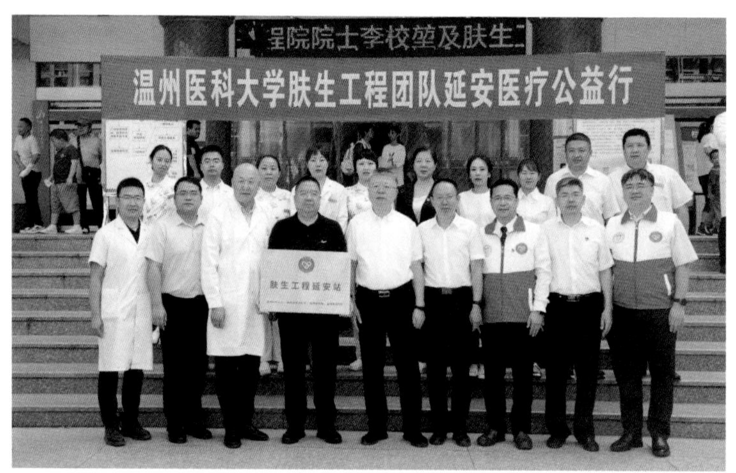

附图 20 "肤生工程"团队延安医疗公益行

温州医科大学药学院党委副书记王建波、阿尔伯塔学院副院长王小尚、附一院副院长陈咨苗、附二院党委副书记陈开亮、附属眼视光医院副院长陈蔚、附属口腔医院副院长刘劲松、校办崔彪等参加活动。

◆ 校地协同四个爱心基地授牌

活动现场举行了"肤生工程"延安创面修复救助站、温州医科大学附二院"童心筑梦"公益志愿服务基地、温州医科大学附属眼视光医院"明眸工程"服务站、温州医科大学附属口腔医院"微笑工程"协力医院等授牌仪式。

李晖说，此次"肤生工程"等团队与延安市人民医院创面修复科、眼科、儿科、口腔科等科室深入开展学科发展交流，并分别授牌建立长远联系机制，搭建起了延安 - 温州医疗事业共同发展的桥梁。他希望在李校堃院士团队和"肤生工程"等团队的帮助下，能够带动医院各专科业务技术的发展及学科建设，从

Wang Xiaoshang, Vice Dean of Alberta College at Wenzhou Medical University, led members of the Norman Bethune Service Society, including Yin Tianran, to participate in volunteer service and presented 10 000 yuan in condolence money and gifts to old party members.

After the public welfare activity ceremony, Academician Li Xiaokun, Zhao Linbin and other leaders visited 11-year-old Shi, who benefited from the Smile Project, and presented him with books, stationery and fruits. Academician Li encouraged him to study hard and make contributions to his hometown and country in the future.

Yan'an Tour of "F&S CHARITY"

On September 3, 2023, Academician Li Xiaokun, academician of the CAE Member and president of Wenzhou Medical University, led medical charity teams such as the "F&S CHARITY" of Wenzhou Medical University to carry out medical charity activities in Yan'an, the revolutionary holy land. Chen Tansheng, a second level researcher from Yan'an Municipal Health Commission, and Li Hui, the director of Yan'an People's Hospital, attended the ceremony.

温州医科大学肤生工程团队延安医疗公益行
肤生工程延安站

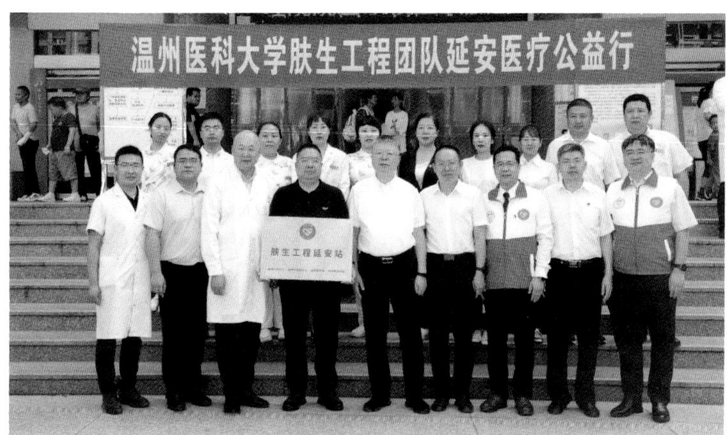

Figure 20 Yan'an Medical Public Welfare Tour of the "F&S CHARITY" Team

Wang Jianbo, Deputy Secretary of the Party Committee of the School of Pharmacy at Wenzhou Medical University, Wang Xiaoshang, Deputy Dean of Alberta College, Chen Zimiao, Deputy Dean of the First Affiliated Hospital, Chen Kailiang, Deputy Secretary of the Party Committee of the Second Affiliated Hospital, Chen Wei, Deputy Dean of the Affiliated Eye and Vision Hospital, Liu Jinsong, Deputy Dean of the Affiliated Stomatological Hospital, Cui Xuan, and others participated in the event.

◆ Four collaborative love bases between the school and the local community were awarded plaques

At the event, award ceremonies were held for the Yan'an Wound Repair and Rescue Station of the "F&S CHARITY", the "Childlike Dream Building" Public Welfare Volunteer Service Base of Wenzhou Medical University Affiliated Second Hospital, the "Bright Eye Project" Service Station of Wenzhou Medical University Affiliated Eye Hospital, and the "Smile Project" Collaborative Hospital of Wenzhou Medical University Affiliated Stomatological Hospital.

Li Hui said that this time, the "F&S CHARITY" and other teams have conducted in-depth exchanges on disciplinary development with departments such as wound repair, ophthalmology, pediatrics, and dentistry at Yan'an People's Hospital, and have been awarded licenses to establish long-term contact mechanisms, building a bridge for the common development of the medical industry between Yan'an and Wenzhou. He hopes that with the help of Academician Li Xiaokun's team and teams such as "F&S CHARITY", it can drive the development of various

而推动延安医疗卫生事业的长足发展。陈探生说，温州医科大学“肤生工程”等医疗团队在延安举行揭牌仪式，充分体现了温州医科大学及各附属医院积极响应“健康中国”战略的高度政治责任感，体现了推动优质资源、精湛技术、先进管理理念下沉的责任担当，以及支持延安卫生事业发展、心系老区百姓健康的深情厚谊，相信必将对大幅提升延安市医疗服务水平、加快健康城市建设产生积极深远影响。“延安宝塔白云牵，革命摇篮聚俊贤”，李校堃院士说，延安是中华民族重要的发祥地，既是民族圣地，也是中国革命圣地，“肤生工程”等团队在延安开展医疗公益活动帮助人民群众，意义非凡。在全校上下深入开展主题教育活动中，医疗公益团队在延安的爱心活动，是发挥学校独特人才优势和优质医疗资源，践行主题教育“惠民生、暖民心、顺民意”要求的生动体现。李校堃院士表示，要用院士团队的科技成果以及温州医科大学的优势医疗资源，为延安的老百姓做点实实在在的事情，要进一步完善医疗帮扶联动工作机制，推进延安市与温州医科大学的情感交流与协同合作，为推动延安的医疗卫生和教育事业发展做出温州医科大学的贡献。

◆ 爱心义诊、公益手术，革命圣地送健康

当天上午 9 时，义诊在延安市人民医院开始，现场人头攒动。

李校堃院士来到义诊现场，与陈咨苗，温州医科大学附一院创面修复科执行主任王健、副主任医师陶克，温州曙光医院业务院长陈善亮等专家共同为创面患者做咨询检查。现场一名 40 岁的患者，左手手背皮肤坏死溃烂，专家们现场讨论治疗方案，帮助患者尽快让伤口痊愈，减轻痛苦；专家们还现场为一名患严重静脉曲张的患者做了检查，并给出治疗方案。

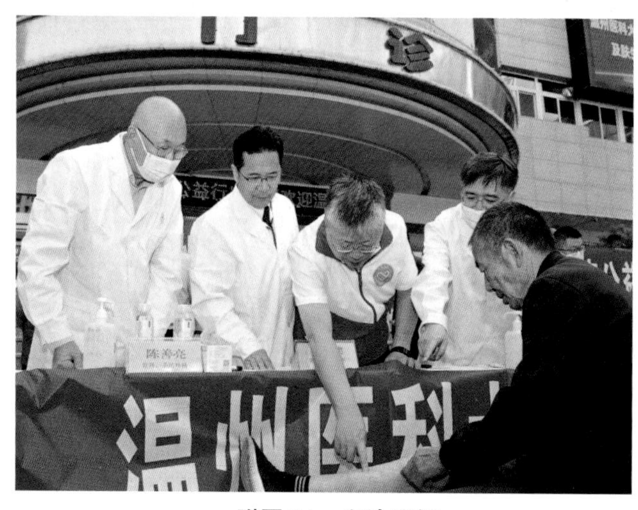

附图 21　义诊现场

specialized business technologies and discipline construction in the hospital, thereby promoting the long-term development of medical and health care in Yan'an. Chen Tansheng said that the unveiling ceremony of the "F&S CHARITY" and other medical teams of Wenzhou Medical University in Yan'an fully reflects the high political responsibility of Wenzhou Medical University and its affiliated hospitals to actively respond to the "Healthy China" strategy, the responsibility to promote the sinking of high-quality resources, exquisite technology, and advanced management concepts, as well as the deep friendship to support the development of Yan'an's health industry and care for the health of the people in the old areas. He believes that it will have a positive and far-reaching impact on significantly improving the level of medical services in Yan'an and accelerating the construction of a healthy city. "Yan'an Pagoda with white clouds, the cradle of revolution gathers talented people", said Academician Li Xiaokun. Yan'an is an important birthplace of the Chinese nation, both a national holy land and a holy land of the Chinese revolution. The" F&S CHARITY "and other teams have carried out medical public welfare activities in Yan'an to help the people, which is of great significance. In the in-depth implementation of theme education activities throughout the school, the love activity of the medical public welfare team in Yan'an is a vivid manifestation of the school's unique talent advantages and high-quality medical resources, and the practice of the theme education's requirements of "benefiting people's livelihood, warming people's hearts, and following public opinion". Academician Li Xiaokun stated that we need to use the scientific and technological achievements of our team and the advantageous medical resources of Wenzhou Medical University to do something tangible for the people of Yan'an. We need to further improve the mechanism of medical assistance linkage, promote emotional exchange and collaborative cooperation between Yan'an City and Wenzhou Medical University, and make Wenzhou Medical University's contribution to promoting the development of medical, health, and education in Yan'an.

◆ Love free clinic, public welfare surgery, revolutionary holy land brings health

At 9:00 am that day, the free clinic began at Yan'an People's Hospital, and the scene was crowded with people.

Academician Li Xiaokun arrived at the free clinic site and, together with experts such as Chen Zimiao, Wang Jian, Executive Director of the Department of Wound Repair at Wenzhou Medical University Affiliated Hospital, Tao Ke, Deputy Chief Physician, and Chen Shanliang, Business Dean of Wenzhou Shuguang Hospital, provided consultation and examination services for wound patients. A 40-year-old patient on site had skin necrosis and ulceration on the back of his left hand. Experts discussed treatment plans on site to help the patient recover from the wound as soon as possible and alleviate the pain; Experts also conducted an on-site examination for a patient with severe varicose veins and provided a treatment plan.

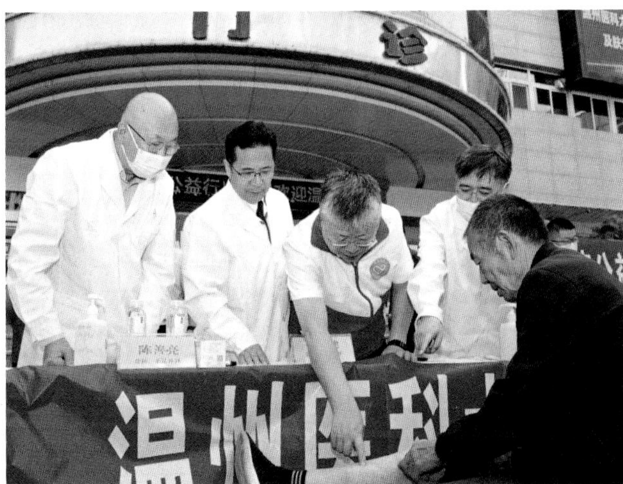

Figure 21 Free clinic site

陈咨苗当天接诊了不少血糖高的患者，这些患者偏胖，不注意饮食，有的甚至不吃药，他一一给予指正。王健教授接诊了不少创面和手外科患者，其中 82 岁的王阿公，左手食指感染，王健给出治疗意见；陶克接诊 18 岁的小苏，他在二三岁时被开水烫伤左手臂，如今起了严重斑痕，因高中毕业后想去当兵，他现场咨询如何把斑痕去掉。超声影像科主任许世豪为当地群众做 B 超检查，解决疑难问题。

温州医科大学附二院团委书记蒋蕾带领“童心筑梦”公益医疗团队参加义诊。当天过来就诊的孩子心脏问题有心包积液、川崎病冠脉扩张、先天性心脏病等。张松跃医生耐心询问患儿病情，详细检查后，对患儿家属的问题一一耐心细致解答；夏天和医生为体检有问题的孩子进行详细心脏超声检查，并为疾病后期随访和保健给予建议。团队还与当地儿科科室建立联络群，方便心脏问题患儿后续跟进。

义诊前一天，陈蔚教授与温州医科大学附属眼视光医院角膜病临床中心副主任郑钦象、公益医疗处副处长李苗苗一行来到延安市人民医院眼科病房查看住院患者，并给出诊疗方案。随后双方还从医、教、研、人才培养、学科建设等方面进行了全面交流。义诊当天，陈蔚一行开展眼科检查并为疑难患者会诊。一名 7 岁孩子眼睛被钢笔划伤引起角膜溃疡，陈蔚针对病情与当地医生进行交流，并给予详细治疗方案；一位 20 岁的小伙子，角膜移植术后再度浑浊，需要进行二次手术，陈蔚表示，后续根据家长意愿，可来温州手术，温州医科大学附属眼视光医院将提供基金救助支持。温州医科大学附属眼视光医院与延安市人民医院一直以来开展眼病、近视防控等相关公益项目，从 2011 首次入延开展“明眸工程”，今年是第三次走进延安。

温州医科大学附属口腔医院的义诊座位前患者络绎不绝，早早过来排在第一位的是 54 岁的李女士，她因右下后牙反复流脓肿痛，久治未愈来就诊。口腔修复专家刘劲松仔细询问病史，反复查体并阅片后给出了专业的治疗方 案。“门牙有缝怎么办？”“虎牙长在外面了要不要拔掉？”……现场有数名家长带着换牙期的孩子前来咨询，赵树蕃耐心地给予指导。

42 岁的刘先生肩膀疼已有四五年时间，一直看不好，找到了陈善亮。经过检查，刘先生患上了肩部肌筋膜炎，陈善亮给他开了处方；48 岁的齐先生左手臂上起了两个包，多年来一直没有治好，陈善亮建议通过手术祛除。义诊当天早上 7 点钟，陶克与陈善亮便来到手术室，为 57 岁的陕北农民李大叔等难愈合创面伤患者实施手术。由于李大叔家庭非常困难，温州都市报陈忠慈善工作室资助他 2 万元。另外一名 70 多岁

Chen Zimiao treated many patients with high blood sugar that day. These patients were overweight, did not pay attention to their diet, and some even did not take medication. He corrected them one by one. Professor Wang Jian has treated many patients with wounds and hand surgery, including 82-year-old Grandpa Wang who had an infection in his left index finger. Wang Jian provided treatment advice; Tao Ke received 18-year-old Xiao Su, who was scalded on his left arm by boiling water when he was two or three years old. He now has severe scars and wants to join the army after graduating from high school. He consulted on-site on how to remove the scars. Director Xu Shihao of the Ultrasound Imaging Department conducted B-ultrasound examinations for local residents to solve difficult problems.

Jiang Lei, Secretary of the Youth League Committee of the Second Affiliated Hospital of Wenzhou Medical University, led the "Childlike Heart Building Dreams" public welfare medical team to participate in free clinics. The child who came for treatment on the same day had heart problems such as pericardial effusion, Kawasaki disease coronary artery dilation, congenital heart disease, etc. Dr. Zhang Songyue patiently inquired about the patient's condition, conducted a detailed examination, and patiently and meticulously answered each question from the patient's family; During the summer, I will conduct detailed cardiac ultrasound examinations with doctors for children who have health problems, and provide recommendations for follow-up and healthcare in the later stages of the disease. The team also established a contact group with the local pediatric department to facilitate follow-up for children with heart problems.

The day before the free clinic, Professor Chen Wei, along with Zheng Qinxiang, Deputy Director of the Corneal Disease Clinical Center at Wenzhou Medical University Affiliated Eye and Vision Hospital, and Li Miaomiao, Deputy Director of the Public Welfare Medical Department, visited the ophthalmology ward of Yan'an People's Hospital to examine hospitalized patients and provide diagnosis and treatment plans. Subsequently, both sides also had comprehensive exchanges in areas such as medicine, education, research, talent cultivation, and discipline construction. On the day of the free clinic, Chen Wei and his team conducted ophthalmic examinations and provided consultations for difficult patients. A 7-year-old child's eyes were scratched by a fountain pen, causing corneal ulcers. Chen Wei communicated the condition with local doctors and provided a detailed treatment plan; A 20-year-old young man, who became cloudy again after corneal transplantation, needs a second surgery. Chen Wei said that according to the wishes of his parents, he can come to Wenzhou for surgery, and Wenzhou Medical University Affiliated Eye and Vision Hospital will provide fund assistance support. Wenzhou Medical University Affiliated Eye and Vision Hospital and Yan'an People's Hospital have been carrying out public welfare projects related to eye disease and myopia prevention and control. Since 2011, they have launched the "Bright Eyes Project" for the first time, and this year is the third time they have entered Yan'an.

In front of the free clinic seats at the Affiliated Stomatological Hospital of Wenzhou Medical University, there is a continuous stream of patients. The first person to come early is 54 years old Ms. Li, who came for treatment due to recurrent pus and swelling in her right lower posterior tooth. Oral restoration expert Liu Jinsong carefully inquired about the medical history, repeated physical examinations, and reviewed the images before providing a professional treatment plan. "What should I do if there is a gap in my front teeth? " "Should I have my tiger teeth pulled out if they grow outside? "Several parents came to consult with their children during the tooth replacement period, and Zhao Shufan patiently provided guidance.

Mr. Liu, who is 42 years old, has been suffering from shoulder pain for four to five years and has been unable to see well. He found Chen Shanliang. After examination, Mr. Liu was diagnosed with shoulder myofascial inflammation, and Chen Shanliang prescribed it to him; Mr. Qi, who is 48 years old, has two bags on his left arm that have not been cured for many years. Chen Shanliang suggests removing them through surgery. At 7 o'clock in the morning on the day of the free clinic, Tao Ke and Chen Shanliang came to the operating room to perform surgery on 57 years old Shaanbei farmer Uncle Li and other patients with difficult to heal wounds. Due to the extreme financial difficulties faced by Uncle Li's family, the Wenzhou City Daily's Chen Zhong Charity Studio provided him

的阿婆臀部溃烂，陈善亮为她做了检查，并给出治疗方案，陈忠慈善工作室也为她资助了 5000 元。

◆ 铭记历史、致敬老兵，时刻牢记延安精神

当天正值抗战胜利纪念日，李校堃院士一行赴八一敬老院看望慰问老红军、老八路，聆听他们的革命故事。

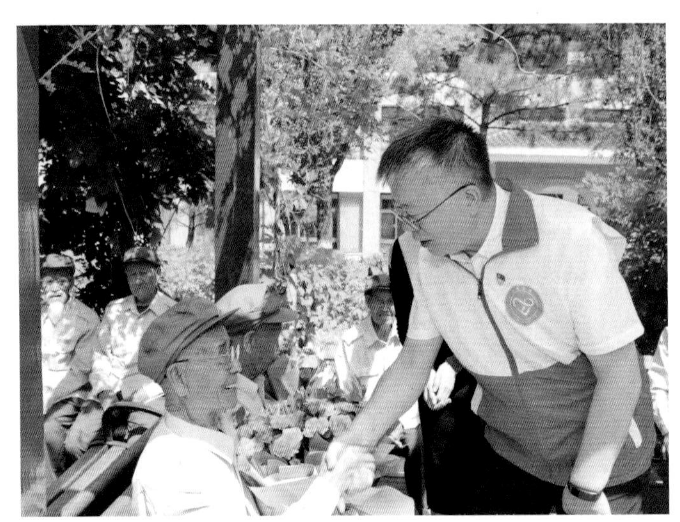

附图 22　赴八一敬老院看望慰问老红军、老八路

团队一行还赴杨家岭革命旧址参观学习，李校堃院士为大家上了一堂生动的主题党课，勉励大家学习延安精神，不忘初心牢记使命。李校堃院士说，这次“肤生工程”团队到延安开展公益活动，在主题教育期间能够为革命老区老百姓做些公益医疗服务，意义重大，既是贯彻落实党的二十大精神，践行总书记重要讲话精神，也是弘扬温州医科大学的大医大爱精神与文化的生动体现。他勉励团队成员，作为教育、医务、科技工作者，应当时刻牢记延安精神，不忘初心、牢记使命，全心全意为人民服务。

“肤生工程”为残疾人服务 >>>

2024 年 3 月 17 日，温州医科大学“肤生工程”闽浙爱心助残公益行在福建福鼎市启动，温州、福鼎两地联动、跨省协作，精准帮扶残障人群。

这是“肤生工程”第一次将创面修复公益帮扶与残疾人群体紧密联结，将利用温州医科大学教育、科技、医疗等优势，联合媒体、慈善组织等，探索打造中国最有温度的科技助残品牌，服务帮助深受创面问题困扰的残疾人，助力乡村振兴和共同富裕。

with a sponsorship of 20 000 yuan. Another elderly woman in her 70s had a sore buttock. Chen Shanliang conducted an examination for her and provided a treatment plan. Chen Zhong Charity Studio also sponsored 5000 yuan for her.

◆ Remembering history, paying tribute to veterans, and always keeping in mind the Yan'an spirit

On the day of the Victory Day of the War of Resistance Against Japanese Aggression, Academician Li Xiaokun and his delegation visited and comforted the old Red Army and the Eighth Route Army at the August 1st Nursing Home, listening to their revolutionary stories.

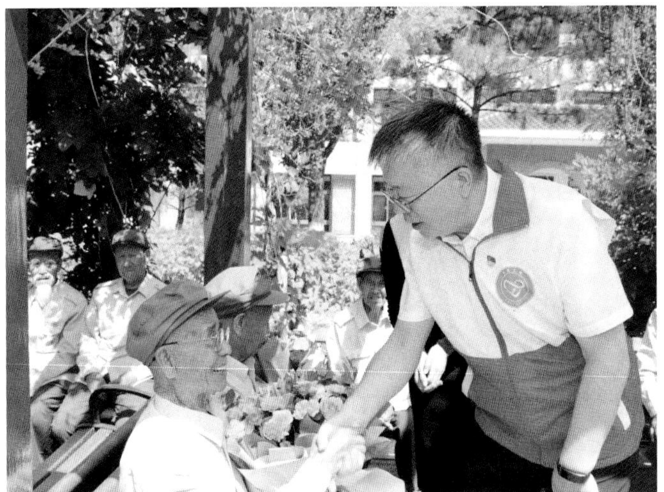

Figure 22 Visiting and sympathizing with the elderly Red Army and Eighth Route Army at the August 1st Nursing Home

Academician Li Xiaokun said that the "F&S CHARITY" team's participation in public welfare activities in Yan'an during the theme education period can provide some public medical services for the people in revolutionary old areas, which is of great significance. It is not only to implement the spirit of the 20th National Congress of the Communist Party of China and the important speech of the General Secretary, but also a vivid embodiment of the spirit and culture of great medical love at Wenzhou Medical University. He encouraged team members, as educators, medical professionals, and technology workers, to always keep in mind the Yan'an spirit, never forget their original aspirations and missions, and serve the people wholeheartedly.

The "F&S CHARITY" serves people with disabilities

On March 17, 2024, the "F&S CHARITY" Fujian Zhejiang Love and Assistance for the Disabled Public Welfare Campaign of Wenzhou Medical University was launched in Fuding City, Fujian Province. Wenzhou and Fuding collaborated and crossed provinces to provide targeted assistance to people with disabilities.

This is the first time that the "F&S CHARITY" has closely linked wound repair public welfare assistance with the disabled population. It will utilize the advantages of education, technology, and medical care at Wenzhou Medical University, and collaborate with media, charitable organizations, etc. to explore and create China's most warm technology assisted disability brand, serving and helping disabled people who are deeply troubled by wound problems, and promoting rural revitalization and common prosperity.

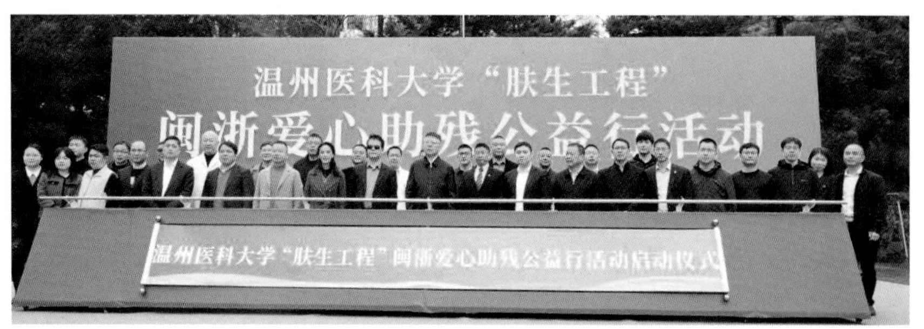

附图 23　“肤生工程”闽浙爱心助残公益行活动启动仪式

启动仪式现场举行了“肤生工程”宁德市爱心助残公益服务站、“肤生工程”福鼎创面修复救助站、温州医科大学附一院全科医学联盟单位、温州医科大学附二院童心筑梦公益志愿服务基地、温州医科大学附属眼视光医院明眸工程福鼎市服务站、温州医科大学附属口腔医院微笑工程福鼎市爱心服务站等授牌仪式。福鼎市残联、慈善总会、市妇联、市医院、龙安医院、同禾医院、微爱行动志愿者协会等单位揭牌。温州一批爱心企业捐赠物资和善款。

作为中国残联副主席，中国工程院院士、温州医科大学校长李校堃院士时刻关注康复医学事业发展，也一直在引导师生参与助残公益实践。

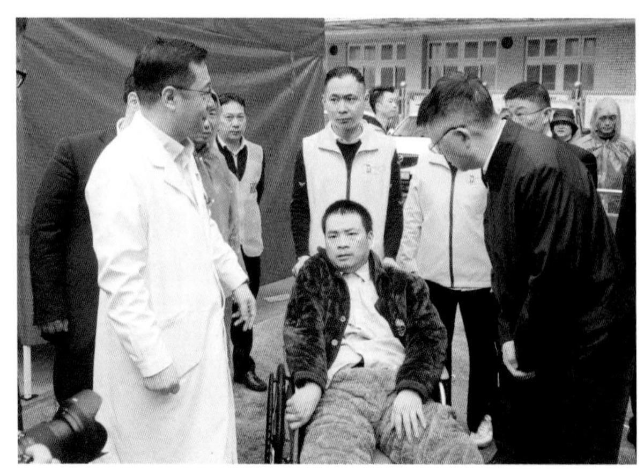

附图 24　师生参与助残公益实践

他表示，希望以这次医疗公益活动为纽带，进一步推进校地合作，利用温州医科大学在医疗卫生、健康产业、人才培养等方面的优势资源，助力福鼎经济社会高质量发展。同时，通过持续帮扶共同打造新时代医疗公益慈善品牌，切实提升医疗卫生水平，让更多老百姓享受到优质的医疗服务。

温州医科大学"肤生工程"
闽浙爱心助残公益行活动
温州医科大学"肤生工程"闽浙爱心助残公益行活动启动仪式

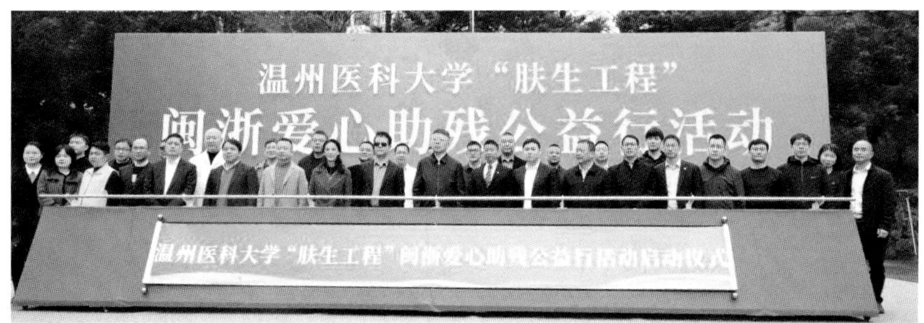

Figure 23 Launch ceremony of the Fujian Zhejiang Love and Assistance for the Disabled Public Welfare Campaign "F&S CHARITY"

At the launch ceremony, the "F&S CHARITY" Ningde Love and Assistance for the Disabled Public Welfare Service Station, "F&S CHARITY" Fuding Wound Repair and Rescue Station, Wenzhou Medical University Affiliated First Hospital General Medicine Alliance Unit, Wenzhou Medical University Affiliated Second Hospital Childlike Dream Public Welfare Volunteer Service Base, Wenzhou Medical University Affiliated Eye Hospital Mingmou Project Fuding City Service Station, Wenzhou Medical University Affiliated Stomatological Hospital Smile Project Fuding City Love Service Station and other awarding ceremonies were held. Fuding Disabled Persons' Federation, Charity Federation, Women's Federation, Municipal Hospital, Long'an Hospital, Tonghe Hospital, Weiai Action Volunteer Association and other units unveiled their plaques. A group of caring enterprises in Wenzhou donated materials and donations.

As the vice chairman of the China Disabled Persons' Federation, academician Li Xiaokun, academician of the CAE Member and president of Wenzhou Medical University, always pays attention to the development of rehabilitation medicine, and has also been guiding teachers and students to participate in the public welfare practice of helping the disabled.

第三部分　附录

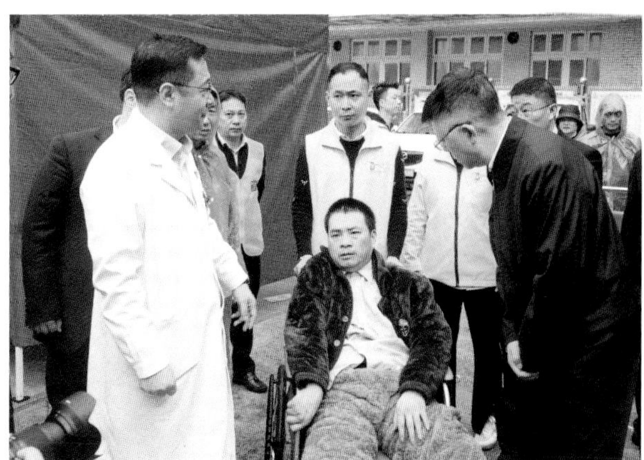

Figure 24 Participation of teachers and students in helping the disabled public welfare practice

He expressed his hope to use this medical public welfare activity as a link to further promote cooperation between the university and the local area, and to leverage the advantageous resources of Wenzhou Medical University in medical and health care, health industry, talent cultivation, and other areas to assist in the high-quality development of Fuding's economy and society. At the same time, through continuous assistance, we will jointly build a new era of medical public welfare and charity brands, effectively improve the level of medical and health care, and enable more people to enjoy high-quality medical services.

参加启动仪式的中国残联副主席王永澄说，“肤生工程”是利国利民的工程，为残疾人健康保驾护航，让人感动和钦佩。宁德市残联主席雷明感谢李校堃院士用高科技成果为残疾人服务。她说，目前，宁德市有残疾人 10 万多人，希望在人才培养、科普知识、康复等方面得到温州医科大学的帮助。

福鼎市委常委、政法委书记郑健瑜，福鼎市副市长陈晓龙等则期待“肤生工程”在闽浙爱心助残公益道路上不断前行，进一步拓宽服务范围、提高服务质量，让更多有需要的人享受到科技进步带来的福祉，助力每一位残疾人过上更有品质、更加美好的生活。

名医义诊送健康，志愿服务暖人心。当天，温州医科大学“肤生工程”“明眸工程”“微笑工程”“童心筑梦”医疗团队，以及温州“道德地标”“红日亭”公益团队，为当地群众进行各项健康检查并送上可口美味的温州名小吃。

李校堃院士一行还慰问了福鼎市自立自强的残疾人代表。

肤生浙里行

2023 年 7 月 1 日，正值中国共产党 102 周年华诞，温州医科大学党委书记吕一军带领温州医科大学“肤生工程”等医疗慈善团队赴丽水景宁开展公益慈善活动，红日亭、温州都市报陈忠慈善工作室、国药控股温州公司、温州曙光医院等单位同行参加活动。现场举行了“肤生工程”丽水景宁创面修复救助站、温州医科大学附一院“众善爱心团”山区二十六县爱心服务团、温州医科大学附二院童心筑梦公益志愿服务基地、温州医科大学附属眼视光医院明眸工程服务站、温州医科大学附属口腔医院微笑工程爱心服务站、温州红日亭景宁县爱心驿站授牌仪式。

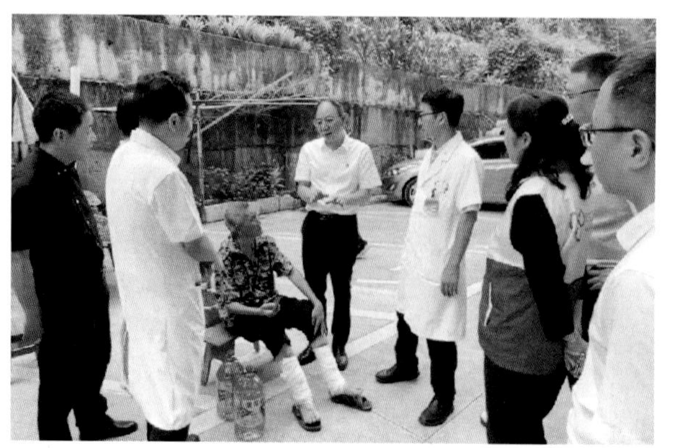

附图 25 “肤生工程”团队赴丽水景宁开展公益慈善活动

Wang Yongcheng, Vice Chairman of the China Disabled Persons' Federation, who attended the launch ceremony, said that the "F&S CHARITY" is a project that benefits the country and the people, and provides protection for the health of people with disabilities, which is touching and admirable. Lei Ming, Chairman of the Disabled Persons' Federation of Ningde City, thanks Academician Li Xiaokun for using high-tech achievements to serve people with disabilities. She said that currently, there are over 100 000 disabled people in Ningde City, and she hopes to receive assistance from Wenzhou Medical University in talent cultivation, popular science knowledge, rehabilitation, and other areas.

Zheng Jianyu, member of the Standing Committee of the Fuding Municipal Party Committee and Secretary of the Political and Legal Affairs Commission, and Chen Xiaolong, Deputy Mayor of Fuding City, are looking forward to the continuous progress of the "F&S CHARITY" on the public welfare road of caring for the disabled in Fujian and Zhejiang, further expanding the scope and improving the quality of services, allowing more people in need to enjoy the benefits brought by technological progress, and helping every disabled person live a better and more quality life.

Famous doctors offer free consultations to promote health, and volunteer service warms people's hearts. On that day, the medical teams of "F&S CHARITY", "Bright Eyes Project", "Smile Project" and "Childlike Dream Building" at Wenzhou Medical University, as well as the public welfare team of "Moral Landmark" and "Red Sun Pavilion" in Wenzhou, conducted various health checks for local residents and delivered delicious Wenzhou snacks.

Academician Li Xiaokun and his delegation also expressed condolences to the independent and self reliant disabled representatives in Fuding City.

Skin Health Tour in Zhejiang

On July 1, 2023, on the occasion of the 102nd anniversary of the CPC, Lv Yijun, Secretary of the Party Committee of Wenzhou Medical University, led medical charity teams such as the "F&S CHARITY" of Wenzhou Medical University to carry out charity activities in Jingning, Lishui. The Red Sun Pavilion, Wenzhou City Daily Chen Zhong Charity Studio, Sinopharm Holdings Wenzhou Company, Wenzhou Dawn Hospital and other units attended the activities. The "F&S CHARITY" Lishui Jingning Wound Repair and Rescue Station, Wenzhou Medical University Affiliated First Hospital "Zhong Shan · Love Team" Mountain 26 County Love Service Team, Wenzhou Medical University Affiliated Second Hospital Childlike Dream Public Welfare Volunteer Service Base, Wenzhou Medical University Affiliated Eye and Vision Hospital Bright Eye Project Service Station, Wenzhou Medical University Affiliated Stomatological Hospital Smile Project Love Service Station, and Wenzhou Hongri Pavilion Jingning County Love Station were awarded plaques on site.

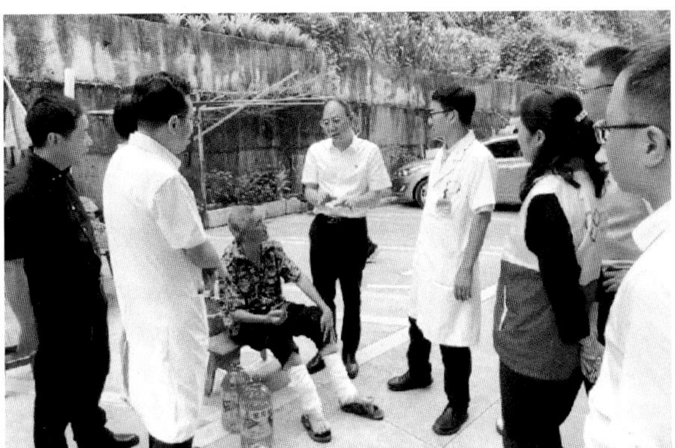

Figure 25 The "F&S CHARITY" team went to Jingning, Lishui to carry out public welfare and charity activities

◆ 山海协作、校地融合、共同发展

景宁县副县长吴海东说，景宁是全国唯一的畲族自治县，华东唯一的少数民族自治县，由于地处山区，乡镇多而分散，县域优质医疗资源较为欠缺，尤其是在皮肤科、眼科、口腔科等多个专科建设上都存在人才、技术方面的不足。2012 年起，温州医科大学与景宁县建立了高校定向培养协作关系，不仅有效缓解了当地卫生健康人才不足的问题，更将温州医科大学的前沿医疗制度、先进医疗手段带到了畲乡景宁。此次，温州医科大学党委书记吕一军带领团队赴畲乡景宁开展义诊，设立服务站，不仅是对十余年精诚合作的再深化，更是帮扶情谊的再延续，相信在温州医科大学及其附属医院的倾力帮扶下，畲乡医疗卫生事业将迎来大跨步、大发展，为 17 万畲汉群众带来健康的新福音。

吕一军说，七一建党节走进景宁这片浙西南革命老区，以医疗公益活动帮助群众，推动畲乡景宁医疗卫生和教育事业发展，助力景宁经济社会高质量发展，这是件十分有意义的事情。“医学是科学，是美学，更是人学。”他希望发挥温州医科大学独特人才优势和优质医疗资源，通过医疗公益团队在景宁的爱心活动，教育引导师生在医疗公益实践中践行主题教育“惠民生、暖民心、顺民意”的要求，以新时代卫生健康事业发展助推中国式现代化建设。

吕一军表示，本次公益活动集聚了温州医科大学最有优势、最具特色的医疗慈善团队：有为难愈合创面患者提供慈善救助的“肤生工程”公益团队，有为困难眼病患者重见光明的“明眸工程”公益团队，有帮助唇腭裂患儿修补缺口重拾灿烂笑容的“微笑工程”公益团队，有为儿童先天性心脏病困难患者提供公益救治的“童心筑梦”公益团队，有专为山区二十六县提供医疗帮扶的“众善·爱心团”公益团队。特别还要感谢有温州“道德地标”之称的“红日亭”公益团队参加本次活动。各支团队在“挂牌”之后，将进一步完善医疗帮扶联动工作机制，建立常态化公益服务模式，把医疗慈善活动做深做实做细，切实为提升景宁医疗卫生服务水平做出贡献。同时，他期待以本次授牌仪式为契机，进一步推进景宁县与温州医科大学的情感交流与协同合作，为下一步的合作交流打下良好基础，推动形成山海协作、校地融合、共同发展的良好局面。

吕一军一行还前往了景宁县鹤溪镇石牛山村慰问创面患者 64 岁的蓝阿公。蓝阿公是孤寡老人，患有糖尿病和心脏病，而且双脚下肢已经开始溃烂。吕一军给他送上了慰问品和慰问金，并详细了解患者的病情及生活情况，表示回去后要研究出最适合患者的治疗方案，为其减轻疾病痛苦。

◆ Mountain sea cooperation, school land integration, and common development

Wu Haidong, Deputy County Mayor of Jingning County, said that Jingning is the only She ethnic autonomous county in China and the only minority autonomous county in East China. Due to its location in a mountainous area with many scattered townships, the county lacks high-quality medical resources, especially in the construction of multiple specialties such as dermatology, ophthalmology, and dentistry, where there are deficiencies in talent and technology. Since 2012, Wenzhou Medical University has established a cooperative relationship with Jingning County for targeted training, which not only effectively alleviates the problem of insufficient local health talents, but also brings Wenzhou Medical University's cutting-edge medical system and advanced medical methods to Jingning, She Township. This time, Lv Yijun, Secretary of the Party Committee of Wenzhou Medical University, led a team to Jingning, She Township to carry out free clinics and set up service stations. This is not only a further deepening of more than ten years of sincere cooperation, but also a continuation of the friendship of assistance. We believe that with the full support of Wenzhou Medical University and its affiliated hospitals, the medical and health care industry in She Township will usher in great strides and development, bringing a new gospel of health to 170 000 She and Han people.

Lv Yijun said that it is very meaningful to visit Jingning, a revolutionary old area in southwestern Zhejiang, on the occasion of the July 1st Party Day, to help the masses through medical public welfare activities, promote the development of medical and health care and education in She Township Jingning, and assist in the high-quality development of Jingning's economy and society. "Medicine is science, aesthetics, and more importantly, human learning." He hopes to give play to the unique talent advantages and high-quality medical resources of Wenzhou Medical University, and through the love activities of the medical public welfare team in Jingning, educate and guide teachers and students to practice the requirements of the theme education "benefiting people's livelihood, warming people's hearts, and following people's will" in the practice of medical public welfare, so as to boost the construction of Chinese path to modernization with the development of health care in the new era.

Lv Yijun stated that this public welfare event has gathered the most advantageous and distinctive medical charity teams from Wenzhou Medical University: the "F&S CHARITY" charity team that provides charity assistance to patients with difficult to heal wounds, the "Bright Eyes Project" charity team that helps patients with difficult eye diseases regain their sight, the "Smile Project" charity team that helps children with cleft lip and palate repair their gaps and regain a bright smile, the "Childhood Dream Building" charity team that provides public welfare treatment for children with congenital heart disease difficulties, and the "Zhong Shan · Love Team" charity team that provides medical assistance to 26 counties in mountainous areas. Special thanks also go to the "Red Sun Pavilion" public welfare team, known as the "moral landmark" of Wenzhou, for participating in this event. After being listed, each team will further improve the linkage mechanism of medical assistance, establish a normalized public welfare service model, deepen and refine medical charity activities, and make practical contributions to improving the level of medical and health services in Jingning. At the same time, he looks forward to taking this award ceremony as an opportunity to further promote emotional exchange and collaborative cooperation between Jingning County and Wenzhou Medical University, laying a good foundation for the next step of cooperation and exchange, and promoting the formation of a good situation of mountain sea cooperation, school local integration, and common development.

Lv Yijun and his delegation also went to Shiniushan Village, Hexi Town, Jingning County to comfort the 64 years old Lan Grandpa, a wounded patient. Lan Ah Gong is a lonely old man, suffering from diabetes and heart disease, and his legs have begun to fester. Lv Yijun presented him with condolence gifts and money, and inquired in detail about the patient's condition and living conditions. He expressed his intention to study the most suitable treatment plan for the patient after returning, in order to alleviate their illness and pain.

On that day, Zheng Feizhong, Director of the Office of Wenzhou Medical University, Lin Li, Dean of the

当天，温州医科大学办公室主任郑飞中、温州医科大学药学院院长林丽、温州医科大学办公室副主任蒋建微、周建国、金剑锋，温州医科大学药学院党委副书记王建波，温州医科大学阿尔伯塔学院副院长王小尚、 温州医科大学附一院副院长陈容苗，国药控股温州有限公司董事长、党总支书记朱宇鸿等参与志愿活动。

◆ 温州医科大学优势、特色医疗慈善团队现场义诊

当天，陈容苗带领温州医科大学附一院医务处负责人暨玲、创面修复科执行主任王健、骨科执行主任滕红林、呼吸与危重症医学科副主任陈彦凡、消化内科副主任李慧萍、急诊科副主任邱俏檬、创伤科副主任吴云刚、眼科医生杨崇猛、康复科主管技师林晓克等10多名医务人员在现场开展义诊。

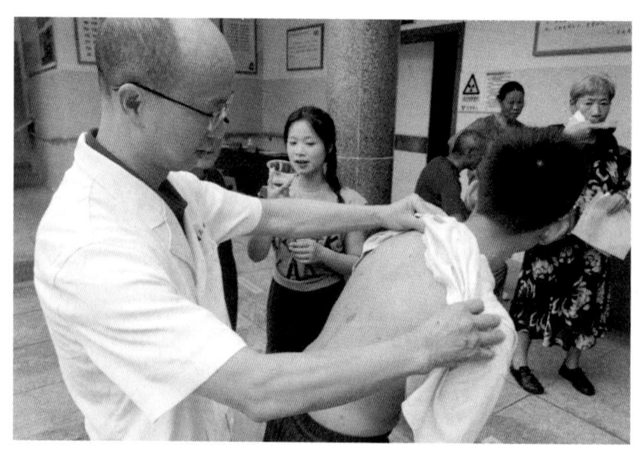

附图 26　医务人员在现场开展义诊

88岁的林阿婆患高血压、糖尿病等多种疾病，当天她带着一袋子药找到陈容苗看病。陈容苗看完后，建议林阿婆胰岛素的用量加一些，有的药不用吃了，并细心地为林阿婆的药一一标出。林阿婆说，温州专家不仅技术好，还很耐心，让她很感动。

现场还有不少创面患者找到王健看病，其中就包括叶女士，她的右手肘关节有明显瘢痕，做了一次手术后还未消除，还影响了肘关节功能。王健建议她可以来温州医科大学附一院创面修复科治疗，为她解决病痛。

16岁的吴同学下半年要上高中，希望在暑假治好脊柱侧弯。滕红林为他做了检查后说，吴同学的脊柱侧弯可以找他做手术，他将帮助吴同学挺直腰杆。

接诊了不少普外科方面疾病患者的暨玲说，当地群众缺乏健康知识的教育，有的群众甚至在没有医生

School of Pharmacy of Wenzhou Medical University, Jiang Jianwei, Zhou Jianguo, Jin Jianfeng, Deputy Director of the Office of Wenzhou Medical University, Wang Jianbo, Deputy Secretary of the Party Committee of the School of Pharmacy of Wenzhou Medical University, Wang Xiaoshang, Deputy Dean of the Alberta School of Wenzhou Medical University, Chen Zimiao, Deputy Dean of the First Affiliated Hospital of Wenzhou Medical University, Zhu Yuhong, Chairman and Secretary of the Party Branch of China National Pharmaceutical Group Wenzhou Co., Ltd., participated in the volunteer activity.

◆ Wenzhou Medical University's Advantage and Characteristic Medical Charity Team conducts on-site free consultations

On that day, Chen Zimiao led more than 10 medical personnel, including Ji Ling, the head of the Medical Department of Wenzhou Medical University Affiliated Hospital, Wang Jian, the executive director of the Wound Repair Department, Teng Honglin, the executive director of the Orthopedics Department, Chen Yanfan, the deputy director of the Respiratory and Critical Care Medicine Department, Li Huiping, the deputy director of the Gastroenterology Department, Qiu Qiaomeng, the deputy director of the Emergency Department, Wu Yungang, the deputy director of the Trauma Department, Yang Chongmeng, an ophthalmologist, and Lin Xiaoke, the chief technician of the Rehabilitation Department, to conduct a free clinic on site.

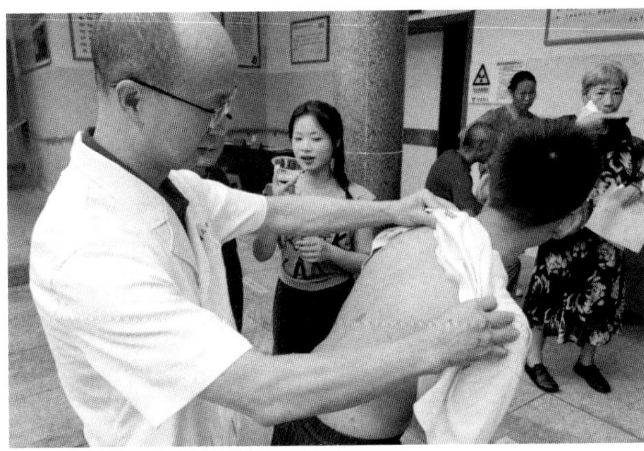

Figure 26 Medical personnel conducting free clinics on site

88 years old Grandma Lin suffered from hypertension, diabetes and other diseases. She took a bag of medicine to see Chen Zimiao the same day. After reading it, Chen Zimiao suggested that Granny Lin increase the dosage of insulin and avoid taking some medications. He also carefully marked Granny Lin's medications one by one. Grandma Lin said that Wenzhou experts are not only skilled, but also very patient, which moved her a lot.

There were still many wound patients who sought medical treatment from Wang Jian on site, including Ms. Ye. Her right elbow joint had obvious scars that had not been eliminated after a surgery, which also affected the function of the elbow joint. Wang Jian suggested that she could come to the Wound Repair Department of Wenzhou Medical University Affiliated Hospital for treatment, to solve her illness.

16-year-old student Wu is going to high school in the second half of the year and hopes to cure scoliosis during the summer vacation. After conducting an examination for him, Teng Honglin said that Wu's scoliosis can be treated with surgery, and he will help Wu straighten his back.

Ji Ling, who has treated many patients with general surgery related diseases, said that the local population lacks education on health knowledge, and some people even use medication without the guidance of doctors, which leads to poor treatment results. Therefore, it is necessary to strengthen health science popularization education and teach them how to use medication correctly.

的指导下用药，这样导致治疗效果不好，因此要加强健康科普知识教育，让他们学会正确用药。

温州医科大学附二院、育英儿童医院儿内党总支书记吴蓉洲主任带领童心筑梦团队5人参加义诊，前来咨询的居民络绎不绝。吴蓉洲耐心为当地儿童进行体检，夏天和医生携带目前最先进的便携式心脏超声仪为体检有问题的孩子进行心脏超声检查，周燕护士长和黄静两位护理专家就家属关于家庭医疗保健给予现场指导。该院超声科医生赵智林放弃休息时间，带着儿子赵恒溢一起来做志愿者。吴蓉洲说，今后“童心筑梦”工程将继续深入基层乡村，为更多儿童先天性心脏病患者提供帮助。

温州医科大学附属口腔医院爱心义诊队伍由口腔颌面外科主任聂鑫、研究生赵烨珂、护士姜爱君、朱凌萱组成，为当地村民进行免费口腔健康检查，并提供专业口腔保健知识指导。

温州医科大学附属眼视光医院公益医疗处处长黄象好、角膜临床中心主任郑钦象、护士潘伟伟等医务人员为村民检查眼睛。当天郑钦象的儿子郑昊乐也来做志愿者。

温州曙光医院业务院长陈善亮带领曹丽、梅运霞等医务人员组成的医疗团队开展义诊。

国药控股温州公司在现场开展党日主题志愿服务，在朱宇鸿的带领下，志愿者一行12人忙前忙后，总共为景宁现场患者送上了价值上万元的药品。

当天，温州红日亭负责人孙兰香带领金光龙、王金元、沙定友、黄加松、张晓萍、黄伟君、汪少华、翁连华等义工，不到7点从温州出发，为当地群众带来了温州名小吃炒粉干、松糕、青草豆腐、伏茶等。

他们一到现场就不停地忙碌着，摆开爱心摊位，在现场炒粉干和蒸松糕，送出丰盛的小吃，被群众团团围住。红日亭义工提前一天准备好了所有食材，他们在现场蒸了200来个松糕，大家现场纷纷夸赞。孙兰香说，红日亭在与温州毗邻的景宁畲族自治县设立爱心驿站，能为当地百姓做点实事，把温州大爱传播畲乡，很有意义。

一批难愈合创面患者得到救助，推动生命健康慈善共同体

2016年，2岁的藏族女孩代吉拉（化名）不慎跌进热水锅中，造成全身严重烫伤。贫困的家庭无力承担高额的治疗费，小姑娘需要进行多年手术治疗。代吉拉的人生转折发生在2020年8月，“肤生工程”团队走进西藏，开展医疗公益行。“小女孩属于重度烫伤，我们通过会诊，为她制订了多达十几次的手术方案，并将她从西藏接到浙江温州治疗。”一位参与救治代吉拉的医生说道。治疗期间，“肤生工程”团队免费为她提供生长因子药物，助力创面修复和愈合，从源头上帮助她解决今后的治疗药物、费用等后顾之忧。如今，她恢复良好，成了一名快乐的小学生。

Director Wu Rongzhou, Secretary of the Pediatric Party Branch of Wenzhou Medical University Affiliated Second Hospital and Yuying Children's Hospital, led a team of five people from Tongxin Dream Building to participate in the free clinic, and residents came in a continuous stream for consultation. Wu Rongzhou patiently conducted physical examinations for local children. During the summer, he and the doctor carried the most advanced portable cardiac ultrasound device to conduct cardiac ultrasound examinations for children with health problems. Nurse Zhou Yan and nursing experts Huang Jing provided on-site guidance to family members on home healthcare. Dr. Zhao Zhilin, an ultrasound specialist at the hospital, gave up his rest time and volunteered with his son Zhao Hengyi. Wu Rongzhou said that in the future, the "Childhood Dream Building" project will continue to penetrate into grassroots rural areas, providing assistance to more children with congenital heart disease.

The Love Clinic Team of Wenzhou Medical University Affiliated Stomatological Hospital is composed of Nie Xin, Director of Oral and Maxillofacial Surgery, Zhao Yeke, a graduate student, Jiang Aijun, and Zhu Lingxuan, nurses. They provide free oral health examinations for local villagers and offer professional guidance on oral health knowledge.

Huang Xianghao, Director of the Public Welfare Medical Department of Wenzhou Medical University Affiliated Eye and Vision Hospital, Zheng Qinxiang, Director of the Corneal Clinical Center, and nurse Pan Weiwei, among other medical staff, conducted eye examinations for villagers. On that day, Zheng Haole, the son of Zheng Qinxiang, also came to volunteer.

Chen Shanliang, the business director of Wenzhou Shuguang Hospital, led a medical team composed of medical personnel such as Cao Li and Mei Yunxia to conduct free clinics.

Guoyao Holdings Wenzhou Company carried out Party Day themed volunteer services on site. Under the leadership of Zhu Yuhong, a team of 12 volunteers worked tirelessly and delivered drugs worth tens of thousands of yuan to patients in Jingning.

On that day, Sun Lanxiang, the person in charge of Wenzhou Hongri Pavilion, led volunteers such as Jin Guanglong, Wang Jinyuan, Sha Dingyou, Huang Jiasong, Zhang Xiaoping, Huang Weijun, Wang Shaohua, Weng Lianhua, etc. to depart from Wenzhou before 7 o'clock, bringing Wenzhou famous snacks such as stir fried noodles, sponge cake, green grass tofu, and Fucha to the local people.

They were busy as soon as they arrived at the scene, setting up a charity booth, stir frying dried noodles and steaming sponge cakes, giving out delicious snacks, and were surrounded by the crowd. Red Sun Pavilion volunteers prepared all the ingredients one day in advance and steamed about 200 sponge cakes on site, which was praised by everyone on site. Sun Lanxiang said that setting up a love station in Jingning She Autonomous County, adjacent to Wenzhou, can do practical things for the local people and spread the love of Wenzhou to She Township, which is very meaningful.

A group of patients with difficult to heal wounds receive assistance, promoting a community of life and health charity

In 2016, a 2-year-old Tibetan girl named Daijila (pseudonym) accidentally fell into a hot water pot, causing severe burns all over her body. Poor families cannot afford the high cost of treatment, and the little girl needs to undergo years of surgical treatment. Daijila's life turning point took place in August 2020, when the "F&S CHARITY" team went to Xizang to carry out medical public welfare activities. "The little girl was severely scalded. Through consultation, we worked out more than a dozen surgical plans for her and sent her from Xizang to Wenzhou, Zhejiang Province for treatment." A doctor who was involved in treating Dejila said. During the treatment period, the "F&S CHARITY" team provided her with free growth factor drugs to assist in wound repair and healing, helping her solve future concerns such as treatment drugs and costs from the source. Now, she has recovered well and become a happy elementary school student.

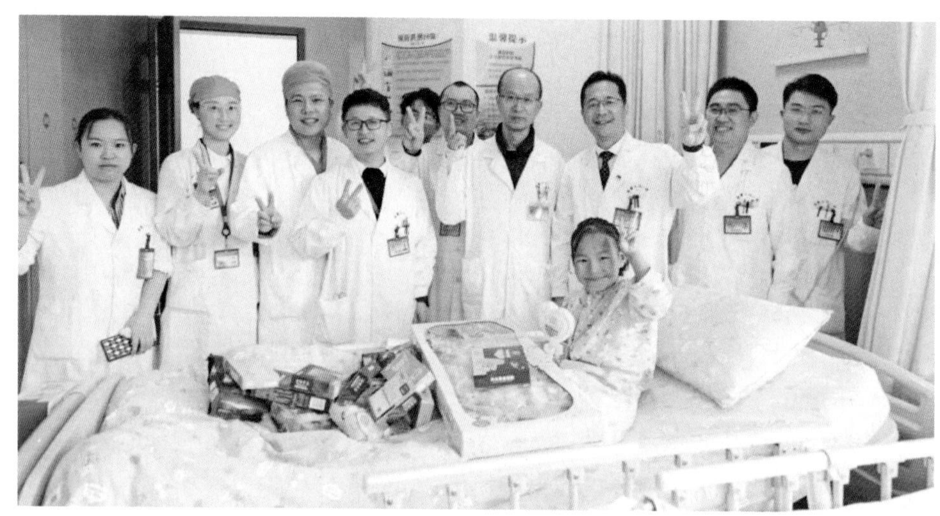

附图 27 被救助的小女孩

对于全国一些难愈合创面伤困难患者，“肤生工程”都出手相救，尤其文成、泰顺等珊溪库区，资助了不少患者。

2022 年 3 月 15 日，在温州 20 多年的甘肃张先生突然休克被送到温州医科大学附一院急救，他的左下肢烂得已经露出骨头，情况非常严重，多处组织坏死，可谓命悬一线。后转到温州曙光医院医治，经过 1 个多月的精心救治，“肤生工程”使他重新站起来，陈忠慈善工作室为他筹集了 10 多万元善款。

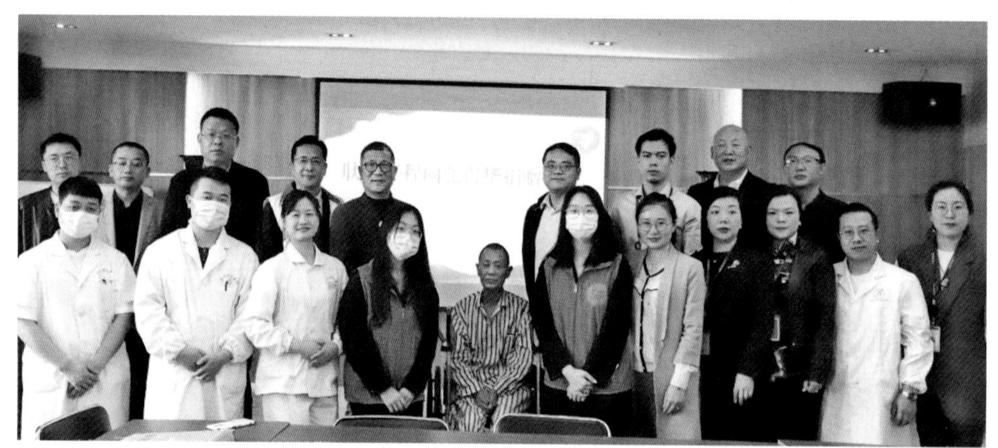

附图 28 被救助患者康复

2022 年 7 月 31 日，“肤生工程”走进泰顺村尾村义诊，发现 93 岁的赖阿公头颈后长了一个排球大的肿瘤，“肤生工程”专家陈善亮给他做了手术，解除了他的 10 多年之痛苦。乐清叶阿公屁股和脚都烂起来，屁股烂了一个 A5 张的大洞，奇臭无比，家人弃他而去，面临着生命危险，在“肤生工程”的帮助下，他被接到温州曙光医院治疗，经过 4 个多月治疗，叶阿公治好了，2021 年 6 月 2 日，叶阿公被亲戚接回乐清，他的

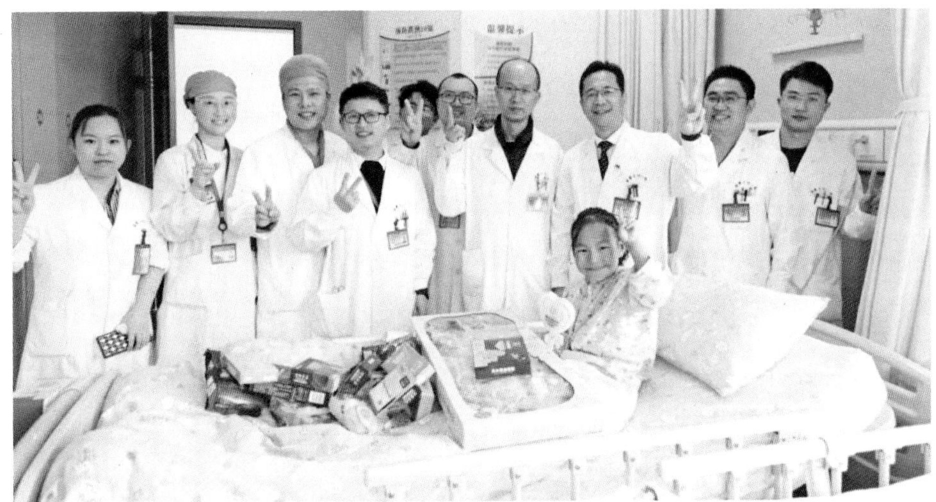

Figure 27 The rescued little girl

For some patients with difficult to heal wounds and injuries across the country, the "F&S CHARITY" has come to the rescue, especially in Shanxi reservoir areas such as Wencheng and Taishun, which have provided financial support to many patients.

On March 15, 2022, Mr. Zhang from Gansu, who had been in Wenzhou for more than 20 years, suddenly went into shock and was sent to the First Affiliated Hospital of Wenzhou Medical University for emergency treatment. His left lower limb was so badly decayed that his bones were exposed, and his condition was very serious, with multiple tissues necrotic and his life hanging in the balance. Later, he was transferred to Shuguang Hospital in Wenzhou for treatment. After more than a month of careful treatment, the "F&S CHARITY" helped him stand up again, and Chen Zhong Charity Studio raised more than 100 000 yuan in donations for him.

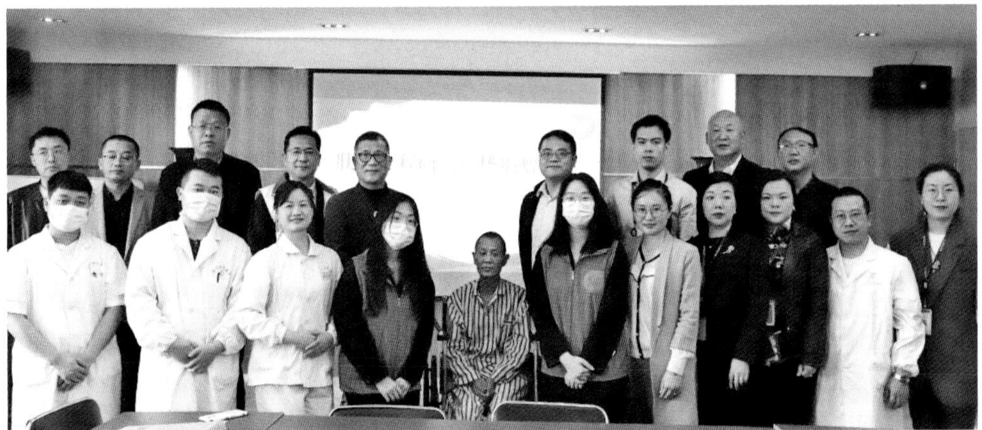

Figure 28 Rehabilitation of rescued patients

On July 31, 2022, "F&S CHARITY" entered the free clinic in Wei Village, Taishun Village and discovered that 93 years old Lai Agung had a volleyball sized tumor on the back of his head and neck. "F&S CHARITY" expert Chen Shanliang performed surgery on him, relieving him of more than 10 years of pain. Yueqing Grandpa Ye's buttocks and feet were both rotten, with a large hole of A5 pieces on his buttocks, which smelled extremely foul. His family abandoned him and he was facing life-threatening situations. With the help of the "F&S CHARITY", he was taken to Wenzhou Shuguang Hospital for treatment. After more than four months of treatment, Grandpa Ye was

姐夫黄连多说，多亏社会各界爱心人士的帮助，救了他的命，非常感谢，为此陈忠慈善工作室为他筹集了10多万元善款。

福建省福鼎市15岁的巨肢少年陈同学，1岁时左脚发现比右脚偏大。家里人曾带他去上海求医，但四五十万的治疗费用对一个普通家庭来说，是一笔天文数字。因为家庭困难，他的病情没有及时得到妥善治疗。陈同学长大后病情越来越严重，生活和学习都受到很大影响。他最大的心愿就是左脚能穿着鞋子，和同学们一起参加体育运动。在“肤生工程”的帮助下，浙、闽、沪当地开展联合救助，被接到温州曙光医院治疗，2023年5月3日，由复旦大学附属华山医院方有生教授、温州医科大学附一院创面修复科执行主任王健、温州曙光医院业务院长陈善亮三方联合为陈同学开展手术。手术过程中发现，陈同学的病情远比想象的复杂。不仅患有巨肢症，还有神经纤维瘤病变，已造成骨头关节病变，决定第一期手术先将左足和下肢减肥。在三方合作下，历时5小时将陈同学的左足重塑，把病变的左脚指头切除。2023年7月16日，陈同学在经历82天4次手术治疗后，成功解除了左脚巨肢症的顽疾，重塑了左足，今后可以正常穿鞋走路。

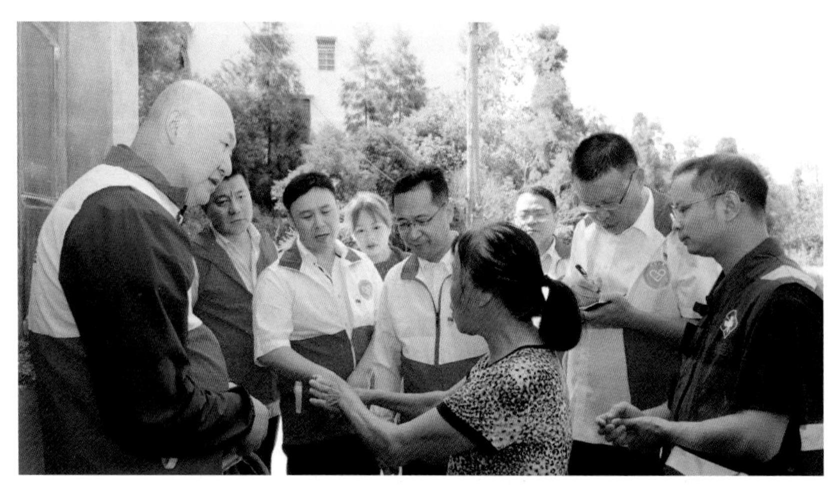

附图29 “肤生工程”团队爱心公益行

踏着乡间泥泞的小路，背着充满温度的药箱，“肤生工程”团队不惧严寒酷暑，持续开展“千村千点”爱心公益行。5年以来，“肤生工程”团队先后在青海玉树、西藏那曲、福建福鼎、陕西富平、衢州开化以及温州永嘉、文成、泰顺等地建立了68个创面修复救助点，与100家志愿者义工组织合作建立公益救助网络，累计捐款捐物1000万元，总公益行程超20多万公里，受益者达5万余人，其中，2021年3月，“肤生工程”福鼎站成立，从三佛塔村双腿溃烂43年的梁先生，到叠石乡臀部溃烂10多年的李先生，目前他

cured. On June 2, 2021, Grandpa Ye was brought back to Yueqing by relatives. His brother-in-law Huang Lianduo said that thanks to the help of kind-hearted people from all walks of life, his life was saved. He was very grateful, and for this, Chen Zhong Charity Studio raised more than 100 000 yuan in donations for him.

Chen, a 15-year-old boy with giant limbs from Fuding City, Fujian Province, discovered that his left foot was larger than his right foot when he was 1 year old. His family once took him to Shanghai for medical treatment, but the cost of four to five hundred thousand yuan is an astronomical figure for an ordinary family. Due to family difficulties, his condition did not receive timely and proper treatment. Chen's condition became increasingly severe as he grew up, greatly affecting his life and studies. His biggest wish is to wear shoes on his left foot and participate in sports with his classmates. With the help of the "F&S CHARITY", joint assistance was carried out in Zhejiang, Fujian, and Shanghai, and the patient was taken to Wenzhou Shuguang Hospital for treatment. On May 3, 2023, Professor Fang Yousheng from Huashan Hospital affiliated with Fudan University, Executive Director of the Wound Repair Department of Wenzhou Medical University Affiliated Hospital Wang Jian, and Business Dean of Wenzhou Shuguang Hospital Chen Shanliang jointly performed surgery for Chen. During the surgery, it was discovered that Chen's condition was much more complex than imagined. Not only does he suffer from gigantism, but he also has neurofibromatosis, which has caused bone and joint lesions. It has been decided that the first surgery will focus on weight loss in the left foot and lower limbs. Under the cooperation of three parties, Chen's left foot was reshaped over a period of 5 hours, and the diseased left toe was removed. On July 16, 2023, after 82 days and 4 surgeries, Chen successfully relieved the stubborn condition of left foot gigantism, reshaped his left foot, and can walk normally wearing shoes in the future.

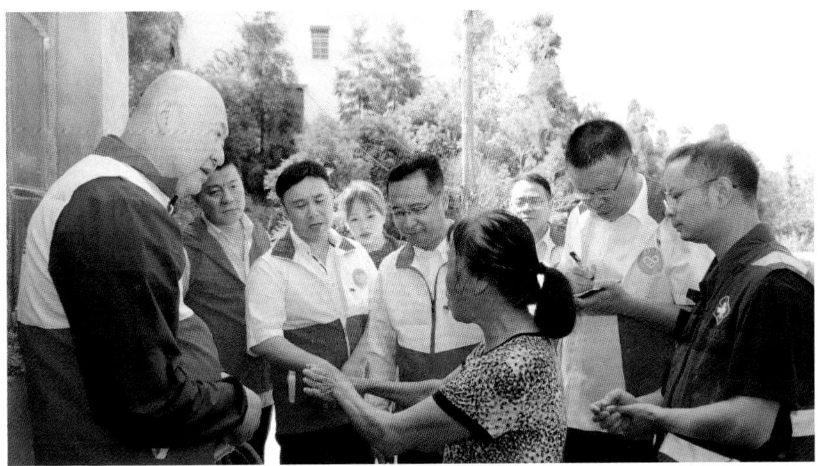

Figure 29 "F&S CHARITY" Team Charity Walk

Stepping on muddy rural roads and carrying medicine boxes filled with warmth, the "F&S CHARITY" team is not afraid of extreme cold and heat, and continues to carry out the "Thousand Villages, Thousand Points" charity walk. Over the past five years, the "F&S CHARITY" team has successively established 68 wound repair and rescue sites in Yushu, Qinghai, Naqu, Xizang, Fuding, Fujian, Fuping, Quzhou, Kaihua, Wenzhou, Yongjia, Wencheng, Taishun and other places, and cooperated with 100 volunteer volunteer organizations to establish a public welfare rescue network. They have donated 10 million yuan in total, with a total public welfare journey of more than 200 000 kilometers, and more than 50 000 beneficiaries. Among them, in March 2021, the "F&S CHARITY" Fuding Station was established. From Mr. Liang, who has suffered from leg ulcers for 43 years in Sanfo Tower Village, to Mr. Li, who has suffered from hip ulcers for more than 10 years in Dieshi Township, their team has now rescued more than 50 patients with refractory wounds in Fuzhou, Ningde, Fuqing, Gutian and other places have contributed

们团队已经救助福州、宁德、福清、古田等地难愈合创面伤患者50多名，共投入善款200多万元。项目先后获人民日报、新华社、央视新闻联播、光明日报、浙江日报等主流媒体关注报道。院士王松灵、付小兵、顾玉东、张志愿、李校堃先后为“肤生工程”题词、点赞，助力项目实施。

在巩固脱贫成果助力乡村振兴的大背景下，“肤生工程”将救助对象锁定为深受创面问题困扰的人群，避免这类人群“因病返贫”。团队在衢州站试点设立全国首家慢性创面精准分级诊疗示范中心，将“市、县、乡”三级卫生机构力量进行整合，推出“分级诊疗、精准帮扶”的肤生慈善救助新模式，充分发挥“国标省统、县管乡用”的基层全科医生力量，以及地级市三甲医院的创面修复学科优势，形成“全专结合”的全新公益救助网络。

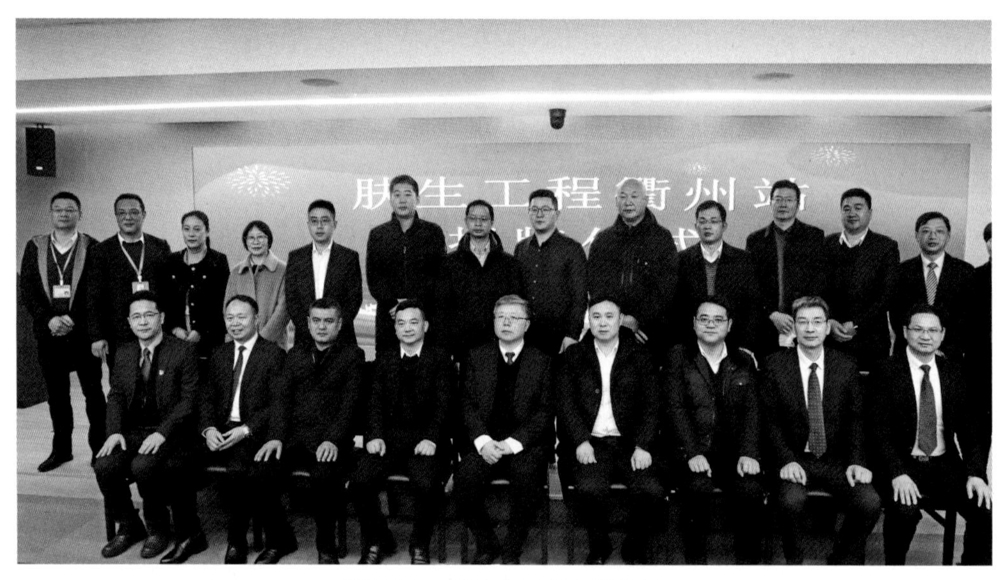

附图 30 “肤生工程”衢州站

肤生工程推动成立生命健康慈善共同体。2021年，“肤生工程”在建党百年之际，联合温州医科大学“明眸皓齿”“童心筑梦”等医疗公益团队，启动温州医科大学共富生命慈善联合体，开展“百年红肤生行”健康中国行大型公益活动，不断在全国扩大“肤生工程”的影响，惠及更多的难愈合伤创面患者。项目团队以“肤生浙里行”结对村帮扶、“肤生中国行”健康公益行、“肤生百年红”宣传教育月等系列子活动为主要载体，走进山西省永和县红军东征纪念地、全国先进基层党组织福建省福鼎市柏洋村、永嘉县红星社区红十三军旧址、平阳县凤林村省一大会址、陕西富平、陕西延安等地，听当地老党员们讲述自己的军

more than 2 million yuan. The project has been reported by mainstream media such as People's Daily, Xinhua News Agency, CCTV News Network, Guangming Daily and Zhejiang Daily. Academicians Wang Songling, Fu Xiaobing, Gu Yudong, Zhang Zhiyuan, and Li Xiaokun have successively inscribed and praised the "F&S CHARITY" to assist in its implementation.

Against the backdrop of consolidating the achievements of poverty alleviation and supporting rural revitalization, the "F&S CHARITY" targets the population who are deeply troubled by wound problems, avoiding them from returning to poverty due to illness. The team has piloted the establishment of the first national demonstration center for precise grading diagnosis and treatment of chronic wounds at Quzhou Station, integrating the strengths of "city, county, and township" health institutions, and launching a new model of skin care charity assistance with "grading diagnosis and treatment, precise assistance". It fully leverages the strength of grassroots general practitioners who are "national standard provincial unified, county managed and township used", as well as the advantages of wound repair disciplines in tertiary hospitals in prefecture level cities, forming a new public welfare assistance network that combines "comprehensive expertise".

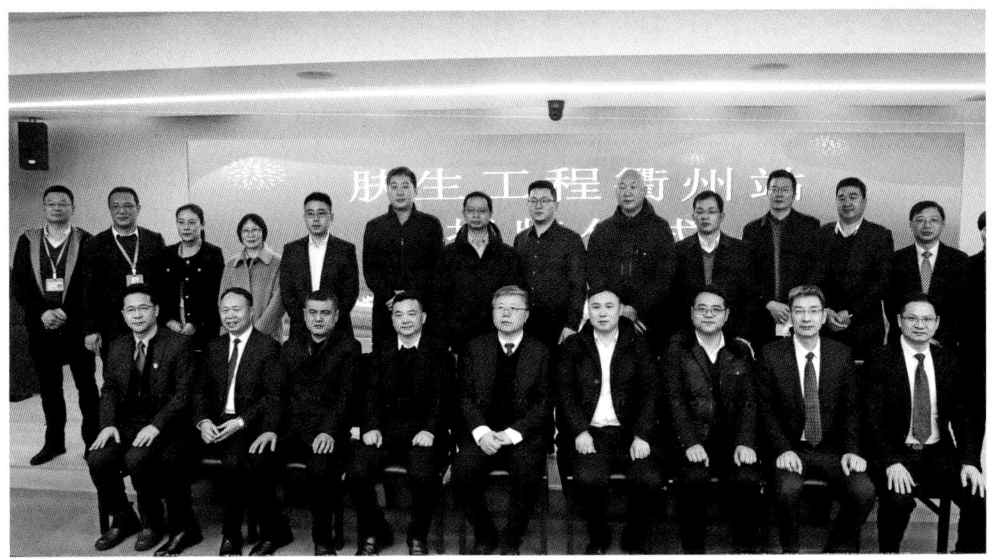

Figure 30 "F&S CHARITY" Quzhou Station

Fusheng Engineering promotes the establishment of a life and health charity community. In 2021, on the occasion of the 100th anniversary of the founding of the Communist Party of China, the "F&S CHARITY" joined forces with medical public welfare teams such as "Bright Eyes and Bright Teeth" and "Childhood Dreams" from Wenzhou Medical University to launch the Wenzhou Medical University Co Prosperity Life Charity Alliance, carrying out the "Century Red Skin Revitalization Campaign" Healthy China Campaign large-scale public welfare activities, continuously expanding the influence of the "F&S CHARITY" nationwide, and benefiting more patients with difficult to heal wounds. The project team mainly carried out a series of sub activities such as the "Skin Born Zhejiang Village Tour" paired village assistance, the "Skin Born China Tour" health public welfare tour, and the "Skin Born Centennial Red" publicity and education month. They visited the Red Army East Expedition Memorial Site in Yonghe County, Shanxi Province, Baiyang Village in Fuding City, Fujian Province, an advanced grassroots party organization in China, the former site of the Red Third Army in Hongxing Community, Yongjia County, the site of the First National Congress in Fenglin Village, Pingyang County, Fuping, Shaanxi Province, Yan'an, and other places. They listened to local veteran party members talk about the spiritual strength and military imprint

旅生活带给他们的精神力量和军旅印记，在陈列馆开展党史学习教育主题党日活动，重温建党伟业，传承红色基因，并为老党员困难户送上慰问品和慰问金，为贫困退伍军人提供免费公益救助手术。活动累计为 3000 多名当地群众提供公益慈善和医疗救助服务，为数百名患有难愈合创面伤的老人提供免费救治。

（陈　忠）